Plumer's
Principles and Practice
of Intravenous Therapy

Plumer's Principles & Practice of Intravenous Therapy

Sixth Edition

Sharon M. Weinstein, RN, CRNI, MS
Director, Office of International Affairs
Premier, Inc. and related companies
Westchester, Illinois

Infusion Therapy Consultant
Former Faculty, Department of Surgery
Finch University of Health Sciences/
The Chicago Medical School
North Chicago, Illinois

Former Vice-Chair, Intravenous Nurses
Certification Corporation,
Executive Board

Past President, The Intravenous Nurses Society, Inc.

Leader, Intravenous Therapy Delegations
to People's Republic of China,
Commonwealth of Independent States, Austria,
and Germany

Lippincott
Philadelphia • New York

Acquisitions Editor: Margaret B. Zuccarini
Editorial Assistant: Emily Cotlier
Project Editor: Amy P. Jirsa/Erika Kors
Production Manager: Helen Ewan
Production Coordinator: Patricia McCloskey
Design Coordinator: Kathy Kelley-Luedtke
Indexer: Alexandra Nickerson

6th Edition

Library of Congress Cataloging-in-Publication Data

Weinstein, Sharon.
    Plumer's principles & practice of intravenous therapy/Sharon M. Weinstein. — 6th ed.
        p.   cm.
    Includes bibliographical references and index.
    ISBN 0-397-55311-0 (alk. paper)
    1. Intravenous therapy. I. Plumer, Ada Lawrence. II. Title.
    [DNLM: 1. Infusions, Intravenous WB 354 W424p 1997]
    RM 170.P57 1997
    6.158'55 — dc20
    DNLM/DLC
    for Library of Congress   96-20620
                                                                          CIP

The material contained in this volume was submitted as previously unpublished material, except in the instances in which credit has been given to the source from which some of the illustrative material was derived.

Any procedure or practice described in this book should be applied by the health-care practitioner under appropriate supervision in accordance with professional standards of care used with regard to the unique circumstances that apply in each practice situation. Care has been taken to confirm the accuracy of information presented and to describe generally accepted practices. However, the authors, editors, and publisher cannot accept any responsibility for errors or omissions or for any consequences from application of the information in this book and make no warranty, express or implied, with respect to the contents of the book.

The authors and publisher have exerted every effort to ensure that drug selection and dosage set forth in this text are in accordance with current recommendations and practice at the time of publication. However, in view of ongoing research, changes in government regulations, and the constant flow of information relating to drug therapy and drug reactions, the reader is urged to check the package insert for each drug for any change in indications and dosage and for added warnings and precautions. This is particularly important when the recommended agent is a new or infrequently employed drug.

Materials appearing in this book prepared by individuals as part of their official duties as U.S. Government employees are not covered by the above-mentioned copyright.

9 8 7 6 5 4 3 2 1

Contributors

Carole DeCicco, RN, MSN, CNSN
Nutrition Support Consultant
and
Former Director, Nutrition Support Services
West Jersey Hospital
Voorhees, New Jersey

Anne Marie Frey, RN, BSN, CRNI
IV Nurse Clinician
Children's Hospital of Philadelphia
Philadelphia, Pennsylvania

Margaret M. McCluskey, RN, OCN, CRNI, MPH, MA
Nurse Coordinator
Cook County Hospital
Chicago, Illinois

Susan Y. Pauley, RN, CRNI
IV Supervisor
Massachusetts General Hospital
Boston, Massachusetts

Barbara St. Marie, RN, CS, MA, ANP, GNP
Adult and Geriatric Nurse Practitioner
Department of Internal Medicine
Park-Nicollet Clinic
Health System Minnesota
Minneapolis, Minnesota

Acknowledgments

Plumer's Principles & Practice of Intravenous Therapy, Sixth Edition, is the result of the collaborative efforts of its original authors, Ada Lawrence Plumer and Faye Cosentino; the outstanding contributors to this edition: Carole DeCicco, RN, MSN, CNSN, Anne Marie Frey, RN, BSN, CRNI, Margaret M. McCluskey, RN, OCN, CRNI, MPH, MA, CHES, Susan Y. Pauley, RN, CRNI, and Barbara St. Marie, CRNI, MS, and myself. I am so grateful to them for their valuable contributions to this text, and for the contributions that they have individually and collectively made to our professional practice. I would also like to thank the manufacturers of infusion products and equipment for their information and assistance, as well as the authors and publishers who permitted use of their copyright materials in producing this text.

A special thank you to Margaret Belcher Zuccarini, Senior Editor, and Emily Cotlier, Editorial Assistant in the Nursing Division, and to Amy Jirsa and Erika Kors, Project Editors in Production at Lippincott-Raven for their encouragement, support, and technical assistance in developing a superior manuscript—one that readily supports the Plumer name.

Thanks are extended to William Eudailey, Pharm D, and to the late David Blaess, RPh, who served as my mentors, and who taught me to apply the principles gleaned from Plumer's book to my daily practice.

A special thank you to Jaclyn Tropp, CRNI, with whom I have had the privilege of working for over 10 years. Jackie has been an inspiration to many IV nurses nationwide . . . her zest for our practice continues to inspire me. She constantly strives to educate IV nurses and to share our specialty practice.

Finally, thanks to my growing family, for understanding and acknowledging my need to share my passion for infusion therapy practice via the written word.

SMW

Special Acknowledgment

The name Ada Plumer is synonymous with infusion therapy. A leader, pacesetter, and cofounder of the professional society, Plumer set the tone for our professional practice, served as a mentor to many nurses, and encouraged excellence in the delivery of intravenous nursing care.

From my first entry into this rapidly changing field to today, I have used Plumer's book as a reference, a guide, a bible for professional practice. The "original" IV reference manual retains its position today as the only complete source of information available to the practicing clinician, student, and educator. The success of the fifth edition is attributed to Plumer . . . the growth of our practice is likewise a result of her initial efforts. Many thanks from all of us in whom you have instilled a passion for excellence in intravenous nursing practice.

Preface

For 26 years, *Plumer's Principles & Practice of Intravenous Therapy* has retained its position as the most reliable complete source of information addressing intravenous therapy for practicing clinicians, educators, and students. Completely updated and revised to meet the changing needs of our professional practice, this sixth edition, like its predecessors, provides the most current base of knowledge available to those who share the responsibility of ensuring high-quality infusion care to patients in a diversity of clinical settings.

Our practice continually changes as a result of changing patient care delivery systems, the impact of managed care on health care reimbursement, constant restructuring of the workforce, and reengineering of the health care system. Mergers and acquisitions have resulted in large networks of acute care facilities, home care agencies, semiacute care settings, and extended care institutions. These changes have had a dramatic impact on our professional practice as we move on the continuum from care delivered in the acute care environment to care delivered in alternative sites. However, one thing remains unchanged, and that is the continuous need for an unprecedented high level of expertise for delivering infusion therapy.

Plumer's Principles & Practice of Intravenous Therapy, Sixth Edition, has been updated and reorganized to create a resource that meets and exceeds these needs. Addition of boxes and tables creates an easy-to-use format and easy-to-access references. A more integrated approach to content results in a five-section organization. Part I reviews the history, legal implications, nursing role, and recent innovations in infusion therapy practice, including credentialing processes for RNs and LP/VNs. Risk management has again been updated to reflect current regulations and process improvement. Nursing role and responsibility includes the most current Standards of Practice. Cost Factors associated with intravenous care have been added.

Part II addresses relevant anatomy and physiology, techniques of therapy, complications and laboratory analysis. Complications has been completely revised to meet the reference needs of clinicians in all settings.

Part III, Principles of Equipment Selection and Clinical Applications, presents state-of-the-art equipment, methods for assessing product and equipment needs, central venous catheterization, and advanced forms of vascular access. This is an area that is constantly changing as manufacturers meet our ongoing needs for advanced methods of vascular access. Troubleshooting techniques are provided. Arterial therapy also has been updated.

The most dramatic changes may be seen in Part IV, Applications of Intravenous Therapy for Homeostasis. Contributing authors make this section the most current and complete source of information available today. The chapters on fluid and electrolyte balance and parenteral fluids are totally updated. A new but seasoned author, Carole DeCicco, has totally revised the chapter on Parenteral Nutrition. DeCicco has over 25 years of experience in this intensive field, is an active educator and practitioner, and brings a new approach to this important subject matter. A renowned expert in Pain Management, Barbara St. Marie, has written the chapter on "Pain," emphasizing practical aspects of care.

Drug administration, pediatrics, transfusion therapy, and antineoplastics have been updated to reflect current practice. The subject of Intravenous Therapy in the Older Adult Patient is a new addition and one that is much needed as we continue to provide care for an aging population. Finally, alternate site care has been reorganized, rewritten, and updated, producing a comprehensive source of information on home care, infusion centers, and reimbursement methodologies.

The sixth edition addresses the revised Standards of Practice throughout. Revised to meet the needs of the clinician responsible for delivering high-quality infusion care, regardless of the clinical setting, *Plumer's Principles & Practice of Intravenous Therapy*, Sixth Edition, retains its place as the most essential tool available in intravenous practice today.

Sharon M. Weinstein, RN, CRNI, MS

Contents

Chapter 5
Cost Factors Associated With Infusion Therapy   42

Part II
Principles of Venipuncture   47

Chapter 6
Anatomy and Physiology Applied to Intravascular Therapy   49

Chapter 7
Techniques of Intravenous Therapy   58

Chapter 8
Complications   84

Chapter 9
Laboratory Tests   111

**Part III
Principles of Equipment Selection
and Clinical Applications   135**

Chapter 10
Intravenous Equipment   137

Part IV
Application of Intravenous Therapy for Homeostasis   285

Chapter 14
Fluid and Electrolyte Balance   287

Chapter 15
Principles of Parenteral Fluid Administration   317

Chapter 16
Parenteral Nutrition   345

$\mathcal{P}$ART I

Practice of Intravenous Therapy

CHAPTER 1

History of Intravenous Therapy

Key Terms

Antisepsis	Experimentation	Parenteral solutions
Blood	History	Quill and bladder
Circulation	Multidisciplinary	Standards of practice

EARLY HISTORY

Methodology

The idea of injecting various substances, including blood, into the circulatory system is not new; it has been in the human mind for centuries. In 1628, William Harvey's discovery of blood circulation stimulated increased experimentation.

Devices

As early as 1656, Sir Christopher Wren, with a quill and bladder, injected opium intravenously into dogs, and 6 years later, J.D. Major made the first successful injection in man.[4] Wren is known as the father of modern intravenous (IV) therapy.

In 1665, an animal near death from loss of blood was restored by infusion of blood from another animal. In 1667, a 15-year-old Parisian boy was the first human to receive a transfusion successfully; lamb's blood was administered directly into the circulation by Jean Baptiste Denis, physician to Louis XIV.[5] The enthusiasm aroused by this success led to promiscuous transfusions of blood from animals to man with fatal results, and in 1687, by an edict of church and parliament, animal-to-man transfusions were prohibited in Europe.

About 150 years passed before serious attempts were again made to inject blood into people. James Blundell, an English obstetrician, revived the idea. In 1834, saving the lives of many women threatened by hemorrhage during childbirth, he proved that animal blood was unfit to inject into man and that only human blood was safe. Nevertheless, complications persisted; infections developed in donors and recipients. With the discovery of the principles of antisepsis by Pasteur and Lister, another obstacle was overcome, yet reactions and deaths continued.

The first attempt, recorded in 1821, to prevent coagulation during transfusion was by Jean Louis Prévost, a French physician, who, with Jean B.A. Dumas, used defibrinated blood in animal transfusions.[5]

TWENTIETH-CENTURY ADVANCES

Blood

In 1900, Karl Landsteiner proved that not all human blood is alike; classifications were made.[4] In 1914, a chemical, sodium citrate, was found to prevent blood from clotting.[5] Since then, rapid advances have been made.

Hugh Leslie Marriot and Alan Kekwick, English physicians, introduced the continuous slow-drip method of blood transfusion; their findings were published in 1935.[5]

Parenteral Solutions

Administration of parenteral fluids by the IV route has become widely used only during the past 40 years. The difficulty in accepting this procedure resulted from the lack of safe solutions. The solutions used contained substances called pyrogens, proteins that are foreign to the body and not destroyed by sterilization. These caused chills and fever when injected into the circulation. About 1923, with the discovery and elimination of these pyrogens, the IV administration of parenteral fluids became safer and more common.

Until 1925, the most frequently used parenteral solution was normal saline solution. Because of its hypotonicity, water could not be administered IV and had to be made isotonic; sodium chloride achieved this effect.[2] After 1925, dextrose was used extensively to make isotonic solutions and to provide a source of calories.[3]

In the middle 1940s, disposable plastic sets became available and eventually replaced the reusable rubber tubings.

A whole new approach to IV therapy and a respite to the starving patient evolved in 1965 when members of the Harrison Department of Surgical Research at the University of Pennsylvania showed that sufficient nutrients could be given to juvenile beagle dogs to support normal growth and development.[2] This led to what is known today as total parenteral nutrition.

In the middle 1960s, Dr. Stanley Dudrick developed the first formula for parenteral nutrition, a method by which sufficient nutrients are administered into the central vein to support life and maintain one's growth and development.

Glass containers were first used for IV solutions. Plastic bags were introduced in the 1970s; because air venting is not required, the risks of air embolism and airborne contamination were reduced. Today, plastic is the primary container for IV solutions. Glass containers are used when stability of the infusate in plastic is a concern.

Manufacturers have continued to keep pace with demands for technologically advanced products that ensure patient safety and reliability in the delivery of infusion therapy.

THE NURSING ROLE

In the early 1930s, administration of an IV injection was a major procedure reserved for the critically ill patient. The physician performed the venipuncture, assisted by a nurse. The success of IV therapy and the great increase in its use led to the establishment of a department of specially trained personnel for infusion therapy. In 1940, the Massachusetts General Hospital became one of the first hospitals to assign a nurse as an IV specialist. The services of the IV nurse consisted of administering IV solutions and transfusions, cleaning infusion sets, and cleaning and sharpening needles. Emphasis was placed on the technical responsibility of maintaining the infusion and keeping the needle patent. The sole requisite of the IV nurse was the ability to perform a venipuncture skillfully.

As knowledge of electrolyte and fluid therapy grew, more solutions became available, and further knowledge was needed to monitor the fluid and electrolyte status of the patient. The nurse assigned to the patient in need of IV therapy was expected to have a working knowledge of fluid and electrolyte balance and to assess the "whole" patient in terms of fluid needs. Normal saline was no longer the only electrolyte solution. Today more than 200 commercially prepared IV fluids are available to meet every need of the patient.

The 1970s brought tremendous scientific, technologic, and medical advances, and IV therapy gained recognition as a highly specialized field. Nurses performed many of the functions formerly reserved for the medical staff—intra-arterial therapy, neonatal therapy, and antineoplastic therapy. Professional organizations were established to provide a forum for the exchange of ideas, information, experiences, and knowledge, with the ultimate goal of raising standards and increasing the level of patient care.

On October 1, 1980, the United States House of Representatives recognized the profession and declared an official day of honor for IV nurses: "Resolved, that IV Nurse Day be nationally celebrated in honor of the National Intravenous Therapy Association, Inc. on January 25 of each year." The proclamation was presented by the Honorable Edward J. Mackey from the Fifth Congressional District of the Commonwealth of Massachusetts.[4,6]

The Intravenous Nurses Society, Inc.

The Intravenous Nurses Society, Inc. (INS) has continued to grow nationwide. Educational offerings have been expanded to include advanced studies in an effort to meet the needs of the advanced practitioner.

Credentialing for RNs and LPNs

The Intravenous Nurses Certification Corporation (INCC) likewise expanded to include the National Board of IV Nurse Examiners, the LP/VN Board of Nurse Examiners, and an Executive Committee. The first examination to become a Certified LPN or LVN in intravenous therapy was offered on September 7, 1996.

Professional IV nurses are encouraged to prepare for the credentialing process through videotapes, a core curriculum, educational programs, the society's professional journal, clinical textbooks, and published Standards of Practice.

Delivery of IV therapy has permeated all clinical settings; the role of the IV nurse is now well established as integral to multidisciplinary, quality care in all practice settings.[1] The growth of this specialty practice has resulted in expanded roles for IV nurses nationally and internationally. IV nurses are constantly striving to find new and more efficient ways to perform their services in a changing health care environment.

REFERENCES

1. Baranowski, L. (1995). Presidential address: Take ownership. *Journal of Intravenous Nursing, 18*(4), 163.
2. Dudrick, S. J. (1971). Rational intravenous therapy. *American Journal of Hospital Pharmacy 28,* 83.
3. Elman, R. (1949). Fluid balance from the nurse's point of view. *American Journal of Nursing 49,* 222.
4. Gardner, C. (1982). United States House of Representatives honors the National Intravenous Therapy Association, Inc. *Journal of the National Intravenous Therapy Association 5*(1), 14.
5. Schmidt, J. E. (1959). *Medical discoveries who and when* (p. 59). Springfield, IL: C. C. Thomas.
6. Editorial. Journal of Intravenous Nursing 5(1).

CHAPTER 2

Risk Reduction and Quality Improvement

Key Terms

Analysis	Criminal law	Quality improvement
Assault	Data analysis	Reevaluation
Battery	Evaluation	Resolution
Benchmarking	Incident reports	Risk
Civil law	Interpretation	Tort
Corrective action plans	Malpractice	Unusual occurrence

LEGAL IMPLICATIONS

Because of the law and its interpretation, doubts and questions exist regarding the legal rights of nurses to administer IV therapy. As the scope of IV therapy has become more complex and specialized, nurses have become more involved in administration procedures formerly performed solely by physicians and considered medical acts. Because violation of the Medical Practice Act is considered a criminal offense, IV nurses should be well versed in such procedures.

Professional and Governmental Regulations

To alleviate the nurse's fears regarding possible liability for claimed violation of the Medical Practice Act, the medical profession has issued joint policy statements with nursing associations on a number of procedures, including IV therapy. These joint statements are written when questions arise regarding the nurse's professional responsibility or obligation to perform specific therapeutic measures and these questions are not answered in existing statutes (ie, nursing practice acts and medical practice acts). This is considered the most useful way to deal with procedures performed by members of both professions.

Sponsors of joint statements are the state nurses' association, which is concerned with the area of nursing practice; the state medical society, which is concerned with therapeutic measures that were formerly considered solely the practice of medicine and that legally must be prescribed by the physician; and the state hospital association, which is concerned with institutional liability for therapeutic measures performed in member health care facilities.

Other ways of dealing with procedures are through rulings made by attorneys general, by state boards of nursing, and by the interpretation of the Nurse Practice Act. In some states, the nurse practice acts relating to the definition of nursing are global and do not refer to specific procedures because it is believed that with frequent changes in professional practice, it would not be feasible to have state legislators review such changes before implementation in a practice setting.

State boards of nursing have sought the input of IV nursing professionals and the professional societies to ensure high levels of care. Professional nursing societies are taking an expanded role in decision making as it pertains to the specialty practice. Standards of practice have been developed that provide criteria for judgment and ensure maximal safety for the patient as well as protection for the physician, nurse, and health care organization.

To answer the question "Can I legally administer IV therapy?" each nurse must ask the following questions:

1. Does the state law delegate this function to the nurse?
2. Does the particular institution's or agency's policy, with the approval of the medical staff, permit the nurse to perform this function?
3. Are nurses limited in the types of fluids and medications they may administer by a list delineated by the hospital?
4. Is the order written by a licensed physician for a specific patient?
5. Is the nurse qualified by education and experience to administer IV therapy?

Nurses may properly refuse to perform IV therapy if in their professional judgment they are not qualified and competent. It has been established by law that in a question of negligence, individuals are not protected because they have "carried out the physician's orders." They are held liable in relation to their knowledge, skill, and judgment.

In hospitals and states in which no written opinion relevant to IV therapy exists, what is the registered nurse's responsibility when ordered by a licensed staff physician to administer IV therapy? "A nurse is legally required to carry out any nursing or medical procedure she is directed to carry out by a duly licensed physician unless she has reason to believe harm will result to the patient from doing so."[1] To meet their legal responsibilities to patients, nurses must be qualified by knowledge and experience to execute the procedure, otherwise they may properly refuse to perform it. "Where there is no medical reason to question a physician's order, the nurse's failure to carry out such an order will subject her to liability for any consequent harm to the patient."[3]

States are recommending that schools of professional nursing include in their curriculum a course that will offer the student nurse clinical instruction and experience in IV therapy. IV nursing specialists have been instrumental in developing the content for such programs.

The Private Duty Nurse

A private duty nurse, who works under the direction, supervision, and control of a hospital and private physician, is subject to the rules and regulations of the hospital concerning all matters relating to nursing care. If the hospital policy-making committee has rules regarding who may and may not give IV therapy, the private duty nurse is subject to the same rules that apply to the staff nurse. To prevent any misunderstanding on the part of the private duty nurse, a specific sentence may be added to the hospital's joint policy statement noting that the private duty nurse who has complied with the criteria applicable to the administration of IV therapy may give an IV infusion.

The Agency Nurse

Temporary staffing agencies continue to proliferate nationwide, providing valuable assistance during times when a shortage of licensed professional personnel occurs. When given responsibility for the administration of intravascular therapies, agency personnel must be oriented to the facility's policies and procedures and the functions performed by a specialized department. Every effort should be made to ensure patient safety, public protection, and viability of the IV program.

GUIDELINES

The IV nurse's fear of involvement in malpractice suits is increasing with the growth in complexity of therapy and delegation of responsibility for infusion therapy in some institutions to less qualified paraprofessionals. In many cases, the professional nurse is legally responsible for the work performed by nonlicensed personnel. Many of the functions performed by the nurse have important legal consequences. An understanding of the legal principles and guidelines involved is necessary if daily professional actions are not to result in unwanted malpractice suits. It will be easier to have a clearer understanding of these guidelines if a few of the legal terms are first defined.

Definitions

Criminal law relates to an offense against the general public because of its harmful effect on the welfare of society as a whole. Criminal actions are prosecuted by a government authority, and punishment includes imprisonment or fine, or both. The administration of IV therapy, if performed in an unlawful manner, can involve the nurse in criminal conduct. Violation of the Nursing Practice Act or the Medical Practice Act by an unlicensed person is considered a criminal offense.

Civil law deals with conduct that affects the legal rights of the private person or corporation. When harm occurs, the guilty party may be required to pay damages to the injured person.

A *tort* is a private wrong, by act or omission, that can result in a civil action by the harmed person. Common torts relevant to professional nursing practice include negligence, assault, battery, false imprisonment, slander, libel, and invasion of privacy. There are some defenses in civil actions, such as contributory negligence on the part of the plaintiff.

Coercion of a rational adult patient to insert a cannula constitutes *assault* (the threat to do harm) and *battery* (actually hitting or forcing). If the patient refuses treatment, and explanation and encouragement fail, the physician should be notified.

Malpractice is the negligent conduct of professional persons. Negligent conduct is not acting in a reasonable and prudent manner, with resultant damage to a person or that individual's property. It is not synonymous with carelessness although a person who is careless is negligent.

If a nurse with no previous training administers an IV infusion, performs an arterial puncture, or adds medications to IV fluids, and does it as carefully as possible but harm results, a civil court may rule such conduct as negligent; that nurse should not have performed the act without previous training and experience. Such a negligent action is considered an act of malpractice because it involves a professional person. However, if the act of malpractice does not create harm, legal action cannot be initiated.

The *rule of personal liability* is "every person is liable for his own tortious conduct" (his own wrongdoing).[1] No physician can protect the nurse from an act of negligence by bypassing this rule with verbal assurance. The nurse involved cannot avoid legal liability even though another person may be sued and held liable. The physician who orders placement of a peripherally inserted central catheter (PICC) cannot assume responsibility for the nurse who is negligent in implementing the procedure. If harm occurs as a result of the action, the nurse is liable for this wrongdoing.

The rule of personal liability is relevant in medication errors. Medication errors are a common cause of malpractice claims against nurses.[6] Negligence results from the administration of a drug to the wrong patient, at the wrong time, in an incorrect dosage, or in an improperly prescribed manner. If the physician writes an incomplete or partially illegible order and the nurse fails to clarify it before administration and harm results, the nurse is liable for negligence. The same applies to the administration of IV fluids. Nurses have a legal and professional responsibility to know the purpose and effect of the IV fluids and medications they administer. They must take care to ensure that patients receive the prescribed volume of fluid at the prescribed rate of flow. Fluid administered in an amount above or below that ordered constitutes an error that can result in fluid and electrolyte imbalances and lead to serious consequences for the patient and litigation for the nurse.

Nursing Role

The act of *observation* is the legal and professional responsibility of the nurse. Frequent observation is imperative for the early detection and prevention of complications. Undetected complications that are allowed to increase in severity because of failure to observe the patient constitute an act of negligence on the part of the nurse.

The rule of personal liability applies to supervisors and nurses under their supervision. Supervisors usually will not be held liable for the negligence of nurses under their supervision because every person is liable for his or her own wrongdoing. However, a supervisor is expected to know if the nurse is competent to perform assigned duties without supervision. Supervisors who are negligent in the assignment of an inexperienced nurse or a nurse who requires supervision may be held liable for the acts of the nurse.[1] Nurses themselves are always held liable.

Nurse–patient relationships play a significant role in influencing patients to initiate legal liability against nurses. Nurses performing IV therapy must be particularly aware of and attentive to the emotional needs of their patients. Inserting cannulas can cause pain and apprehension in patients. Specialists must develop appropriate interpersonal relationships. Nurses who are impersonal, aloof, and so busy with the technical process of starting an IV infusion that they have no time for establishing kindly relationships with patients are the suit-prone nurses whose personalities may initiate resentment and later malpractice suits. Patients most likely to sue are those who are resentful, frequently hostile, uncooperative, and dissatisfied with the nursing care. By demonstrating respect, care, and concern for all patients, as well as rendering skilled, efficient nursing care, nurses may avoid malpractice claims.

Policies and procedures should be detailed, and all nurses practicing infusion therapy should be required to know them and review them periodically. Policies and procedures should follow national guidelines established by the Centers for Disease Control and Prevention (CDC) and Standards of Practice established by the Intravenous Nurses Society (INS). These guidelines provide a model for IV nurses and foster optimal care for the patient receiving IV therapy.

Credentialing

Credentialing of IV nurses nationwide began with the first certification examination in 1985. The credentialing process consists of three components: licensure, accreditation, and certification. *Licensure* represents the entry into practice level afforded to all professional nurses who successfully complete the registered nurse examination. *Accreditation* reflects a program or service meeting established guidelines. Accreditation is offered to facilities, agencies, and other health care providers by groups such as the Joint Commission on Accreditation of Healthcare Organizations (JCAHO) and the Community Health Accreditation Program (CHAP), administered by the National League for Nursing (NLN).

Certification is the highest level attainable by the professional IV nurse. It is the process by which a society attests to the professional and clinical competence of the individual who successfully completes the process.

Evaluation of Adequate Performance

A standard must be carefully defined for the health care institution or the nurse to evaluate adequate performance. Tools useful in this process include the following:[6]

1. INS Standards of Practice[7]
2. State Board of Nursing regulations for registered nurses and licensed practical/vocational nurses

3. American Nurses Association Standards of Nursing Practice

4. Policies and procedures of the employing health care institution or agency

PLACEMENT OF THE PERIPHERALLY INSERTED CENTRAL CATHETER

The placement of a PICC requires special training and demonstrated competency on the part of the professional registered nurse. Each state sets its own practice guidelines, and not all states consider the placement of PICC catheters to be within the scope of professional nursing practice. The INS has assembled a task force to standardize the usage, terminology, and adjunctive guidelines for the insertion of PICCs. Still, it is incumbent on the institution or facility to contact the respective state Board of Nursing to determine policy. Each health care facility must establish criteria for qualification within its own legal guidelines. Such a program should include:

- Indications
- Advantages
- Placement technique
- Complications
- Care and maintenance
- Legal issues
- Product education

Minimal standards for successful completion of an educational program include:

- Satisfactory performance during initial probationary/review period
- Successful completion of inhouse IV certification course
- Clinical competency evidenced by actual practice
- Successful completion of inhouse requirements for PICC insertion

RISK MANAGEMENT

Given the continued growth of infusion therapy practice and the shift to alternative care settings, the potential for associated risks is more intense than ever before. The institution is responsible for the quality of care delivered by its agents.

Malpractice Claims

The hospital or involved professional person (or both) may be charged with malpractice if an injury occurs *and* 1) a standard of care or duty can be established; 2) the standard of care or duty was not met; 3) the patient was harmed or injured because the standard was not met; and 4) it was possible to foresee that injury or harm would result from not meeting the standards (depending on state law).

Incident Reports

An *incident report* is required for any accident or error resulting in actual or potential injury or harm. The report should contain only factual statements regarding the incident. Each report must be immediately followed by a full investigation into all possible causes, and corrective action must be taken immediately to prevent its recurrence.

Unusual Occurrence Report

Some institutions require that staff complete an *unusual occurrence report* when an untoward outcome follows administration of infusion therapy. This type of a report may be used to help identify problem patterns and institute corrective actions. Surveillance programs can be effective in preventing unsafe or insecure environments that can result in injuries to the patient.

QUALITY ASSURANCE

The JCAHO previously mandated an ongoing program for monitoring quality based on outcomes. The trend now is toward process.

Opportunities to improve the quality of care and to ensure positive patient outcomes should be pursued. Quality assurance has typically focused on:

- Identification
- Evaluation
- Analysis and interpretation
- Corrective action
- Reevaluation
- Resolution

This pattern has typically been useful in improving the quality of care to patients receiving IV therapies.

Identification

Problems may be readily identified through incident reports, patient complaints, employee complaints, questionnaires, patient satisfaction surveys, and suggestions from patients, visitors, or other staff.

To determine if a problem warrants further investigation, the following questions need to be answered:

1. Is the problem related to quality of patient care?
2. Does the problem arise frequently enough to require correction?
3. Can the problem be solved?
4. Are the benefits to patient care from solving the problem worth the cost of investigation and solution?

Evaluation

Methods used for problem evaluation may include criterion-based studies, interviews with patients and staff members, survey instruments, and observations. Experimental designs can be an excellent method for problem evaluation. However, such designs can be complex and costly.

Analysis and Interpretation

Study methodology and criteria must be established before data can be collected, analyzed, and interpreted. The Standards of Practice of the INS and guidelines of the CDC, American Association of Blood Banks, and JCAHO may all be beneficial in developing IV practice standards by which to measure performance.[1,4,8]

In analyzing and interpreting data, *compliance* refers to those situations in which the criteria are met. *Noncompliance* refers to the situations in which the criteria are not met. Both compliance and noncompliance are usually expressed in percentages. The expected compliance rate should be reasonable and achievable.

Descriptive statistics allow for meaningful reporting of findings in a small amount of space and are used to calculate: 1) the average result; 2) the difference between individual results and the average; and 3) the relationship between the average result on one part of the study and the average result on another part.[5]

Arithmetic Mean
In statistical analysis, the average result is the mean. To determine the mean, simply total all results and divide the answer by the total number in the study.

Median
Median is the result that falls exactly in the middle of all the score results.

Mode
In any test or study situation, several people can achieve the same score or test result. The score seen most frequently is called the mode.

Standard Deviation
The difference between individual results and the mean indicates the extent to which figures in a given set vary from the mean. This tells how much variation is present between the group and the individual. To calculate this figure:

1. Calculate the mean for each score.
2. Subtract the mean from each score and square the answer.
3. Add all the squares together.
4. Divide the sum by the total number of scores.
5. Take the square root of that value.

In most quality assurance studies, it is sufficient to know that normally 68% of the scores will fall, plus or minus, within a given range from the mean. Only from a well designed experimental study can one expect to find that one thing causes another to occur.

Corrective Action

Factors to consider when choosing a corrective action include: 1) areas for change that the environment can best accommodate; 2) areas of potential barriers or constraints; 3) areas of potential support; and 4) the needed resources.

The best method of corrective action depends on each particular problem and individual situation. Methods may include policy or procedure revision, equipment change, a new information system, continuous monitoring, or on-site education.

Reevaluation

After corrective action has been implemented, a reevaluation is necessary to determine if the applied corrective action resolves the problem. Frequently, reevaluation is performed by repeating the first evaluation and comparing preaction data with postaction data.

Resolution

The final step in the process is the development of a plan to ensure the maintenance of the quality of care achieved with the corrective action. Periodic or continuous screening may be required.

QUALITY IMPROVEMENT

The greatest impact on quality within health care organizations has been the influence of Deming and others who introduced the concept of Total Quality Improvement (TQI) or Continuous Quality Improvement (CQI). Such processes provide a mechanism for examining the process, rather than the individual involved, and encourage participation across interdepartmental lines to improve the process itself. Quality improvement teams within an organization are appointed and study areas are identified; process improvement is the direct result of the CQI program.

Outcome Measurement and Improvement

Interest in patient outcomes and their improvement has continued to escalate. One reason for this growth is mounting evidence of wide and perplexing variations in outcomes of care, use of resources, and costs of care.[9,10] Patient outcomes may include physiologic values (vital signs, chemical results), physical values (ability to self-administer IV therapy), mental or psychological terms (cognitive skill, affective interactions), social terms (ability to assume responsibility for self-care), and other health-related quality of life parameters (pain level, energy, sleep).

The quality assurance technique: 1) operates on the assumption that the professional or institution is the sole cause of adverse outcomes; and 2) ignores the reality that sources of adverse outcomes are complex and include variations in policies, procedures, equipment, and techniques, as well as people (patients, professionals, support staff) and their interactions.

Process Improvement

Process improvement may follow this pattern: basic process flowchart → detailed process flowchart → identify/rework errors → redesign processes.[2]

The basic flowchart begins with admission to the institution; the detailed flowchart highlights areas of possible duplication, complexity, and sources of error.[2] Using the flowchart as a basic tool, many institutions have developed methods of managing the process by incorporating the Plan-Do-Check-Act (PDCA) improvement trial. Those who use this model proceed through the following sequence: state aim → identify measures of improvement → plan—do pilot test → check and study results → act to improve → reflect on learning.[2]

- *Aim*—What are we trying to accomplish?
- *Measure*—How will we know that a change is an improvement?
- *Possible changes*—What changes can we make that we predict will lead to improvement?
- *Plan*—How shall we plan the pilot? Who? Does what? When? With what tools and training? Baseline data to collect?
- *Do*—What are we learning as we do the pilot?
- *Check*—As we check and study what happened, what have we learned?
- *Act*—As we act to hold the gains or abandon the pilot, what needs to be done?[2]

A multidisciplinary quality council may be appointed within an organization to determine the best institution-wide approach to managing quality. A technique such as process management—merging comparative data analysis, operational and clinical analysis, benchmarking (comparing an institution with the best institutions nationwide), quality methods, and simulation methods—results in improvements in quality.

REFERENCES

1. American Association of Blood Banks. (1993). Technical manual (11th ed.). Bethesda, MD: Author.
2. Baltalden, P. B., Nelson, E. C., Roberts, J. S. (1994). Linking outcomes measurement to continual improvement: The serial "V": Way of thinking about improving clinical care. *Journal on Quality Improvement* 20(4), 168–169.
3. Bernzweig, E. P. (1981). Nurse's liability for malpractice (3rd ed., p. 68). New York: McGraw–Hill.
4. Centers for Disease Control and Prevention. (1994). Guidelines for the prevention and control of nosocomial infections. Atlanta, GA: Author.
5. Colton, T. (1974). Statistics in medicine. Boston: Little, Brown.
6. Guarriello, D. L. (1983). Intravenous therapy and the law. *Journal of the National Intravenous Therapy Association, 6,* 278.
7. Revised intravenous nursing standards of practice. (1990). *Journal of Intravenous Nursing* (Suppl.), S3–S11.
8. Joint Commission on Accreditation of Healthcare Organizations. (1995). Accreditation manual for hospitals. Chicago: Author.
9. Tarlov, A. R., et al. (1989). The medical outcomes study: An application of methods for monitoring the results for medical care. *Journal of the American Medical Association, 262,* 925–930.
10. Wennberg, J. E., et al. (1989). Hospital use and mortality among Medicare beneficiaries in Boston and New Haven. *New England Journal of Medicine, 321,* 1168–1173.

BIBLIOGRAPHY

Revised intravenous nursing standards of practice. (1990). *Journal of Intravenous Nursing* (Suppl.), S17.

REVIEW QUESTIONS

1. Which of the following rules indicates that "every person is liable for his own tortious conduct"?
   a. negligent action
   b. personal liability
   c. tortious conduct
   d. wrongdoing act

2. Coercion of a rational adult patient to insert a cannula is which of the following?
   a. assault
   b. battery
   c. a only
   d. a and b

3. The credentialing process consists of which of the following components?
   a. licensure
   b. accreditation
   c. certification
   d. all of the above

4. An incident report should contain what type of information?
   a. factual
   b. anecdotal
   c. editorialized
   d. subjective

5. A PICC training program should include which of the following?
   a. practicum
   b. technique
   c. a and b
   d. b only

6. Researchers who have influenced the quality improvement process include:
   a. Deming
   b. Evanson
   c. Riding
   d. Colton

7. The process of benchmarking denotes comparing:
   a. institution to like institutions
   b. institution to the best institutions
   c. practitioner to practitioner
   d. practitioner to the best practitioner

8. Quality improvement is a way of looking at:
   a. individuals
   b. processes
   c. a and b
   d. b only

CHAPTER 3

Organization of an Intravenous Department

Key Terms

Complexities	Performance	Scope of practice
Functions	Policies	Skills
IV nursing	Preventive measures	Standards of practice
IV teams	Procedures	

INTRAVENOUS NURSING TEAMS

It is now well established that an IV nursing team enhances the level of care that an organization may provide. The quality of patient care is improved because specialized nurses, freed from other responsibilities, are able to focus their attention on developing high standards of performance. Such nurses, cognizant of the inherent risks of infusion therapy, are vigilant and meticulous in performing and maintaining IV therapy. Their high standards of performance contribute to atraumatic venipunctures, conservation of veins for future use, and reduction of routine complications. The knowledge, skills, and abilities of these specialized nurses ensure patient safety. The IV nursing teams continue to proliferate nationwide as more health care institutions recognize their value.

With the increasing complexity of IV therapies and the potential dangers associated with this practice, hospitals have recognized the value of IV therapy teams. Parenteral departments have been established in many hospitals and home care programs nationwide.

LEADERSHIP

Because the functions performed by the IV department are not generally classified as nursing procedures, the responsibility for this department is often allocated to the head of another department directly involved in the functions of IV therapy, such as the director of the blood bank, the pharmacy, or the anesthesia department. The IV department fulfills an important function of the blood bank, administering bloods and blood components; is in close alliance with the pharmacy, administering infusions of which 50% to 80% contain drugs; and executes many of the functions performed by the anesthesiologist. IV departments may also function as self-contained cost centers within the institution's infrastructure.

PHILOSOPHY AND OBJECTIVES

In organizing a department, the first consideration should be to establish a philosophy and the objectives necessary to support such a philosophy. An example follows:

Philosophy

To administer safe and successful IV therapy in the best interests of the patient, the hospital, and the nursing profession.

Objectives

The objectives of an IV department are:

1. To develop skills and impart knowledge that will provide a high level of safety in the practice of IV therapy (embodies administration of solutions and drugs, administration of blood and blood components, placement of IV cannulas, and withdrawal of blood samples)
2. To encourage further education and knowledge in the field of IV therapy
3. To assist in keeping the nursing staff educated in the maintenance of IV therapy and other nursing needs relevant to IV therapy
4. To collaborate with orientation personnel in the development and implementation of continuing education in IV therapy
5. To develop nursing judgment in IV therapy
6. To keep abreast of the latest scientific and medical advances and their implications in the practice of IV therapy

FUNCTIONS OF THE DEPARTMENT

In organizing an IV department, the functions to be performed must be delineated. They may include:

1. Administration of parenteral fluids
2. Preparation and administration of drugs in solution
3. Administration of blood and blood components

4. Routine inspection and daily change of all infusion tubings and dressings

5. Therapeutic phlebotomy

6. Collection of venous blood samples for all laboratories: chemistry, bacteriology, hematology, blood bank, and so on. This includes:

    a. Collection of blood samples from central lines

    b. Knowledge of the requirements of the various laboratory tests, including the proper collection and handling of blood samples

7. Total parenteral nutrition

8. Antineoplastic therapy

9. Intra-arterial therapy

10. Pediatric IV therapy

11. Home infusion therapy

12. Outpatient procedures

13. Pain management

14. Placement of peripherally inserted central catheters

15. Maintenance of intra-arterial lines, Ommaya reservoirs, and other alternative accesses

16. Development of departmental policies and procedures in collaboration with other hospital departments to meet patient care needs

Policies and Procedures

Policies and procedures play a vital role in the functioning of a department, serving as a guide to its operations, providing the nurse with adequate instruction, and ensuring the patient of a high level of nursing care. They may also provide legal protection in determining whether an individual involved in negligent conduct has had adequate instruction in performing the act.

Policies and procedures should comply with state and federal laws, and national guidelines should be followed. The Joint Commission on Accreditation of Healthcare Organizations (JCAHO) publishes a manual for both hospital and home care accreditation. The American Association of Blood Banks (AABB) provides a technical manual with standards for care and administration of blood and component therapy. The Centers for Disease Control and Prevention (CDC) and Intravenous Nurses Society (INS) provide guidelines as well as Standards of Practice.[2]

Policies describing the responsibilities of the IV nurse vary significantly among hospitals and should be outlined to prevent confusion or misunderstanding. Examples of a few such policies follow.

Administration of Parenteral Fluids

1. IV nurses will, on written order, initiate all infusions, with the exception of those not approved for administration by the nurse.

2. No more than two attempts at venipuncture will be allowed.

3. Venipunctures should be avoided in the lower extremities except when the pa-

tient's condition may necessitate this use and this location has specifically been ordered by the physician.

Preparation and Administration of Intravenous Drugs

1. Nurses will, on written order, prepare and administer only those solutions, medications, and combinations of drugs approved in writing by the pharmacy and the therapeutics committee.
2. Nurses must check the patient's clinical record and question the patient regarding sensitivity to drugs that may cause anaphylaxis. They must observe the patient after initial administration of such drugs.

Use of Force in Performing Venipuncture

No coercion will ever be used on a rational adult patient. A patient may refuse treatment.

Patency Flushing

Flushing with heparinized saline solution to ensure and maintain patency of an intermittent IV cannula shall be accomplished at established intervals.[2] The concentration of heparinized saline used should not alter the patient's clotting factors.

Incompatibility Flushing

Flushing with 0.9% sodium chloride shall be done prior to and following administration of medications and solutions that are incompatible.

Product Integrity

All IV therapy products are to be checked for integrity before use.

Nursing Care Plan

A nursing care plan should be established within 24 hours of date/time of admission.

Peripheral Cannula Selection

The cannula selected should be of the smallest gauge and shortest length to accommodate the prescribed therapy. Only radiopaque catheters may be used.

Personnel Qualifications

Because IV therapy involves specialized judgment and skills, the IV nurse must be qualified to meet the job requirements and scope of practice.[2] Because of the highly specialized therapy and the responsibility involved, the success of the department depends on the selection of its personnel.

The nurse, who will be drawing blood samples and giving transfusions where carelessness can mean a patient's life, must be conscientious. The importance of the job, the importance of being accurate, and the importance of careful patient identification must be realized by the nurse. Duties include mixing and administering drugs which, given IV, act rapidly. There is no margin for error.

Collaboration and teamwork are essential to the success of the department. No one individual's job is finished until the entire department has completed its work. If one nurse becomes involved in a time-consuming emergency, the others must be ready and willing to assist and accomplish the remaining work.

Mental and emotional stability are important in the nurse's success as an IV specialist. Manual dexterity, necessary in administering an IV infusion, is greatly affected by the mental and emotional attitude of the nurse. The performance of few procedures is so easily affected by stress as is the execution of a difficult venipuncture.

Outstanding verbal and written communication skills are other assets necessary to the success of the individual and the department. The nurse has unpleasant functions to perform, which are better tolerated by the patient if the nurse is empathic.

Tact is important. The nurse works in close conjunction with the hospital nursing staff, ancillary departments, and the patient. An inappropriate attitude and uncooperative personality can do much to impair harmony and disrupt care.

The nurse in charge of the IV department, who must assume responsibility for the teaching, training, and successful functioning of this department, should have a voice in selecting its personnel.

Once the functions of this department are classified, the work load should start at a reasonable level. It may be desirable to start by performing only a few designated functions, such as the administration of blood and fluids. After this program has been successfully organized, other functions may be added. By so doing, the problems that may arise when initiating such a program can be met and remedied, and the success of the department may be guaranteed from the outset.

Before this department can be operational, the hospital nursing staff must first be apprised of its functions.

Call System

A system for receiving calls must be organized, with special emphasis on emergency calls. Some systems work better than others under various conditions. The size of the hospital, number of patients, size and location of the department, and the functions to be performed must be considered when deciding which system would be most adaptable. Voicemail may be used for routine scheduling and non-emergencies.

Requisitions
Requests for parenteral administrations and other functions may be filled out on requisitions and sent to the department. This system has the drawbacks of added paperwork, lost time involved, and the necessity of the IV nurse having to return to the department to pick up the requisitions. It may prove successful in a smaller hospital, where calls are not as numerous as in a large hospital and where the nurses are stationed in the blood bank or pharmacy. Facsimile transmissions are also frequently used to save time and ensure accuracy.

Page System
The page operator lists the floor extensions as they are received. The IV nurse calls in every half hour to pick up calls. Any emergency call may be put through by means of voice page or by means of a radio pager.

Routine Rounds

Routine rounds may be made twice a day by the IV nurse. The requests for services are listed on a clipboard with the patient's name and room number. When orders have been filled, they are checked off by the IV nurse. Emergencies are handled by pager.

This system involves less expenditure of time by the nursing staff. It eliminates the necessity for placing calls or sending out requisitions. The IV department is freed from unnecessary phone calls. The charge nurse, with a glance at the board, immediately knows what procedures have been performed.

Preparation of Equipment

Setting up the necessary equipment for procedures to be performed must be allotted to either the IV department or the nursing staff.

Preparation of Equipment by the Intravenous Department

When preparation of equipment becomes the responsibility of the IV department, an equipment cart must be provided on each floor. This cart carries all necessary equipment for parenteral administration as follows:

IV solutions	Alcohol, povidone prep pads
Venous access devices	Syringes
Armboards	Sterile sponges
Administration sets	Antiseptic swabs and ointment
Filters	Transparent dressings
Tourniquet	IV start kits
Tape	Gloves

The professional IV nurse ascertains the accuracy of the physician's order and assembles supplies from the cart maintained on each nursing unit or from alternative means.

Other Systems

Regardless of the method of securing equipment for venipuncture, the IV nurse has a crucial role in determining accuracy of the order, assembling the appropriate equipment consistent with the therapy that has been ordered, and using the equipment in a safe manner.

Patients with infusions in progress may visit ancillary hospital departments during their hospital stay, including medical imaging, nuclear medicine, surgery, and others. To ensure the success and viability of an IV therapy department/team, other departments within the institution must be oriented to the team's functions. If orders are written early in the day, it will be easier to meet all requests and to ensure timely delivery of therapy to each patient under the team's care.

DIDACTIC PROGRAM

An adequate teaching program and criteria for the evaluation of the IV nurse must be established. The criteria depend on the role of the IV nurse as dictated by hospital policies. The competency of the nurse must be evaluated and maintained. The IV nurse receives on-the-job training. The length of time involved in teaching depends on the individual and may range from 6 to 8 weeks. The following is a suggested outline for teaching IV, drug, and transfusion therapy.

Suggested Teaching Outline

I. Legal implications of IV therapy
  A. State policy
    1. Review state rulings, joint policies related to IV therapy.
  B. Hospital policy
    1. Review health institution's or agency's policy, which has been approved by the medical staff.
    2. Responsibilities of nurse in administering IV therapy
    3. List of fluids and drugs delineated by the hospital for administration by the nurse
  C. National standards
    1. CDC
    2. INS
  D. Legal requirements
    1. Qualification by education and experience
    2. Adherence to hospital policy
    3. Thorough knowledge of fluids and drugs: their effects, limitations, and dosages
    4. Order by licensed physician for specific patient
    5. Skilled judgment
  E. Review of policy and procedure books
    1. Policy statements do not provide immunity if the nurse is negligent.
    2. The nurse is legally responsible for own actions.

II. Equipment
  A. Review all types of equipment, their characteristics and usage.
  B. Review procedures for the proper handling of equipment, changing of administration sets, use of products.
  C. Adhere to established infection control procedures and guidelines in the use of equipment.
    1. Aseptic technique in manipulation of equipment
    2. Inspection of parenteral fluids and containers
    3. Scheduled change of administration sets

III. Anatomy and physiology as applied to IV therapy
  A. Review names and locations of peripheral veins of the upper extremity.
  B. Differentiate between arteries and veins. Recognize an inadvertent arterial puncture.
  C. Recognize dangers associated with the use of veins of the lower extremities.

   D. Understand factors that influence the size and condition of the vein.
      1. Trauma
      2. Temperature
      3. Diagnosis of the patient
      4. Psychological outlook of the patient
   E. Choose veins suitable for venipuncture
      1. To infuse various fluids and medications, with preservation of veins in mind
      2. To draw blood samples
      3. To administer blood
IV. IV therapy
   A. Methods of infusion
      1. Continuous
      2. Intermittent
      3. Electronic infusion device
   B. Manner and approach to the patient
      1. Explain the vasovagal reaction (an undesirable autonomic nervous system response).
      2. Alleviate fears.
         a. Make patient comfortable.
         b. Explain procedure.
         c. Reassure patient.
         d. Appear confident.
   C. Methods of venous distention
      1. Apply a broad tourniquet above selected site.
      2. Apply a blood pressure cuff inflated to 50 to 60 mm Hg or to just below diastolic pressure.
      3. Have patient clench fist periodically.
      4. Allow arm to hang dependent over the side of the bed.
      5. Tap lightly slightly distal to the proposed venipuncture site.
      6. Apply moist heat to entire extremity.
   D. Antiseptic and aseptic technique. Skin flora have been implicated as an important source of organisms responsible for catheter-associated infection. Stress importance of handwashing. Adherence to aseptic technique is imperative, especially during preparation of the venipuncture site.
   E. Choice of cannula (steel needle, catheter)
      1. Purpose of the infusion
      2. Condition and availability of the vein
      3. Gauge and length of cannula depend on:
         a. Location of the vein
         b. Fluid used
         c. Purpose of the infusion
         d. Available venous access
   F. Techniques of venipuncture
      1. Steel needle
      2. Syringe and needle
      3. Vacuum tube and needle holder (commercially supplied)

4. Catheters (over-the-needle, through-the-needle). Complications associated with catheters include mechanical and chemical thrombophlebitis, infection, and catheter embolism.

G. Hazards and complications. Observing the patient, reporting reactions, and taking measures to prevent complications are the nurse's legal and professional responsibilities.

1. Systemic complications

a. Infections (septicemia, fungemia)

Preventive measures:

(1) Use aseptic technique.

(2) Inspect all fluids and containers before use.

(3) Use fluids within 24 hours.

(4) Change administration sets consistent with published standards.

(5) Do not irrigate plugged cannulas.

(6) Remove nonfunctioning sets and needles.

b. Pulmonary embolism (occurs when a substance, usually a clot, becomes free floating and is propelled by the venous circulation to the right side of the heart and into the pulmonary artery)

Preventive measures:

(1) Use clot filters for infusing blood and blood components.

(2) Use special blood filters of micropore size for infusing several units of stored bank blood.

(3) Avoid using veins of the lower extremities.

(4) Avoid irrigating plugged cannulas.

c. Air embolism (may be fatal when small bubbles accumulate dangerously and form tenacious bubbles that block the pulmonary capillaries)

Preventive measures:

(1) Vigilance in preventing fluid containers from emptying. Infusions through a central venous catheter carry greater risk of running dry because a negative venous pressure is more likely.

(2) Vented Y-type infusions or piggyback infusions allowing solutions to run simultaneously may introduce air into line if container empties. Check valves, safety valves, and micropore filters (wet) to reduce this risk.

d. Circulatory overload (a real hazard in patients with impaired renal and cardiac functions)

Preventive measures:

(1) Maintain infusion at prescribed flow rate. Do not play "catch-up" if infusion is behind schedule.

(2) Never apply positive pressure when infusing fluids and blood.

(3) Do not administer fluids in excess of quantity ordered to maintain a keep-open infusion.

(4) Be alert to signs of circulatory overload.

e. Speed shock (systemic reaction occurring when a substance foreign to the body is rapidly introduced into the circulation)

Preventive measures:
    (1) Slow injection of drugs
    (2) Use of controlled-volume chambers
    (3) Use of microbore drip sets
    (4) Use of double clamps—an extra clamp ensures greater safety should the initial clamp let go.
    (5) Ensure that IV fluid is flowing freely before regulating flow.
  f. Fluid and medication error
Preventive measures:
    (1) Be familiar with IV fluids.
    (2) Know drug, dosage, and rate of administration.
    (3) Clarify orders.
    (4) Verify identity of the patient and the admixture.
 2. Local complications
  a. Phlebitis (mechanical, chemical, and septic)
Preventive measures:
    (1) Do not use veins located over an area of joint flexion.
    (2) Anchor cannulas well to prevent motion and reduce the risk of introducing microorganisms into puncture wound.
    (3) Adequately dilute medications.
    (4) Use a cannula relatively smaller than the vein.
    (5) Use aseptic and antiseptic technique.
    (6) Remove cannula within 48 hours.
    (7) Remove cannula for:
      (a) Erythema
      (b) Induration
      (c) Tenderness by palpation of venous cord
      (d) Nonfunctioning needle
  b. Infiltration (recognize extravasation)
    (1) Check questionable extremity against normal extremity.
    (2) Apply a tourniquet tightly enough to restrict venous flow proximal to the injection site. If infusion continues regardless of this venous obstruction, extravasation is evident.
 H. Intra-arterial therapy
  1. Arterial puncture
    a. Syringe and needle
    b. Indwelling catheter
  2. Constant arterial pressure monitoring
    a. Set-up procedure
  3. Arterial blood gases
    a. Collection
    b. Interpretation
  4. Swan-Ganz catheter
    a. Basic knowledge
    b. Insertion
    c. Complications
V. Rationale of fluid and electrolyte therapy
 A. Fundamentals of fluid and electrolyte metabolism

       1. Body fluid compartments
       2. Electrolyte composition
       3. Acid–base balance
   B. Principles of fluid therapy
       1. Deficit
       2. Maintenance
       3. Replacement
   C. IV fluids
       1. Classification and effect
          a. Isotonic
          b. Hypotonic
          c. Hypertonic
       2. Parenteral fluids

VI. Drug therapy
   A. Hazards
       1. Incompatibilities
          a. Therapeutic (undesirable reaction from overlapping effect of two drugs)
          b. Physical (interaction that leads to a visible change such as color, precipitate, or gas bubbles)
          c. Chemical (invisible interaction, with degradation of drug and loss of therapeutic activity)
       2. Vascular trauma
       3. Speed shock
       4. Bacterial and fungal contamination
       5. Particulate contamination
       6. Medication errors
   B. Knowledge of the drug
       1. Dose and effect
       2. Recommended rate of infusion
       3. Reactions
       4. Contraindications
   C. Factors controlling stability and compatibility of admixtures
       1. Pharmaceutical agents in drug formation (buffers, preservatives, and stabilizers)
       2. Brand of drug (formulation varies)
       3. pH of drug, pH of IV fluid
       4. Concentration (degree of dilution)
       5. Order of mixing
       6. Diluent
       7. Period of time solution stands
       8. Light
       9. Temperature
   D. Preparation of admixture
       1. Procedure for transcribing orders on medication label
       2. Frequency with which medication order should be renewed
       3. Reconstitution of drug using aseptic and antiseptic technique
          a. Correct diluent

          b. Correct volume

          c. Absence of particulate matter

     4. Procedure for adding drug to fluid container

     5. Stability of the admixture

     6. Labeling

  E. Administration of drugs

     1. Verify identity of patient and admixture.

     2. Check for sensitivities of patient to any drug that may cause anaphylaxis.

     3. Observe patient for untoward reactions when administering an initial dose of an antibiotic.

     4. Patients known to be sensitive to a drug require the presence of a physician.

     5. Inspect admixture each time before administration.

     6. Record drug, dosage, and amount of fluid on fluid intake chart and medication sheet.

VII. Transfusion therapy

  A. Principles of immunohematology

     1. Factors governing red blood cell destruction

     2. ABO compatibility

     3. Rh compatibility

     4. Handling and storage of blood

  B. Blood and blood components

     1. Uses

     2. Methods of administration

     3. Reactions and protocol to follow

  C. Administration of blood and blood components

     1. Order for the transfusion must be written on the day the transfusion is scheduled.

     2. Substantiate identity of patient and blood.

     3. Inspect blood before administration.

     4. Follow proper technique in administration.

     5. Observe patient.

     6. Document in patient's record.

IMPACT OF COST CONTAINMENT ON INFUSION TEAMS

In today's managed care environment, it is becoming increasingly difficult for established IV teams to justify their existence and for new teams to gain approval. The hospital setting has changed dramatically; fiscal constraints are often overwhelming, forcing institutions to scrutinize methods of therapy delivery for efficiency and cost effectiveness.

As a result, hospitals have downsized, restructured the workplace, and developed new patient care delivery models. Such models have had a significant impact on IV teams because ancillary services are not regarded as appropriate to the new, centralized, unit-based approach to patient care. In all practice settings, IV teams must be innovative and adaptable while maximizing capabilities and analyzing complimentary practice roles and multidisciplinary care.[1] The teams must work with their professional society to lead the way toward designing new directions for IV nursing practice.[1]

Recently, the Centers for Disease Control and Prevention (CDC) released the draft, "Guidelines for Prevention of Intravascular Device-Related Infections: An Overview and Part 2, Recommendations for Prevention of Intravascular Device-Related Infections." The draft was published in the September 27, 1995 Federal Register (Vol. 60, No. 187). The final document will be published in Infection Control and Hospital Epidemiology as well as the American Journal of Infection Control. The revised guidelines are expected to advise hospitals that eliminating IV teams downgrades patient care by raising the risk of infection. The new document will upgrade the CDC recommendation that IV teams be used in hospitals from a category 3 rating (weak) to a category 1 rating (strongest).[4]

REFERENCES

1. Baranowski, L. (1995). Presidential address: Take ownership. *Journal of Intravenous Nursing* 18(4), 163.
2. Centers for Disease Control and Prevention. (1994). *Guidelines for prevention of intravascular infection.* Atlanta, GA: Author.
3. Revised intravenous nursing standards of practice. (1990). *Journal of Intravenous Nursing,* (Suppl.), S7.
4. *Nursing Spectrum,* April 22, 1996, 9(9), p.3.

REVIEW QUESTIONS

1. Parenteral infusion teams are a part of the program in which of the following?
   a. home care companies
   b. acute care hospitals
   c. clinics
   d. all of the above

2. Leadership of the IV department may be:
   a. self-directed
   b. pharmacy
   c. administration
   d. any of the above

3. Policies and procedures should comply with which of the following?
   a. state and federal laws
   b. local ordinances
   c. county rules and regulations
   d. local law

4. Concentration of heparinized saline used should:
   a. not alter patient's clotting factors
   b. alter patient's clotting factors
   c. minimally alter patient's bleeding time
   d. not alter patient's bleeding time

5. A cannula selected for peripheral infusion therapy should be:
   a. largest gauge and longest length
   b. smallest gauge and shortest length
   c. largest gauge and shortest length
   d. smallest gauge and longest length

CHAPTER 4

Nursing Roles and Responsibilities

Key Terms

Assessment	Nursing care plan	Role
Complications	Responsibility	Standards of practice
Hazards		

Administration of safe, high-quality infusion therapy in the health care organization depends on the contributions of many members of the health care team. The nurse plays a primary role in maintaining the infusion and in protecting the patient from the hazards and complications associated with routine IV therapy. Policies regarding the responsibilities of staff nurses vary significantly among health care institutions and are often influenced by the presence or absence of a full-service IV team.

National standards of practice and guidelines have been established to protect the patient. Each nurse within an organization must be cognizant of the policies and procedures relevant to infusion therapy and be familiar with nursing responsibilities to provide a safe level of care for the patient.

The role of an IV team and delineation of responsibilities must be part of the orientation program and ongoing education for all nurses to provide a team approach to safe IV care. Specialized teams of IV nurses provide clinical expertise and cost-effective care and decrease the risk of complications associated with infusion therapy. Ideally, registered nurses with clinical and theoretical expertise should be responsible for administering IV therapy. All nurses responsible for administering IV therapy should be familiar with established Standards of Practice.

STANDARDS OF PRACTICE

The Intravenous Nurses Society's (INS) Standards of Practice is an authoritative document that outlines the nurse's scope of practice and educational requirements and defines autonomy, accountability, and responsibility for the specialty practice of infusion therapy. Institutional policies and procedures should be developed and implemented based on these standards and interpretations, regardless of the clinical setting in which care is delivered.

NURSING CARE PLAN

A nursing care plan should be established within 24 hours of completion of the initial nursing assessment. The care plan should:

- Reflect nursing diagnosis
- Evaluate progress and effectiveness of care
- Include time frames for goal achievement
- Be modified consistent with the patient's clinical progress

ASSESSMENT

Initial assessment of the patient for whom IV therapy has been ordered includes a review of body systems, underlying illnesses that may have an impact on the results of infusion therapy, and the status of the patient's vascular system. A thorough assessment enables the clinician to select a site appropriate for the type of therapy ordered and ensures positive IV therapy patient outcomes.

INITIATION

Intravenous therapy is initiated for therapeutic or diagnostic purposes on the order of a licensed physician. Consent should be confirmed before therapy is initiated. The physician's order should include:

- Volume
- Rate
- Frequency
- Route

SITE SELECTION

Site selection ensures the most appropriate vascular access for delivery of the prescribed therapy. For peripheral and arterial therapy, the selection process includes:

- Patient's condition
- Age
- Diagnosis
- Vein condition
- Size
- Location
- Type and duration of therapy
- Other therapies in progress

Vein selection for placement of peripherally inserted central catheters (PICCs) includes:

- Patient's condition
- Age
- Diagnosis
- Vein condition
- Size
- Location
- Type and duration of therapy
- Anatomic measurements to ensure full advancement of the catheter and catheter tip placement in a central vein

Site selection of central catheters, other than for PICCs, is a medical act.

CANNULA SELECTION

Proper cannula selection is imperative to accommodate the prescribed therapy and to minimize potential complications. The cannula selected for peripheral and arterial therapy should be the smallest gauge and length that will accommodate the therapy required. All catheters should have radiopaque properties.

The catheter selected for PICC placement should be radiopaque, designed for central placement by peripheral access; the length should be sufficient to enable the tip to reside in the superior vena cava.

Selection of central catheters is consistent with the patient's condition and prescribed therapies.

HAIR REMOVAL

Excess hair is removed to enhance access; hair should be clipped with safety scissors.

SITE PREPARATION

Aseptically cleaning the peripheral or arterial site before cannula insertion reduces the potential for infection by minimizing microbial flora on the skin. Unusually dirty skin may be cleansed with soap and water initially. Antimicrobial solutions that may be used to prepare the cannula site include:

- Tincture of iodine 1% to 2%
- Iodophors
- 70% isopropyl alcohol
- Chlorhexidine

When isopropyl alcohol is used, it should be applied with friction for a minimum of 30 seconds or until the final applicator is visually clean.[2]

CANNULA PLACEMENT

The cannula should be placed for a specific therapeutic or diagnostic indication. Aseptic technique should be used. A device may be used one time only. When aseptic technique has been compromised, as in an emergency, the line is considered compromised, and another cannula should be placed as soon as the patient stabilizes but within 24 hours. The contaminated line should then be removed.

Cannulas should be stabilized so that the nurse is able to monitor and assess the site. Tape or securement devices are generally used.[2]

Junction Securement

Junctions may be secured with Luer locking devices, clasps, and tape.[2]

Dressings

A sterile, occlusive dressing is used to ensure integrity of the IV site. The dressing may be tape and gauze or semipermeable membrane material.[2]

Needle/Stylet Disposal

Recapping of used devices increases potential risk to the nurse. Needles and stylets should be disposed of in nonpermeable tamperproof containers. Use of needleless systems minimizes risk of needlestick injuries.[2]

INTRAVENOUS ADMINISTRATION SET CHANGE

Routine changing of administration sets is an infection control measure. Administration sets are changed consistent with the type of set used and the specific therapy ordered for the patient.[2]

Primary Continuous

1. Change every 48 hours and immediately on suspected contamination or when the integrity of the product has been compromised.
2. Avoid touch contamination.
3. Use aseptic technique.

Secondary

1. Change every 48 hours and immediately on suspected contamination or when the integrity of the product has been compromised.
2. Avoid touch contamination.
3. Use aseptic technique.

Primary Intermittent

1. Change every 24 hours and immediately on suspected contamination or when the integrity of the product has been compromised.
2. Remove attached needles after each use, and aseptically attach a new, sterile needle.
3. Maintain asepsis.
4. Avoid touch contamination.
5. Change of add-on devices should coincide with changing of the administration set.

Total Parenteral Nutrition

1. Change every 24 hours and immediately on suspected contamination or when the integrity of the product has been compromised.
2. Use aseptic technique.
3. Sets specific for electronic infusion devices should be changed every 24 hours unless physical properties or visual inspection requires more frequent set change.

Lipid Emulsion

1. Discard after each use unless additional units are added consecutively.
2. If consecutive administration is used, change every 24 hours.
3. Change immediately on suspected contamination or when the integrity of the product has been compromised.

Blood/Blood Components

1. Change after each unit given.
2. Change immediately on suspected contamination or when the integrity of the product has been compromised.
3. Use aseptic technique.
4. Do not use for more than 4 hours.
5. Change add-on filters consistent with set change.
6. Use each set for only one unit to identify the unit responsible for a possible reaction.

Hemodynamic and Arterial Pressure Monitoring

1. Change set, dome, and pressure tubing every 48 hours and immediately on suspected contamination or if the integrity of the product has been compromised.
2. Use aseptic technique.
3. Change of add-on devices should coincide with set change.

INTRAVENOUS CONTAINERS

The risk of infection is great if aseptic technique is not observed.

1. Wash hands before parenteral fluids are opened and administered.
2. Inspect fluid containers before use for cracks, leaks, damaged caps, and expiration date.
3. Inspect fluid for discoloration, turbidity, and evidence of particulate matter.
4. Check label to ensure evidence of time and date opened, any additives, and appropriateness of infusate for the patient for whom ordered.

DRESSING CHANGES

A sterile, occlusive dressing is an appropriate infection control measure.

1. Gauze dressings should be applied aseptically and securely taped.
2. Change every 48 hours and immediately if the integrity of the dressing has been compromised.
3. When a transparent semipermeable membrane (TSM) is used over gauze, it is considered a gauze dressing and should be changed every 48 hours.
4. Do not cover site dressings with roller bandages.
5. TSM dressings should be changed at established intervals using aseptic technique or when the integrity of the dressing has been compromised.

AMBULATING THE PATIENT

Special precautions must be taken when ambulating patients with infusions. The fluid container must be kept sufficiently high at all times to maintain a constant flow. Any cessation in the rate must be detected immediately and remedied before a clot is allowed to plug the needle.

FREQUENT OBSERVATION

Fluid maintenance requires frequent observation of patients receiving infusions. The attending nurse should visit the patient frequently, checking the rate of flow, the amount of solution remaining, and the site of infusion, as described in the following sections.

Rate of Flow

Because the rate of flow, once established, is often difficult to maintain, the staff nurse should check and readjust the flow whenever necessary. Flow control devices may be used to assist in regulating a prescribed administration rate. Electronic infusion devices may be used when warranted by the patient's age, condition, and prescribed therapy.

When Infusion Stops

When an infusion stops, the cause must be immediately investigated and remedied. The following procedure is to be used:

1. Check for infiltration.
2. Check the fluid level in the bottle.
3. Check for kinking of the tubing.
4. Open the clamp.
5. Check air vent. Has it been inserted if required and is it patent?
6. Check the cannula for patency by kinking the tubing a few inches from the cannula while pinching and releasing the tubing between the cannula and the kinked tubing. Resistance, if encountered, should be treated with caution because a clot may have plugged the cannula. If the patient complains of pain, a sclerosed vein may be the cause of the cessation of flow. In either case, the cannula must be removed.
7. Is the cannula in line with the vein or up against the wall of the vein? A slight adjustment, by moving the cannula, may remedy the problem.
8. If the IV solution is cold, as in the case of blood, venous spasm may result. Heat placed directly on the vein will relieve the spasm and increase the flow of the infusion.
9. If the infusion is blood, check the filter; heavy sediment may be slowing the flow. Replace the filter if necessary.
10. Increase the height of the bottle to increase gravity.
11. If unable to restart the flow after these procedures have been followed, restart the infusion.

Amount of Solution in the Container

Air embolism and *blood embolism* are significant hazards of infusion therapy and may be associated with delay in changing solution containers. Subsequent solutions should be added before the level of fluid falls in the drip chamber. Failure to do this results in the following problems.

Plugged Cannula

Intravenous solutions flow into the vein by means of gravity. Once the fluid level has dropped in the tubing to about the level of the patient's chest, the blood will be forced back into the cannula, occluding the lumen of the cannula. Occluded cannulas should be removed, not irrigated. Fibrinous material injected into the vein can propagate a thrombus, possibly resulting in an infarction. Irrigation may embolize small infected cannula thrombi, which could result in septicemia. Aspiration aimed at dislodging the fibrin may cause the vein to collapse around the cannula point, traumatizing the vessel wall.

Trapped Air

If the bottle (in an air-venting system) is changed after the level of fluid drops in the tubing and before the cannula plugs, the air is trapped in the tubing and forced into the patient by pressure of the fresh solution. Fatal air embolism can result. The use of plastic bags, containers that contain no air, and administration sets that have no junctions through which air can leak have reduced the risk of introducing air into the patient's veins. Air can be introduced at the beginning of an infusion by not completely clearing the set of air or when changing containers. Infusions through a central venous catheter carry an even greater risk of air embolism than do those through a peripheral vein. Air embolism can occur during tubing changes involving the central venous catheter. It has been suggested, through animal experimentation, that a normal adult should tolerate air embolism of as much as 200 mL, but for persons in poor health smaller amounts may be fatal; less than 10 mL might be fatal in a gravely ill person.[1]

Before the flow ceases and the bottle empties, replace the empty bottle with fresh solution using the following procedure:

1. Vent fresh bottle if vent is required.
2. Kink tubing to prevent air from being introduced into the flowing solution.
3. Change container. Hang solution bottle before unkinking tubing.
4. Readjust rate if necessary.

Nonfunctioning (leaking or plugged) sets should be removed.

The 0.2-μm Air-Eliminating Filter

A 0.2-μm air-eliminating filter protects the patient from air embolism, bacteria, and particulate matter. The INS advocates the use of the 0.2-μm air-eliminating filters for routine administration of IV fluids.[2]

Recommendations for the Use of 0.2-μm Air-Eliminating Filters[2]

1. The filter should be placed at the terminal end of the administration set, that is, as close to the cannula as possible.
2. The filter should be changed at the time of administration set change.
3. Lipid emulsions, blood, and blood products should not be administered through the filter.
4. Consideration must be made to the administration of some drugs because their dosage may be affected by the filter; follow the manufacturer's recommendations.
5. The psi of the filter must be compatible with the electronic infusion device in use.

Infiltration or Inflammation at Injection Site

Failure to recognize an infiltration before the swelling has increased to a sizable degree may:

1. Cause damage to the tissues.
2. Prevent the patient from receiving necessary and urgent medication.
3. Limit veins available for future therapy.

If the question of infiltration exists, compare the questionable extremity with the normal extremity. An infusion has infiltrated if:

1. Swelling occurs about the site of the cannula.
2. A tourniquet applied above the cannula does not stop the flow of fluid.

Checking for an infiltration by a backflow of blood into the adapter is not a reliable method because:

1. In small veins, the cannula may approach the size of the vein, occluding the lumen and obstructing the flow of blood; the solution flows undiluted so that no backflow of blood is obtained.
2. The cannula may have punctured the vein, causing an infiltration, and at the same time be within the lumen of the vein, or the bevel may be only partially within the lumen of the vein, causing a swelling and still producing a backflow of blood on test.

Inspect the injection site for erythema, induration, or tenderness by palpating the venous cord. If any of these signs occur, remove the cannula. When replacing it, sterile equipment should be used and the site changed, preferably to the opposite arm. Should infection be noted, the cannula and the infusate should be cultured and lot numbers of sets and infusions recorded.

MONITORING

Ongoing monitoring provides information regarding a patient's response to the prescribed therapies. Patients receiving IV therapies should be monitored at frequent, established intervals based on practice setting, prescribed therapy, condition, and age. Monitoring should:

- Be established in policies and procedures
- Minimize risk of potential complications of routine IV therapy
- Include cannula site, flow rate, clinical data, patient response[2]

DOCUMENTATION

Documentation of care provides written affirmation of the level of care provided and should include the following:

- Cannula
- Site
- Patient's response to treatment
- Type of treatment
- Date, time
- Name of professional providing care

Documentation should provide sufficient information to identify procedures, prescribed treatments, complications, and nursing interventions.[2]

DISCONTINUATION OF THERAPY AND CANNULA REMOVAL

To discontinue an infusion, use the following procedure:

1. Stop flow by clamping off tubing.

2. Remove all tape from cannula. Do not use scissors.

3. With a dry sterile sponge held over the injection site, remove cannula. The cannula must be removed nearly flush with the skin. This prevents the point from damaging the posterior wall of the vein, thus encouraging the process of thrombosis. Visually ascertain that the length of the cannula removed corresponds with length inserted. Information should be noted on the dressing.

4. Apply pressure instantly and firmly. Do not rub. Hematomas occur from cannulas carelessly removed and render veins useless for future cannulation.

Small adhesive bandages, such as Band-Aids, should not be used unless specifically ordered. It must be emphasized that such a bandage is not used to stop bleeding and does not take the place of pressure. If ordered, it should be applied only after pressure has been applied and the bleeding stopped.

REFERENCES

1. Fireitag, J., & Miller L. (Eds.). (1980). *Manual of medical therapeutics* (23rd ed., p. 293). Boston: Little, Brown.

2. *Revised intravenous nursing standards of practice.* (1990). *Journal of Intravenous Nursing* (Suppl.), S20, 27-31, 33, 35, 57.

BIBLIOGRAPHY

Alfaro, R. (1986). *Application of nursing process: A step-by-step guide* (p. 108). Philadelphia: J. B. Lippincott.

Hogan, G. F. (1986). Signature requirements for drug orders in medical records. *American Journal of Hospital Pharmacy, 43*(5), 1152.

REVIEW QUESTIONS

1. The INS Standards document defines:
   a. scope of practice
   b. educational requirements
   c. a only
   d. a and b

2. Ongoing monitoring provides information regarding:
   a. care plan
   b. set change
   c. patient's response to therapy
   d. family's feelings about therapy

3. To minimize the risk of phlebitis, routine IV tubing should be changed at what frequency?
   a. 24 hours
   b. 36 hours
   c. 48 hours
   d. 72 hours

4. Tubing used to administer total parenteral nutrition should be changed at what frequency?
   a. 24 hours
   b. 36 hours
   c. 48 hours
   d. 72 hours

5. Which of the following is an appropriate occlusive dressing?
   a. adhesive strip
   b. gauze and tape
   c. transparent semipermeable membrane
   d. elastoplast

6. The 0.2-μm filter protects the patient from which of the following?
   a. air
   b. bacteria
   c. particulate matter
   d. all of the above

7. Which of the following is NOT true of failure to recognize an infiltration?
   a. damage to the tissues occurs
   b. patient prevented from receiving medication
   c. limited access available
   d. patient's care will not be compromised

8. Which of the following is NOT a sign of infusion phlebitis?
   a. redness
   b. swelling
   c. tenderness
   d. pus

9. An IV nursing care plan should reflect which of the following?
   a. nursing diagnosis
   b. time frames for goal achievement
   c. evaluation of process and effectiveness of care
   d. all of the above

10. Monitoring of infusion therapy:
    a. minimizes risk
    b. eliminates risk
    c. maximizes risk
    d. produces risk

Chapter 5

Cost Factors Associated With Infusion Therapy

Key Terms

Alternate site	Capitation	Health care reform
Case management	Cost cutting	Managed care

Hospitals and other health care providers today face an increasing complex dilemma—that of providing the highest quality of care at the lowest price.[1] Cost-cutting measures have enhanced the growth of new ways to provide IV services, such as outpatient centers, physicians' offices, infusion centers, and home care. Hospitals nationwide have used the specter of impending national health care reform to justify downsizing and reorganization. IV nurses must assess the level of skills and services currently being provided and determine avenues to best use their skills, including, but not limited to:

- Outpatients
- Physicians' offices
- Rural settings
- Other hospitals within their system
- Home care agencies
- Surgicenters
- Peripherally inserted central and midline catheter insertions

- Nursing homes and long-term care facilities
- Workshops for other staff and community[2]

Adding to this problem is the influx of managed care programs and a case management approach to patient care.

MANAGED CARE

Managed care is a system of controls to manage access, cost, and quality of health care services. The controls may include any or all of the following:

- Preferred provider contracts
- Prior approval/authorization
- Patient education/incentives
- Utilization review/quality assurance
- Case management

Case Management

Case management is a program to manage high-cost health care cases by exploring alternative care options to achieve the same patient outcomes while better controlling costs.

Capitation

Capitation is a system of prepayment for health care in which providers receive a flat monthly fee for agreeing to provide specified services to health maintenance organization (HMO) members assigned to them for a contracted length of time, usually a year. Unlike traditional fee-for-service (FFS) systems, capitated systems pay providers, either individually or collectively, the same amount per member each month, in advance, regardless of how many times members use their services. Usually, risk sharing is involved and the HMO and contracted provider share the financial risks and rewards to provide cost-effective care.

IMPACT OF MANAGED CARE ON INFUSION THERAPY

Under the auspices of the "managed care umbrella":

- Payers are changing.
- New delivery systems are designed around risk sharing.
- Payers/providers are competing for managed care savings (profits).
- Competition is increasing.
- Risk is shifting (in both directions).
- Attitudes of providers/payers/employers are changing.

Under the "old" system, providers were paid on a FFS basis; they are now paid discounted FFS or by capitation. Under the old system, the patient base was the local community; now it is covered lives. Under the old system, the philosophy of care was to "treat the disease and restore wellness"; now it is to maintain health.

Alternate Site

Incentives have changed for providers. When home care providers are reimbursed on a per diem rate, the incentive is to decrease costs, manage case mix and length of stay on service, and decrease utilization. Referrals to home infusion companies proliferate, however, with the top patient needs being in:

- Obstetrics/neonatal care
- Outpatient surgery
- Ventilator care and dependency
- Antibiotics
- Nutritional support
- Antineoplastics
- Pain management

This results in a greater influx of patients to the home care setting and increases the need for highly qualified, independent providers of home infusion therapy. Chapter 24 fully addresses the subject of Alternate Site Therapies.

Inpatient

When providers are reimbursed under bundling or capitated contracts, the incentive is to keep healthy, provide care in the least costly setting, and decrease total costs.

Shorter lengths of stay in hospitals have dramatically decreased the number but not the complexity of IV nurses' patient caseloads. Patients who are admitted to the hospital for short stays generally require the services of an IV nurse. Those who are confined for longer periods are often receiving more complex therapies, multiple IV accesses, and intensive treatment. Never before have the opportunities been greater for IV nurses in the inpatient environment to become involved in provision of direct services to patients and their families and in staff and community education.

REFERENCES _____

1. Abernathy, R. (1993). Special report healthcare reform. *RN 56*(10), 15–16.
2. Anderson D., & Anderson C. (1994). Market your expertise for the changing future of intravenous therapy. *Journal of Intravenous Nursing 17*(6), 291–294.

REVIEW QUESTIONS

1. Frequent discharges to home include patients in need of which of the following therapies?
   a. antineoplastics
   b. nutrition support
   c. antibiotics
   d. all of the above

2. Which of the following is true under managed care?
   a. payers are changing
   b. risk is shared and increasing
   c. a only
   d. a and b

3. Capitation involves
   a. prepayment on a monthly basis
   b. prepayment on a quarterly basis
   c. payment based on utilization
   d. increased payment for decreased utilization

PART II

Principles
of Venipuncture

CHAPTER 6

Anatomy and Physiology Applied to Intravascular Therapy

Key Terms

Arterial spasm	Superficial fascia	Valves
Diagnostic	Tunica	Vascular
Radiopaque		

ANATOMY AND PHYSIOLOGY

Intravascular therapy consists of the introduction of fluids, blood, and drugs directly into the vascular system, that is, into arteries, bone marrow, and veins. The *arteries* are used as a route to introduce radiopaque material for diagnostic purposes, such as arteriograms for cerebral disorders, as well as for monitoring blood pressure, determining arterial blood gases, and administering chemotherapy. The dangers of arterial spasm and subsequent gangrene present problems that make this type of therapy hazardous for therapeutic use. The *bone marrow*, because of its venous plexus, is used for intravascular therapy, by the intraosseous route. The *veins*, because of their abundance and location, present the most readily accessible route.

Applied to intravascular therapy, knowledge of the anatomy and physiology of veins and arteries is essential to the proficiency of the clinician and to ensure a positive patient outcome. Through a study of the superficial veins, the nurse acquires a sense of discrimination in the choice of veins for IV use. Many factors must be considered in selecting a vein; the anatomic characteristics offer a basis for good judgment. The size, location, and resilience of the vein affect its desirability for infusion purposes.

Familiarity with the principles underlying venous physiology is also of prime value to the nurse. An understanding of the reaction of veins to the nervous stimulation of the vasoconstrictors and vasodilators enables the clinician to 1) increase the size and visibility of a vein before attempting venipuncture and 2) relieve venous spasm and thus assist in infusion maintenance. The primary goal of therapy is to provide a positive outcome for the patient. Painless and effective therapy is desirable, promoting the patient's comfort, well-being, and often complete recovery from disease or trauma. An integral part of this goal is the recognition and prevention of complications. Through their knowledge of anatomy and physiology, clinicians can minimize this risk.

Phlebitis and *thrombosis* are by far the most common complications resulting from parenteral therapy. Although seemingly mild, they do present serious consequences: 1) they cause moderate to severe discomfort, often taking many days or weeks to subside; and 2) they limit the veins available for further therapy. Injury to the endothelial lining of the vein contributes to these local complications. A thorough understanding of the peripheral veins alerts the clinician to observe precautions in performing venipunctures. Proper technique minimizes the trauma to the vessel wall and provides an entry as painless and safe as possible. Examination of the superficial veins of the lower extremities alerts the nurse to the dangers resulting from their use. By avoiding venipunctures in veins susceptible to varicosities and sluggish circulation, the likelihood of phlebitis and thrombosis is decreased and the secondary risk of *pulmonary embolism* is reduced.

Awareness of the characteristics that differentiate veins from arteries assists the clinician in reducing the risk of *necrosis* and *gangrene*; these serious complications occur when a medication is inadvertently injected into an artery.

An understanding of the anatomy and physiology of the veins and arteries enables the clinician to recognize the existence of an *arteriovenous anastomosis*; failure to recognize this condition results in repeated and unsuccessful venipunctures performed in an attempt to initiate the infusion. These repeated punctures compound the trauma to the inner lining of the vein and increase the risk of the local complications already described, any one of which limits the number of available veins, interrupts the course of therapy, and causes unnecessary pain and even dire consequences for the patient.

THE VASCULAR SYSTEM

The circulatory system is divided into two main systems, the pulmonary and the systemic, each with its own set of vessels. The *pulmonary system* consists of the blood flow from the right ventricle of the heart to the lungs, where it is oxygenated and returned to the left atrium. The *systemic system*, the larger of the two, is the one that concerns the IV nurse. It consists of the aorta, arteries, arterioles, capillaries, venules, and veins through which the blood must flow. The blood leaves the left ventricle, flows to all parts of the body, and returns to the right atrium of the heart via the vena cava. The *systemic veins* are divided into three classes: 1) superficial, 2) deep, and 3) venous sinuses.[2]

Superficial Veins

The superficial or cutaneous veins are those used in venipuncture. They are located just beneath the skin in the superficial fascia. These veins and the deep veins sometimes unite; in the lower extremities they unite freely.[1] For example, the small saphenous vein, a superficial vein, drains the dorsum of the foot and the posterior section of the leg; it ascends the back of the leg and empties directly into the deep popliteal vein. Before the small saphenous vein terminates in the deep popliteal, it sends out a branch that, after joining the great saphenous vein, also terminates in a deep vein, the femoral vein. Because of these deep connections, great concern arises when it becomes necessary to use the veins in the lower extremities. Thrombosis may occur, which could easily extend to the deep veins and cause pulmonary embolism. Understanding this, the nurse should refrain from using these veins.

Varicosities occurring in the lower extremities, although readily available to venipuncture, are not a satisfactory route for parenteral administration. The relatively stagnant blood in such veins is likely to clot, resulting in a superficial phlebitis. Medication injected below a varicosity may result in another potential danger, a collection of the infused drug in the varicosity. This is caused by the stagnant blood flow. This "pocket" of infused medication may delay the effect of the drug when immediate action is desired; another concern is the danger of untoward reactions to the drug, which may occur when this accumulation reaches the general circulation.

Arteriovenous Anastomosis

Deep veins are usually enclosed in the same sheath with the arteries. Occasionally an arteriovenous anastomosis may occur congenitally or as the result of past penetrating injury of the vein and adjacent artery. When such trauma occurs, the blood flows directly from the artery into the vein; as a result, the veins draining an arteriovenous fistula are overburdened with high-pressure arterial blood. These veins appear large and tortuous. In these unusual circumstances, the nurse's quick recognition of an arteriovenous fistula may prevent pain, complications, and loss of time resulting from repeated unsuccessful attempts to start the infusion.

Arteries and Veins

Knowledge of the characteristics differentiating veins from arteries and the position of each is important so that the nurse may avoid the complications of an inadvertent arterial puncture. Arteries and veins are similar in structure; both are composed of three layers of tissue. A close examination of these layers reveals their differing characteristics.

Tunica Intima or the Inner Layer

The first layer consists of an inner elastic endothelial lining, which also forms the valves in veins. These valves are absent in arteries. The endothelial lining is identical in the arteries and the veins, consisting of a smooth layer of flat cells. This smooth surface allows the cells and platelets to flow through the blood vessels without interruption under normal conditions. Care must be taken to avoid roughening this surface when performing a venipuncture or removing a needle from a vein. Any trauma that roughens the endothelial lining encourages the process of thrombosis, whereby cells and platelets adhere to the vessel wall.

Many veins contain valves, which are semilunar folds of the endothelium. These valves are found in the larger veins of the extremities; their function is to keep the blood flowing toward the heart. Where muscular pressure would cause a backing up of the blood supply, these valves play an important role. They occur at points of branching and often cause a noticeable bulge in the veins. Applying a tourniquet to the extremity impedes the venous flow. When suction is applied, as occurs in the process of drawing blood, the valves compress and close the lumen of the vein, preventing the backward flow of blood. Thus, these valves interfere with the process of withdrawing blood. Recognizing the presence of a valve, the nurse may resolve the difficulty by slightly readjusting the needle.

These valves are absent in many of the small veins, which can therefore be used when, because of obstruction from a thrombus in the ascending vein, they would otherwise prove useless. The cannula may be inserted below the thrombosis, with its direction toward the distal end of the extremity; this results in a rerouting of the fluid and avoidance of the thrombosed portion.

Tunica Media or the Middle Layer

The second layer consists of muscular and elastic tissue. The nerve fibers, both vasoconstrictors and vasodilators, are located in this middle layer. These fibers, constantly receiving impulses from the vasoconstrictor center in the medulla, keep the vessels in a state of tonus. They also stimulate both arteries and veins to contract or relax. The middle layer is not as strong and stiff in the veins as in the arteries, and therefore the veins tend to collapse or distend as the pressure within falls or rises. Arteries do not collapse.

Stimulation by a change in temperature or by mechanical or chemical irritation may produce spasms in the vein or artery. For instance, interrupting a continuous infusion to administer a pint of cold blood may produce vasoconstriction; this results in spasm, impedes the flow of blood, and causes pain. Application of heat to the vein promotes vasodilation, which will relieve the spasm, improve the flow of blood, and relieve the pain. The same results are obtained by heat when an irritating drug has caused vasoconstriction. In this situation, heat relieves the spasm and increases the blood flow and protects the vessel wall from inflammation caused by the medication—with heat dilating the vein and increasing the flow of blood, the drug becomes more diluted and less irritating. The use of heat to achieve vasodilation is also an aid when it is necessary to use small and poorly filled veins.

Spasms produced by a chemical irritation in an artery may have dire consequences. A single artery supplies circulation to a particular area. If this artery is damaged, the related area will suffer from impaired circulation and possibly from necrosis and gangrene. If a chemical agent is introduced into the artery, a spasm may result—a contraction that could shut off the blood supply completely. This problem is not as serious when veins are used because many veins supply a particular area; if one is injured, others will maintain the circulation.

Tunica Adventitia or the Outer Layer

The third layer consists of areolar connective tissue; it surrounds and supports the vessel. In arteries this layer is thicker than in veins because it is subjected to greater pressure from the force of blood within.

Arteries need more protection than veins and are so placed that injury is less likely to occur. Whereas veins are superficially located, most arteries lie deep in the tissues and are protected by muscle. Occasionally an artery is located superficially in an unusual place; this artery is then called an *aberrant artery*. An aberrant artery must not be mistaken for a vein. If a chemical that causes spasm is introduced into an aberrant artery, permanent damage may result.

Arteries pulsate and veins do not, a helpful differentiating characteristic.

Superficial Veins of the Upper Extremities

The superficial veins of the upper extremities are shown in Figures 6-1 and 6-2. They consist of the following: digital, metacarpal, cephalic, basilic, and median veins.

The Digital Veins

The dorsal digital veins flow along the lateral portions of the fingers and are joined to each other by communicating branches.[2] At times, these veins are available as a last resort for fluid administration. In some patients, they are prominent enough to accommodate a small-gauge needle. With adequate taping the fingers can be completely immobilized, thereby preventing the needle from puncturing the posterior wall of the vein and causing extravasation of fluid.

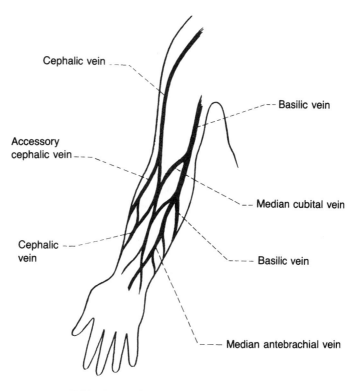

FIGURE 6-1   Superficial veins of the forearm.

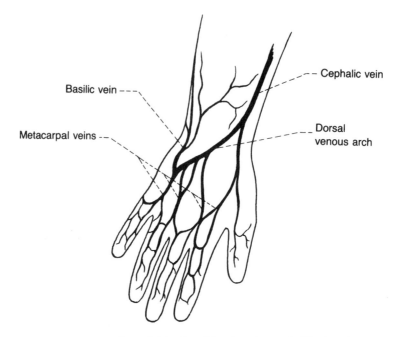

FIGURE 6-2   Superficial veins of the dorsal aspect of the hand.

The Metacarpal Veins

The three metacarpal veins are formed by the union of the digital veins.[2] The position of these veins makes them well adapted for IV use; in most cases, the needle and adapter lie flat between the joints and the metacarpal bones of the hand, the bones themselves providing a natural splint. The early use of the metacarpal veins is important in a course of parenteral therapy. Irritating fluid passing through a vein traumatized by previous puncture causes inflammation and pain. Therefore, performing venipunctures for fluid administration at the distal end of the extremity, early in the course of therapy, is beneficial; it enables the nurse to initiate each successive venipuncture above the previous puncture site. Unnecessary inflammation and pain are avoided and opportunity for multiple venipunctures is provided.

Occasionally the use of the metacarpal veins in the elderly is contraindicated. Because of inadequate tissue and thin skin in this area, extravasation of blood on venipuncture may readily occur.

The Cephalic Vein

The cephalic vein has its source in the radial part of the dorsal venous network formed by the metacarpal veins. Receiving tributaries from both surfaces of the forearm, it flows upward along the radial border of the forearm.[2] Because of its size and position, this vein provides an excellent route for transfusion administration. It readily accommodates a large cannula and, by virtue of its position in the forearm, a natural splint is provided for the cannula and adapter.

The *accessory cephalic vein* originates from either one of two sources—a plexus on the back of the forearm or the dorsal venous network. Ascending the arm, it joins the cephalic vein below the elbow. Occasionally it arises from that portion of the cephalic vein just above the wrist and flows back into the main cephalic vein at some higher point.[2] The accessory cephalic vein readily receives a large cannula and is a good choice for use in blood administration.

The Basilic Vein

The basilic vein has its origin in the ulnar part of the dorsal venous network and ascends along the ulnar portion of the forearm. It diverges toward the anterior surface of the arm just below the elbow, where it meets the median cubital vein. During a course of IV therapy, this large vein is often overlooked because of its inconspicuous position on the ulnar border of the hand and forearm; when other veins have been exhausted, this vein may still be available. By flexing the elbow and bending the arm up, the basilic vein is brought into view.

The Median Veins

The *median antebrachial vein* arises from the venous plexus on the palm of the hand and extends upward along the ulnar side of the front of the forearm; it empties into the basilic vein or the median cubital vein. This vein, when prominent, affords a route for parenteral fluid administration. However, there are frequent variations of the superficial veins of the forearm, and this vein is not always present as a well defined vessel.

The *median cephalic* and *median basilic veins* in the antecubital fossa are the veins most generally used for withdrawal of blood. Because of their size and superficial location, they are readily accessible for venipuncture. They accommodate a large cannula, and because of the muscular and connective tissue supporting them, they have little tendency to roll.

The median cephalic vein crosses in front of the brachial artery; therefore, care must be taken during venipuncture to avoid puncturing the artery. Accidental intra-arterial injection of a drug could result in permanent damage.

The basilic vein, outside the antecubital fossa on the ulnar curve of the arm, is the least desirable for venipuncture. When the cannula is removed, a hematoma may readily occur if the patient flexes the elbow to stop the bleeding rather than elevating the arm in the preferred manner.

THE SKIN

The skin is made up of two layers, the epidermis and the dermis. The *epidermis* is the uppermost layer, which forms a protective covering for the dermis. Its degree of thickness varies in different parts of the body. It is thickest on the palms of the hands and the soles of the feet and thinnest on the inner surface of the limbs. Its degree of thickness also varies with age. In an elderly patient, the skin on the dorsum of the hand may be so thin that it does not adequately support the vein for venipuncture when parenteral infusions are required.

The *dermis*, or underlayer, is highly sensitive and vascular. It contains many capillaries and thousands of nerve fibers. These nerve fibers are of different types and include those that react to temperature, touch, pressure, and pain. The number of nerve fibers varies in different areas of the body. Some areas of the body skin are highly sensitive; other areas are only mildly sensitive. The insertion of a needle in one area may cause a great deal of pain, yet another area may be virtually painless. In my experience, the inner aspect of the wrist is a highly sensitive area. Venipunctures are performed here only when other veins have been exhausted.

SUPERFICIAL FASCIA

The superficial fascia, or subcutaneous areolar connective tissue, lies below the two layers of skin and is, in itself, another covering. It is in this fascia that the superficial veins are located. It varies in thickness. When a cannula is inserted into this fascia, there is free movement of the skin above. Great care in aseptic technique must be observed because an infection in this loose tissue spreads easily. Such an infection is called *cellulitis*.[1]

REFERENCES

1. Kimber, D. C., Gray, C. E., & Stackpoles, C. E. (1966). *Textbook of anatomy and physiology* (15th ed., pp. 69, 398, 423–431). New York: Macmillan.

2. Warwick, R., & Williams, P. L. (Eds.). (1973). *Gray's anatomy of the human body* (28th ed., pp. 700–703). Philadelphia: Lea & Febiger.

REVIEW QUESTIONS

1. Layers of the skin include:
   a. dermis
   b. epidermis
   c. fascia
   d. tunica intima

2. Which veins are most useful for venous sampling?
   a. median cephalic
   b. cutaneous
   c. median basilic
   d. accessory cephalic

3. An infection involving connective tissue is known as:
   a. cellulitis
   b. phlebitis
   c. thrombophlebitis
   d. phlebothrombosis

4. Superficial veins of the upper extremity include which of the following:
   a. digital
   b. metacarpal
   c. cephalic
   d. median basilic

5. An artery located superficially in an unusual location is known as:
   a. aberrant
   b. arteriovenous
   c. residual
   d. superficial

6. The basilic vein originates in which part of the dorsal venous network?
   a. radial
   b. ulnar
   c. metacarpal
   d. dorsal digital

7. The systemic system contains:
   a. aorta
   b. arteries
   c. ligaments
   d. veins

8. The pulmonary system contains:
   a. blood flow from right ventricle to lungs
   b. blood flow from left ventricle to lungs
   c. blood flow to the body
   d. blood flow from the body

9. A medication inadvertently injected into an artery may result in:
   a. necrosis
   b. gangrene
   c. cellulitis
   d. pustule formation

10. The bone marrow, because of its venous plexus, may be used for intravascular therapy via which route of administration?
    a. intravenous
    b. intramuscular
    c. subcutaneous
    d. intraosseous

CHAPTER 7

Techniques of Intravenous Therapy

Key Terms

Approach	Flexion	Palpation
Fear	Hemochromatosis	Syncope

APPROACH TO THE PATIENT

The nurse's approach to the patient may have a direct bearing on that patient's response to IV therapy. Because an undesirable response can affect the patient's ability to accept treatment, the nurse's manner and attitude are significant factors.

Although routine for the nurse, IV therapy may be a new and frightening experience to the patient unfamiliar with the procedure. Patients may have heard rumors of fatalities associated with infusions or may misinterpret the treatment. By explaining the procedure, the nurse will alleviate fears and help the patient to accept therapy.

Clinical Condition

The critically ill patient is particularly susceptible to fears, which can at times become exaggerated, triggering an undesirable autonomic nervous system response usually known as a *vasovagal reaction*. Such a reaction may manifest itself in the form of syncope and can be prevented if the nurse appears confident and reassures the patient. Sympathetic reaction may follow syncope and result in vasoconstriction. Peripheral collapse then limits available veins, complicating the venipuncture. Repeated attempts at venipuncture can result in an experience so traumatic as to affect the further course of fluid therapy. Only a skilled clinician should perform a venipuncture on an anxious patient with limited and difficult veins. (See Chapter 21 for special considerations in the pediatric patient.)

Reactions to exaggerated fear may not only make therapy difficult, but they may constitute a real threat to the patient with severe cardiac disease. Fear stimulates the adrenal medulla to secrete the vasopressors, which help maintain blood pressure and increase the work of the heart. Increased adrenal cortical secretions result in sodium and chloride retention, which causes water retention, and loss of cellular potassium, which draws water with it into the intravascular system. Increased antidiuretic hormone secretions cause a decreased urinary output, which results in retention of fluids and an increase in blood volume.[6] Such an increase may be sufficient to send a patient with an overburdened vascular system into pulmonary edema.

Type of Therapy Ordered

The type of therapy ordered often dictates the approach to providing care. The ambulatory surgical patient will have decidedly different educational needs than the critically ill patient with multiple IV accesses. If the patient will be involved in self-care and self-administration of IV medications and solutions, the approach must encourage and support the patient's independence and confidence. Considerations include:

- Type of therapy
- Duration of treatment
- Patient's past IV history
- Patient's clinical condition
- Patient's experience level
- Available IV access

SELECTING THE VEIN

The selection of the vein may be a deciding factor in the success of the infusion and in the preservation of veins for future therapy. The most prominent vein is not necessarily the most suitable for venipuncture; prominence may be from a sclerosed condition, which occludes the lumen and interferes with the flow of solution, or the prominent vein may be located in an area impractical for infusion purposes. Scrutiny of the veins in both arms is desirable before a choice is made. The prime factors to be considered in selecting a vein are suitable location, condition of the vein, purpose of the infusion, and duration of therapy.

Location

Most superficial veins are accessible for venipuncture (Fig. 7-1), but some of these veins, because of their location, are not practical. The antecubital veins are such veins, located over an area of joint flexion where any motion could dislodge the cannula and cause infiltration or result in mechanical phlebitis. If these large veins are impaired or damaged, phlebothrombosis may occur, which can limit the many available hand veins. The antecubital veins offer excellent sources for withdrawing blood and may be used numerous times without damage to the vein, provided good technique and sharp needles are used. But one infusion of long duration may traumatize the vein, limiting these vessels that most readily provide ample quantities of blood when needed.

IV PLACEMENT CHART

Cephalic Vein

Basilic Vein

Brachial Artery

Accessory
Cephalic Vein

Median Cubital Vein

Radial Artery

Basilic Vein

Cephalic
Vein

Cephalic
Vein

Ulnar
Artery

Dorsal
Venous
Arch

Basilic
Vein

Metacarpal
Veins

Median
Antebrachial
Vein

Digital Veins

Superficial Veins of the Forearm

**Superficial Veins of the
Dorsal Aspect of the Hand**

FIGURE 7-1 IV placement chart. (Courtesy: Becton Dickinson Vascular Access, Sandy, UT)

Because of the close proximity of the arteries to the veins in the antecubital fossa, special care must be taken to prevent intra-arterial injection when medications are introduced. An artery can generally be detected by the thicker and tougher wall, the brighter red blood, and usually the presence of a pulse. Aberrant arteries in the antecubital area are present in 1 of 10 people. When a patient complains of severe pain in the hand or arm on infusion, an arteriospasm caused by an intra-arterial injection is to be suspected, and the infusion must be stopped immediately.

Surgery often dictates which extremity can be used. Veins should be avoided in the affected arm of an axillary dissection, such as a radical mastectomy; the circulation may be impaired, affecting the flow of the infusion and increasing the edema. When the patient is turned sideways during the operation, the upper arm is used for the IV infusion; increased venous pressure in the lower arm may interfere with the free flow of the solution.

The use of the veins in the lower extremities is frequently challenged. These objections arise from the danger of pulmonary embolism caused by a thrombus extending into the deep veins. Complications may also arise from the stagnant blood in varicosities; pooling of infused medications can cause untoward reactions when a toxic concentration reaches the circulating blood. Because of the stagnant blood, varicosities are susceptible to trauma. Phlebitis interferes with ambulation of the patient.

The Centers for Disease Control and Prevention (CDC) guidelines strongly recommend that "in adults, the upper extremity (or if necessary, subclavian and jugular sites) should be used in preference to lower extremity sites for IV cannulation. All cannulas inserted into a lower extremity should be changed as soon as a satisfactory site can be established elsewhere."[3]

Condition of the Vein

Frequently, the dorsal metacarpal veins provide points of entry that should be used first to preserve the proximal veins for further therapy. The use of these veins depends on their condition. In some elderly patients, the dorsal metacarpal veins may be a poor choice; blood extravasation occurs more readily in small thin veins, and difficulty may be encountered in adequately securing the cannula because of thin skin and lack of supportive tissue. At times these veins do not dilate sufficiently to allow for successful venipuncture; when hypovolemia occurs the peripheral veins collapse more quickly than do the large ones.

Palpation of the vein is an important step in determining the condition of the vein and in differentiating it from a pulsating artery. A thrombosed vein may be detected by its lack of resilience, by its hard, cordlike feeling, and by the ease with which it rolls. Use of such traumatized veins can result only in repeated venipunctures, pain, and undue stress.

Occasionally, when thrombosis from multiple infusions interferes with the flow of solution and limits available veins, the venipuncture may be performed with the cannula inserted in the direction of the distal end; lack of valves in these small peripheral veins permits rerouting of the solution and bypassing of the involved vein.

Often, large veins may be detected by palpation and offer advantages over the smaller but more readily discernible veins. Because of the small blood volume, the more superficial veins may not be easily palpated and may not make a satisfactory choice for venipuncture.

Continual use by the nurse of the same fingers for palpation will increase their sensitivity. The thumb should never be used because it is not as sensitive as the fingers; also, a pulse may be detected in the nurse's thumb, and this may be confused with an aberrant artery.

Although not apparent, edema may conceal an available vein; application of finger pressure for a few seconds often helps to disperse the fluid and define the vein.

Purpose of the Infusion

The purpose of the infusion dictates the rate of flow and the solution to be infused—two factors that inherently affect the selection of the vein. When large quantities of fluid are to be rapidly infused, or when positive pressure is indicated, a large vein must be used. When fluids with a high viscosity such as packed cells are required, a vein with an adequate blood volume is necessary to ensure flow of the solution.

Large veins are used when hypertonic solutions or solutions containing irritating drugs are to be infused. Such solutions traumatize small veins; the supply of blood in these veins is not sufficient to dilute the infused fluid.

Duration of Therapy

A prolonged course of therapy requires multiple infusions, which makes preservation of the veins essential. Performing the venipuncture distally with each subsequent puncture proximal to the previous one and alternating arms will contribute to this preservation.

The patient's comfort should also be considered when infusions are required over an extended period of time; avoiding areas over joint flexion and performing venipunctures on veins located on the dorsal surface of the extremities will provide more freedom and comfort to the patient.

SELECTING THE CANNULA

Infusions may be administered through a cannula or steel needle (Figs. 7-2, 7-3, and 7-4).

Typical cannulas include:

1. Over-the-needle catheter (ONC). Once the venipuncture is made, the catheter is slipped off the needle into the vein and the steel needle removed. The Intravenous Nurses Society (INS) does not recommend the use of obturators, which are inserted into the catheter to maintain patency for intermittent infusion.

2. Inside-the-needle catheter (INC). The venipuncture is performed and the catheter is then pushed through the needle until the desired length is within the lumen of the vein; the cutting edge is then protected by a shield to prevent the catheter from being severed.[4]

The choice of catheter depends on the purpose of the infusion and the condition and availability of the veins. The ONCs are used routinely today to ensure a ready route for the administration of blood and fluid. The INCs are used when a longer catheter is desired. They afford less risk of infiltration than does the steel cannula, often being used for administering drugs or hypertonic solutions that may cause necrosis if extravasation occurs.

FIGURE 7-2   Protectiv™ IV cannula. (Courtesy: Critikon, Inc., Tampa, FL)

FIGURE 7-3 Over-the-needle IV catheter. (Courtesy: Abbott Laboratories, North Chicago, IL)

Catheter Materials

Catheters are made of a diversity of materials; for many years polyvinylchloride was used almost exclusively. Ideally, to reduce the risk of thrombi formation on the catheter, the catheter should be of a hemorepellant material. Silicone catheters are thought to be helpful in this respect. Catheters should be radiopaque for detection by x-ray in the event the catheter is severed and lost in the circulation.

Steel needles are of two types, the steel cannula (not recommended for infusion purposes) and the winged infusion device or small-vein needle. The gauge refers to both the inside and the outside diameters of the lumen—the smaller the gauge, the larger the lumen. Steel needles are often thin walled. Because the wall of the needle is thinner than that of the standard needle, a larger lumen is obtained for the same external diameter, offering the advantage of enhanced flow rates. Today, the steel needle is most commonly used for venous sampling purposes.

The winged infusion device or small-vein needle is similar to the steel cannula, with the hub replaced with two flexible wings. Originally designed for pediatric and geriatric use, it has been used in prolonged therapy for all ages. Two types of small-

FIGURE 7-4 Venipuncture with over-the-needle catheter. (Courtesy: Critikon, Inc., Tampa, FL)

vein needles are available, one with a short length of plastic tubing and a permanently attached resealable injection site, the other with a variable length of plastic tubing permanently attached to a female Luer adapter that accommodates an administration set. The small-vein needle with the resealable injection site offers a method for the intermittent administration of medications or fluids. A dilute solution of heparin maintains patency of the needle when it is not in use.

The small-vein needle is approximately ½ inch long and ranges in size from a 27-gauge bore to a 16-gauge bore. It has definite advantages: the short bevel reduces the risk of infiltration from puncture to the wall of the vein, and the plastic wings provide a firm grip for inserting the needle and better control in performing the venipuncture. The wings fold flat against the skin, affording better anchoring power than the straight steel needle with a bulky hub.

The factors to be considered in selecting a steel needle are length of bevel, gauge, and length of the needle.

A short *bevel* reduces the risk of 1) trauma to the endothelial wall; 2) infiltration from a puncture to the posterior wall; and 3) hematoma or extravasation occurring when the steel needle enters the vein. When a steel needle with a long bevel is inserted into the vessel, blood may leak into the tissues before the entire bevel is within the lumen of the vein.

Whenever possible, the *gauge* of the needle should be appreciably smaller than the lumen of the vein to be entered; when the gauge of the needle approaches the size of the vein, trauma may occur. When a large needle occludes the flow of blood, irritating solutions flowing through the vein with no dilution of blood may cause chemical phlebitis. Mechanical phlebitis may result from motion and pressure exerted by the needle on the endothelial wall of the vein.

When large amounts of fluid are required, a needle of adequate size must be used; a small lumen interferes with the flow of solution. As Adriani stated,[1]

> The flow of blood varies inversely as the fourth power of the radius of the lumen of the needle. Thus, a needle with an internal radius of 1 mm. delivering 1 cc. of blood with a fixed pressure on the plunger or in the infusion bottle delivers only 1/16 of a cc. when the radius is reduced to ½ mm.

A large needle is also required with fluids of high viscosity. The rate of flow of the solution decreases in proportion to the viscosity of the fluid.

The flow of the solution varies inversely with the *length of the needle shaft*. If the length of the needle is increased, other conditions being equal, the volume flowing will be reduced.[1] Use of a short needle for infusions reduces the risk of infiltration. Because a short needle affords more play than a long needle, more motion is needed to puncture the vessel wall.

SECURING AN APPROPRIATE ENVIRONMENT

The importance of proper lighting should not be overlooked. A few extra seconds spent in obtaining adequate light may actually save time and free the patient from unnecessary venipunctures. The ideal light is either an ample amount of daylight or a spotlight that does not shine directly on the vein but leaves enough shadow for clearly defining the vessel.

VENOUS DISTENTION

Special care must be taken to distend the vein adequately. To achieve this, a soft rubber tourniquet is applied with enough pressure to impede the venous flow while the arterial flow is maintained; if the radial pulse cannot be felt, the tourniquet is too tight. To fill the veins to capacity, pressure is applied until radial pulsation ceases and then released until pulsation begins. A blood pressure cuff may be used; inflate the cuff and then release it until the pressure drops to just below the diastolic pressure.

The tourniquet is applied to the mid-forearm if the selected vein is in the dorsum of the hand. If the selected vein is in the forearm, the tourniquet is applied to the upper arm.

Very little pressure is applied when performing venipunctures on patients with sclerosed veins. If the pressure is too great or the tourniquet is left on for an extended length of time, the vein will become hard and tortuous, causing added difficulty when the cannula is introduced. For some sclerosed veins, a tourniquet is unnecessary and only makes the phlebotomy more difficult.

If pressure exerted by the tourniquet does not fill the veins sufficiently, the patient may be asked to open and close his or her fist. The action of the muscles will force the blood into the veins, causing them to distend considerably more. A light tapping will often fill the vein. It may be helpful, before applying the tourniquet, to lower the extremity below the heart level to increase the blood supply to the veins. Occasionally, these methods are inadequate to fill the vein sufficiently. In such cases, application of heat helps. To be effective, the heat must be applied to the entire extremity for 10 to 20 minutes and retained until the venipuncture is performed.

PREPARATION

Check Solution and Container

Careful inspection must be made to ensure that the fluid is clear and free of particulate matter and that the container is intact—there are no cracks in the glass bottle or holes in the plastic bag. The label must be checked to verify that the correct solution is being used and that the container is not outdated. Indicate the time and the date the bottle is opened; after 24 hours the fluid is outdated and should not be used.

Attach Administration Set to Fluid Container

The set is attached to the container by closing the roller clamp to equalize pressure, squeezing the drip chamber, and entering the bottle with a thrust, not a twisting motion. The chamber is released, causing immediate function of the air vent and filling of the drip chamber on the suspension of the bottle. This prevents leakage of fluid through the air vent and expedites clearing the infusion set of air, thus preventing bubbles from entering the tubing. In systems that do not require air venting—plastic bags and semirigid bottles—squeezing the drip chamber before insertion avoids the introduction of air into the container.

Height of the Fluid Container

The fluid container is suspended at approximately 3 feet above the injection site. At this height, adequate pressure is provided to achieve a maximum flow rate. The greater the height of the container, the greater the force with which the fluid will flow into the vein should the adjusting clamp release, and the greater the risk of speed shock.

Preparing the Patient and Providing Privacy

Visitors should be asked to leave the room during the procedure; curtains should be pulled if a roommate is present. The patient should be in a comfortable position with the arm on a flat surface. If necessary, a strip of tape is used to secure the arm to an armboard to prevent an uncooperative or disoriented patient from jerking the arm while the cannula is being inserted.

If the area selected for venipuncture is hairy, clipping the hair will permit better cleansing of the skin and make removal of the cannula less painful when the infusion is terminated. Shaving is not recommended, consistent with INS standards. Products such as Skin-Prep decrease bacterial flora and should be considered for use before venipuncture.

PROCEDURE

Direct Method or One-Step Entry

This method is performed with a thrust of the cannula through the skin and into the vein with one quick motion. The cannula enters the skin directly over the vein. This technique is excellent as long as large veins are available. However, because often one must resort to the use of small veins, this is not the preferred technique. Such an attempt at entry into the small veins will result in hematomas.

Indirect Method

This method consists of two complete motions:

1. Insertion of the cannula through the skin. The cannula enters the skin below the point where the vein is visible; entering the skin above the vein tends to depress the vein, obscuring its position.
2. Relocation of the vein and entry into the vein.

Recommended Skin Preparation[3]

The injection site should be scrubbed with an antiseptic and allowed to remain in contact for at least 30 seconds before venipuncture.

1. Tincture of iodine 1% to 2%, iodophor, or chlorhexidine may be used.
2. Isopropyl 70% alcohol is recommended if the patient is sensitive to iodine.

The basic venipuncture is performed as follows:

1. Put on gloves.

2. Apply tourniquet and select vein.

3. Prepare skin according to recommendations.

4. After establishing a minimum rate of flow by adjusting the clamp, kink the infusion tubing between the third and little fingers of the right hand. When the kinked tubing is released, the minimum rate of flow will prevent a rapid infusion of fluid and drugs with the potential danger of speed shock. Obstructing the flow of solution manually expedites the procedure and leaves the hands free for anchoring the steel cannula and caring for any collected blood samples.

5. Hold the patient's hand or arm with the left hand, using the thumb to keep the skin taut and to anchor the vein to prevent rolling.

6. Place the steel cannula in line with the vein, about ½ inch below the proposed site of entry (see Figure 7-4). The bevel-up position of the cannula facilitates venipuncture and produces less trauma to the skin and the vein on puncture.

To prevent extravasation in small veins, it is often necessary to enter the vein with the bevel down; any readjustment of the cannula should be made before releasing the tourniquet to prevent puncturing the vein and producing a hematoma.

7. Insert the cannula through skin and tissue at a 45° angle.

8. Relocate the vein and decrease the cannula angle slightly.

9. Slowly, with downward motion followed at once by raising point, pick up vein, leveling cannula until almost flush with skin.

10. On entering the vein there may be a flashback of blood, which indicates successful entry (Fig. 7-5). With experience, the fingers will become sensitive to the cannula's entering the vein—the resistance encountered as the cannula meets the wall of the vein and the snap felt at the loss of resistance as the cannula enters the lumen. This is more difficult to discern on thin-walled

FIGURE 7-5   Evidence of flashback. (Courtesy: Critikon, Inc., Tampa, FL)

FIGURE 7-6   Catheter is advanced and the introducer is removed. (Courtesy: Critikon, Inc., Tampa, FL)

veins with small blood volume. To prevent a through puncture, advance the cannula slowly, checking at each movement for a flashback of blood.

11. Release the tourniquet and remove the introducer (Fig. 7-6).

12. Release the pressure exerted by the little finger, connect administration set to hub, and allow the solution to flow (Fig. 7-7).

13. Check carefully for any signs of swelling.

FIGURE 7-7   Primed administration set is connected to the catheter hub. (Courtesy: Critikon, Inc., Tampa, FL)

If the vein has sustained a through puncture (evidenced by a developing hematoma) and the venipuncture is unsuccessful, the cannula should be immediately removed and pressure applied to the site. Never reapply a tourniquet to the extremity immediately after a venipuncture; a hematoma will occur, limiting veins and providing an excellent culture medium for bacteria.

ANCHORING THE DEVICE

The Cannula

1. Use ½-inch wide tape over the hub. Tape the cannula flush with the skin; no elevation of the hub is necessary, and it would only increase the risk of a through puncture from the point of the cannula.

2. Place a ½-inch strip of tape—adhesive up—under the hub of the cannula. Place one end tightly and diagonally over the cannula. Repeat with the other end, crossing the first. This secures the cannula firmly and prevents any sideward movement. Avoid placing tape directly over the actual injection site.

3. Loop the tubing and secure it with tape independently of the cannula. This eliminates dislodging the cannula by an accidental pull on the tubing.

4. Apply an occlusive dressing over the cannula entrance site to allow for routine, standardized inspection.

5. Indicate type, gauge, insertion date, and initials near the dressing and in the clinical record. Variations in taping are shown in Figures 7-8 and 7-9.

An armboard may be helpful for immobilizing the extremity when undue motion can result in infiltration or phlebitis. It is a valuable aid in restraining the arm when infusions are initiated on uncooperative, disoriented, or elderly patients or children, or when the cannula is inserted on the dorsum of the hand or in an area of joint flexion. When the metacarpal veins are used, the fingers should be immobilized to prevent any movement of the cannula that could result in phlebitis.

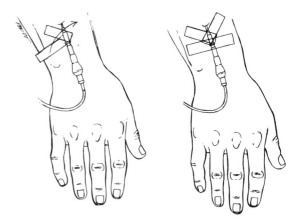

FIGURE 7-8 Chevron taping technique.

FIGURE 7-9 Variations in taping of over-the-needle cannula.

The function of the hand may be endangered and even permanently impaired by the widespread hospital practice of flattening the hand on an armboard during IV therapy. This complication results from failure to recognize that the hand has both transverse and longitudinal arches and that if the knuckle joints (metacarpophalangeal) are immobilized in a straight position, they will develop contracture that will prevent motion. Patients on long-term therapy with edema or muscular weakness are particularly vulnerable. Intensive physical therapy, splinting, and even surgery may be required to restore mobility.

To preserve maximal function, the hand should be immobilized in a functional position on the armboard.

If a plastic armboard is used, cover it with absorbent paper or bandage to prevent the arm from perspiring and sticking to the board. Make certain that any tape placed on the cannula is independent of the board so that a motion of the arm on the board will not cause a pull on the cannula. If restraint of the arm is necessary, the restraint is secured to the board, not to the patient's arm above the puncture area; such restraint might act as a tourniquet, causing a backflow of blood into the cannula, resulting in clotting and obstruction of the flow.

Armboards have changed dramatically, and many manufacturers now provide sophisticated devices aimed at ensuring patient comfort.

APPLICATION OF DRESSINGS

Consistent with INS Standards of Practice, an occlusive dressing should be applied over the infusion site. The occlusive dressing may be either gauze and tape or a transparent semipermeable membrane (TSM) dressing.

The following procedure is applicable to the Tegaderm pouch dressings manufactured by 3M Healthcare (Fig. 7-10). The professional is encouraged to follow the manufacturer's recommendations for the use of a specific product.

Infusion sites should be labeled with type of cannula (Fig. 7-11), length and size, date, time, and initials of individual who initiated the infusion. Many labels are available to facilitate this practice (Fig. 7-12).

How to Apply 3M Tegaderm Transparent Dressings

1. Thoroughly read Contraindications, Warnings and Precautions before beginning.

2. Prepare skin according to institution protocol. Allow all prep liquids to dry completely. If antimicrobial ointment is used, apply the recommended amount directly to the puncture site. Excess ointment can melt and spread, and compromise dressing adhesion.

3. Peel the printed liner from the dressing (**Figure 1**), and view the IV site through the film. Line up the slit in the frame with the catheter hub. (**Figure 2**) Apply the dressing just to top edge of the hub.

4. Do not stretch the dressing during application. Relax the film around the hub, so the dressing edges can be pinched together under the catheter to assure a good seal. (**Figure 3**)

5. Firmly smooth down the dressing edges as the frame is slowly removed. (**Figure 4**)

6. Gently pinch and seal the dressing snugly around the catheter. (**Figure 5**)

7. Smooth down the entire dressing from the center out to the edges, using firm pressure to enhance adhesion.

8. Document catheter insertion or dressing change information before removing the identification label from the frame. Apply the label to the edge of the dressing or directly on the skin. (**Figure 6**)

Dressing Removal

Support the skin and the catheter with your fingers while removing the dressing. Use one of the following removal techniques based on your patient's skin condition and your own personal preference.

1. Gently grasp one edge and slowly peel the dressing from the skin in the direction of hair growth. Try to peel the dressing back, rather than pulling it up from the skin.

   or

2. Grasp one edge of the dressing and gently pull it straight out to stretch and release adhesion. (**Figure 7**)

   or

3. Apply an adhesive remover suitable for use on skin to the adhesive edge while gently peeling from skin.

HINT: To aid in lifting a dressing edge, secure a piece of surgical tape to one corner and rub firmly. Use the tape as a tab to help you slowly peel back the dressing. (**Figure 8**)

FIGURE 7-10   Applications and special techniques for 3M Tegaderm Transparent Dressings on IV Catheters. (Courtesy: 3M Health Care, St. Paul, MN. Reprinted with permission.)

FIGURE 7-11 Labeling of the venipuncture site consistent with INS standards. (Courtesy: United Ad Label Co., Inc., Brea, CA)

OTHER TECHNIQUES

The Inside-the-Needle Catheter

Because this type of catheter is associated with a higher incidence of serious complications, it is seldom used. The inherent danger of infection from bacteria invading the vein through the cutaneous opening and being carried along the plastic cannula makes thorough skin preparation necessary. Trauma caused by the insertion of a large catheter is increased when the procedure is performed by an inexperienced clinician.

A catheter severed by the cutting edge of the needle can result in a serious complication when lost in the bloodstream. A catheter introduced into a vein over a joint flexion increases the risk of complication if the extremity is not immobilized.

An INC facilitates prolonged therapy but increases the risk of thrombophlebitis. Limiting the length of time the catheter is in use reduces the incidence of phlebitis; a time limit is sometimes difficult to enforce, however, because veins may be exhausted in a critically ill patient whose life depends on infusion therapy.

Insertion of the Inside-the-Needle Catheter

1. Put on gloves.
2. Apply a tourniquet and select the vein.
3. Prepare the injection site area according to recommendations.
4. Make the venipuncture.
5. Gently thread the catheter through the lumen of the needle into the vein until the desired length has been introduced.
6. Apply digital pressure on the vein to hold the catheter in place; withdraw the needle.
7. Apply pressure with a sterile sponge for 30 seconds to minimize bleeding through the puncture site.

PCA
Patient Controlled
Analgesia

PCA
Patient Controlled
Analgesia

IV256 Fl. Yellow

DATE:
TIME:
GAUGE:
NAME:

IV251 White

HEPARIN FLUSH
_____ UNITS

IV111 Fl. Red

SALINE FLUSH

IV110 Fl. Green

SALINE FLUSH

IV254 Fl. Green

IV Dressing Changed
Date _____Initial _____
Catheter size_____
Next change due_____

IV246 Fl. Pink

Saline Lock
Device _____ Size _____
Inserted: Date _____ Time _____
Nurse ____ _____

IV250 Fl. Green

HEPARIN LOCK
Device_____Size: _____
Inserted: Date _____Time: _____
Init _____

IV214 Fl. Yellow

**Intrathecal
Catheter
No IV Access**

**Intrathecal
Catheter
No IV Access**

IV247 Fl. Green

I.V. SET–_____Hours Only
RN initial _____
START-date/hr. _____
DISCARD-date/hr. _____

IV201 Fl. Green

**CAUTION
Epidural Catheter
No IV Access**

**CAUTION
Epidural Catheter
No IV Access**

IV248 Fl. Red

**PROXIMAL
PORT**

**PROXIMAL
PORT**

LI210 Fl. Green

P.I.C.C.
Peripherally
Inserted Central
Catheter

P.I.C.C.
Peripherally
Inserted Central
Catheter

IV249 Fl. Yellow

**DISTAL
PORT**

**DISTAL
PORT**

LI211 Tan

**WRAP
AROUND
IV
TUBING**

IV TUBING CHANGED
Date _____ Hr. _____

By_____

IV407 Fl. Orange

FIGURE 7-12 Variety of site, tubing, and chart labels available. (Courtesy: United Ad Label Co., Inc., Brea, CA)

8. Attach the needle to the infusion set, and regulate the flow rate. Never withdraw the catheter back through the needle. If the venipuncture is unsuccessful, the needle and catheter must be removed together; to pull the catheter back through the needle may sever the catheter and result in its loss in the circulation.

9. Slip the shield from the base of the needle over the bevel and tape; the shield must be kept in place to protect the cutting edge of the needle and prevent its severing the catheter. A tongue depressor is frequently used to secure the needle and catheter to further guard against kinking and breaking of the catheter at the junction of the needle.

10. Tape the catheter to prevent motion.

11. Ascertain the patency and position of the catheter in the vein.

12. Topical antibiotic or antiseptic ointment should be applied to the injection site.

13. Apply a sterile gauze or TSM dressing; the puncture made by the needle is larger than the in-lying catheter, and seepage of fluid and infection can occur.

14. Indicate length, gauge, and type of catheter, initials of nurse, and date of insertion on tape near dressing and in medical record.

15. Use an armboard if the catheter lies over a point of flexion—motion contributes to phlebitis. The arm must not be fastened tightly to the armboard; vascular occlusion results in a plugged catheter, and stasis edema may occur.

16. Remove gloves. Wash hands.

The Over-the-Needle Catheter

Venipuncture and Insertion

1. Put on gloves.

2. Apply a tourniquet and select the vein.

3. Prepare the injection site according to recommendations. If palpation of the vein is necessary, prepare the fingertip in the same manner. Do not touch the proposed insertion site.

4. Perform the venipuncture in the usual manner. When the needle has punctured the venous wall, introduce it ½ inch farther to ensure entry of the catheter into the lumen of the vein.

5. Hold the needle in place and slowly slide the catheter hub until the desired length is in the vein. If the venipuncture is unsuccessful, do not reinsert the needle into the catheter. To do so can sever the catheter.

6. Remove the needle by holding the catheter hub in place. To minimize leakage of blood while removing the needle and connecting the infusion set, apply pressure on the vein beyond the catheter with the little finger.

7. Attach the administration set, which has been previously cleared of air, and regulate the rate of flow.

8. Topical antiseptic iodophor ointment should be considered or a broad-spectrum antiseptic ointment for patients sensitive to iodine.

9. Tape catheter securely to prevent motion that could contribute to phlebitis. Avoid taping over injection site; cover site with sterile sponge or TSM dressing.

10. Loop the tubing and tape independent of the catheter to prevent an accidental pull from withdrawing the catheter.

11. Indicate the length, gauge, and type of catheter, the date of insertion, and the initials of the nurse on the tape, close to the dressing, and again in the clinical record.

12. Remove gloves and wash hands.

Midline Catheter Insertion

The midline catheter has been designed for peripheral infusion of general IV solutions and medications and venous sampling. Indications for midline IV therapy include antibiotics, hydration, pain medication, peripheral nutrition solutions of 12.5% or less final glucose concentration, and selected antineoplastic agents (excluding vesicants, which the Oncology Nursing Society generally recommends be infused through a central line).

The procedure should be performed only by trained clinical staff and after careful consideration of the possible risks, including thrombosis, phlebitis, air embolism, infection, vascular perforation, bleeding, and catheter transection.

As with any venipuncture, adequate assessment of the patient and the venous status is essential to ensure success. The basilic vein is the vein of choice for longer line IV insertions because of its larger size, straighter course, and adequate hemodilution capability.

Before insertion, the clinician should carefully select the vessel site and aseptically prepare it consistent with institutional policy and recommended INS Standards of Practice, then establish a sterile field and apply gloves.

HYPODERMOCLYSIS _____

Although seldom used, the IV nursing professional should be familiar with the terminology *hypodermoclysis* and its clinical applications. When performing a hypodermoclysis, the subcutaneous route is used as a vehicle for absorption of IV isotonic hydration fluids, usually lactated Ringer's solution. One-half ampule of Wydase is added to each 500 mL of IV solution to enhance absorption of the solution within the subcutaneous tissue.

A clysis needle, resembling the standard winged infusion needle, is entered into the lateral aspect of the patient's thigh and the infusion is initiated. Standard skin preparation consistent with INS Standards of Practice should be followed before the procedure and for removal of the needles at the completion of the clysis.[5] Some manufacturers provide therapy-specific clysis administration sets. In lieu of such a set, a standardized 78-inch administration set may be used.

PHLEBOTOMY

Phlebotomy is performed in many institutions by the professional IV nurse. The phlebotomy, a bleeding of between 400 and 500 mL blood, is performed for transfusion purposes, as well as therapeutically for acute pulmonary congestion, polycythemia vera, hemochromatosis, and porphyria cutanea tarda.

Blood for Transfusion Purposes

Routine Blood Bank Blood

When the bleeding is performed for routine bank blood, donor selection is based on the medical history and the physical examination (weight, temperature, pulse, blood pressure, and hemoglobin). The technique is according to the standards of the American Association of Blood Banks (AABB).[2]

Autotransfusion

Autotransfusion is used to return the patient's own blood to the circulation. The phlebotomy may be either:

1. *Blood bank procedure.* When the phlebotomy is performed in the blood bank, the usual blood bank procedure is followed. The blood can be stored at 4°C or the red cells can be frozen.

2. *Non-blood bank procedure.* When the bleeding is performed outside the confines of the blood bank, the same technique (according to the standards of the AABB) is used. However, the donor criteria can be modified; for example, a person with a history of cancer cannot make a routine donation but may donate for himself. Blood, which is suitable only for the donor, must be labeled with the person's name, hospital number or Social Security number, and segregated from other donor bloods. The ABO type is confirmed just before transfusion.

An important fact to bear in mind is the possibility of sepsis; clinically undetected bacteremia may exist in the patient with a catheter, a tracheostomy, or a disease process.

Blood for Therapeutic Purposes

The therapeutic phlebotomy is a valuable means by which a quantity of blood is removed to promote the health of the donor. It requires a written order by the physician specifying the date, the amount of blood to be drawn, the frequency of bleeding, and the hemoglobin or hematocrit at which the patient should be bled. If the recipient's physician approves and if the label conspicuously indicates the diagnosis and a therapeutic bleeding, the blood may be used for transfusion.

Acute Pulmonary Congestion (Inpatient)

The phlebotomy is performed to reduce venous pressure and to relieve the workload on the heart of a patient suffering from acute pulmonary edema of cardiac failure or overtransfusion. Overtransfusion is much less likely to occur today because central venous pressure monitoring provides a valuable guide for fluid administration; also, drugs are available to increase cardiac output and lower the central venous pressure.

Because the patient with acute pulmonary congestion is critically ill, the phlebotomy should probably be done by, or in the presence of, the patient's physician.

Polycythemia Vera (Inpatient or Outpatient)
The therapeutic phlebotomy is most frequently performed on the hospital patient for the production of remissions in the treatment of polycythemia vera, a disease characterized by a striking increase in the number of circulating red blood cells. It is used to reduce the red cell mass, either alone or in combination with radioactive phosphorus (^{32}P), lowering the blood volume, reducing blood viscosity, and improving circulatory efficiency. The number of and interval between phlebotomies should be specified by the physician and the hematocrit value determined after the blood donation.

Hemochromatosis (Usually Outpatient)
Hemochromatosis is characterized by excessive body stores of iron. The phlebotomy is performed to reduce the total body iron concentration. Because these patients usually have a hematocrit value in the normal range, periodic checks on the hematocrit value are desirable.

Porphyria Cutanea Tarda (Usually Outpatient)
The mechanism of relief of these skin lesions by phlebotomy is not clear. Because these patients have a normal hematocrit reading, they are most likely to be bled too much; periodic hematocrit checks are desirable.

Procedure for Bleeding

To allay apprehension and to avoid a vasovagal reaction, the procedure should be explained and the patient reassured and put at ease.

Identification
1. Identify donor with the record and the order for the phlebotomy.
2. Make sure that identically numbered labels to donor record are attached to the blood collection container and to test tubes for donor blood samples.
3. Make sure that the processing tubes are correctly numbered and kept with the container during the collection of blood.

Donor Arm Preparation
Adequate preparation of the skin is vital in providing an aseptic site for venipuncture to protect both the donor and the recipient. In preparing the area, always start at the venipuncture site and move outward in concentric spirals for at least 1½ inches; use sterile materials and instruments.

1. Put on gloves
2. Using a 15% aqueous (not alcoholic) soap or detergent solution, scrub vigorously for at least 30 seconds with gauze or 60 seconds with cotton balls.
3. Apply 10% acetone in 70% isopropyl alcohol to remove the soap; let dry.

4. Apply tincture of iodine (3% in 70% ethyl alcohol) and allow to dry.

5. Use 10% acetone in 70% isopropyl alcohol to remove the iodine; allow to dry.

6. Place a dry sterile gauze over the site until ready to perform the venipuncture.

Alternative procedure:

1. Put on gloves

2. Use 0.7% aqueous scrub solution of iodophor compound (povidone-iodine or poloxamer-iodine complex), scrubbing the area for 30 seconds. Remove the foam; it is not necessary to dry the arm.

3. Prepare with iodophor complex solution (eg, 10% povidone-iodine); allow to stand 30 seconds. The solution need not be removed.

4. Place a dry sterile gauze sponge over the site until ready to perform the venipuncture. Do not repalpate vein.

Collection of Blood

The following procedure for the collection of blood using the plastic bag is reproduced from the AABB's *Technical Manual*.[2] This procedure may be modified when the blood is to be discarded.

1. Inspect bag for any defects. Apply pressure to check for leaks. The anticoagulant solution must be clear.

2. Position bag carefully, being sure it is below the level of the donor's arm.

   a. If balance system is used, be sure counterbalance is level and adjusted for the amount of blood to be drawn. Unless metal clips and a hand sealer are used, make a very loose overhand knot in tubing. Hang the bag and route tubing through the pinch clamp.

   b. If balance system is not used, be sure there is some way to monitor the volume of blood drawn.

   c. If a vacuum-assist device is used, the manufacturer's instructions should be followed.

3. Reapply tourniquet or blood pressure cuff. Have donor open and close hand until previously selected vein is again prominent.

4. Uncover sterile needle and do venipuncture immediately. A clean, skillful venipuncture is essential for collection of a full, clot-free unit. Tape the tubing to hold needle in place and cover site with sterile gauze.

5. Open the temporary closure between the interior of the bag and the tubing, if present.

6. Have donor open and close hand, squeezing a rubber ball or other resilient object slowly every 10 to 12 seconds during collection. Keep the donor under observation throughout phlebotomy. The donor should never be left unattended during or immediately after donation.

7. Mix the blood and anticoagulant gently and periodically (approximately every 30 seconds) during collection. Mixing may be done by hand, by placing bag on a mechanical agitator, or by using a rocking vacuum-assist device.

8. Be sure blood flow remains fairly brisk, so that coagulation activity is not triggered. Rigid time limits are not warranted if there is continuous agitation, although units requiring more than 8 minutes to draw may not be suitable for preparation of platelet concentrates, fresh frozen plasma, or cryoprecipitate.

9. Monitor volume of blood being drawn. If a balance or vacuum-assist device is used, blood flow will stop after the proper amount has been collected. One mL of blood weighs 1.053 g, the minimum allowable specific gravity for female donors. A convenient figure to use is 1.06 g; a unit containing 405 to 495 mL should weigh 425 to 520 g plus the weight of the container with its anticoagulant.

10. Clamp tubing temporarily using a hemostat, metal clip, or other temporary clamp. Next, collect blood-processing sample by a method that precludes contamination of the donor unit. This may be accomplished in several ways.

    a. If the blood collection bag contains an in-line needle, make an additional seal with a hemostat, metal clip, hand sealer, or a tight knot made from previously prepared loose knot just distal to the in-line needle. Open the connector by separating the needles. Insert the proximal needle into a processing test tube, remove the hemostat, allow the tube to fill, and reclamp tubing. Carefully reattach slide connector. Donor needle is now ready for removal.

    b. If the blood collection bag contains an in-line processing tube, be certain that the processing tube, or pouch, is full when the collection is complete and the original clamp is placed near the donor needle. Entire assembly may now be removed from donor.

    c. If a straight-tubing assembly set is used, there are two alternative procedures. In the first method, remove the needle from the donor's arm as soon as the tubing is clamped. Take bag and assembly to sealer area or collect processing tube at the donor chair by placing a hemostat close to where donor tubing enters the bag, leaving the tubing full of blood. Remove the clamp next to donor needle, empty contents of donor tubing into the processing test tube, reapply clamp or permanently seal next to donor needle, remove hemostat next to donor bag, and allow the donor tubing to refill with blood, well mixed, from donor bag.

    In the second method, place two hemostats or temporary seals on the tubing. Cut tubing between the seals, put cut end of the tubing into the processing test tube, remove the proximal hemostat, allow tube to fill, and reclamp tubing.

11. Deflate and remove tourniquet. Remove needle from arm. Apply pressure over gauze and have donor raise arm (elbow straight) and hold gauze firmly over phlebotomy site with the other hand.

12. Discard needle assembly into rigid container designed to prevent accidental injury to and contamination of personnel.

13. Strip donor tubing as completely as possible into the bag, starting at seal. Work quickly, to avoid allowing the blood to clot in the tubing. Invert bag several times to mix thoroughly, then allow tubing to refill with anticoagulated blood from the bag. Repeat this procedure a second time.

14. Seal the tubing left attached to the bags into segments on which the segment number is clearly and completely readable. Knots, metal clips, or a dielectric sealer may be used to make segments suitable for crossmatching. It must be possible to separate segments from the container without breaking sterility of the container.

15. Reinspect container for defects.

16. Recheck numbers on container, processing tubes, and donation record. Be sure the expiration date of the unit is on the container label.

17. Place blood at appropriate temperature. Unless platelets are to be removed, whole blood should be placed at 1° to 6°C immediately after collection. If platelets are to be harvested, blood should not be chilled but should be maintained at room temperature (about 20°–24°C) until platelets are separated. Platelets should be separated within 6 hours after collection of the unit of whole blood.

Treatment of Adverse Donor Reactions

Stop the phlebotomy at the first sign of reaction and call the physician.

1. *Fainting*
   a. Elevate the donor's feet above head level.
   b. Loosen tight clothing.
   c. Ascertain that the donor has adequate airway.
   d. Apply cold compresses to forehead and back of neck.
   e. Check and record blood pressure, pulse, and respiration periodically.

2. *Nausea and vomiting*
   a. Instruct the donor to breathe slowly.

3. *Muscular twitching* or tetanic spasms of hands or face
   a. Instruct donor to rebreathe into a paper bag. Do not give oxygen.

4. *Convulsions* (rare)
   a. Call for assistance.
   b. Prevent the donor from injuring himself or herself by turning the patient on the left side.

5. *For more serious reactions* or if donor does not respond
   a. Call for medical assistance.

Record the nature and treatment of all reactions on the donor's record; include opinion as to the future use of the donor for blood donations.

Suggested Procedure for Therapeutic Phlebotomy

The blood must be discarded. This procedure is not adequate for recipient protection.

Equipment

Phlebotomy pack (obtained from blood bank); if only double pack is available, ignore the satellite pack.

Counterbalance stand (obtained from blood bank) or small spring scale

Blood pressure cuff or tourniquet

Tincture of iodine (3% in 70% ethyl alcohol) or iodophor complex solution (10% povidone-iodine)

10% acetone in 70% isopropyl alcohol for use with tincture of iodine

Sterile sponges

Technique

Preparation

1. Put on gloves

2. Select the most suitable vein. Apply a tourniquet or a blood pressure cuff inflated to 50 to 60 mm Hg. Opening and closing the fist will make the vein more prominent. Remove the tourniquet.

3. Prepare the venipuncture site. Always start at the puncture site and move out in concentric spirals for 1½ inches.
   a. Apply tincture of iodine; allow to dry. *Question patient before applying; some patients may be allergic to iodine.*
   b. Apply 10% acetone in 70% isopropyl alcohol to remove iodine. Allow to dry. Iodophor complex (10% povidone-iodine) may be substituted for iodine. It does not cause skin reactions even in iodine-sensitive individuals. Do not wash off iodophor complex. Cover the site with dry sterile gauze to prevent contamination until the phlebotomy is begun.

Collection of Blood

1. Suspend bag from donor scale as far below donor's arm as possible.

2. If counterbalance scales are used, adjust the balance for amount of blood to be drawn.

3. Make loose overhand knot in donor tube near needle.

4. Apply tourniquet (do not impair arterial circulation).

5. *Do not touch or repalpate vein.*

6. Perform phlebotomy.

7. Tape needle in place and cover with sterile sponge.

8. Pinch bead into bag from junction of donor tube and bag to open lumen and allow blood to flow.

9. Instruct patient to open and close fist slowly.

10. Collect blood until bag falls on scale. If spring scales are used, collect until prescribed amount has been withdrawn.

11. Pull knot tight.

12. Release tourniquet, withdraw needle, and apply pressure with gauze pad until bleeding has stopped. *Do not flex arm.* The arm may be elevated while applying pressure.

13. Dispose of blood and equipment as directed by hospital procedure.

14. Record procedure in clinical record.

REFERENCES

1. Adriani, J. (1962). Venipuncture. *American Journal of Nursing, 62,* 66.
2. American Association of Blood Banks. (1994). *Technical manual* (11th ed., pp. 11–15). Washington, DC: Author.
3. Centers for Disease Control and Prevention. (1994). *Guidelines for prevention of intravascular infection.* Atlanta, GA: Author.
4. Dudley, H. A. (1960). Modified technique for intravenous cannulation. *Surgery, Gynecology and Obstetrics, 111,* 513.
5. *Revised intravenous nursing standards of practice.* (1990). *Journal of Intravenous Nursing* (Suppl.), S41.
6. Metheny, N. M. (1996). *Fluid and electrolyte balance* (3rd ed., pp. 8, 10). Philadelphia: J. B. Lippincott.

BIBLIOGRAPHY

Jemison-Smith, P., & Thrupp, L. D. (1982). Phlebitis, infections and filtration. *Journal of the National Intravenous Therapy Association, 5*(5), 329–335.
Turco, S. J. (1987). Infusion phlebitis: A review of literature. *Parenterals, 5*(3), 1–8.

Zenowich, D. (1981). Physics of maintaining I.V. flow. *Journal of the National Intravenous Therapy Association, 4*(3), 212–214.

REVIEW QUESTIONS

1. The term "vasovagal reaction" refers to an autonomic nervous system response to:
   a. stress
   b. fluid resuscitation
   c. sudden hydration
   d. circulatory overload

2. Veins used initially to preserve future venous access include which of the following?
   a. cephalic
   b. metacarpal
   c. basilic
   d. digital

3. Prime factors to be considered in selecting a vein for infusion include which of the following?
   a. location
   b. condition
   c. purpose
   d. duration

4. Application of digital pressure applied to disperse fluid denotes presence of:
   a. hypertension
   b. edema
   c. circulatory collapse
   d. hypotension

5. The catheter most frequently used today is:
   a. through the needle
   b. cutdown
   c. over the needle
   d. subclavian

6. A needle commonly used for venous sampling is:
   a. steel
   b. aluminum
   c. Silastic
   d. polyethylene

7. Trauma to the endothelial wall is minimized by use of:
   a. long bevel
   b. short bevel
   c. thin wall
   d. large needle

8. The basilic vein is the vein of choice for longer line IV insertions because of its:
   a. larger size
   b. straighter course
   c. adequate hemodilution
   d. density

9. Indications for midline therapy include which of the following?
   a. hydration
   b. antibiotics
   c. pain medication
   d. peripheral nutrition

10. Therapeutic phlebotomy may be performed for which of the following reasons?
    a. polycythemia vera
    b. hemochromatosis
    c. acute pulmonary congestion
    d. thrombocytopenia

CHAPTER 8

Complications

Key Terms

Air embolism	Infiltration	Speed shock
Catheter embolism	Local	Systemic
Culturing	Microbial pathogens	Thrombosis
Extravasation	Phlebothrombosis	Thrombophlebitis
Host	Practice setting	

Intravenous therapy subjects the patient to numerous potential hazards, many of which can be avoided if the nurse understands the risks involved and uses all available measures to prevent their occurrence. Local complications occur frequently but are rarely serious. Systemic complications, though rarer, are serious and frequently life-threatening, requiring immediate recognition and medical attention.

LOCAL COMPLICATIONS

Occasionally local complications are not recognized until considerable damage is done. Early recognition may prevent 1) extensive edema that deprives the patient of urgently needed fluid and medications; 2) necrosis; and 3) thrombophlebitis with the subsequent danger of embolism. The local complications occur as the result of trauma to the wall of the vein.

Thrombosis

Any injury that roughens the endothelial cells of the venous wall allows platelets to adhere and a thrombus to form. Because the point of the cannula traumatizes the wall of the vein where it touches, thrombi form on the vein and at the tip of the cannula. Thrombosis occurs when a local thrombus obstructs the circulation of blood. It must be remembered that thrombi form an excellent trap for bacteria, whether carried by the bloodstream from an infection in a remote part of the body or introduced through the subcutaneous orifice.[7]

Thrombophlebitis

Thrombophlebitis is the term used to denote a twofold injury—thrombosis plus inflammation. The development of thrombophlebitis is easily recognized. A painful inflammation develops along the length of the vein. If the infusion is allowed to continue, the vein progressively thromboses, becoming hard, tortuous, tender, and painful.[15] Early detection may prevent an obstructive thrombophlebitis, which causes the infusion to slow and finally stop. This condition is most painful, persisting indefinitely, incapacitating the patient, and limiting valuable veins for future therapy.

Usually a sterile inflammation develops from a chemical or mechanical irritation. When the inflammation is the result of sepsis, it is much more serious and carries with it the potential danger of septicemia and acute bacterial endocarditis.

There is always the inherent danger of embolism when thrombosis occurs. The more pronounced the inflammation and the more intense the pain, the more organized the thrombus is likely to become. Embolism is less likely to occur from the well attached clot of thrombophlebitis than from phlebothrombosis.[11]

Phlebothrombosis

Phlebothrombosis denotes thrombosis and usually indicates that the inflammation is relatively inconspicuous. It is thought to give rise to embolism because the thrombus is poorly attached to the wall of the vein.[11] Both thrombophlebitis and phlebothrombosis have a degree of inflammation and are associated with potential embolism.

Contributing Factors

Any irritation involving the wall of the vein predisposes the patient to thrombophlebitis. Inflammation to the vein will occur from any foreign body and is mediated by the following:

- Duration of the infusion
- Composition of the solution
- Site of the infusion
- Technique
- Method used

Duration of the infusion is a significant factor in the development of thrombophlebitis. As the duration of time is lengthened, the incidence and degree of inflammation increase.

The *composition of the solution* may play a role. Venous irritation and inflammation may result from the infusion of hypertonic glucose solutions, certain drug additives, or solutions with a pH significantly different from that of the plasma. Solutions of dextrose are irritating to the vein.[9,10] The United States Pharmacopeia specifications for pH of dextrose solutions range from 3.5 to 6.5; acidity is necessary to prevent "caramelization" of the dextrose during autoclaving and to preserve the stability of the solution during storage. Studies have shown a significant reduction in thrombophlebitis when buffered glucose solutions have been infused.[9] Neut, a sodium bicarbonate 1% solution, may be added to increase the pH of acid IV solutions. This additive, however, poses a problem of incompatibility when added to solutions containing drugs. The largest number of incompatibilities may be produced by changes in pH.[17] As an example, tetracycline hydrochloride, with a pH of 2.5 to 3.0, is unstable in an alkaline environment.

The *site of infusion* can be a factor contributing to thrombophlebitis. The veins in areas over joint flexion undergo injury when motion of the cannula irritates the venous wall. The veins in the lower extremities are especially susceptible to trauma, enhanced by the stagnant blood in varicosities and the stasis in the peripheral venous circulation.

Small veins are subject to inflammation when used to infuse an irritating solution. The infusion cannula may occlude the entire lumen of the vein, obstructing the flow of circulating blood; the solution then flows undiluted, irritating the wall of the vein.

Technique can mean the difference between a successful infusion and the complication of thrombophlebitis. Only minimal trauma results from a skillfully executed venipuncture, whereas a carelessly performed venipuncture may seriously traumatize the venous wall.

Phlebitis associated with sepsis may be related to the technique of the operator. Infection is always a risk if sterile technique is not zealously observed. Thorough cleansing of the skin is important in preventing infections. Maintenance of asepsis is essential during long-term therapy, particularly in the use of the through-the-needle cannula.[4]

Methods used to infuse parenteral solutions may foster septic thrombophlebitis. This complication is most often associated with the through-the-needle cannula. The cannula threaded through the needle remains sterile and does not come in contact with the skin, but provides a large subcutaneous orifice facilitating entry of bacteria around the catheter and seepage of fluid.

The over-the-needle cannula is not without fault because it comes in direct contact with the skin before being introduced into the vein. However, the tight fit through the skin may bar further bacterial entry.

Preventive Measures

In performing venipunctures, the nurse should exercise every caution to avoid injuring the wall of the vein needlessly. Multiple punctures, through-and-through punctures, and damage to the posterior wall of the vein with the point of the cannula can cause thrombosis. The risk of phlebitis may be minimized if the nurse:

1. Refrains from using veins in the lower extremities.
2. Selects veins with ample blood volume when infusing irritating substances.
3. Avoids veins in areas over joint flexion; uses an armboard if the vein must be located in an area of flexion.
4. Anchors cannulas securely to prevent motion.

To prevent septic phlebitis, thorough preparation of the skin, together with aseptic technique and maintenance of asepsis during infusion, is imperative.

Periodic inspection of the injection site will detect developing complications before serious damage occurs. Complaints of a painful infusion make it necessary to differentiate between early phlebitis and venospasm from an irritating solution. If the latter is present, slowing the solution and applying heat to the vein will dilate the vessel and increase the blood flow, diluting the solution and relieving the pain. Following hypertonic solutions with isotonic fluids will flush the vein of irritating substances.

If inflammation accompanies the pain, a change in the injection site should be considered. To continue the infusion will only bring progressive trauma and limit available veins. Adherence to time limits for removal of the cannula reduces the incidence of phlebitis.[9]

Phlebitis is often graded using a set scale:

1+ = pain at site; erythema and/or edema; no streak; no palpable cord

2+ = pain at site; erythema and/or edema; streak formation; no palpable cord

3+ = pain at site; erythema and/or edema; streak formation; palpable cord[9]

During removal of the infusion cannula, care must be taken to prevent injury to the wall of the vein; the cannula should be removed at an angle nearly flush with the skin. Pressure should be applied for a reasonable length of time to prevent extravasation of blood.

Infiltration

Dislodgment of the cannula with consequent infiltration of fluid is common and frequently is considered of minor significance. With the increasing numbers of irritating solutions and the frequency with which potent drugs are infused in IV solutions, serious problems may occur when the fluid invades the surrounding tissues. Hypertonic, acid, and alkaline solutions are contraindicated for hypodermoclysis and are not intended for other than venous infusions. If they are allowed to infiltrate, necrosis may occur.

If necrosis is avoided, edema may nevertheless:

1. Deprive the patient of fluid and drug absorption at the rate essential for successful therapy.
2. Limit veins available for venipuncture, complicating therapy.
3. Predispose the patient to infection.

Extravasation

Extravasation can easily be recognized by the increasing edema at the site of the infusion. A comparison of the infusion area with the identical area in the opposite extremity assists in determining whether swelling is present.

Frequently the edema is allowed to increase to great proportions because of a misconception that a backflow of blood into the adapter is significant proof that the infusion is entering the vein. This is not a reliable method for checking a possible infiltration. The point of the cannula may puncture the posterior wall of the vein, leaving the greater portion of the bevel within the lumen of the vein. Blood return will be obtained on negative pressure, but if the infusion is allowed to continue, fluid will seep into the tissues at the point of the cannula, increasing the edema.

Occasionally, a blood return is not obtained on negative pressure. This may occur when the needle occludes the lumen of a small vein, obstructing the flow of blood.

To confirm an infiltration, apply a tourniquet proximal to the injection site tightly enough to restrict the venous flow. If the infusion continues regardless of this venous obstruction, extravasation is evident.

Once an infiltration has occurred, the cannula should be removed immediately.

Drugs that contribute to extravasation necrosis are most often osmotically active or ischemia inducing, or they cause direct cellular toxicity. Mechanical compression within the infiltrated tissue can increase the extent of damage, as can infection of the resulting wound. If only superficial tissue loss occurs and remains free of infection, debridement will yield a clean bed capable of granulating. If deep structures are involved, spontaneous wound healing may be averted, resulting in the need for wide excision, debridement, grafting, or amputation to restore tissue integrity.

SYSTEMIC COMPLICATIONS

Septicemia

Septicemia is caused by invasion of the bloodstream by microorganisms or their by-products, including bacteria, fungi, mycobacteria, and rarely viruses. Certain predisposing factors put the infusion therapy patient at risk:

- Age less than 1 year or greater than 60 years
- Presence of granulocytopenia
- Immunocompromised state
- Loss of skin integrity
- Presence of a distant infection that might contribute to hematogenous seeding

Cannula factors can also contribute to development of septicemia, including the size of the cannula, the number of lumens, the function and use of the cannula, catheter material and bacterial adherence, and thrombogenicity.

Clinical manifestations of septicemia include chills, fever, general malaise, and headache. Supportive therapy for the patient with septicemia includes fluid replacement, blood pressure maintenance, oxygenation, cardiac output maintenance, nutritional support, and preservation of acid–base balance. Ancillary treatments involve administration of steroids, naloxone, and endotoxin vaccination.

Prevention programs support the use of 0.2-μm air-eliminating, bacterial-retentive filters. Intravascular systems should be considered potential portals for infection. Good handwashing techniques; line care protocols; and adherence to the Intravenous Nurses Society (INS) Standards of Practice for monitoring, maintenance of infusion, tubing changes, and catheter care all contribute to an environment that will not readily support development of septicemia in patients receiving infusion therapies.

Pulmonary Embolism

Pulmonary embolism occurs when a substance, usually a blood clot, becomes free floating and is propelled by the venous circulation to the right side of the heart and into the pulmonary artery.[6] Emboli may obstruct the main pulmonary artery or the arteries to the lobes, occluding arterial apertures at major bifurcations.[10] Obstruction of the main artery results in circulatory and cardiac disturbances. Recurrent small emboli may eventually result in pulmonary hypertension and right heart failure.[10]

Preventive Measures
Certain precautions must be taken to prevent this serious complication.

1. Blood or plasma must be infused through an adequate filter to remove any particulate matter that could result in small emboli.

2. Veins on the lower extremities should be avoided when venipunctures are performed. These veins are particularly susceptible to trauma, predisposing the patient to thrombophlebitis. Although superficial veins rarely seem to be the source of emboli consequence,[10] a thrombus may extend into the deep veins, resulting in a potentially viable clot; superficial and deep veins unite freely in the lower extremities.

3. Positive pressure should not be used to relieve clot formation. To check for patency of the lumen of the cannula, kink the infusion tubing about 8 inches from the cannula. Then kink and release the tubing between the cannula and the pinched tubing—if the tubing becomes hard and meets with resistance, obstruction is evident, necessitating removal and reinstatement of the infusion.

4. Special precautions should be observed in the drug-additive program. Reconstituted drugs must be completely dissolved before being added to parenteral solutions; it is the inherent nature of red cells to adhere to particles, adding to the danger of clot formation.

5. Solutions should be examined to detect any particulate matter.

Air Embolism

Although air embolism is a significant possible complication with air-dependent containers, it is much more frequently associated with central venous lines. There is a potential risk for air embolism on the insertion of a central venous catheter, on inadequate sealing of the tract subsequent to disconnection of a central venous catheter, with disconnection of central lines, and with bypassing the "pump housing" of an electronic volumetric pump with an IV piggyback connection. Fatal embolism may occur when small bubbles accumulate dangerously and form tenacious bubbles that block the pulmonary capillaries.[1] Recognition of the circumstances that contribute to this hazard and measures taken to prevent their occurrence are imperative for safe fluid therapy.

Gravity Infusions
If a vented container is allowed to run dry, air enters the tubing and the fluid level drops to the proximity of the patient's chest. The pressure exerted by the blood on the walls of the veins controls the level to which the air drops in the tubing. A negative pressure in the vein may allow air to enter the bloodstream. A negative pressure occurs when the extremity receiving the infusion is elevated above the heart.[17] Infusions flowing through a central venous catheter carry an even greater risk of air embolism when the container empties than those flowing through a peripheral vein; be-

cause the central venous pressure is less than the peripheral venous pressure, there is more apt to be a negative pressure that could suck air into the circulation. The nurse should take precautions while changing the administration set of a central venous infusion. The patient should be lying flat in bed and should be instructed to perform the Valsalva maneuver (forced expiration with the mouth closed) immediately before and during the time that the catheter is open to the air.

If the fluid container on a continuous infusion should empty, fresh solution will force the trapped air into the circulation. To remove the air from the administration set:

1. Place a hemostat close to the infusion cannula.
2. Hang the fresh solution.
3. With an antiseptic, clean the rubber section of the tubing proximal to the hemostat and below the air level in the tubing.
4. Insert a sterile needle to allow the air to escape.
5. Remove clamp and readjust flow.

The Y-type infusion set used with vented containers (Fig. 8-1) is a less obvious source but one by which great quantities of air can be drawn into the bloodstream.

FIGURE 8-1 (**A**) The container runs dry during simultaneous infusion of fluids through a Y-type administration set. Pressure below the partially constricted clamp is less than atmospheric, allowing air from the empty container (atmospheric) to enter infusion. (**B**) A secondary infusion "piggybacked" through the injection site of a primary IV set. Lacking an automatic shut-off valve, air from the empty container will enter the circulation. The same principle is involved as in the Y-type set.

Running solutions simultaneously is the contributing factor. If one vented container empties, it becomes the source of air for the flowing solution. This is explained by the fact that the atmospheric pressure is greater in the open tubing to the empty container than below the partially restricted clamp on the infusion side. Recurrent small air bubbles are constantly aspirated into the flowing solution and on into the venous system. The introduction of air may be prevented by running one solution at a time. Vigilance is imperative if vented solutions are ordered to run simultaneously. The tubing must be clamped off completely before the solution container is allowed to empty.[20]

This same principle is involved in the piggyback setup for secondary infusions. The potential danger of air embolism exists whenever solutions from two vented sets run simultaneously through a common cannula. Advanced technologies have minimized the use of piggyback setups.

All connections of an infusion set must be tight. Any faulty opening or defective hole in the set allows air to be emitted into the flowing solution. If a stopcock is used, the outlets not in use must be completely shut off.

The regulating clamp on the infusion set should be located no higher than the chest level of the patient. Because the pressure exerted by the blood on the venous wall will normally raise a column of water from 4 to 11 cm above the heart, a restricting clamp placed above this point will result in a negative pressure in the tubing.[17] If great enough, the pressure can suck air into the flowing solution should a loose connection or a faulty opening exist between the clamp and the cannula.[17] The lower the clamp, the greater is the chance of any defects occurring above the clamp, where positive pressure can force the solution to leak out.[20]

An infusion set long enough to drop below the extremity gives added protection against air being drawn into the vein should the infusion bottle empty. In-lying pressure chambers on administration sets should be kept filled at all times. Manual compression of an empty chamber will force air into the bloodstream.

Occurrence of an Air Embolism

The nurse should be familiar with the symptoms associated with air embolism that arise from sudden vascular collapse: cyanosis, drop in blood pressure, weak rapid pulse, rise in venous pressure, and loss of consciousness. If air embolism occurs, the source of air entry must be immediately rectified. The patient should be turned on his left side with his head down.[17] This causes the air to rise in the right atrium, preventing it from entering the pulmonary artery. Oxygen is then administered and the physician notified.

Catheter Embolism

Catheter embolism may occur during the insertion of a through-the-needle catheter if strict adherence to the proper procedure is not followed. The catheter should never be pulled back through the needle. If it becomes necessary to remove the catheter, the entire unit should be removed and a new catheter inserted. Catheter embolism may also occur during the insertion of an over-the-needle catheter if the needle is either partially or totally withdrawn and then reinserted. If the catheter is sheared off and embolized, the intervention of cardiac catheterization with shearing the catheter under the fluoroscope may be necessary.

Pulmonary Edema

Overloading the circulation is a real hazard to elderly patients and to patients with impaired renal and cardiac function. Fluids too rapidly infused increase the venous pressure, with the possibility of cardiac dilation and subsequent pulmonary edema.

Preventive Measures

These measures should be taken to prevent pulmonary edema.

1. Infusions should be maintained at the flow rate prescribed.
2. Positive pressure, using the pressure-chamber administration sets, should never be applied by the nurse to infuse solutions. If the patient requires fluids at such rapidity that positive pressure is required, infusion then becomes the physician's responsibility.
3. Controlled-volume infusion sets give added protection by preventing large quantities of fluid from being accidentally infused. These sets control the volume from 10 to 150 mL.
4. Solutions not infused within the 24-hour period ordered should be discarded and not infused with the following day's solutions; fluids administered in excess of the quantity ordered can overtax the homeostatic controls, increasing the danger of pulmonary edema.

The attending nurse must be alert to any signs or symptoms suggestive of circulatory overloading. Venous dilation, with engorged neck veins, increased blood pressure, and a rise in venous pressure, should alert the nurse to the danger of pulmonary edema. Rapid respiration and shortness of breath may occur. The infusion should be slowed to a minimal rate and the physician notified. Raising the patient to a sitting position may facilitate breathing.

Speed Shock

Speed shock is the term used to denote the systemic reaction that occurs when a substance foreign to the body is rapidly introduced into the circulation. Caution must be observed in the administration of IV push injections. Rapid injection permits the concentration of a medication in the plasma to reach toxic proportions, flooding the organs rich in blood—the heart and the brain. As a result, syncope, shock, and cardiac arrest may occur.[1]

Preventive Measures

Certain precautions can minimize the potential danger of speed shock.

1. By reducing the size of the drop, pediatric-type infusion sets provide greater accuracy, thereby reducing the risk of rapid administration. These sets are valuable when solutions containing potent drugs must be maintained at a minimal rate of flow.
2. Electronic flow-control devices control the rate of infusion, an asset imperative to the administration of IV medications.
3. On initiating the infusion, ascertain that the solution is flowing freely before adjusting the rate. Movement of a cannula in which the aperture is partially

obstructed by the wall of the vein can cause an increase in the flow, contributing to the danger of speed shock.

INTRAVENOUS-ASSOCIATED INFECTIONS

Cannula-Related

Infections may be cannula or solution related. Cannula-related infections are those that generate from the cannula material itself or from migration of organisms through the open skin along the cannula.

Solution-Related

Solution-related infections are those that result from contaminated IV solutions, either in the manufacturing process or in use. This subject has been discussed in great detail.

SOURCES OF BACTERIA

Three main sources yield the bacteria responsible for IV-associated infection: the air, the skin, and the blood. Microorganisms (flora and fauna) characteristic of a given location are referred to accordingly, thus the terms *skin flora*, *intestinal flora*, and so on. Table 8-1 lists microbial pathogens associated with infusion-related septicemia.

The Air

The number of microbes per cubic foot of air varies, depending on the particular area involved. Where infection is present, bacteria escape in body discharges, contaminating clothing, bedding, and dressings. Activity, such as making a bed, sends bacteria flying into the air on particles of lint, pus, and dried epithelium.[12] Increased activity causes a rise in the number of airborne particles and provides an environment that interferes with aseptic technique and potentially contributes to contamination. Airborne microorganisms may be plentiful in patient areas and utility rooms. These contaminants find easy access to unprotected IV fluids.

The Skin

The skin is the main source of bacteria responsible for IV-associated infection. The bacteria found on the skin are referred to as *resident* or *transient*. Resident bacteria are those normally present, and they are relatively constant in a given individual. They adhere tightly to the skin and usually include *Staphylococcus albus* as well as diphtheroids and *Bacillus* species.[12] Because not all bacteria are removed by scrubbing, meticulous care must be observed to avoid touching sterile equipment.

The transient bacteria are responsible for infection carried from one person to another. Touch contamination is a potential hazard of infection because hospital personnel move about frequently, touching patients and objects. Frequent handwashing is imperative.

The skin of the patient offers fertile soil for bacteria growth. It has been estimated that a minimum of 10,000 organisms are present per square centimeter of normal

TABLE 8-1
Microbial Pathogens Associated With Infusion-Related Septicemia

Source of Septicemia	Major Pathogens
Conventional infusion therapy Cannula	Coagulase-negative *Staphylococcus* (>50%)
	Staphylococcus aureus
	Enterococcus
	Klebsiella-Enterobacter
	Serratia marcescens
	Candida species
	Pseudomonas aeruginosa
	Pseudomonas cepacia
	Corynebacterium species (diphtheroids), JK-1
Contaminated infusate	Tribe Klebsielleae (90%)
	Klebsiella
	Enterobacter*
	Serratia
	P. cepacia*
	Citrobacter freundii
	Flavobacterium
Hyperalimentation, Hickman-Broviac catheters (most, catheter-related)	Coagulase-negative *Staphylococcus* (>50%)
	Candida species, *Torulopsis glabrata*
	S. aureus
	Klebsiella-Enterobacter
	Enterococcus
Contaminated blood products (contaminated infusate)	Pseudomonads other than *P. aeruginosa* (>50%)*
	S. marcescens
	Achromobacter
	Salmonella choleraesuis
	Citrobacter
	Flavobacterium
Arterial pressure monitoring	*P. cepacia**
	Serratia
	P. acidovorans
	P. aeruginosa
	Enterobacter
	Flavobacterium
	Candida (very rare)
Regional intra-arterial cancer chemotherapy (catheter-related)	*S. aureus*

*Septicemia caused by *E. cloacae, E. agglomerans,* or *P. cepacia,* in particular, should prompt investigations for contaminated infusate.

Source: Adapted from Maki, D. G. (*1976*). Growth properties of microorganisms in infusion fluid and methods of detection. In I. Phillips, P. D. Meers, & P. F. D'Arcy (Eds.), *Microbiological hazards of infusion therapy.* Lancaster, England: MTP Press.

skin.[23] A square centimeter is equal to 0.155 square inches. Organisms such as *Staphylococcus epidermidis*, *S. aureus*, gram-negative bacilli (especially *Klebsiella*, *Enterobacter*, and *Serratia*), and enterococci are ubiquitous on the skin of hospitalized patients.[16]

The Blood

The blood may harbor potentially dangerous microorganisms. Therefore, care must be taken to prevent bacterial contamination from blood spills when drawing samples and performing venipuncture. Refer to Chapter 17 for a discussion of bloodborne pathogens.

See Box 8-1 for the Occupational Safety and Health Administration (OSHA) guidelines to prevent the spread of human immunodeficiency virus.

FACTORS INFLUENCING THE SURVIVAL OF BACTERIA

Infection depends on the ability of bacteria to survive and proliferate. The factors that influence their survival are: 1) the specific organisms present, 2) the number of such organisms, 3) the resistance of the host, and 4) the environmental conditions.[14]

The Specific Organisms

Bacteria are referred to as *pathogenic* or *nonpathogenic*. Pathogenic bacteria are capable of producing disease. All bacteria should be considered pathogenic. Reports show that bacteria previously considered nonpathogenic may produce infection. In one study, *Serratia* was implicated in 35% of cases of gram-negative septicemia resulting from IV therapy.[2,3,5]

Bacteria are classified as *gram-positive* and *gram-negative*. In recent years gram-negative bacteria have replaced gram-positive bacteria as the leading cause of death from septicemia.[18] The single most important reason for the intensity of the problem is probably the increased usage of antibiotics highly effective against gram-positive organisms but only selectively effective against gram-negative organisms. With the competitive inhibition of gram-positive bacteria eliminated, the more resistant gram-negative organisms have proliferated in the hospital environment.[13]

Number of Organisms

The number of contaminants present influences the probability of production of an infection. The power of bacteria to proliferate must not be underestimated. It is simply *not true* that a small amount of bacteria from touch contamination is harmless. Contamination of IV fluids and bottles with even a few organisms is extremely dangerous because some fungi and many bacteria can proliferate at room temperature in a variety of IV solutions to more than 105 organisms/mL within 24 hours.[8]

Host Resistance

The resistance of the host influences the development and course of septicemia. Underlying conditions such as diabetes mellitus, chronic uremia, cirrhosis, cancer, and leukemia may adversely affect the patient's capacity to resist infection. Treatments such as

Box 8-1
Precautions to Prevent Transmission of HIV*

Universal Precautions

Because medical history and examination cannot reliably identify all patients infected with human immunodeficiency virus (HIV) or other blood-borne pathogens, blood and body fluid precautions should be consistently used for *all* patients. This approach, previously recommended by the CDC and referred to as *universal blood and body-fluid precautions* or *universal precautions*, should be used in the care of *all* patients, especially those in emergency care settings in which the risk of blood exposure is increased and the infection status of the patient is usually unknown.

BARRIER PRECAUTIONS

Health care workers should always use appropriate barrier precautions to prevent exposure of skin and mucous membranes when contact with blood or other body fluids of any patient is anticipated.

1. Gloves should be worn when touching blood and body fluids, mucous membranes, or non-intact skin of all patients, for handling items or surfaces soiled with blood or body fluids, and for performing venipuncture and other vascular access procedures.

2. Gloves should be changed after contact with each patient.

3. Masks and protective eyewear or face shields should be worn during procedures that are likely to generate droplets of blood or other body fluids to prevent exposure of mucous membranes of the mouth, nose, and eyes.

4. Gowns or aprons should be worn during procedures likely to cause splashes of blood body fluids.

HAND WASHING

1. Hands and other skin surfaces should be washed immediately and thoroughly if contaminated with blood or other body fluids.

2. Hands should be washed immediately after gloves are removed.

PROTECTION AGAINST INJURY

1. All health care workers should take precautions to prevent injuries caused by needles, scalpels, and other sharp instruments or devices
   (a) During procedures
   (b) When cleaning used instruments
   (c) During disposal of used needles
   (d) When handling sharp instruments after procedures

2. To prevent *needlestick injuries*, needles should not be recapped, purposely bent or broken by hand, removed from disposable syringes, or otherwise manipulated by hand.

3. After they are used, disposable syringes and needles, scalpel blades, and other sharp items should be placed in puncture-resistant containers for disposal. The puncture-resistant containers should be located as close as practical to the use area.

4. Large-bore reusable needles should be placed in a puncture-resistant container for transport to the reprocessing area.

SALIVA

Although saliva has not been implicated in HIV transmission, to minimize the need for emergency mouth-to-mouth resuscitation, mouthpieces, resuscitation bags, or other ventilation devices should be available for use in areas in which the need for resuscitation is predictable.

EXUDATE

Health care workers who have exudative lesions or weeping dermatitis should refrain from all direct patient care and from handling patient-care equipment until the condition resolves.

PREGNANCY

1. Pregnant health care workers are not known to be at greater risk of contracting HIV infection than health care workers who are not pregnant.

(continued)

Box 8-1
Precautions to Prevent Transmission of HIV* *(Continued)*

PREGNANCY

2. If a health care worker develops HIV infection during pregnancy, the infant is at risk of infection resulting from perinatal transmission.

3. Because of this risk, pregnant health care workers should be especially familiar with and strictly adhere to precautions to minimize the risk of HIV transmission.

ISOLATION

1. Implementing universal blood and body fluid precautions for *all* patients eliminates need for use of the isolation category of "blood and body fluid precautions" previously recommended by the CDC for patients known or suspected to be infected with blood-borne pathogens.

2. Isolation precautions (e.g., enteric, AFB) should be used as necessary if associated conditions, such as infectious diarrhea or tuberculosis, are diagnosed or suspected.

Precautions for Invasive Procedures

In this document, an invasive procedure is defined as surgical entry into tissues, cavities, or organs, or repair of major traumatic injuries.

1. In an operating or delivery room, emergency department, or outpatient setting, including both physicians' and dentists' offices

2. Cardiac catheterization and angiographic procedures

3. A vaginal or cesarean delivery or other invasive obstetric procedure during which bleeding may occur

4. The manipulation, cutting, or removal of any oral or perioral tissues, including tooth structure, during which bleeding occurs or the potential for bleeding exists

The universal blood and body fluid precautions listed previously, combined with the precautions listed in the following section, should be the minimum precautions for *all* such invasive procedures.

BARRIER PROTECTION

1. All health care workers who participate in invasive procedures must routinely use appropriate barrier precautions to prevent skin and mucous membrane contact with blood and other body fluids of all patients.

2. Gloves and surgical masks must be worn for all invasive procedures.

3. Protective eyewear or face shields should be worn for procedures that commonly result in the generation of droplets, splashing of blood or other body fluids, or the generation of bone chips.

4. Gowns or aprons made of materials that provide an effective barrier should be worn during invasive procedures that are likely to result in the splashing of blood or other body fluids.

5. All health care workers who perform or assist in vaginal or cesarean deliveries should wear gloves and gowns when handling the placenta or the infant until blood and amniotic fluid have been removed from the infant's skin. They should also wear gloves during post-delivery care of the umbilical cord.

6. If a glove is torn or a needle stick or other injury occurs, the glove should be removed and a new glove used as promptly as patient safety permits. The needle or instrument involved in the incident should also be removed from the sterile field.

immunosuppressive drugs, corticosteroids, anticancer agents, and extensive radiation therapy may depress immunologic response and permit the invasion of infection. Therapy may mask infection so that septicemia may be unrecognized until autopsy.[2]

Environmental Factors

Environmental factors that affect the survival and propagation of bacteria in IV fluids are 1) the pH; 2) the temperature; and 3) the presence of essential nutrients in the infusion.

Some organisms grow rapidly in a neutral solution and are less likely to grow in an acid medium. Buffering of acidic dextrose solutions has been recommended for prevention of phlebitis,[10] but at the same time, the neutral environment provided by the buffer may enhance the survival and proliferation of bacteria.

The temperature of the fluid may affect the ability of bacteria to multiply. At room temperatures, strains of *Enterobacter cloacae*, *E. agglomerans*, and other members of the tribe Klebsiellae proliferate rapidly in commercial solutions of 5% dextrose in water.[6,16] Total parenteral nutrition fluids should be used as soon as possible after preparation, and when it becomes necessary to store them temporarily they should be refrigerated at 4°C; at this temperature growth of *Candida albicans* is suppressed.[16]

The presence of certain nutrients is essential to the growth of bacteria. Blood and crystalloid solutions provide nutrients that broaden the spectrum of pathogens capable of proliferation. Maki and associates stated that the administration of blood or reflux of blood into the infusion system may provide sufficient nutrients to broaden this spectrum.[16] The American Association of Blood Banks requires blood to be stored at a constant controlled refrigeration of 1° to 6°C.

Saline solutions are likely to contain enough biologically available carbon, nitrogen, sulfur, and phosphate together with traces of other material to support, under favorable conditions, the survival and multiplication of any gram-negative bacillus introduced to as many as a million organisms per milliliter.[16]

FACTORS CONTRIBUTING TO INFECTION

Faulty Handling

Faulty handling and procedures contribute to contamination. Containers of parenteral fluid are accepted as being sterile and nonpyrogenic on arrival from the manufacturer. The potential risk of contamination occurring in transit or in use is frequently overlooked by hospital personnel. However, through faulty handling or carelessness, glass containers may become cracked or damaged and plastic bags punctured. Bacteria and fungi may penetrate a hairline crack in an IV container, even though the crack is so fine that fluid is not lost from the container.

Intravenous solutions of dextrose, as well as providing carbon and an energy source, include the extra nutrients needed to support the growth of 10 million organisms per milliliter. If the fluid is not examined closely, its opalescence may be overlooked, and subsequent infusion of a few hundred milliliters of such contaminated fluid will result in deep shock or possibly death.[16]

Before use, containers of fluid should be examined, preferably against a light and dark background, for cracks, defects, turbidity, and particulate matter; plastic containers should be squeezed to detect any puncture hole. Accidental puncture may occur without being evident and provide a point of entry for microorganisms.[16] Any container with a crack or defect must be regarded as suspect and not used. Any glass container lacking a vacuum when opened should not be used.

Airborne Contamination

When a 1-liter glass container is opened, approximately 100 mL of air rushes in to replace the vacuum. In areas with a high concentration of airborne particles, contamination of unprotected fluids is a potential risk. The sterile environment of a laminar flow hood prevents this problem.

Outdated Intravenous Solutions

The longer the container is in use, the greater the proliferation of bacteria and the greater the infection should contamination inadvertently occur.[6] The risk of infusing outdated fluids can be avoided by adhering to special limits, supported by a strong monitoring policy. Every container should be labeled with the time it is opened. The guidelines of the Centers for Disease Control and Prevention (CDC) and INS Standards of Practice should be followed.

Admixtures

Allowing untrained hospital personnel to add drugs to IV containers potentially contributes to the risk of contamination. This risk is reduced when admixtures are prepared under laminar flow hoods by trained personnel adhering to strict aseptic technique as provided by a pharmacy additive program. The necessity for nurses and physicians to prepare admixtures in an emergency does arise. All personnel involved in the preparation and administration of IV drugs should receive special training in the preparation of admixtures and the handling of IV fluids and equipment. Adherence to strict aseptic methods is vital. It must be understood that touch contamination is the primary source of infection and that although laminar flow hoods prevent airborne contamination, they do not ensure sterility when a break in aseptic technique occurs.

Manipulation of In-Use Intravenous Equipment

Intravenous fluids can be inadvertently contaminated by faulty techniques in the manipulation of equipment. In open systems, where solutions are not protected by air filters, the simple procedure of hanging the container may be taken for granted and the risk of contamination overlooked. When an administration set is inserted into the container and the container is inverted, the fluid tends to leak out the vent onto the unsterile surface of the container. Regurgitation of the contaminated fluid into the container occurs when the container vents. Instructions in the use of the equipment often go unread and unheeded. Squeezing the drip chamber of the administration set before inserting it into the container and releasing it when the container is inverted will prevent regurgitation of fluid and minimize the risk of contamination.

Injection Ports

Meticulous aseptic technique must be observed in the use of injection ports because they are a potential source of contamination when used to piggyback infusions. The injection port location, at the distal end of the tubing, exposes it to patient excreta and drainage, which enhance the growth of microorganisms and contribute to contamination. The injection port must be *scrubbed* at least 1 minute with an accepted antiseptic; 70% isopropyl alcohol is commonly used. Scrubbing the injection cap for 30 seconds with an antimicrobial (povidone-iodine) solution provides good protection. The needle should be firmly engaged up to the hub in the injection site and securely taped to prevent an in-and-out motion of the needle from introducing bacteria into the infusion. The use of needleless systems minimizes risk (see Chapter 10).

Three-Way Stopcocks

Three-way stopcocks are potential mechanisms for transmission of bacteria to the host because their ports, unprotected by sterile covering, are open to moisture and contaminants. Connected to central venous catheters and arterial lines, they are frequently used for drawing blood samples. Aseptic practices are vital in preventing the introduction of bacteria into the line. A sterile catheter plug attached at the time the stopcock is added and changed after each use will reduce the risk of contamination. Whenever fluid leakage is discovered at injection sites, connections, or vents, the IV set should be replaced.

Cannula-Associated Infection

Following insertion of a plastic cannula into a vessel, a loosely formed fibrin sheath forms around the intravascular portion of the device within 24 to 48 hours (Fig. 8-2), forming a nidus within which microorganisms can multiply and that shields them to an extent from host defenses and antibiotics. Thrombogenesis of cannula materials may play a role in vulnerability to cannula-related infections. Again, careful adherence to policies and procedures, based on INS standards, with respect to site rotation and indwell time, may reduce the inherent problems of cannula-associated infection.

Most device-related septicemias are actually caused by the patient's own skin flora or by microorganisms transmitted from the hands of the health care professional.

Antibiotic Lock Technique

The antibiotic lock technique has met with favorable response from the health care community as a means to lessen the potential for central venous cannula-related infection in the immunocompromised patient. Vancomycin, amphotericin B, and fluconazole have all been successfully used as flush solutions. A small amount of concentrated antibiotic/antifungal agent is instilled within the catheter and capped (Table 8-2).

Skin Preparation

Microbes on the hands of health care personnel contribute to hospital-associated infection. Too often breaks in sterile technique occur from failure to wash the hands before changing containers or sets or preparing admixtures. Besides the usual skin

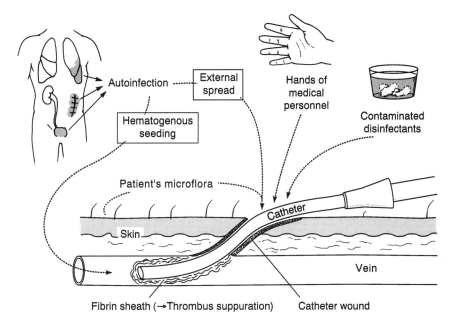

FIGURE 8-2 Sources of vascular cannula-related infection. (Modified from Maki, D. G. [1976]. In I. Phillips, P. D. Meers, & P. F. D'Arcy [Eds.]. *Microbiological hazards of infusion therapy* [p. 106]. Lancaster, England: MTP Press.)

flora, antibiotic-resistant gram-negative organisms frequently contaminate the hands of hospital personnel.[16]

To maintain asepsis, the CDC recommends that the hands be thoroughly washed for insertion of central venous catheters.[5] OSHA guidelines support the use of sterile gloves.

Adequate and reliable preparation of the patient's skin and maintenance of asepsis are imperative when a catheter is used for IV therapy. The skin, the first defense barrier of the body, is broken, providing a vulnerable port for the migration of bacteria. Skin flora has been implicated as a source of contamination of catheters. In a study made of 118 patients receiving IV therapy through an indwelling polyvinyl catheter, 53 catheters were found to be contaminated with bacteria; in 28 of these,

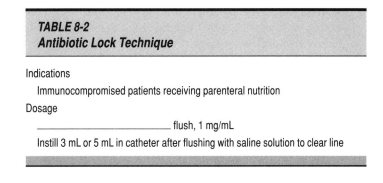

TABLE 8-2
Antibiotic Lock Technique

Indications

Immunocompromised patients receiving parenteral nutrition

Dosage

_____ flush, 1 mg/mL

Instill 3 mL or 5 mL in catheter after flushing with saline solution to clear line the organisms were comparable to those cultured from the skin of the patient before the skin was cleaned with iodine.[3]

Frequently the question arises of whether to shave the skin. The need to remove the hair is not substantiated by scientific evidence; antiseptics used to clean the skin also clean the hair. Shaving may produce microabrasions, which enhance the proliferation of bacteria.[16]

Alcohol 70% frequently is used to prepare the skin site for venipuncture. Studies show that ethyl alcohol, 70% by weight, is an effective germicide for the skin when *applied with friction for 1 minute*; INS standards support its use. It is as effective as 12 minutes of scrubbing and reduces the bacterial count by 75%.[23] Because a minimum of 10,000 organisms/cm^2 is present on normal skin, the count would be reduced to 2500. Too frequently the use of alcohol consists of a quick wipe, which fails to reduce the bacterial count significantly.

Iodine and iodine-containing disinfectants are still the most reliable agents for preparing the skin for venipuncture because they provide bactericidal, fungicidal, and sporicidal activity. Because of occasional patient allergy to iodine, the possibility of sensitivity should be investigated before its use. Tincture of iodine (2% iodine in 70% alcohol) is inexpensive and well tolerated. Solution should be liberally applied, allowed to dry for at least 30 seconds, and washed off with 70% alcohol. Both agents should be applied with friction, working from the center of the field to periphery.[9,16] Iodophor preparations, when used for patients with sensitive skin, should not be washed off because the sustained release of free iodine may be necessary for germicidal action. Iodophor preparations require 30-second contact time.

Quaternary ammonium compounds such as aqueous benzalkonium chloride are inactivated by organic debris, are ineffective against gram-negative organisms, and should not be used for skin disinfection.[16]

The tourniquet itself may be a source of cross-infection and contamination because it is used repeatedly from patient to patient and handled just before venipuncture. This possibility should be kept in mind and the tourniquet disinfected periodically; consideration should be given to the use of start-kits.

Once the venipuncture is completed and it is within the lumen of the vein, the cannula must be securely anchored; to-and-fro motion of the catheter in the puncture wound may irritate the intima of the vein and introduce cutaneous bacteria. Thought should be given to the possible contamination of the adhesive tape used to secure the cannula. Rolls of tape last indefinitely and may be a source of contamination; they are transported from room to room, placed on patients' beds and tables, and frequently roll to the floor. Furthermore, before venipuncture, strips of tape often are torn off the roll and placed in convenient locations on the bed, table, and uniform. These facts should be kept in mind. Adhesive tape should not be applied over the puncture wound. The puncture wound must be considered an open wound and asepsis must be maintained.

CARE OF THE VENOUS ACCESS DEVICE

The CDC recommends the use of a topical antibiotic or antiseptic ointment at the IV site after cannula insertion. The wound should be protected by a sterile dressing. Dressing change should be consistent with INS standards. The same applies to catheter site rotations. Frequent observations should be made for signs of malfunction of the cannula, infiltration, and phlebitis characterized by erythema, induration, or tenderness. Such signs require immediate removal of the cannula. Fuchs has noted that the major factor influencing the frequency of catheter colonization is the presence of other catheter complications such as subcutaneous infiltration and phlebitis.[9,10] He defined *colonization* as positive culture of the catheter tip without evidence of local or systemic infection.

Irrigation of a plugged catheter may embolize small catheter thrombi, some of which are infected. Contamination of the catheter may result from a break in aseptic technique, from contaminated fluid or set, from bacterial invasion of the puncture wound, or from clinically undetected bacteremia arising from an infection in a remote area of the body, such as a tracheostomy, the urinary tract, or a surgical wound. The clot around or in the catheter serves as an excellent trap for circulatory microorganisms and as a nutrient for bacterial proliferation.[21]

INTRAVENOUS-ASSOCIATED INFECTIONS

Intravenous-associated sepsis is not always accompanied by phlebitis. Symptoms of infection consist of chills and fever, gastric symptoms, headache, hyperventilation, and shock. Should infection develop from an unknown source in a patient receiving IV therapy, the IV system should be suspected and the entire system, including the cannula, removed. The catheter and the infusion fluid should be cultured.

The following procedure should be used for culturing the catheter.[9]

1. Cleanse the skin about the cannula site with alcohol, allowing the alcohol to dry before removing the cannula.
2. Maintaining asepsis, remove the catheter and with sterile scissors snip 1 cm of the catheter tip into blood culture or other appropriate culture medium.

The following procedure should be used for culturing the infusion fluid.[11]

1. Aseptically withdraw 20 mL fluid from the IV line: 1 mL is used to prepare a pour plate; the remaining fluid is used to inoculate two blood culture containers.
2. Add to the remaining IV fluid in the container an equal volume of brain–heart infusion broth enriched with 0.5% beef extract. Inoculate at 37°C; this is a more sensitive culture for detecting low-level contamination.

All containers of fluid previously administered to the patient should be suspected and, if possible, retained and cultured. All information and identification, including the lot number of the suspected solution, should be recorded on the culture requisition and the patient chart. The United States Food and Drug Administration, the CDC, and the local health authorities should be notified if contamination during manufacturing is suspected; fluids bearing implicated lot numbers should be stored for investigation.

PARTICULATE MATTER

Particulate matter is defined as the mobile, undissolved substances unintentionally present in parenteral fluids. Such foreign matter may consist of rubber, glass, cotton fibers, drug particles, molds, metal, or paper fibers.

Vascular Route of Infused Particles

The pulmonary vascular bed acts as a filter for infused particles. Particles introduced into the vein travel to the right atrium of the heart, down through the tricuspid valve, and into the right ventricle. From there they are pumped into the pulmonary artery and on through branches of arteries that decrease in size until the particles are trapped in the massive capillary bed in the lungs, where the capillaries measure 7 to 12 µm in diameter.

Five microns, the size of an erythrocyte suspended in fluid, has been suggested as the largest allowable size for a particle in the pulmonary capillary bed. Particles larger than 5 µm are recognized as potentially dangerous because they are likely to become lodged. Particles as large as 300 µm can pass through an 18-gauge cannula, and much larger particles may pass through an indwelling catheter with a larger lumen. Table 8-3 lists particle size comparisons. If occlusion of a small arteriole inhibits oxygenation or normal metabolic activities, cellular damage or tissue death may result. Where there is ample collateral circulation, the occlusion would have no appreciable biologic effect. However, a particle that is not biologically inert may incite an inflammatory reaction, a neoplastic response, or an antigenic, sensitizing response.[14,16]

Particles may gain access to the systemic circulation, where occlusion of a small arteriole in the brain, kidney, or eye can be serious, in one of the following ways:

TABLE 8-3
Particle Size Comparisons

Microns		Inches
175	=	.007
150	=	.006
125	=	.005
100	=	.004
75	=	.003
50	=	.002
25	=	.001

Source: Contamination Control Laboratories. *Particle Size Comparisons* (information circular). Livonia, MI, 1970.

Note: One micron equals 40 millionths of an inch (approx.). A human hair is approximately 125 µm in thickness. Bacteria range in size from 0.3 to 0.5 µm. We cannot see a particle or hole smaller than 20 µm. A hole 25 µm in diameter in a HEPA filter is more than 75 times larger than the contaminants and bacteria passing through.

1. The pulmonary vascular bed does not filter out all particles. Prinzmetal and associates demonstrated that glass beads up to 390 µm may pass through the pulmonary capillary bed and reach the systemic circulation.[14,16]

2. Large arteriovenous shunts exist in the human lung.[12,14,16] Particles bypass the pulmonary capillary bed and enter the systemic circulation, where a systemic occlusion could be serious.

3. Particles larger than 5 µm may reach the systemic circulation by interarterial injection or infusion.

Sources of Contamination

The United States Pharmacopeia has established an acceptable limit of particles for single-dose infusion as not more than 50 particles/mL that are equal to or larger than 10.0 µm, and not more than 5 particles/mL that are equal to or larger than 25.0 µm in effective linear dimension (see Chapter 10.) Great efforts are being made by manufacturers to produce high-quality IV injections. Their efforts are defeated by numerous manipulations before final infusion.

Medication Additives

Drugs constitute a major source of contamination. Improper technique in the preparation of drugs results in the formation of insoluble particles. An IV additive service is recommended.

Glass Ampules

Glass ampules may be responsible for the injection of thousands of glass particles into the circulation. Turco and Davis, in a study prompted by the frequency of high-dose administration of furosemide, showed that a dose of 400 mg, which at that time required the breaking of 20 ampules, could add 1085 glass particles larger than 5 µm to the injection. A dose of 600 mg, requiring 30 ampules, could result in 2387 particles larger than 5 µm.

Antibiotic Injectables

Particulate contamination levels of bulk-filled antibiotics may be 2 to 10 times greater than those of stable antibiotic solutions and lyophilized antibiotics. Filtration is impossible because packaging by the sterile bulk-fill method involves extracting and processing the antibiotic in sterile bulk powder form and then aseptically placing the bulk antibiotic into dry presterilized vials. In the lyophilized and the stable liquid packaging processes, the particulate matter can be terminally removed by filtration directly into presterilized vials. The majority of the antibiotics are packed by the bulk-fill method.

Particulate matter in IV injections may be responsible for much of the phlebitis that so often occurs with the infusion of these drugs. Russell listed the major pathologic conditions caused by particulate matter as 1) direct blockage of vessels; 2) platelet agglutination leading to formation of emboli; 3) local inflammation caused by impaction of particles; and 4) antigenic reactions with subsequent allergic consequence.[19]

Intravenous Fluids

Walter noted that critically ill patients who had received large amounts of IV fluid died of pulmonary insufficiency characterized by increased venous pressure and pulmonary hypertension. He observed that the lungs looked like leather and speculated that the cause of death might be the result of accumulated matter from the many liters of infused fluids.[22]

Reducing the Level of Contamination

Because particulate matter infused through IV fluids may produce pathologic changes that can have an adverse effect on critically ill patients, every effort must be made to reduce the particulate count in IV injections. Nurses and doctors in general have been unaware of the potential dangers that exist and have unknowingly added to the contamination. Official agencies have developed standards for an acceptable limit for particles in IV fluids. Industry has provided the medical profession with filters to limit direct access of bacteria, fungi, and particulate matter to the bloodstream.

Filters

A filter aspiration needle specially designed to remove particulate matter from IV medicaments is available. With this device attached to a syringe, the medication is drawn from the vial or glass ampule, filtering out the particles. The filter needle must then be discarded to prevent the particles trapped on the filter from being injected when the medication is added to the IV fluid.

Final Filters

The National Coordinating Committee on Large Volume Parenterals has recommended the in-line filter that is both particulate and microbe retentive for the following: hyperalimentation patients and immunodeficient or immunocompromised patients. The particulate-retentive IV filter is generally recommended for patients receiving IV infusions with many additives, when drugs requiring constitution are known to be heavily particulated, or to minimize particulate matter in infusions to which additives have been introduced.

The INS policy advocates the routine use of 0.2-μm air-eliminating filters in delivering routine IV therapy because these filters remove particulates, bacteria, and air, and some remove endotoxins as well.[9]

Filters are manufactured in a variety of forms, sizes, and materials. Some block the passage of air under normal pressure when wet. Used in conjunction with electronic infusion devices, they play an important role in preventing air from being pumped into the bloodstream should the fluid container become empty.

A knowledge of filter characteristics, use, and proper handling is important for patient safety. Faulty handling can cause plugging of the filter, resulting in the patient not receiving prescribed fluids and the necessity of performing a venipuncture to insert a new line. A ruptured filter may go undetected and introduce filter fragments, bacteria, and possibly air into the IV system. A thorough discussion of IV filtration and its benefits may be found in Chapter 10.

CULTURING

Culture Profile

The process of culturing identifies the presence of microorganisms in suspected IV infections. Prior to removing a cannula for culture, the surrounding skin should be cleansed with 70% isopropyl alcohol and allowed to air dry. If purulent drainage is present, a culture of the drainage should be taken prior to cleansing the skin.

When line sepsis is suspected, three blood cultures should be drawn, ideally from separate venipuncture sites. Deep candidal sepsis—systemic candidiasis—is often associated with negative blood cultures. It is common practice in a number of clinical settings to develop a culture profile for the patient with suspected sepsis and to routinely culture, in intensive care units, blood of patients receiving multiple infusion therapies. Quantitative blood cultures, using pour plates, provide an excellent method for diagnosis of catheter-related infection.

Semiquantitative Technique for Culturing Cannulas

Before removing a cannula, the skin around the insertion site is cleansed with an alcohol-impregnated pad to reduce contaminating skin flora and to remove any residual antibiotic ointment. After drying, the cannula is withdrawn, taking care to avoid contact with the surrounding skin. If pus can be expressed from the cannula wound, it is Gram stained and cultured separately. For short indwelling catheters, the entire length of the cannula is cut from the skin-catheter junction (Fig. 8-3) using sterile scissors. With longer catheters, a 2-inch segment is cultured: the tip and the intracutaneous segment. Segments are cultured as soon as possible following removal and within 2 hours. In the laboratory, the segment is rolled back and forth across the surface of a 100-mm 5% blood agar plate four times. Plates are then incubated aerobi-

FIGURE 8-3 Segments of vascular cannulas cultured semiquantitatively. (From Maki, D. G., et al. [1977]. *Journal of Surgical Research, 22,* 513. Reprinted with permission of D. G. Maki and Little, Brown & Co. © 1986.)

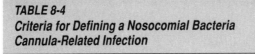

TABLE 8-4
Criteria for Defining a Nosocomial Bacteria Cannula-Related Infection

- Isolation of the same species in significant numbers on semiquantitative culture of the cannula and from blood cultures obtained by separate venipunctures with negative culture of infusate
- Clinical and microbiologic data disclosing no other apparent source of septicemia
- Clinical features consistent with bloodstream infection

cally at 37°C for at least 72 hours. This technique has outstanding sensitivity and specificity in the diagnosis of cannula-related infections. Table 8-4 lists criteria for defining a nosocomial bacteremia as cannula related.

PRACTICE SETTING

The practice setting in which care is delivered has no relevance to the level of diligence needed to provide quality infusion therapy. This theory is based on the fact that the patient is accustomed to the flora in his own environment. In any clinical environment, principles of asepsis must be adhered to in an effort to minimize the risk of IV catheter-related infection and to ensure a high level of IV patient care.

REFERENCES

1. Adriani, J. (1962). Venipuncture. *American Journal of Nursing 62,* 66–70.
2. Altemeier, W. A., Todd, J. C., & Inge, W. W. (1967). Gram-negative septicemia: A growing threat. *Annals of Surgery, 166,* 530–542.
3. Banks, D. C., Cawdreys, H. M., Yates, D. B., & Harries, M. G. (1970). *Lancet 1,* 443.
4. Bennett, J. V., & Brachman, P. S. (1986). *Hospital infections* (2nd ed., pp. 562, 563, 567–569). Boston: Little, Brown.
5. Centers for Disease Control. (1982). Guidelines for prevention of intravascular infection. *Journal of the National Intravenous Therapy Association, 5*(1), 39–50.
6. Centers for Disease Control. (1971). Nosocomial bacteremias associated with intravenous fluid therapy. *Morbidity and Mortality Weekly Report, 20*(Special Suppl.), no. 9.
7. Druskin, M. S., & Siegel, P. D. (1963). Bacterial contamination of indwelling intravenous polyethylene catheters. *Journal of the American Medical Association, 185,* 966–968.
8. Felts, S. K., Shaffner, W., Melly, M. A., & Koenig, M. G. (1972). Sepsis caused by contaminated intravenous fluids: Epidemiological clinical and laboratory investigation of an outbreak in one hospital. *Annals of Internal Medicine, 77,* 881.
9. *Revised intravenous nursing standards of practice.* (1990). *Journal of Intravenous Nursing* (suppl.), S42, S43.
10. Fonkalsrud, E. W., Pederson, B. M., Murphy, J., & Beckerman, J. H. (1968). Reduction of infusion thrombophlebitis with buffered glucose solutions. *Surgery, 63,* 280–284.
11. Hickan, J. B., & Sieker, H. O. (1959). Pulmonary embolism and infarction. *Disease-A-Month,* January.
12. Hirshfield, J. W. (1941). Bacterial contamination of wounds from the air, from the skin of the operator, and from the skin of the patient. *Surgery, Gynecology and Obstetrics, 73,* 72–78.
13. Lillehei, R. C., Dietzman, R., Moras, S., & Block, J. H. (1967). Treatment of septic shock. *Modern Treatment, 4*(2), 342–346.

14. McGaw Laboratories. (1969). *McGaw technical information bulletin #16.* Glendale, CA.
15. McNair, T. J., & Dudley, H. A. F. (1959). The local complications of intravenous therapy. *Lancet, 2,* 365–368.
16. Maki, D. G., Goldman, D. A., & Rhama, F. S. (1973). Infection control in intravenous therapy. *Annals of Internal Medicine, 79,* 869, 870, 872, 875, 876, 878, 880.
17. Metheny, N. M. (1992). *Fluid and electrolyte balance* (2nd ed., pp. 164–165). Philadelphia: J. B. Lippincott.
18. Motsay, G. J., Dietzman, R. H., Ersek, R. A., & Lillehei, R. C. (1970). Hemodynamic alterations and results of treatment in patients with gram-negative septic shock. *Surgery 67,* 577–583.
19. Russell, J. H. (1970). Pharmaceutical application of filtration, part 2. *American Journal of Hospital Pharmacy, 28,* 125–126.
20. Tarail, R. (1950). Practice of fluid therapy. *Journal of the American Medical Association, 171,* 45–49.
21. Tropp, J. [Speaker]. (1992). Central venous thrombosis. Audiotape of presentation to Annual Meeting of Intravenous Nurses Society, May, 1992. Alexandria, VA: Audio Transcripts Ltd., 40–729-92.
22. Walter, C. W. (1967). *FDA Symposium on Safety of Large Volume Parenteral Solutions.* Washington, DC: U.S. Government Printing Office.
23. Walter, C. W. (1956). *The aseptic treatment of wounds.* New York: Macmillan.

BIBLIOGRAPHY

Bivins, B. A., Rapp, R. P., Deluca, P. P., McKean, H., & Ward, O. G., Jr. (1979). Fluid inline filtration: A means of decreasing the incidence of infusion phlebitis. *Surgery, 85*(4), 388–394.

Buxton, A. E., Highsmith, A. K., Garner, J. S., West, C. M., Stamm, W. E., Dixon, R. E., & McGowan, J. E. (1979). Contamination of intravenous infusion fluid: Effects of changing administration sets. *Annals of Internal Medicine, 90,* 764–768.

Contamination Control Laboratories. (1970). *Particle size comparisons* [information circular]. Livonia, MI.

Crossley, K., & Matsen, J. M. (1972). The scalp-vein needle: A prospective study of complications. *Journal of the American Medical Association, 220,* 985.

Davis, N. M., & Turco, S. (1971). A study of particulate matter in I.V. infusion fluids—phase 2. *American Journal of Hospital Pharmacy, 28,* 620–623.

Dudrick, S. J. (1974). Article in *Hospital Tribune.* University and Hospital Edition of *Medical Tribune and Medical News, 8*(3), 1.

Jemison-Smith, P. (1984). Understanding the acquired immune deficiency syndrome. *Journal of the National Intravenous Therapy Association, 7*(2), 115.

Moseley, R. V., & Doty, D. B. (1970). Death associated with multiple pulmonary emboli soon after battle. *Annals of Surgery, 171,* 336.

National Coordinating Committee on Large Volume Parenterals. (1976, March). Recommendations to pharmacists for solving problems with large volume parenterals. *American Journal of Hospital Pharmacy, 33,* 231–236.

Thomas, E. T., Evers, W., & Racz, C. B. (1970). Post infusion phlebitis. *Anesthesia and Analgesia, 49,* 150–159.

REVIEW QUESTIONS

1. Thrombophlebitis involves what two injuries to the vein?
   a. inflammation
   b. irritation
   c. thrombosis
   d. infection

2. Factors that may contribute to thrombophlebitis include which of the following?
   a. viscosity of solution
   b. pH of solution
   c. type of cannula
   d. all of the above

3. To prevent septicemia, which of the following precautions are needed?
   a. Examine solutions carefully.
   b. Observe maximum hang time.
   c. Mix solutions at bedside.
   d. Mix solutions in laminar flow.

4. In the event of a suspected air embolism, the appropriate nursing intervention is to:
   a. turn patient on left side, head down
   b. turn patient on right side, head down
   c. turn patient on left side, head raised
   d. turn patient on right side, head raised

5. To prevent the incidence of pulmonary edema, it is necessary to do which of the following?
   a. Maintain prescribed rate of flow.
   b. Avoid positive pressure.
   c. Administer total volume within 24-hour time frame.
   d. Avoid negative pressure.

6. To minimize the danger of speed shock, it is necessary to:
   a. control volume
   b. avoid free flow
   c. catch up all solutions
   d. use positive pressure

7. Symptoms of air embolism include which of the following?
   a. cyanosis
   b. drop in blood pressure
   c. weak, rapid pulse
   d. drop in venous pressure

8. Primary sources of bacteria responsible for IV-associated infections include all EXCEPT:
   a. air
   b. skin
   c. blood
   d. mucous membrane

9. Extrinsic contamination may occur in all of the following areas EXCEPT:
   a. administration sets
   b. additive ports
   c. manufacturing process
   d. cannulas

10. The use of iodophor preparations for skin prep before venipuncture is based on what theory?
    a. disinfectant quality
    b. release of free iodine
    c. presence of skin germs
    d. prevention of cross-infection

CHAPTER 9

Laboratory Tests

Key Terms

Arterial	Collection	Liver function
Blood urea nitrogen	International unit	Venous
Cannula	Kidney function	

In the past, IV departments included the collection of venous blood samples as one of their functions. Although collection of venous blood now is usually delegated to a team of laboratory phlebotomists or technologists, in many instances the IV nurse will be involved:

- In critical care units
- When veins have become exhausted
- When the patient is to receive an IV infusion
- When the specimen is to be obtained from a central venous cannula that is to be removed, from a multilumen central venous cannula, from a Hickman-Broviac catheter, or from an implanted vascular access device

Definite advantages are gained when this nurse is involved in collecting venous blood.[1] The nurse, understanding the importance of the preservation of veins for infusion therapy, is cautious when choosing veins and in applying blood-drawing techniques.[2] Frequently, one venipuncture permits both the withdrawal of blood and the initiation of the infusion, thereby preserving veins, reducing discomfort, and avoiding undue distress of the patient.[3] The patient–blood identification is of paramount importance in preventing the error of infusing incompatible blood. Because the department assumes responsibility for patient–blood identification in administering blood and is aware of existing hazards, its personnel are well qualified and trained in the collection of samples for typing and crossmatching.

The nurse in any clinical setting is often faced with the problem of collecting blood with little or no knowledge of the tests to be performed other than the amount of blood needed and the type of tube required. This chapter is intended primarily to provide the nurse with information concerning the most commonly performed laboratory tests—their purpose and normal values—and the collection and proper handling of the specimens. No attempt is made to explain laboratory procedures.

VENOUS SAMPLING

Collection of Blood

The collection of blood samples for certain tests must meet special requirements. Some tests call for whole blood, whereas others require components such as plasma, serum, or cells. The proper requirements must be met to prevent erroneous or misleading laboratory analysis.

Serum consists of plasma minus fibrinogen and is obtained by drawing blood in a dry tube and allowing it to coagulate. Serum is required by the majority of laboratory tests in common use.

Plasma consists of the stable components of blood minus the cells and is obtained by using an anticoagulant to prevent the blood from clotting. Several anticoagulants are available in color-coded tubes. Choice of the anticoagulant depends on the test to be performed. Most of the anticoagulants, including sodium or potassium oxalate, citrate, and ethylenediaminetetraacetic acid (EDTA), prevent coagulation by binding the serum calcium. Other anticoagulants, such as heparin, are valuable in specific tests but are not commonly used. Heparin prevents coagulation for only limited periods of time.

Whole blood is required for many tests, including blood counts and bleeding time. Potassium oxalate is commonly used to preserve whole blood.

Hemoconcentration through venous stasis should be avoided or inaccurate results will occur in some tests. Hemoconcentration increases proportionally with the length of time the tourniquet is applied. Once the venipuncture has been made, the tourniquet should be removed. This is a simple but important precaution, ignored by many. Carbon dioxide and pH are examples of tests affected by hemoconcentration. If the tourniquet is required to withdraw the blood, it should be noted on the requisition that the blood was drawn with stasis.

Hemolysis causes serious errors in many tests in which lysis of the red blood cells (RBCs) permits the substance being measured to escape into the serum. When erythrocytes rich in potassium rupture, the serum potassium level rises, giving a false measurement. To avoid hemolysis, the following special precautions should be observed:

1. Dry syringes and dry tubes must be used.

2. Excess pressure on the plunger of the syringe should be avoided; such pressure collapses the vein and may cause air bubbles to be sucked from around the hub of the needle into the blood.

3. Clotted blood specimens should not be shaken unnecessarily.

4. Force should be avoided in transferring blood to a container or tube; force of the blood against the tube results in rupture of the cells. In transferring blood to a vacuum tube, no needle larger than 20 gauge should be used.

Intravenous Solutions

Intravenous solutions may contribute to misleading laboratory interpretations. Blood samples should never be drawn proximal to an infusion but preferably from the contralateral extremity. If the solution contains a substance that may affect the analysis, an indication of its presence should be made on the requisition—for example, potassium determination during an infusion of electrolyte solution.

Special Handling

Special handling is required with some samples when a delay is unavoidable. Some determinations, such as the pH, must be done within 10 minutes after the blood is drawn. When a delay is inevitable, the sample is placed in ice, which partially inhibits *glycolysis*, the production of lactic acid by the glycolytic enzymes of the blood cells, resulting in a rapid lowering of pH on standing.

Blood gases also require special handling and must be analyzed as soon as blood is collected. When the carbon dioxide content of serum is to be determined, the blood must completely fill the tube or carbon dioxide will escape. Several procedures are currently in use; in each, the escape of carbon dioxide must be prevented.

Fasting

Because absorption of food may alter the blood, test results often depend on the patient's fasting. Blood glucose and serum lipid levels are increased by ingestion of food. Serum inorganic phosphorous values are depressed after meals.

Promptness of Examination

Immediate dispatch of blood samples to the laboratory is vital to the accurate determination of some blood tests; promptness in examining blood samples is necessary in the analysis of labile constituents of blood. In certain tests, such as potassium, the substance being measured diffuses out of the cells into the serum being examined and gives a false measurement. To prevent this rise in serum concentration, the cells must be separated from the serum promptly.

Infected Samples

Special caution must be observed in the care of all blood specimens because blood from all patients is to be considered infective. Specimens should not be allowed to spill on the outside of the containers. Contaminated material should be placed in bags and treated according to institutional policies for disposal of infectious material. Cannulas should not be recapped or broken but disposed of intact in cannula-proof containers. All personnel handling blood should wear gloves.

Emergency Tests

Blood tests ordered as emergencies must be sent directly to the laboratory. Red cellophane tape or other alert-type stickers, according to facility preference, may be used to indicate a state of emergency. Tests most likely to be designated as emergencies include amylase, blood urea nitrogen (BUN), carbon dioxide, potassium, prothrombin, sodium, sugar, and blood typing.

THE VACUUM SYSTEM

The vacuum system has increased the efficiency of the process. It consists of a plastic holder into which screws a sterile disposable double-ended needle. A rubber-stoppered vacuum tube slips into the barrel. The barrel has a measured line denoting the distance the tube is inserted into the barrel; at this point the needle becomes embedded in the stopper. The stopper is not punctured until the needle has been introduced into the vein.

After entry into the vein, the rubber-stoppered tube is pushed the remaining distance into the barrel. As the needle is pushed into the vacuum tube, a rubber sheath covering the shaft is forced back, allowing the blood to flow. The tourniquet is released and several specimens may be obtained by simply removing the tube containing the sample and replacing it with another tube. As the tube is removed, the rubber sheath slips back over the needle, preventing blood from dripping into the holder.

If the vein is not located, removing the tube before the needle is withdrawn will preserve the vacuum in the tube.

At times it becomes necessary to draw blood from small veins. If suction from the vacuum tube collapses the vein, difficulty will be encountered in drawing the blood. By pressing the finger against the vein beyond the point of the needle or by placing the bevel of the needle lightly against the wall of the vein, suction is reduced and the vein allowed to fill. In the latter process, particular caution should be exercised to prevent injury to the endothelial lining of the vein. The pressure is intermittently applied and released, filling and emptying the vein. A small-gauge winged infusion needle with vacuum adapter may also be used; the smaller needle reduces the amount of suction and may prevent collapse of the vein. A syringe is often used to draw blood from small veins because the amount of suction can be more easily controlled.

PERIPHERAL VENIPUNCTURES

A venipuncture, when skillfully executed, causes the patient little discomfort. The numerous blood determinations necessary for diagnosis and treatment make good technique imperative.

The one-step entry technique should be avoided because too often it results in through-and-through punctures, contributing to hematoma formation. The needle should be inserted under the skin and then, after relocation of the vein, into the vessel.

The veins most commonly used are those in the antecubital fossa. The median antecubital vein, though not always visible, is usually large and palpable. Because it is well supported by subcutaneous tissue and least likely to roll, it is often the best choice for venipuncture. Second choice is the cephalic vein. The basilic vein, though often the most prominent, is likely to be the least desirable. This vein rolls easily, making the venipuncture difficult, and a hematoma may readily occur if the patient is allowed to flex the arm, which squeezes the blood from the engorged vein into the tissues.

Sufficient time should be spent in locating the vein before attempting venipuncture. Whenever the veins are difficult to see or palpate, the patient should lie down. If the patient is seated, the arm should be well supported on a pillow.

Complications

Hematomas

Hematomas are the most common complication of routine venipuncture for withdrawing blood, and they contribute more to the limitation of available veins than any other complication. They may result from through-and-through puncture to the vein or from incomplete insertion of the needle into the lumen of the vein, which allows the blood to leak into the tissues through the bevel of the needle. In the latter case, correction may be made by advancing the needle into the vein. At the first sign of uncontrolled bleeding, the tourniquet should be released and the needle withdrawn.

Hematomas also result from the application of the tourniquet after an unsuccessful attempt has been made to draw blood. The tourniquet should never be applied to the extremity immediately after a venipuncture.

Hematomas most frequently result from insufficient time spent in applying pressure and from the bad habit of flexing the arm to stop the bleeding. Once the venipuncture is completed, the patient should be instructed to elevate the arm; elevation causes a negative pressure in the vein, collapsing it and facilitating clotting. With cardiac patients, elevation of the arm should be avoided. Constant pressure is maintained until the bleeding has stopped. Pressure is applied with a dry sterile sponge; a wet sponge encourages bleeding. Band-Aids do not take the place of pressure and, if ordered, are not applied until the bleeding has stopped. Ecchymoses on the arm indicate poor technique or haphazard manner.

Bloodborne Disease

Special caution must be exercised in the care of needles used to draw blood from patients suspected of harboring microorganisms. Contaminated needles should be placed immediately in a separate container for disposal. A vacuum tube with stopper provides adequate protection against accidental puncture from the contaminated needle until proper disposal can be made. Any needle puncture should be reported at once.

Other Complications

Other complications of venipuncture include syncope, continued bleeding, and thrombosis of the vein.

Syncope is rarely encountered when the clinician is confident and skillful and reassures the patient.

Continued bleeding is a complication that may affect the patient receiving anticoagulants, the patient with a blood dyscrasia, or the oncology patient undergoing chemotherapy. To prevent bleeding and to preserve the vein, pressure to the site may be required for an extended period. The nurse should remain with the patient until the bleeding has stopped.

Thrombosis in routine venipuncture occurs from injury to the endothelial lining of the vein during the venipuncture. Antecubital veins may be used indefinitely if the clinician uses good technique.

CENTRAL VENIPUNCTURES

Occasionally it is desirable to draw blood samples through the central venous catheter. Such occasions include difficulty in obtaining an adequate vein, cases in which the avoidance of stress is imperative, and situations in which blood tests are ordered frequently and repeatedly.

Aseptic technique is vital in preventing the introduction of bacteria into the catheter. A sterile IV catheter cap reduces the risk of bacterial invasion.

Procedure

Follow this procedure in drawing blood by way of the central venous catheter from a patient not on drug therapy:

1. Put on gloves. Clamp off the infusion.
2. Remove catheter plug and, with a sterile syringe, withdraw 4 mL blood; discard it.
3. Using a sterile syringe, withdraw the required amount of blood. If difficulty is encountered in drawing blood samples, raise patient's arm to shoulder level or higher to reduce axillary pressure on catheter.
4. Recap stopcock with a sterile plug.
5. Open clamp and flush catheter with about 5 mL infusion fluid to maintain catheter patency.
6. Adjust flow to prescribed flow rate. After contact with patient, remove gloves and wash hands.

If the patient is receiving drug therapy, follow the same procedure, except *use a hemostat* to stop the infusion temporarily; after the blood is drawn, the control clamp maintains the prescribed rate of flow without readjustment. *Note*: Only a jawless clamp should be used on a Silastic tunneled catheter.

Precaution

Patients receiving vasopressors may not tolerate an interruption of medication. Check with the charge nurse before stopping the infusion; extra caution may be required.

INITIATING AN INFUSION

Drawing blood samples and initiating an infusion can be efficiently accomplished by a single venipuncture in the following way:

1. Put on gloves. Fill IV set with solution.
2. Regulate the flow to a minimum rate.
3. Clamp tubing manually by kinking between third and little fingers.
4. Hold adapter between the forefinger and second finger, leaving the hand free for holding the syringe and cannula and collecting blood.
5. Draw blood.

6. Remove syringe; attach the infusion set to the cannula, releasing little finger; solution will flow at the previously adjusted rate.

7. Secure cannula with a piece of tape.

8. Attach syringe to needle, previously imbedded in stopper of vacuum tube, and transfer blood. Vacuum will cause tube to fill—never apply force. Use needle no larger than 20 gauge; lysis of cells can occur.

9. Remove gloves and wash hands.

COMMON LABORATORY TESTS

Laboratory tests are performed for several reasons:

- To indicate relatively common disorders
- To make a diagnosis
- To follow the course of a disease
- To regulate therapy

Standard laboratory values are listed in Table 9-1; examples of conversions of those values to Système International (SI) units are given in Table 9-2.

Blood Cultures

In cases of suspected bacteremia, blood cultures are performed to identify the causative microorganisms. Isolation of the organism is necessary to enable the physician to direct proper antimicrobial therapy. Blood cultures are performed during febrile illnesses or when the patient is having chills with spiking fever. Intermittent bacteremia accompanies such infections as pyelonephritis, brucellosis, cholangitis, and others. In such cases, repeated blood cultures are usually ordered to be performed when the fever spikes. In other infections, such as subacute bacterial endocarditis, the bacteremia is more constant during the 4 to 5 febrile days. Usually four or five cultures are obtained over a span of 1 to 2 days, and antimicrobial therapy is initiated with the realization that the majority of cultures harbor the offending microorganism. If antimicrobial therapy is administered before the blood culture or before the patient's admittance to the hospital, the bacteremia may be suppressed, rendering isolation difficult.

Penicillinase may be ordered to be added to the blood culture medium to neutralize the existing penicillinemia and to recover the organism. Usually antimicrobial therapy must be withheld to await report of culture to make a precise diagnosis. The penicillinase is added to the culture medium before or immediately after the blood sample is drawn.

Some bacteriology laboratories routinely culture blood under both aerobic and anaerobic conditions. If this is not done routinely and bacteremia with strict anaerobes is suspected, the laboratory should be notified because a special culture broth is necessary.

Extreme care must be observed in preparing the area for venipuncture because the skin affords a fertile field for bacterial growth. *Staphylococcus albus*, diphtheroids, and yeast (common skin or environment contaminants) usually indicate

TABLE 9-1
Selected Laboratory Values

Parameter		Parameter	
Blood chemistry/electrolytes	*Normal values*	*Blood chemistry/electrolytes*	*Normal Values*
Blood urea nitrogen (BUN)	10–20 mg/dL	Magnesium	1.3–2.1 mEq/L or 1.8–3.0 mg/dL
Serum creatinine	0.7–1.5 mg/dL	Chloride	97–110 mEq/L
Creatinine clearance	Male: 110–150 mL/min	Carbon dioxide	24–30 mmol/L
	Female: 105–132 mL/min	Phosphate	Adults: 2.5–4.5 mg/dL (1.8–2.6 mEq/L)
BUN:creatinine ratio	10:1		Children: 4.0–7.0 mg/dL (2.3–4.1 mEq/L)
Hematocrit	Male: 44–52%		
	Female: 39–47%	Zinc	77–137 µg/dL (by atomic absorption)
Hemoglobin	Male: 13.5–18.0 g/dL		
	Female: 12.0–16.0 g/dL	Lithium	0.8 mEq/L (therapeutic level 8–12 h after administration)
Red blood cells	Male: 4600–6000/mm³		
	Female: 4200–5400/mm³	Serum proteins	
Mean corpuscular volume	80–95 mm³	Total	6.0–8.00 g/dL
Mean corpuscular hemoglobin	26–34 pg	Albumin	3.5–5.5 g/dL
Mean corpuscular hemoglobin concentration	32–36%	Globulin	1.5–3.0 g/dL
Complete blood count		Lactate (arterial blood)	4.5–14.4 mg/dL
Total leukocytes	4500–11,000/mm³	Serum ketones	Often >50 mg/dL in diabetic ketoacidosis. Usually under 20 mg/dL in salicylate intoxication
Myelocytes	0		
Band neutrophils	150–400/mm³ (3–5%)		
Segmented neutrophils	3000–5800/mm³ (54–62%)	Serum salicylates	Therapeutic range: 20–25 mg/dL
Lymphocytes	1500–3000/mm³ (25–33%)		
Monocytes	300–500/mm³ (3–7%)		Toxic range: >30 mg/dL
Eosinophils	50–250/mm³ (1–3%)	Anion gap	12–15 mEq/L
Basophils	15–50/mm³ (0–0.75%)	Aspartate aminotransferase (AST)	7–40 mµ/mL (30 C)
Platelets	150,000–300,000/mm³		
Reticulocytes	0.5–1.5%	Alanine aminotransferase (ALT)	5/35 mµ/mL (37 C)
Red cell volume	Male: 20–36 mL/kg		
	Female: 19–31 mL/kg	Alkaline phosphatase	20–90 mµ/mL (30 C)
Plasma volume	Male: 25–43 mL/kg	Serum bilirubin	
	Female: 28–45 mL/kg	Total	0.3–1.1 mg/dL
Clotting time	8–18 min	Direct	0.1–0.4 mg/dL
Prothrombin time	11–15 s	Indirect	0.2–0.7 mg/dL (total minus direct)
Iron	60–90 µg/dL		
Total iron-binding capacity (TIBC)	250–420 µg/dL	Lactate dehydrogenase [LOW]	100–190 mµ/mL

(continued)

TABLE 9-1 (Continued)

Parameter		Parameter	
Blood chemistry/electrolytes	**Normal Values**	**Blood chemistry/electrolytes**	**Normal Values**
Serum transferrin	>200 mg/dL (measured directly)	Urine chemistry/electrolytes*	
		Sodium	80–180 mEq/24 h (varies with Na+ intake)
	(0.8 TIBC) –4.3 estimates from TIBC)	Potassium	40–80 mEq/24 h (varies with dietary intake)
Partial thromboplastin time	Standard: 68–82 s		
	Activated: 32–46 s	Chloride	100–250 mEq/24 h
Fibrinogen	160–415 mg/dL	Calcium	100–150 mg/24 h (if on average diet)
Serum osmolality	280–295 mOsm/kg		
Serum amylase	25–125 mµ/ml		Varies with dietary intake
Serum glucose	70–110 mg/dL	Osmolality	Typical urine is 500–800 (mOsm/L [extreme range is 50–1400 mOsm/L])
Serum electrolytes			
Sodium	135–145 mEq/L		Usually about 1½–3 times greater than serum osmolality
Potassium	3.5–5.0 mEq/L		
Calcium	Total: 8.9–10.3 mg/dL or 4.6–5.1 mEq/L	Specific gravity (SG)	1.002–1.030 (most random samples have an SG of 1.012–1.025)
	Ionized: 4.6–5.1 mg/dL		
		pH	4.5–8.0
		Arterial blood gases	
		pH	7.35–7.45
		PaO$_2$	80–100 mm Hg
		PaCO$_2$	38–42 mm Hg
		Bicarbonate	22–26 mEq/L
		Base excess	–2 to +2

*Measurement of electrolytes may be of limited value because of recent administration of diuretics and/or lack of knowledge of dietary intake.

contamination, whereas *S. aureus* presents a greater problem by indicating either a contaminant or the presence of a serious pathogen.

Procedure

Several procedures are currently in use. Newer methods for collecting the blood sample use special vacuum tubes containing prepared culture media. The amount of blood required depends on the laboratory and procedure used. All require thorough preparation of the puncture area with an effective antiseptic. An iodine preparation followed by 70% isopropanol is a highly recommended preparation; question the patient about iodine sensitivity. Gloves should be worn by all personnel performing venipuncture.

Text continues on p. 122

TABLE 9-2
Examples of Conversions to Système International (SI) Units

		Present Reference	Present	Conversion	SI Reference	SI Unit
Alanine aminotransferase (ALT)	Serum	5–40	U/L	1.0	5–40	U/L
Albumin	Serum	3.9–5.0	mg/dL	10	39–50	g/L
Alkaline phosphatase	Serum	35–110	U/L	1.00	35–110	U/L
Aspartate aminotransferase (AST)	Serum	5–40	U/L	1.00	5–40	U/L
Billirubin	Serum					
Direct		0–0.2	mg/dL	17.10	0–4	μmol/L
Total		0.1–1.2	mg/dL	17.10	2–20	μmol/L
Calcium	Serum	8.6–10.3	mg/dL	0.2495	2.15–2.57	mmol/L
Carbon dioxide, total	Serum	22–30	mEq/L	1.00	22–30	mmol/L
Chloride	Serum	98–108	mEq/L	1.00	98–108	mmol/L
Cholesterol	Serum					
Age <29 y		<200	mg/dL	0.02586	<5.15	mmol/L
30–39 y		<225	mg/dL	0.02586	<5.80	mmol/L
40–49 y		<245	mg/dL	0.02586	<6.35	mmol/L
>50 y		<265	mg/dL	0.02586	<6.85	mmol/L
Complete blood count	Blood					
Hematocrit						
Men		42–52	%	0.01	0.42–0.52	1
Women		37–47	%	0.01	0.37–0.47	1
Hemoglobin						
Men		14.0–18.0	g/dL	10.0	140–180	g/L
Women		12–16	g/dL	10.0	120–160	g/L
Red cell count						
Men		$4.6–6.2 \times 10^8$	/mm³	10^6	$4.6–6.2 \times 10^{12}$/L	
Women		$4.2–5.4 \times 10^8$	/mm³	10^6	$4.2–5.4 \times 10^{12}$/L	
White cell count		$4.5–11.0 \times 10^3$	/mm³	10^6	$4.5–11.0 \times 10^9$/L	
Platelet count		$150–300 \times 10^3$	/mm³	10^6	$150–300 \times 10^9$/L	
Cortisol	Serum					
8 AM		5–25	μg/dL	27.59	140–690	nmol/L
8 PM		3–13	μg/dL	27.59	80–360	nmol/L
Cortisol	Urine	20–90	μg/24 h	2.759	55–250	nmol/24 h
Creatine kinase (CK)	Serum					
High CK group (black men)		50–520	U/L	1.00	50–520	U/L
Intermediate CK group (nonblack men, black women)		35–345	U/L	1.00	35–345	U/L
Low CK group (nonblack women)		25–145	U/L	1.00	25–145	U/L

(continued)

TABLE 9-2   *(Continued)*

Component	System	Present Reference Intervals	Present Unit	Conversion Factor	SI Reference Intervals	SI Unit Symbol
Creatinine kinase isoenzyme, MB fraction	Serum	>5	%	0.01	>0.05	1
Creatinine	Serum	0.4 –1.3	mg/dL	88.40	35–115	µmol/L
Men		0.7–1.3	mg/dL	88.40		
Women		0.4–1.1	mg/dL	88.40		
Digoxin, therapeutic	Serum	0.5–2.0	ng/mL	1.281	0.6–2.6	nmol/L
Erythrocyte indices	Blood					
Mean corpuscular volume (MCV)		80–100	microns³	1.00	80–100	fL
Mean corpuscular hemoglobin (MCH)		27–31	pg	1.00	27–31	pg
Mean corpuscular hemoglobin concentration (MCHC)		32–36	%	0.01	0.32–0.36	1
Ferritin	Serum					
Men		29–438	ng/mL	1.00	29–438	µg/L
Women		9–219	ng/mL	1.00	9–219	µg/L
Folate	Serum	2.5–20.0	ng/mL	2.266	6–46	nmol/L
Follicle-stimulating hormone (FSH)	Serum					
Children		12 or <	mIU/mL	1.00	12 or <	IU/L
Men		2.0–10.0	mIU/mL	1.00	2.0–10.0	IU/L
Women, follicular		3.2–9.0	mIU/mL	1.00	3.2–9.0	IU/L
Women, midcycle		3.2–9.0	mIU/mL	1.00	3.2–9.0	IU/L
Women, luteal		2.0–6.2	mIU/mL	1.00	2.0–6.2	IU/L
Gases arterial	Blood					
pO_2		80–95	mm Hg	0.1333	10.7–12.7	kPa
pCO_2		37–43	mm Hg	0.1333	4.9–5.7	kPa
Glucose	Serum	62–110	mg/dL	0.05551	3.4–6.1	mmol/L
Iron	Serum	50–160	µg/dL	0.1791	9–29	µmol/L
Iron-binding capacity (IBC)	Serum					
Total IBC		230–410	µg/dL	0.1791	41–73	µmol/L
Saturation		15–55	%	0.01	0.15–0.55	1
Lactic dehydrogenase	Serum	120–300	U/L	1.00	120–300	U/L
Luteinizing hormone	Serum					
Men		4.9–15.0	mIU/mL	1.00	4.9–15.0	IU/L
Women, follicular		5.0–25	mIU/mL	1.00	5.0–25	IU/L
Women, midcycle		43–145	mIU/mL	1.00	43–145	IU/L
Women, luteal		3.1–31	mIU/mL	1.00	3.1–31	IU/L

(continued)

TABLE 9-2 *(Continued)*

Component	System	Present Reference Intervals	Present Unit	Conversion Factor	SI Reference Intervals	SI Unit Symbol
Magnesium	Serum	1.2–1.9	mEq/L	0.4114	0.50–0.78	mmol/L
Osmolality	Serum	278–300	mOsm/kg	1.00	278–300	mmol/kg
Osmolality	Urine	None defined	mOsm/kg	1.00	None defined	mmd/kg
Phenobarbital, therapeutic	Serum	15–40	μg/mL	4.306	65–175	μmol/L
Phenytoin, therapeutic	Serum	10–20	μg/mL	3.964	40–80	μmol/L
Phosphate (phosphorus, inorganic)	Serum	2.3–4.1	mg/dl	0.3229	0.75–1.35	mmol/L
Potassium	Serum	3.7–5.1	mEq/L g/mL	1.00	3.7–5.1	mmol/L
Protein, total	Serum	6.5–8.3	g/dL	10.0	65–83	g/L
Sodium	Serum	134–142	mEq/L	1.00	134–142	mmol/L
Theophylline, therapeutic	Serum	5–20	μg/mL	5.550	28–110	μmol/L
Thyroid-stimulating hormone (TSH)	Serum	0–5	μIU/mL	1.00	0–5	mIU/L
Thyroxine	Serum	4.5–13.2	μg/dL	12.87	58–170	nmol/L
T_3-uptake ratio	Serum	0.88–1.19	I	1.00	0.88–1.19	1
Triiodothyronine (T_3)	Serum	70–235	ng/mL	0.01536	1.1–3.6	nmol/L
Triglycerides	Serum	50–200	mg/dL	0.01129	0.55–2.25	mmol/L
Urate (uric acid)	Serum					
Men		2.9–8.5	mg/dL	59.48	170–510	μmol/L
Women		2.2–6.5	mg/dL	59.48	130–390	μmol/L
Urea nitrogen	Serum	6–25	mg/dL	0.3570	2.1–8.9	mmol/L
Vitamin B$_{12}$	Serum	250–1000	pg/mL	0.7378	180–740	pmol/L

From Fischbach, F. T. (1992), *A manual of laboratory and diagnostic tests* (4th ed., pp. 951–955). Philadelphia: J. B. Lippincott.

MEASUREMENTS OF ELECTROLYTE CONCENTRATION

Electrolyte imbalances are serious complications in the critically ill patient. Such imbalances must be recognized and corrected at once. Frequently electrolyte determinations are ordered on an emergency basis. Accurate measurement is essential and to a large degree depends on the proper collection and handling of blood specimens.

Potassium

Potassium is an electrolyte essential to body function. About 98% of all body potassium is found in the cells; only small amounts are contained in the serum.

The kidneys normally do not conserve potassium. When large quantities of body fluid are lost without potassium replacement, a severe deficiency occurs. Chronic kidney disease and the use of diuretics may cause a potassium deficit. Adrenal steroids play a major role in controlling the concentration of potassium: hyperadrenalism causes increased potassium loss, with deficiency resulting; steroid therapy promotes potassium excretion.

An elevated potassium level results from potassium retention in renal failure or in adrenal cortical deficiency. Hypoventilation and cellular damage also result in an elevated potassium level.

Because intracellular ions are not accessible for measurement, determination must be made on the serum. Because the concentration of potassium in the cells is roughly 15 times greater than that in the serum, the blood for potassium determination must be carefully drawn to prevent hemolysis.

Blood Collection

Blood (2 mL) is drawn in a dry tube and allowed to clot or, preferably, placed under oil; oil minimizes friction and hemolysis of the RBCs. The blood should be sent to the laboratory immediately because potassium diffuses out of the cells and gives a falsely high reading.

Normal serum range is 3.5 to 5.0 mEq/L.[2,4]

Sodium

The main role of sodium is the control of the distribution of water throughout the body and the maintenance of a normal fluid balance.

The excretion of sodium is regulated to a large degree by the adrenocortical hormone aldosterone. Water excretion is regulated by antidiuretic hormone (ADH), and as long as these two systems are in harmony, the sodium and water remain in isosmotic proportion. Any change in the normal sodium concentration indicates that the loss or gain of water and sodium is in other than isosmotic proportion. Increased sodium levels may be caused by excessive infusions of sodium, insufficient water intake, or excess loss of fluid without a sodium loss, as in tracheobronchitis. Decreased sodium levels may be caused by excessive sweating accompanied by intake of large amounts of water by mouth, adrenal insufficiency, excessive infusions of nonelectrolyte fluids, or gastrointestinal suction accompanied with water by mouth.

Blood Collection

Blood (3 mL) is drawn carefully to prevent hemolysis and placed in a dry tube or a tube with oil.

Normal serum range is 135 to 145 mEq/L.[1]

Chlorides

Chlorides are usually measured along with other blood electrolytes. The measurement of chlorides is helpful in diagnosing disorders of acid–base balance and water balance of the body. Chloride has a reciprocal power of increasing or decreasing in concentration whenever changes in concentration of other anions occur. In metabolic acidosis, a reciprocal rise in chloride concentration occurs when the bicarbonate concentration drops.

Elevation in the blood chloride level occurs in such conditions as Cushing's syndrome, hyperventilation, and some kidney disorders. A decrease in blood chloride levels may occur in diabetic acidosis, heat exhaustion, and after vomiting and diarrhea.

Blood Collection
Venous blood (5 mL) is withdrawn and placed in a dry tube to clot.
Normal serum range is 97 to 110 mEq/L.

Calcium

Calcium, an essential electrolyte of the body, is required for blood clotting, muscular contraction, and nerve transmission. Only ionized calcium is useful but, because it cannot be satisfactorily measured, the total amount of body calcium is determined; 50% of the total is believed to be ionized.[2] In acidosis there is a higher level of ionized calcium; in alkalosis, a lower level.

Hypocalcemia (decrease in normal blood calcium) occurs whenever impairment of the gastrointestinal tract, such as sprue or celiac disease, prevents absorption. Deficiency also occurs in hypoparathyroidism and in some kidney diseases and is characterized by muscular twitching and tetanic convulsions.

Hypercalcemia (excess of calcium in the blood) occurs in hyperparathyroidism and in respiratory disturbance where carbon dioxide blood content is increased, such as in respiratory acidosis.

Blood Collection
Venous blood (5 mL) is placed in a dry tube and allowed to clot. Analysis is performed on the serum.
Normal serum range in adults is 8.9 to 10.3 mg/100 mL.[1] The range is slightly higher in children.

Phosphorus

Phosphorus metabolism is related to calcium metabolism and the serum level varies inversely with calcium.

Increased concentration of phosphorus may occur in such conditions as hypoparathyroidism, kidney disease, or excessive intake of vitamin D. Decreased concentrations may occur in hyperparathyroidism, rickets, and some kidney diseases.

Blood Collection
Because RBCs are rich in phosphorus, hemolysis of the blood must be avoided. Analysis is performed on the serum; 4 mL blood is placed in a dry tube to clot.
Normal serum range is 2.5 to 4.5 mg/100 mL.[1] In infants in the first year, the range is up to 6.0 mg/100 mL.

VENOUS BLOOD MEASUREMENTS OF ACID–BASE BALANCE

Acid–base balance is maintained by the buffer system, carbonic acid–base bicarbonate at a 1:20 ratio. When deviations occur in the normal ratio, a change in pH results and is accompanied by a change in bicarbonate concentration.

Carbon Dioxide Content

Carbon dioxide content is the measurement of the free carbon dioxide and the bicarbonate content of the serum, which provides a general measure of acidity or alkalinity. An increase in carbon dioxide content usually indicates alkalosis; a decrease indicates acidosis. This test, along with clinical findings, is helpful in surmising the severity and nature of the disorder. Measurement of pH is necessary for accuracy—a change in carbon dioxide does not always signify a change in pH because pH depends on the ratio and not the carbon dioxide content. When the carbon dioxide and pH are known, the buffer ratio can be determined.

An elevated carbon dioxide content is present in metabolic alkalosis, hypoventilation, loss of acid secretions such as occurs in persistent vomiting or drainage of the stomach, and excessive administration of corticotropin or cortisone. A low carbon dioxide content usually occurs in loss of alkaline secretions such as in severe diarrhea, certain kidney diseases, diabetic acidosis, and hyperventilation.

Blood Collection

Several procedures are now in use: 1) collection in a heparinized syringe with immediate placement on ice; 2) collection in a heparinized vacuum tube; or 3) collection in a dry tube without an anticoagulant. The procedure used depends on the laboratory's routine. The containers must always be filled with blood to prevent carbon dioxide from escaping. In all methods, it is important that the patient avoid clenching the fist; excess muscular activity of the arm can increase the carbon dioxide level in the blood.

Normal serum range is 22 to 31 mEq/L.[1]

Acidity (pH) Content

The pH, a symbol for acidity, indicates the serum concentration of hydrogen ions. The pH becomes lower in acid conditions such as hypoventilation, diarrhea, and diabetic acidosis. The pH rises in alkaline conditions such as hyperventilation and excessive vomiting.

Blood Collection

The blood is collected *without stasis* in a heparinized 2-mL syringe; the syringe is then capped. The blood may be drawn with a small-vein needle, the needle discarded, and the tubing tied off. The specimen is left in the syringe and packed in ice. Loss of carbon dioxide from contact with the air is thus avoided and excess production of lactic acid by enzymic reaction reduced. Blood (5 mL) may also be collected in a green-stopped vacuum tube containing heparin.

Normal blood range is 7.35 to 7.45.

ENZYMES

Amylase

Amylase determination is helpful in the diagnosis of acute pancreatitis or the acute recurrence of chronic pancreatitis. Amylase is secreted by the pancreas; a rise in the serum level occurs when outflow of pancreatic juice is restricted. This test is usually performed on patients with acute abdominal pain or on surgical patients in whom questionable injury may have occurred to the pancreas. Amylase levels usually remain elevated for only a short time—3 to 6 days.

Blood Collection
Venous blood (6 mL) is allowed to clot in a dry tube.

Normal serum range is 4 to 25 U/mL. The range may depend on the normal values established by clinical laboratories because the method may be modified.

Lipase

Lipase determination is used for detecting damage to the pancreas and is valuable when too much time has elapsed for the amylase level to remain elevated. When secretions of the pancreas are blocked, the serum lipase level rises.

Blood Collection
The test is performed on serum from 6 mL of clotted blood. *Normal serum range* is 2 U/mL or less.

Phosphatase, Acid

Acid phosphatase is useful in determining metastasizing tumors of the prostate. The prostate gland and carcinoma of the gland are rich in phosphatase but do not normally release the enzyme into the serum. Once the carcinoma has spread, it starts to release acid phosphatase, increasing the serum concentration.[2] In addition to carcinoma of the prostate, other conditions that produce increased serum acid phosphatase levels are Paget's disease, hyperparathyroidism, metastatic mammary carcinoma, renal insufficiency, multiple myeloma, some liver disease, arterial embolism, myocardial infarction, and sickle cell crisis.[2]

Blood Collection
Blood (5 mL) is allowed to clot in a dry tube. Hemolysis should be avoided. Analysis should be done immediately, or the serum should be frozen.

Normal serum range:

1. Male: Total, 0.13 to 0.63 Sigma U/mL
2. Female: Total, 0.01 to 0.56 Sigma U/mL
3. Prostatic: 0 to 0.5 Fishman-Lerner U/100 mL[1]

Phosphatase, Alkaline

Alkaline phosphatase is a useful test in diagnosing bone diseases and obstructive jaundice. In bone diseases, the small amount of alkaline usually present in the serum rises in proportion to the new bone cells. When excretion of alkaline phosphatase is impaired, as in some disorders of the liver and biliary tract, the serum level rises and may give some evidence of the degree of blockage in the biliary tract.[2]

Blood Collection
Blood (5 mL) is drawn and the test is performed on the serum. Sodium sulfobromophthalein dye should be avoided.

Normal serum range is 13 to 39 U/mL.[1]

TRANSAMINASE

The transaminases are enzymes found in large quantities in the heart, liver, muscle, kidney, and pancreas cells. Any disease that causes damage to these cells will result in an elevated serum transaminase level; clinical signs and other tests are used in diagnosis.

Aspartate Aminotransferase (AST)

(Also known as serum glutamic-oxaloacetic transaminase [SGOT].)

The AST level is used to distinguish between myocardial infarction and acute coronary insufficiency without infarction. It is also useful as a liver function test in following the progression of liver damage or in ascertaining when the liver has recovered.

Blood Collection

The test is performed on serum from 5 mL clotted blood.

Normal serum range is 10 to 40 U/mL. In myocardial infarction, the level is increased 4 to 10 times, whereas in liver involvement a high of 10 to 100 times normal may occur. The serum level remains elevated for about 5 days.

Alanine Aminotransferase (ALT)

(Also known as serum glutamic-pyruvic transaminase [SGPT].)

Alanine aminotransferase is another transaminase that is more specific for hepatic malfunction than AST.

Blood Collection

The test is performed on serum from 5 mL blood. *Normal serum range* is 6 to 36 Karmen U/mL.[2]

Serum Lactate Dehydrogenase (LDH)

The transaminase LDH is present in all tissues and in large quantities in the kidney, heart, and skeletal muscles. Elevated serum levels usually parallel the AST levels. Elevation occurs in myocardial infarction and may continue through the sixth day. Elevations have been found in lymphoma, disseminated carcinoma, and some cases of leukemia.

Blood Collection

Blood (3 mL) is collected and allowed to coagulate. Care must be taken to avoid hemolysis because only a slight degree may give an incorrect reading.

Normal serum range is 60 to 120 U/mL.[1]

LIVER FUNCTION TESTS

Albumin, Globulin, Total Protein, and Albumin/Globulin Ratio

These tests may be useful in diagnosing kidney and liver disease or in judging the effectiveness of treatment. The chief role of serum albumin is to maintain osmotic pressure of the blood; globulin assists. The globulin molecule, being larger than the albumin, is less efficient in maintaining osmotic pressure and does not leak out of the blood. With the loss of albumin through the capillary wall, the body compensates by producing more globulin. The osmotic pressure is reduced and may result in some edema. Certain conditions, such as chronic nephritis, lipoid nephrosis, liver disease, and malnutrition result in a lowered albumin concentration.[2]

Blood Collection

The test is performed on serum from 6 mL clotted blood.
Normal serum range:

1. Total protein: 6.0 to 8.0 g/100 mL
2. Albumin: 3.2 to 5.6 g/100 mL
3. Globulin: 1.3 to 3.5 g/100 mL

Bilirubin (Direct and Indirect)

The bilirubin test, which is becoming less common, differentiates between impairment of the liver by obstruction and hemolysis. Bilirubin arises from the hemoglobin liberated from broken-down RBCs. It is the chief pigment of the bile, excreted by the liver. If the excretory power of the liver is impaired by obstruction, there is an excess of circulatory bilirubin and it is free of any attached protein. Measurement of free bilirubin (direct) usually indicates obstruction.

When increased red blood cell destruction (hemolysis) occurs, the increased bilirubin is believed to be bound to protein (indirect).

A *total bilirubin* determination detects increased concentration of bilirubin before jaundice is seen.

Blood Collection

The test is performed on serum from 5 mL clotted blood.
Normal serum range is 0.1 to 1.0 mg/100 mL.[2]

Cephalin Flocculation

This test is being replaced in many hospitals by more specific tests. In diagnosing liver damage, it frequently detects damage before jaundice becomes evident. It is also useful in following the course of liver disease such as cirrhosis. The serum of patients with damaged liver cells flocculates a colloidal suspension of cephalin and cholesterol, whereas the serum of normal patients does not clump the suspension. Abscesses and neoplasms do not damage liver cells and therefore give negative results.[2]

Blood Collection

The test is performed on serum from 5 mL of clotted blood.
Normal serum range is either negative or 1+. Reports are delayed 24 to 48 hours.

Cholesterol

Cholesterol, a normal constituent of the blood, is present in all body cells. In various disease states the cholesterol concentration in the serum may be raised or lowered. Cholesterol is transported in the blood by the low-density lipoproteins (LDLs; 60%–75%) and high-density lipoproteins (HDLs; 15%–35%).

Blood Collection

The test is performed on serum from 5 mL of clotted blood.
   Normal serum range is 120 to 260 mg/100 mL.

High-density Lipoprotein

A high level of HDL is indicative of a healthy metabolic system in a patient free of liver disease.

Very Low-density Lipoproteins (VLDL) and Low-density Lipoproteins

The VLDLs are major carriers of triglyceride. Degradation of VLDL is a major source of LDL.

Prothrombin Time

The prothrombin time, considered one of the most important screening tests in coagulation studies, indirectly measures the ability of the blood to clot. During the clotting process, prothrombin is converted to thrombin. It is thought that when the prothrombin level is reduced to below normal, the tendency for the blood to clot in the blood vessel is reduced. It is an important guide in controlling drug therapy and is commonly used when anticoagulants are prescribed. The prothrombin content is reduced in liver diseases.

Blood Collection

Venous blood (4 mL) is collected, added to the coagulant, and quickly mixed. It is important to avoid clot formation and hemolysis. The blood should be examined as soon as possible.
   The *normal value* is between 11 and 18 seconds, depending on the type of thromboplastin used.

Thymol Turbidity

Thymol turbidity detects damaged liver cells and differentiates between liver disease and biliary obstruction. Turbidity is usually increased when the serum of patients with liver damage is mixed with a saturated solution of thymol. Turbidity is usually normal in biliary obstruction without liver damage.

Blood Collection

The test is performed on serum from 5 mL of clotted blood.
   Normal serum range is 0 to 4 U.[1]

KIDNEY FUNCTION TESTS

Creatinine

The creatinine test measures kidney function. Creatinine, the result of a breakdown of muscle creatine phosphate, is produced daily in a constant amount in each individual. A disorder of kidney function prevents excretion and an elevated creatinine value gives a reliable indication of impaired kidney function. A normal serum creatinine value does not indicate unimpaired renal function, however.

Blood Collection

The test is performed on serum from 6 mL of clotted blood.
Normal serum range is 0.6 to 1.3 mg/100 mL.

Blood Urea Nitrogen (BUN)

The BUN is a measure of kidney function. Urea, the end product of protein metabolism, is excreted by the kidneys. Impairment in kidney function results in an elevated concentration of urea nitrogen in the blood. Rapid protein metabolism may also increase the urea nitrogen above normal limits. The *nonprotein nitrogen* is a similar test for measuring kidney function.

Blood Collection

The test is performed on blood or serum. Blood (5 mL) is added to an oxalate tube and shaken or placed in a dry tube to clot.
Normal range is 10 to 20 mg/100 mL.

BLOOD SUGAR TESTS

The test for blood sugar is used to detect a disorder of glucose metabolism, which may be the result of any one of several factors, including 1) inability of pancreas islet cells to produce insulin; 2) inability of intestines to absorb glucose; and 3) inability of liver to accumulate and break down glycogen.

An elevated blood sugar level may indicate diabetes, chronic liver disease, or overactivity of the endocrine glands. A decrease in blood sugar concentration may result from an overdose of insulin, tumors of the pancreas, or insufficiency of various endocrine glands.

Fasting Blood Sugar

A fasting blood sugar test requires that the patient fast for 8 hours.

Blood Collection

Venous blood (3–5 mL) is collected in an oxalate tube and shaken to prevent microscopic clots.
Normal serum range is 70 to 100 mg/100 mL (true blood sugar method). The normal value depends on the method of determination. Values greater than 120 mg/100 mL on several occasions may indicate diabetes mellitus.

Postprandial Blood Sugar Determinations

The postprandial sugar test is helpful in diagnosing diabetes mellitus. Blood is drawn 2 hours after the patient has begun to eat. If the blood sugar value is above the upper limits of normal for fasting, a glucose tolerance test is performed.

Glucose Tolerance

The glucose tolerance test is indicated:

1. When the patient shows glycosuria
2. When fasting or 2-hour blood sugar concentration is only slightly elevated
3. When Cushing's syndrome or acromegaly is a questionable diagnosis
4. To establish the cause of hypoglycemia

Blood Collection

A fasting blood sugar sample is drawn. The patient drinks 100 g glucose in lemon-flavored water (some laboratories use 1.75 g glucose/kg ideal body weight). Blood and urine samples are collected at 30, 60, 90, 120, and 180 minutes after ingestion of glucose.

Normal (true blood sugar) values are:

1. Fasting blood sugar below 100 mg/100 mL
2. Peak below 160 mg/100 mL in 30 or 60 minutes
3. Two-hour value returning to fasting level

The values depend on the standards used.

BLOOD TYPING

Blood typing is one of the most common tests performed on blood, being required by all donors and by all patients who may need blood. The ABO system denotes four main groups: O, A, B, and AB. The designations refer to the particular antigen present on the RBCs: group A contains RBCs with the A antigen, B with B antigen, AB with A and B antigens, and O erythrocytes contain neither A nor B antigens.

When erythrocytes containing antigens are placed with serum containing corresponding antibodies under favorable conditions, agglutination (clumping) occurs. Therefore, an antigen is known as an agglutinogen and an antibody as an agglutinin.

An individual's serum contains antibodies that will react to corresponding antigens not usually found on the individual's own cells. For instance, serum of group O contains antibodies A and B, which will react with the corresponding antigens A and B found on the RBCs of group AB.

Although agglutination occurs in antigen–antibody reactions in the laboratory, hemolysis occurs in vivo; antibody attacks RBCs, causing rupture with liberation of hemoglobin. Hemolysis results from infusing incompatible blood and may lead to fatal consequences.

Rh Factor

The antigens belonging to the Rh system are D, C, E, c, and e; they are found in conjunction with the ABO group. The strongest of these factors is the $Rh_o(D)$ factor, found in about 85% of the white population. Therefore the $Rh_o(D)$ factor is often the only factor identified in Rh typing. When not present, further typing may be done to identify any of the less common Rh factors.

Blood Collection

Venous blood is collected and allowed to clot. Usually one tube (10 mL) will set up 4 to 5 U blood. Positive patient identification must be made before the blood is drawn; the name and number on the identification bracelet must correspond to that on the requisition and label. Identity should never be made by addressing the patient by name and awaiting the response. The label is placed on the blood tube at the patient's bedside.

Blood Typing

Various methods are used in typing blood, but all involve the same general principle. The patient's cells are mixed in standard saline serum samples of anti-A and of anti-B. The type of serum, A or B, which agglutinates the patient's cells indicates the blood group. As a double check, the patient's serum is mixed with saline suspensions of A and of B erythrocytes. The ABO group is determined on the basis of agglutination or absence of agglutination of A and of B cells.

Coombs' Test

Not all antibodies cause agglutination in saline; some merely coat the RBCs by combining with the antigen, which is not a visible reaction. The Coombs' test is performed to detect antibodies that cannot cause agglutination in saline; these are known as *incomplete antibodies*. Antihuman globulin serum is used. This serum is obtained by the immunization of various animals, usually rabbits, against human gamma globulin by the injection of human serum, plasma, or isolated globulin. This antiserum, when added to sensitized RBCs (erythrocytes coated with incomplete antibody), causes visible agglutination.

The Coombs' test is performed in two ways. The *direct Coombs' test* is performed when the patient's RBCs have become coated in vivo. This test is a valuable procedure in:

1. Diagnosis of erythroblastosis fetalis. The erythrocytes of the baby are tested for sensitization.
2. Acquired hemolytic anemia. The patient may have produced an antibody that coats his or her own cells.
3. Investigation of reactions. The patient may have received incompatible blood that has sensitized his RBCs.

The *indirect Coombs' test* detects incomplete antibodies in the serum of patients sensitized to blood antigens. It involves use of the patient's serum, in contrast to the use of the patient's RBCs in the direct Coombs' test. When pooled, normal erythrocytes containing the most important antigens are exposed in a test tube to the patient's serum and to Coombs' serum, agglutination of the RBCs occurs and indicates the incomplete antibody present. This test is valuable in:

1. Detecting incompatibilities not found by other methods
2. Detecting weak or variant antigens

3. Typing with certain antiserums, such as anti-Duffy or anti-Kidd, which require Coombs' serum to produce agglutination

4. Detecting antiagglutinins produced by exposure during pregnancy

REFERENCES

1. Castleman, B., & McNeeley, B. (1986). Case records of the Massachusetts General Hospital: Normal laboratory values. *New England Journal of Medicine, 314*, 39–49.
2. Garb, S. (1976). *Laboratory tests in common use* (6th ed., pp. 23–123). New York: Springer.
3. Grove-Rasmussen, M., Lesses, M. F., & Anstall, H. B. (1961). Transfusion therapy. *New England Journal of Medicine, 264*, 1089.
4. Fischbach, F. (1996). *A manual of laboratory and diagnostic tests* (4th ed., pp. 370–371). Philadelphia: J. B. Lippincott.

REVIEW QUESTIONS

1. Serum consists of:
   a. plasma minus fibrinogen
   b. plasma plus fibrinogen
   c. plasma minus fibrin
   d. plasma plus fibrin

2. Glycolysis refers to production of glycolytic enzymes causing which of the following?
   a. rise in pH on standing
   b. drop in pH on standing
   c. rise in blood pressure
   d. orthostatic hypotension

3. Hemolysis refers to:
   a. lysis of cells
   b. lysis of enzymes
   c. clysis of cells
   d. clysis of enzymes

4. Pressure should be applied to a puncture site:
   a. for 1 minute
   b. for 3 minutes
   c. until bleeding stops
   d. until bleeding slows

5. The most important factor in drawing blood for blood grouping and typing is:
   a. preservation of specimen
   b. method used
   c. positive identification
   d. use of OSHA standards

6. BUN is a measure of what function?
   a. liver
   b. kidney
   c. cardiac
   d. lung

7. Which of the following is closely related to body water status?
   a. potassium
   b. calcium
   c. magnesium
   d. sodium

8. Amylase determination is useful in diagnosis of which of the following diseases?
   a. acute gastritis
   b. acute pancreatitis
   c. metastasizing tumors of prostate
   d. primary alkalosis

9. Acid–base balance is maintained by what system?
   a. buffer
   b. neutral
   c. pulmonary
   d. cardiac

10. Erythrocytes are rich in:
    a. calcium
    b. magnesium
    c. phosphorus
    d. sodium

PART III

Principles of Equipment Selection and Clinical Applications

CHAPTER 10

Intravenous Equipment

Key Terms

Bubble point	Hydrophilic	Spring-coil container
Controllers	Monitors	Spring-coil piston
Elastomerics	Needleless	Syringe pump
Electronic infusion devices	Pressure	Tapering
Free flow	Pumps	Volumetric
Gravity	Ramping	Wetted
Hydrophobic		

Rapidly changing technology has kept pace with advances in medical science and has provided many improved, sophisticated devices for the administration of IV therapy. Specialized equipment is available to meet the patient's every need: positive-pressure pumps for IV and intra-arterial therapy; controllers and monitors for regulating and monitoring the rate of infusion; ambulatory infusion devices; and air-venting microbe-retentive filters, catheters, and administration sets. A nurse's knowledge of the selection and use of these devices is vital for the patient's comfort and safety. Even in today's clinical environment with purchasing decisions increasingly being made by groups, nurses may be involved in equipment selection for IV use as members of a product evaluation committee or equipment task force.

SOLUTION CONTAINERS

Glass Containers

Sterile evacuated glass containers with premixed fluids first became available in 1929. Glass remains the container of choice for those solutions that may not be administered in plastic because of incompatibility problems, such as those associated with nitroglycerin or lipid emulsions.

A glass bottle with a partial vacuum requires air vents. The closed system admits only filtered air to the container; the air vent, containing the filter, is an integral part of the administration set. The open system allows air to enter through a plastic tube in the container and collect in the airspace in the bottle.

Plastic Bags

Baxter was the first to develop the plastic bag for parenteral fluids. The plastic container is easily transported with minimal risk of damage and is easily disposed of. Because it contains no rubber bushings, coring is eliminated and particulate matter is reduced. Air venting is not required; thus, the risk of air embolism and airborne contamination is reduced.

Plastic bags are susceptible to accidental puncture, which creates a port of entry for microorganisms. Because punctures may not be evident, the container should be squeezed before use and visually checked for leakage. Today, plastic containers are used for most infusions unless contraindicated because of the type of drug additive.

The plastic bag and plastic bottle contain no vacuum, and because the containers are flexible and collapsible, they need no air to replace fluid flowing from the containers.

Semirigid Containers

Semirigid containers, although not as popular as plastic bags, are as safe for most solutions as glass. The container is lightweight and durable and adapts well to alternative care settings such as home care and ambulatory clinics. However, because of the semirigid nature of the material, the container is not easily adapted to patient-worn pouches and other ambulatory packs. It is also not well suited to freezing.

Syringes

A syringe is also a form of solution container when used with a syringe-loaded electronic infusion device (EID). The limiting feature of the syringe for the adult patient is the limited volume capacity. In neonatology and pediatrics, the syringe becomes an ideal vehicle for infusates.

Use-Activated Containers

A use-activated container is compartmentalized and includes premeasured ingredients that form an admixture when combined in solution. To activate the container, the nurse must rupture a seal or diaphragm within the container by compressing opposing parts or by applying pressure to rupture an internal reservoir. Useful in emergency situations and for patient transport, the system has become popular although it is expensive for routine use.

DELIVERY SYSTEMS

Medication Additives

Methods for adding medications to the fluid containers vary with each system. The plastic bag contains a resealable latex medication port through which the medication is injected. Because the plastic bag lacks a vacuum, medications must be added with a syringe and needle or additive needle. A unit for creating a vacuum in the container is available to the pharmacist and provides speed and ease to the admixture program. When medications are added to the plastic containers during the infusion, special precautions must be taken to ensure that the clamp on the administration set is completely closed and the flow interrupted before the medication is added. This prevents an undiluted, toxic dose of medication from entering the administration set and being infused. Medications and solutions should always be mixed thoroughly before administration, regardless of the system used.

In the closed system, medication may be added to the solution bottle during the infusion by using the air vent located in the administration set as a medication port. The 5-μm filter is removed and the syringe is attached. Meticulous care must be used to maintain sterility of the filter when removing the filter, adding the medication, and replacing the filter. The fluid bottle contains a solid rubber stopper through which medications may be added before infusion.

In the open system, bottles have a removable metal disk under which a sterile latex disk provides a closed method for aseptically adding a medication and for visibly checking for a vacuum. The vacuum is noted by the depression in the seal and must be present to ensure sterility. Before the latex disk is removed, the medication is added through the outlet port with a syringe and needle; the vacuum draws the medication into the bottle. During infusion, the medication may be added through the designated area on the rubber bushing after the clamp on the administration set has been closed. The medication and solution must be mixed thoroughly by agitating the fluid before administration.

ADMINISTRATION SETS

An important factor in the administration set is the rate of flow that the given set is gauged to produce. Commercial sets vary—they may deliver from 10 to 15 drops/mL, depending on the nature of the fluid. Increased viscosity causes the size of the drop to increase, so that a set that delivers 15 drops/mL may deliver 10 drops/mL when blood is administered. This information is of vital concern to the accurate control of the rate of infusion.

Most conventional sets use the roller clamp or slide clamp for controlling the flow rate (Fig. 10-1). Changes in the drop rate invariably occur after the rate is regulated and require time-consuming readjustments of the clamp to establish and maintain flow rates. Alternatives to the roller clamp that save nursing time and that are valuable in maintaining the rate of parenteral solutions are also available.

Another method uses a flow-metering system that eliminates drifting flow rates. The metering device consists of "an adjustable dam" controlled by a knob. Because it is connected on the entry and exit ports, the IV tubing is isolated from the metering device and does not affect changes in the flow rate. The rate can be set and it will stay until the infusion is complete, eliminating "free flow" runaway IVs and helping prevent IV flow rate variations. Refinements in infusion technology continue to provide alternative means by which rate of flow is regulated.

FIGURE 10-1 (**A**) Standard administration set in-line filter. (**B**) Primary venoset, macrodrop. (Courtesy: Abbott Laboratories, North Chicago, IL)

Special-Use Sets

Nonpolyvinylchloride IV administration sets are available for gravity infusion and for volumetric pumps. Nitroglycerin, fat emulsions, and other drugs can be administered without altering the dosage of the drug through absorption into the walls of the polyvinylchloride (PVC) tubing.

Frequently the flow must be maintained at a minimal rate. One method is to reduce the size of the drop by using special sets, originally designed for pediatric infusions. These sets are valuable in parenteral therapy for adults as well because by reducing the size of the drop, a constant IV flow may be maintained with a minimal amount of fluid. These sets deliver 60 drops/mL; at the rate of 60 drops/min, it would take 1 hour to infuse 60 mL. A variety of commercial sets are available for alternate or simultaneous infusion of two solutions. Some sets contain a filter (Fig. 10-2A).

A significant hazard of air embolism may occur when the Y-type administration set is used ignorantly or carelessly with vented containers. Constant vigilance is necessary if both solutions are administered simultaneously. If one container is allowed to empty, large quantities of air can be sucked into the tubing; the empty bottle becomes the vent because of the greater atmospheric pressure in the empty bottle and tube over the pressure below the partially constricted clamp in the tubing of the flowing solution.[7]

Positive-pressure sets are designed to increase the rapidity of infusions and are an asset when rapid replacement of fluid becomes necessary. They permit fluid to be administered by gravity, with a built-in pressure chamber available for rapid administration of blood should an emergency arise. When used with the collapsible plastic blood unit, this system avoids the danger of air embolism; because the bag collapses,

FIGURE 10-2 (**A**) Primary venoset with IVEX-2 integral filter. (**B**) Secondary venoset with hook and needle for piggybacking. (Courtesy: Abbott Laboratories, North Chicago, IL)

the need for air is eliminated. In contrast to the collapsible bag, the glass container must be vented to allow the fluid to flow; air pressure must be used when blood or fluid is forced into the bloodstream. As the last portion of blood from the container is forced into the bloodstream, the air under pressure may rapidly enter the vein before the clamp can be applied, resulting in a fatal embolus. According to Adriani, "Air pressure should not be used to force blood and other fluids into the blood stream."[1]

The pump chamber must be filled at all times. The nurse should never apply positive pressure to infuse fluids.

Check-Valve Sets

Sets are available with an in-line check valve, which provides a more convenient and safer method for administering medications and fluids. A secondary infusion or a single dose of medication can be administered "piggyback" into the injection site located below the check valve. The valve automatically shuts off the main-line infusion while the admixture is running and automatically allows the main infusion to start when the medication has run in. This valve prevents mixing of the two fluids, eliminates the risk of air entering the line when the secondary bottle empties, and prevents the cannula from becoming occluded by an interruption in the infusion. Because the rate of flow must be regulated by one clamp, the rate of administration remains the same for both fluids (see Figure 10-2).

Volume-Controlled Sets

With the increasing use and number of solutions containing drugs and electrolytes, greater accuracy in controlling the volume of IV fluids is necessary. Several available devices permit accurate administration of measured volumes of fluids (Fig. 10-3A, B).

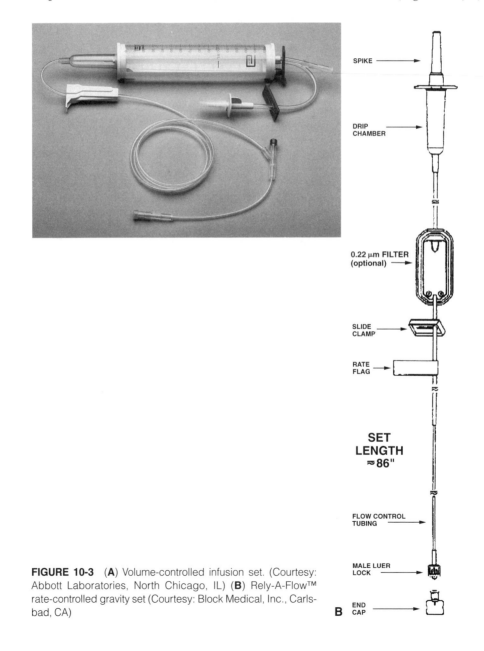

FIGURE 10-3 **(A)** Volume-controlled infusion set. (Courtesy: Abbott Laboratories, North Chicago, IL) **(B)** Rely-A-Flow™ rate-controlled gravity set (Courtesy: Block Medical, Inc., Carlsbad, CA)

Sets contain vented, calibrated burette chambers that control the volume from 100 to 150 mL. The burette chamber of some sets contains a rubber float that prevents air from entering the tubing once the infusion is completed.

Some calibrated burette chambers contain a microporous filter to block the passage of air when the chamber empties. Refilling these chambers requires a specific procedure. The word oscar will help recall the procedure: O—open clamp; S—squeeze drip chamber and hold; C—close clamp close to drip chamber; A—and; R—release drip chamber.

The Rely-A-Flow™ Rate Controlled Set utilizes flow control tubing to administer an infusion at a preset rate with ± 10% accuracy.

Pump-Specific Sets

Some sets are made specifically for use with EIDs. These sets also come in a number of configurations. Such sets and their respective electronic delivery systems ensure safe delivery of infusion therapy to patients of all ages in a variety of clinical settings.

RATE OF FLOW

Pressure and Infusion Therapy

Pressure is the principle of physics underlying fluid therapy. Pressure enables us to overcome the natural resistance to flow created by the administration set, in-line filters, narrow-gauge needles, and venous or arterial backpressure. The human body adapts to changes in pressure, which enables clinicians to deliver IV therapy safely.

Pressure in the arterial system ranges from 80 mm Hg in the aorta to a low of 5 to 10 mm Hg in the venous return system. Intravenous pressure is created by the weight of a column of fluid in the tubing—the weight is due to gravity—and we know it as *hydrostatic pressure*. Fluid always flows from an area of higher pressure to one of lower pressure. To infuse by gravity, it is necessary to create a pressure only slightly more than normal or 40 mm Hg in a peripheral line.

A number of resistance factors may interfere with or inhibit fluid flow. These factors include the patient's own vascular pressure, internal diameter of the tubing, in-line filters, viscosity of fluid, narrow-gauge needles, and the length of the tubing. Resistance to flow is determined by the smallest component in the IV system; this is usually the cannula.

The EIDs have incorporated the concept of pressure to deliver precise amounts of drug and solution. Most recently, differential pressure has been a component of such devices. With a range of two or three levels, such equipment may sense a change in pressure, usually 5 psi over baseline, and some devices monitor and read out line pressure. *Operating* or *line pressure* is the pressure generated by a pump to cause fluid to flow at a predetermined rate. *Maximum occlusion pressure* is the limit to operating pressure at which an occlusion alarm is triggered. *Needle pressure* is the same as venous pressure, and, during an infusion, pressure at the tip of the cannula is only slightly more than the pressure within that vein or artery regardless of the output pressure of the pump. The pressure at the needle tip needs to be slightly higher than vascular pressure for fluid to flow. An understanding of pressure and psi is essential to safely use EIDs, filters, and other components of the IV system.

Gravity Flow

Gravity flow depends on head pressure; roller clamps and screw clamps used to adjust and to maintain rates of flow on gravity infusions vary considerably in their efficiency and accuracy.

Rate minders or flow-control mechanisms may also be used to regulate and adjust flow. The rate minder is added to the IV administration set. The desired flow rate may be preset. Levels of accuracy vary with the type of device used. Factors such as venous spasm, venous pressure changes, patient movement, manipulations of the clamp, and bent or kinked tubing may cause variations in the flow rate.

Either preprinted or self-made time tapes may be used on the IV container to determine consistency with prescribed rate of flow. Attach the time tape to the container and mark hourly increments on the tape or strip, beginning with the time the infusion was hung. Various time tapes and preprinted labels are available to assist with this process (Fig. 10-4).

Rate of Administration

To determine the flow rate intelligently, the nurse must have a knowledge of parenteral solutions, their effect, and rate of administration. The nurse must also understand other factors that influence the speed of the infusion. These factors include 1) body surface area; 2) patient's condition; 3) patient's age; 4) composition of the fluid; and 5) patient's tolerance to the infusion.

Body Surface Area

The body surface area is proportionate to many essential physiologic processes (organ size, blood volume, respiration, and heat loss) and therefore to the total metabolic activity. It provides a helpful guide for determining the amount of fluids and electrolytes and for computing the rates of infusion. The larger an individual, the more fluid and nutrients are required and the faster they can be used. The usual infusion rate is 3 mL/m^2 body surface per minute (see nomograms for determining surface area in Figure 10-5). This rate applies to maintenance and replacement fluids. However, the speed must be carefully adjusted to each individual.

Patient's Condition

Because the heart and kidneys play a vital role in the utilization of infused solutions, the cardiac and renal status of the patient affects the desired rate of administration. An expanded blood volume may occur when fluids, rapidly infused, overtax an impaired heart and renal damage causes retention of fluid. Patients suffering from hypovolemia must receive plasma and blood rapidly, but the desired speed of the infusion should be specified by the physician. Vital signs must be carefully observed and the speed of the infusion decreased as the blood pressure rises.[4]

Patient's Age

The patient's age has a specific effect on patient outcomes.[4] For age-specific parameters, refer to Chapters 21 and 22.

FIGURE 10-4 Time tapes. (Courtesy: United Ad Label Co., Inc., Brea, CA)

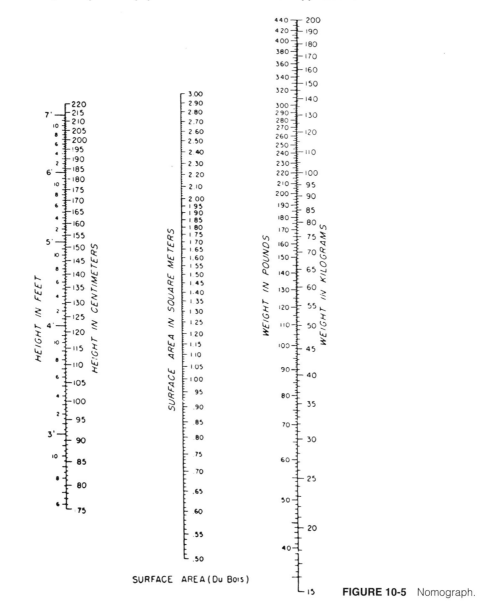

SURFACE AREA (Du Bois)

FIGURE 10-5 Nomograph.

Composition of Fluid

The composition of the fluid affects the rate of flow. When the solution is used as a vehicle for administering drugs, the speed of the infusion depends on the drug and the effect the physician wishes to produce. Because of its deleterious effect on the heart when infused at a rapid rate, potassium should be administered with caution. About 20 to 40 mEq potassium in a liter of solution infused over an 8-hour period is an average rate for administering potassium parenterally.

Concentration of solutions must be considered because the flow rate may alter the desired effect. When dextrose is administered for caloric benefits, it is infused at a rate that will ensure complete utilization. Dextrose has been administered at a maximum rate of 0.5 g/kg body weight per hour without producing glycosuria in a normal individual. At this rate, it would take approximately 1.5 hours to administer a liter of 5% dextrose to an individual weighing 70 kg or twice as long for a liter of 10% dextrose. This maximum rate is faster than usual and is not customarily used except in an emergency.

When a diuretic effect is desired, a more rapid infusion is necessary. If the solution is too rapidly infused for complete metabolism, the glucose accumulates in the bloodstream, increases the osmolality, and acts as a diuretic.

When oliguria or anuria occurs, the status of the kidneys must be determined before solutions containing potassium can be administered. Urinary suppression may be caused by a blood volume deficit or kidney damage. An initial hydrating solution, to test kidney function, is usually administered at a rate of 8 mL/m² body surface per minute for 45 minutes. If urinary flow is not accomplished, the rate is slowed to about 2 mL/m² body surface per minute for another hour. If urinary output has not occurred after this period, it is presumed that kidney damage is present[4] (see Chapters 14 and 15).

Patient's Tolerance

Tolerance to solutions varies with individuals and influences the rate of infusion. A 5% solution of alcohol has been administered at the rate of 200 to 300 mL/h to sedate without intoxication in an average adult.[1] However, when such a solution is to be administered, the rate must be titrated to the individual and prescribed by the physician.

Factors Affecting Rate

The infusion should be checked frequently to maintain the required rate of flow. Because of certain factors, the rate is subject to change.

Height of the Solution Bottle

Intravenous fluids run by gravity. Any change in gravity by raising or lowering the infusion container will alter the rate of flow. When patients receiving infusions are ambulated or transported to ancillary departments, the containers should be retained at the same height, or the speed of the infusion should be readjusted to maintain the prescribed rate of flow.

Clot in the Cannula

Any temporary stoppage of the infusion, such as a delay in hanging subsequent solutions, may cause a clot to form in the lumen of the cannula, partially or completely obstructing it. Clot formation may also occur when an increase in venous pressure in the infusion arm forces blood back into the cannula. This results from restriction of the venous circulation and is most commonly caused by 1) the blood pressure cuff on the infusion arm; 2) restraints placed on or above the infusion cannula; and 3) the patient's lying on the arm receiving the infusion.[2]

Change in Position of the Cannula

A change in the cannula's position may push the bevel of the cannula against or away from the wall of the vein. Special precautions should be taken to prevent speed shock or overloading of the vascular system by making sure that the solution is flowing freely before adjusting the rate.

Other Changes

Stimulation of the vasoconstrictors from any infusion of cold blood or irritating solution may cause venous spasm, impeding the rate of flow. A warm pack placed on the vein proximal to the infusion cannula will offset this reaction.

Trauma to the Vein

Any injury, such as phlebitis or thrombosis, that reduces the lumen of the vein will decrease the flow of the solution.

Clogged Vent

A clogged air vent in the administration set used with air-dependent containers will cause the infusion to stop.

If there is any question as to the rate of administration, the nurse should check with the physician. This applies to IV administration of drugs in solution. The rates should also be established on patients receiving two or more infusions simultaneously. Any change in the rate from that normally used should be ordered by the attending physician. The nurse should never exert positive pressure (manual pressure) to infuse solutions or blood.

Computation

When determining drops per minute the drop rate must be rounded to a whole number. The milliliters per hour also must be rounded to a whole number when gravity sets are being used.

Flow rate calculations require the following base of information: amount of solution to be infused, duration of the administration, and drop factor of the set to be used. First, determine the amount of solution to be administered; then divide that number by the delivery time[8]:

$$\frac{1000 \text{ mL}}{8 \text{ hr}} = 125 \text{ mL/hr}$$

Next, note the drop factor of the set being used. A macrodrip set takes 10, 15, or 20 drops to deliver 1 mL of solution.

$$\frac{\text{No. drops/mL of set}}{60 \text{ (min in an hr)}} \times \text{total hourly volume} = \text{no. drops/min}$$

$$\frac{\text{mL/hr} \times \text{drop factor of set}}{60} = \text{drops/min}$$

For microdrip or pediatric systems, the equation is:

$$\frac{\text{mL/h} \times \text{drop factor}}{60} = \text{drops/min}$$

INTRAVENOUS ACCESSORIES

In addition to the plethora of injection caps, latex ports, and needleless systems available, today's manufacturers also provide the safety of self-contained IV start kits such as SafeStart™ by Becton Dickinson's Vascular Access (Fig. 10-6) and IV loops, extension sets, Y adapters, obturators, and T connectors (Fig. 10-7). Systems such as Abbott's ADD-Vantage® unit dose system (Fig. 10-8) have simplified the administration of IV piggyback medications. Although standard systems still exist, the ADD-Vantage® unit incorporates a single-dose method of touch-free drug delivery.

FINAL INTRAVENOUS FILTERS

Filters prevent passage of undesirable substances into the vascular system (Fig. 10-9). Particulate filters of 1 or 5 μm are recommended when IV medications are being prepared. A bacteria-retentive filter, 0.2 μm in range, is recommended for the routine delivery of IV therapies. The time of change should coincide with the changing of the administration set.

Filters today come in diverse configurations, including add-on and integral units. Add-on filters should be securely connected to the administration set and treated as a part of that set. Integral filters are attached by the manufacturer to the administration set. To achieve final filtration, the filter should be located as close to the cannula site as possible. A 0.2-μm filter is considered an absolute, bacteria-retentive, air-eliminating filter and decreases the complications of infection and the potential for air embolism.

The industry standard is a membrane filter. Membrane filters are screen-type filters with uniformly sized pores that provide an absolute rating. A 0.2-μm screen-type filter will retain on the flat surface membrane all particles greater than 0.2 μm in size.

The United States Pharmacopeia (USP) has established an acceptable limit of particles for single-dose infusion as not more than 50 particles/mL that are equal to

FIGURE 10-6 SafeStart™ IV Start Pak™ components, with gloves. (Courtesy: Becton Dickinson Vascular Access, Sandy, UT)

FIGURE 10-7 (**A**) IV accessories. (Courtesy: Becton Dickinson Vascular Access, Sandy, UT) (**B**) Y connector. (Courtesy: Abbott Laboratories, North Chicago, IL)

FIGURE 10-8 ADD-Vantage® system for single-dose drug delivery. (Courtesy: Abbott Laboratories, North Chicago, IL)

FIGURE 10-9 (**A**) Air-eliminating properties of an IV filter. (**B**) Hydrophilic/hydrophobic membrane properties of an IV filter. (**C**) Optimal IV filter for add-on or in-line use. (Courtesy: Abbott Laboratories, North Chicago, IL)

or larger than 10.0 μm and not more than 5 particles/mL that are equal to or larger than 25.0 μm in effective linear dimension.

Pressure and Air

All filters have a certain pressure value at which they will allow the passage of air from one side of a wetted hydrophilic membrane to the other. This pressure valve is called the *bubble point* of that particular membrane. Because different filter materials (eg, hydrophobic, hydrophilic, depth, screen) have different wetting or nonwetting characteristics, both the pressure value of the material and the test liquid must be specified when bubble points are discussed. Water or saline solution, for example, would be the test fluid of choice when testing hydrophilic membranes for IV filters because solutions given IV are primarily water. Water is inexpensive, can be filtered easily for control of particulates and microorganisms, and is readily available. There are other advantages to using water as a bubble point test fluid. Water will test the wetting characteristics of hydrophilic membrane filters. To further define this point, an explanation of bubble point tests in relation to membranes is required.

Bubble Point Tests

Bubble point tests are conducted in a specific way. The material being tested is first wetted in the solution designated for performing the test. For example, if a flat membrane is being tested, the material would be soaked in the liquid until it has "wetted out." Then the material would be sealed into a holder that has a reservoir constructed over the membrane. More liquid would be poured on top of the membrane. Air pressures would then be applied to the other side of the membrane from below. As the air pressure increased, eventually a *steady* stream of bubbles would be seen rising through the liquid on top of the membrane. The pressure at which this happens is the bubble point of the material. This is called an *open bubble point* because the bubbles can be seen in real time or the time at which the bubble point actually happened.

Testing involves encapsulation of the membrane within an integral housing. Two different types of bubble point tests may be performed: open bubble and closed bubble point. An open bubble point can only be performed if the direction of normal flow is such that the bubbles produced can be seen as they are formed. This means that the housing of the filter must be transparent and the "downstream side" of the membrane can be observed. This test is performed by first flowing the test liquid through the device at low pressures until it is wetted out. Usually, this pressure is the same as that used in administering solution by gravity feed pressures (36–39 inches of water). Then, after the membrane is wetted out, air pressure is applied as before. The bubble point has been reached when a steady stream of bubbles is seen on the downstream side of the membrane.

A *closed bubble point* must be performed when the downstream side of the membrane may not be visualized. The general manipulations of the test are the same, but because the bubbles are not visible as they occur, the distal (outlet) port of the device must be observed. When a steady stream of bubbles exits at the distal port, this is the closed bubble point. Closed bubble points will result in slightly higher values than open bubble points because the air pressure during the test is steadily increasing, and it will take more time for the air bubbles to escape through the distal port. If the pressure is increased slowly, the test will be more accurate.

Testing of membranes and filter devices used in IV therapy with water is significant. Most hydrophilic membranes incorporate either external (applied after they are made) or internal (in the base formula) wetting agents to render them more wettable with water. It is particularly important in IV therapy because it is critical that the membrane should wet properly so that air will not pass the membrane at low pressures.

The 0.2-μm air-venting filters automatically vent air through a nonwettable (hydrophobic) membrane and permit uniform high gravity flow rates via large wettable (hydrophilic) membranes. They prevent an air block, which could ultimately result in a plugged cannula.

Filters are also rated according to the psi of pressure they will withstand, an important consideration in selecting the proper filter. The filter should withstand the psi exerted by the infusion pump or rupture may occur. If the psi rating of the housing is less than that of the membrane, excess force will break the housing, leaving the filter intact.

Optimal filters should 1) automatically vent air; 2) retain bacteria, fungi, and endotoxins; 3) be nonbinding of drugs; 4) allow high gravity flow rates; and 5) have a pressure tolerance to withstand the psi of the infusion pump. Pressure rating of the housing, when less than that of the filter membrane, may provide added protection.

LATEX INJECTION PORTS

The latex injection port or catheter cap (Fig. 10-10) may be used to adapt any indwelling device to an intermittent infusion device. Available either as an individual unit, or incorporated within the design of an over-the-needle (ONC) or winged infusion set, the use of the latex injection port has simplified the administration of intermittent therapies. Intermittent devices may also be called "heparin locks," "INTS," or "PRN adapters" because heparin or saline is routinely instilled into the cap and its housing to maintain patency. Most products now include a Luer lock device to prevent accidental dislodgment of the cap.

Burron Medical features the Safsite® injection cap. Becton Dickinson's Vascular Access Division provides a number of injection caps to meet all clinical needs.

The Click-Lock™ is a product of ICU Medical and was the first positive-locking IV catheter-connecting device (Fig. 10-11). It uses a removable stainless steel needle in a clear plastic housing that snap locks onto the injection port.

NEEDLELESS SYSTEMS

On ongoing technology is that of the needleless system, which has revolutionized infusion therapy. Consisting of a blunt-tipped plastic insertion device and an injection port that opens and immediately reseals, this system was developed to re-

FIGURE 10-10 (**A**) PRN Adapters, used to convert indwelling IV catheters or infusion sets to intermittent administration devices. (Courtesy: Becton Dickinson Vascular Access, Sandy, UT) (**B**) Burron Safsite® injection cap. (Courtesy: Burron Medical Inc., Bethlehem, PA)

duce the incidence of accidental needlestick injuries and to promote safety in infusion practice. Again, diverse systems are available to meet clinical needs in many settings.

Baxter Healthcare's InterLink™ IV Access System (Fig. 10-12) eliminates needlestick risks in a wide range of applications, requiring minimal change in technique. The system includes a vial access cannula for single-dose vial access and a lever lock cannula securely locking all injection site connections.

Abbott Laboratories provides a LifeShield Connector/Docking Station with prepierced reseals and a blunt cannula (Fig. 10-13, p. 156). The system is compatible with Abbott and most competitive standard Y sites and male adapter plugs.

The Centurion® Kleen-Needle® is a low-profile recessed needle that luer locks onto a latex post for safe IV pushes, flushes, blood draws and secure tape-free line connections (Fig. 10-14, p. 157).

Quest Medical features a product known as the "No Needles" set (Fig. 10-15, p. 157) in which all ports are Luer lock, back-check valves prevent retrograding of drug or solution, syringes may be left attached throughout a procedure, and one-handed injection is possible. The set is adaptable to a wide number of clinical settings, including anesthesia. ICU Medical's Clave™ Needleless Connector is a recent addition to the field of needless systems (Fig. 10-16, p. 158).

Acme United manufactures an IV bubble/board system for use in stabilizing infusion sites. The bubble provides a cushion and protection to the IV site, catheter, hub, and tubing to help prevent dislodgment. The anatomically molded board provides enhanced comfort and support for the site (Fig. 10-17, p. 159).

PERIPHERAL VASCULAR ACCESS DEVICES

Innovations in catheter technology have produced catheters to meet the patient's every need, from peripheral infusion to the most sophisticated therapy. Catheters vary in gauge, length, composition, and design. The composition may be PVC, polyurethane, or silicone. Thin-walled catheters provide increased flow rates, which allow smaller-sized catheters to be used. Most catheters are radiopaque or contain a stripe of radiopaque material for radiographic visualization.

Catheters may be ONC, where the catheter, mounted on the needle, is slipped off the needle into the vein and the needle is removed; or inside-the-needle (INC), where the catheter is pushed through the needle until the desired length is in the vein, and the cutting edge is protected by a shield.

Some catheters are provided with wings and all the advantages of a small-vein needle on insertion and on taping. The adapter of the IV set connection is located a few inches from the catheter and provides ease and better technique when changing sets, reducing the potential for mechanical phlebitis and contamination. Such catheters are available with injection sites as an integral part of the catheter; the mixing of drugs or blood components with primary parenteral fluid is reduced to a minimum (0.4 mL), minimizing the potential of incompatibilities.

Over-the-Needle Catheter

The ONC is the most widely used device for peripheral infusion therapy. The introducer needle, or stylet, is removed once successful cannulation is accomplished. The flexibility of this device, diversity of size and length ranges, and its safety offer patients freedom of

FIGURE 10-11 Click-Lock™ locking (junction securement) device. (Courtesy: ICU Medical, San Clemente, CA)

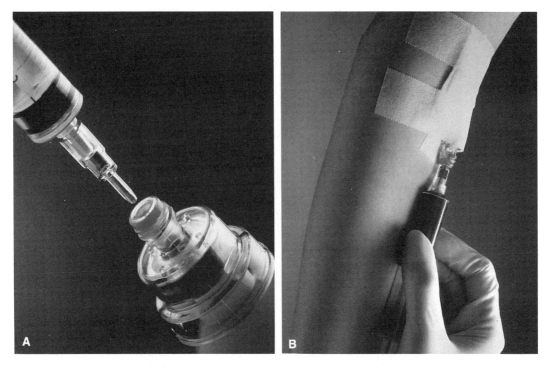

FIGURE 10-12 (**A**) Interlink™ IV Access System components. (**B**) Venous sampling using the Interlink™ IV Access System. (Courtesy: Baxter Healthcare, Deerfield, IL)

FIGURE 10-13   Abbott Laboratories LifeShield needleless system with prepierced reseals and blunt cannula. (Courtesy: Abbott Laboratories, North Chicago, IL)

movement. Consistent with Intravenous Nurses Society (INS) Standards of Practice, the cannula should be placed for a definitive therapeutic or diagnostic indication. Practice dictates using the smallest gauge, shortest length cannula capable of accomplishing the prescribed therapy. All such catheters should be radiopaque and only one device should be used for each attempt at venipuncture. All products should be inspected for integrity before use. Peripheral venous cannulas should be removed every 48 hours and immediately on suspected contamination or complication. Manufacturers' guidelines for the use of their specific products should be adhered to at all times. New technology offers protection against accidental needle sticks. Insyte Auto Guard instantly encases the needle inside a tamper-resistant, transport safety barrel. (Fig. 10-18, p. 160)

Through-the-Needle Catheters

The through-the-needle catheter (TNC) combines an 8- to 12-inch catheter with an introducer needle, which should be protected by a shield after insertion. Historically, these catheters have been used when venous access has been poor and when administration of caustic drugs or hypertonic solutions is required. They are rarely used today and have been replaced in many clinical settings by the peripherally inserted central catheter (PICC).

FIGURE 10-14   The Centurion® Kleen-Needle® System is safe, simple, and universally adaptable. (Courtesy: Tri-State Hospital Supply, Howell, MI)

FIGURE 10-15   "No Needles" set. Check-valve extension sets (**A** and **B**) simplify drug administration with syringes and/or pumps (**C**) (Courtesy: Quest Medical, Inc., Dallas, TX)

FIGURE 10-16 (**A**) Piggy Safe Needless Connector. (**B**) Clave™ Needleless Connector. (Courtesy: ICU Medical, Inc., San Clemente, CA)

Today's catheters are clearly designed for central and peripheral placement. Although they use a through-the-needle concept, the needles are of steel or plastic that splits or peels away, leaving only a pliable catheter exiting the skin's surface.

Winged Infusion Needle

The winged infusion needle (Fig. 10-19, p. 161) is available as an ONC or steel needle. Flexible wings are a part of both devices and are easily grasped during the insertion technique. Once the device is placed within the lumen of the vessel, the wings are flattened against the skin and provide an anchor for stabilization.

Again, manufacturers have kept pace with demands for advanced product concepts, and a variation of the ONC winged infusion needle incorporates a Y-shaped design with a latex cap to permit intermittent infusion of subsequent medications or solutions and protection against accidental needle sticks (Fig. 10-20, p. 161). The thin-walled design of the winged infusion needle facilitates placement; however, the risk of infiltration with the steel needle type deters many professionals from using this product for any other than short-term use.

INSTRUCTIONS FOR USE

I.V. Board

1 Place armboard in correct position. The raised ball of the armboard should rest comfortably in the palm of the hand.

2 Secure in place with cohesive tape.

I.V. Bubble

1 Inflate the Bubble by covering the hole in the center of the foam with your thumb; pump and release until firmly inflated.

2 Position window over the I.V. insertion site, placing the foam next to the skin.

3 Position tubing at the crease.

4 Secure around limb with velcro straps. Trim straps to desired length.

FIGURE 10-17 IV boards and IV bubble use. (Courtesy: United Corp., Fairfield, CT)

CATHETER MATERIALS

Polytetrafluoroethylene (Teflon) is less thrombogenic and less inflammatory than polyurethane or PVC. Vialon is a new advancement in material. Nonhemolytic and free of plasticizers, it is slick when wetted and softens after insertion, minimizing vein trauma and clot induction.

Aquavene is an elastomeric hydrogel that undergoes softening and changes in dimension on contract with aqueous fluids (blood). The complete softening and expansion process takes approximately 90 minutes. Aquavene cannulas expand precisely two gauge sizes—they do not continue to expand beyond this fixed unit. Catheter cannulas consist of an Aquavene outer layer and thin polyurethane inner lining. The polyurethane lining is impermeable and prevents hydration from the inner lumen. The outer Aquavene layer hydrates by absorbing water and electrolytes from the blood and plasma. This type of product permits long-term placement when venous access is limited or when therapy is ordered for a specific period of time. Considered

FIGURE 10-18   Insyte® AutoGuard IV catheter. (Courtesy: Becton Dickinson Vascular Access, Sandy, UT)

a peripheral venous catheter according to the INS standards, professionals are encouraged to develop policies and procedures relevant to indwell time consistent with those standards and institutional guidelines.

ELECTRONIC INFUSION DEVICES

Standards of Practice for Flow-Control Devices

Consistent with the INS Standards of Practice, the rate of IV infusions should be routinely regulated by manual flow-control devices to ensure accurate delivery of the prescribed therapy. Electronic infusion devices should be used when warranted by the patient's age and condition, setting, and prescribed therapy. The nursing professional is responsible and accountable for the use of EIDs. Use of EIDs, deployment of them, selection criteria, and classifications should be outlined in institutional policy and procedure manuals. The nurse's knowledge base concerning EIDs should include at the minimum:[5]

- Indications for use
- Mechanical operation
- Troubleshooting
- The psi rating
- Safe usage

The EIDs are invaluable in neonatal, pediatric, and adult intensive care units, where critical infusions of small volumes of fluid or doses of high-potency drugs are required. These devices have increased the level of safety in parenteral therapy. Today, the risk of air embolism is reduced by alarm systems and by the automatic inter-

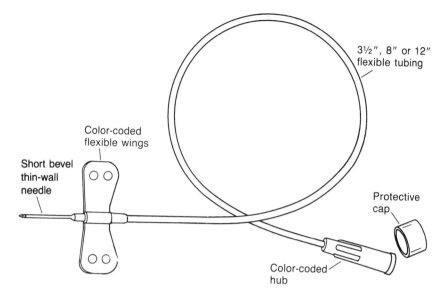

FIGURE 10-19 Winged infusion needle. (Courtesy: Terumo, Inc., Somerset, NJ)

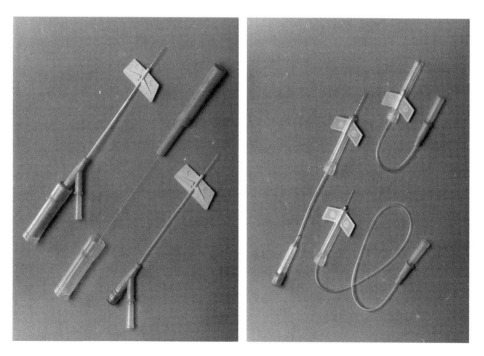

FIGURE 10-20 (**A**) Saf-T-Intima™ IV catheter system. (**B**) Saf-T E-Z Set® winged infusion set. (Courtesy: Becton Dickinson Vascular Access, Sandy, UT)

ruption of the infusion when a container empties. A controlled rate of flow reduces the risk of circulatory overload.

The devices have saved valuable nursing time; uniform control of fluid eliminates the need to count drops and continually adjust flow rates. Plugging of the cannula, which occurs when blood backs into the cannula because of an increase in venous pressure from coughing, crying, or straining, is eliminated. The pressure generated by the EID pump may exceed the maximum venous pressure.

AMBULATORY INFUSION DEVICES

Self-care is an important component of our health care delivery system. The development of compact, battery-driven EIDs has simplified care in diverse ambulatory clinical settings (Tables 10-1 and 10-2).

External Infusion Pumps

The size, weight, and portability of the unit are important considerations in choosing a system. An active patient must be comfortable wearing the lightest pump possible; a sedentary patient may prefer the advantages of a larger device. Accessories and loading procedures vary with the manufacturer and the product selected. Infusion capacity may dictate the choice of the system. Pump-specific sets may be required, as seen in the patient receiving nutritional support or pain medication.

Integral safety features include:

- Occlusion alarm
- Low-volume safety alarm
- Low-battery alarm

Competition in this exciting area of growth has stimulated many new companies to enter the electronic infusion market, resulting in greater availability of more sophisticated products for the professional IV nurse.

Elastomeric Balloon Devices

An elastomeric device is made of a soft, rubberized material capable of inflating to a predetermined volume. The balloon deflates at a rate determined by the diameter of the restricting outlet located in the preattached tubing or in the neck of the container. The size of the tunnel controls the passage of solution. The balloon, safely encapsulated inside a rigid, transparent container, becomes the reservoir for solution. The shape of this device is manufacturer specific and may be round, disk shaped, or cylindrical. A tamper-proof port for injecting medication into the balloon is attached. Typically, the capacity is 50 to 100 mL and the devices are for one-time use only.

Baxter's Intermate® (Fig. 10-21, p. 168) provides fixed rates to ensure accurate dosages and pharmacokinetic consistency. No IV pole or electric cord is needed. The design, in various configurations, is small and lightweight. As a single-use disposable item, it simplifies single-dose infusion therapies.

Spring-Coil Piston Syringes

The syringe volume ranges from 30 to 60 mL and has a spring with which to power the plunger in the absence of manual pressure. Like the elastomeric balloon, this device has limited applications and is for one-time use only. The syringe is filled by withdrawing the piston and overextending the spring. As the spring regains its shape, it forces the piston down, expelling its contents.

Spring-Coil Container

This device combines the principles of the spring-coil piston syringe. The container is multiuse, small volume. An overextended spring in an enclosed space between two disks seeks to collapse, pulling the top and bottom together and forcing the fluid contents out of the restricting orifice. Handy and convenient for the ambulatory patient, it is ideal for home use.

THERAPY-SPECIFIC DEVICES

The EIDs are finding increasing uses in keep-open arterial lines and infusion of drugs, blood, and viscous fluids such as hyperalimentation solutions. Advances in technology have provided us with more sophisticated devices. Many types and models are available. In general, pumps are devices that generate flow under positive pressure. Such devices may be peristaltic, syringe, and pulsatile. Controllers are devices that generate flow by gravity and are capable of either drop counting or volumetric delivery.

Syringe Pumps

Many manufacturers have met the demand for syringe infusion systems. Syringe pumps are calibrated in mL/h, are used with standard disposable syringes, and provide smooth and precise delivery of low volumes of solution to specific patient populations (Table 10-3, p. 170).

Controllers

Controllers do not exert positive pressure greater than the head height of the infusion container, which is generally 2 psi. The controller is used to monitor the infusion for accuracy, to sound an alarm if flow is interrupted, and to provide even, consistent delivery of fluid. A controller uses drop-sensor technology. Manufacturers have developed variations on this theme, specific to patient populations and institutional needs.

For example, Abbott's LifeCare® 75 BREEZE is a controller that uses a standard administration set, is easily set up, and incorporates graphics on a screen (Fig. 10-22, p. 172).

Positive-Pressure Infusion Pumps

A positive-pressure device overcomes vascular resistance, tubing compromises, such as excessive length, and the normal elements of physics that cause an IV to improperly function (see rate of flow discussion).

Text continues on p.169

TABLE 10-1
Rate-Restricted IV Administration Set Infusion Systems

Manufacturer	Product	Therapies Delivered	Pumping Mechanism	Product Size	Product Weight
Abbott Laboratories	Snap Dose™	Antibiotics, intermittent medications	Chemical reaction	4" × 6"	68 g
Baxter Healthcare	Intermate™	Antibiotics, intermittent medications	Elastomeric mechanical device	5" × 2.5" 7" × 2.5"	Not stated Not stated
	Infusor	Chemotherapy, longer term continuous infusions	Elastomeric mechanical device	6.5" × 1.2" Not stated 7" × 2.5"	4 oz Not stated 307 g
Block Medical	Homepump®	Antibiotics, intermittent medications	Elastomeric mechanical device	Not stated Not stated Not stated	Not stated 6 oz Not stated
	Homepump Eclipse™	Antibiotics, intermittent medications	Elastomeric mechanical device	Not stated Not stated Not stated Not stated Not stated Not stated	Not stated 5 oz 5 oz Not stated Not stated Not stated
I-Flow/Solo Pak Pharmaceuticals	SideKick™	Antibiotics, intermittent medications	Coiled spring drive	1.9" × 3.7" 2.1" × 4.0"	8.7 oz 11.5 oz
	Paragon™	Short-term, intermittent, or long-term continuous infusions	Precision, multiple spring drive	2.3" × 4.0"	13 oz
	Elite™	Short-term, intermittent, or long-term continuous infusions	Precision, multiple spring drive	2.3" × 4.0"	13 oz
McGaw	ReadyMED™	Antibiotics, intermittent medications	Elastomeric mechanical device	Not stated Not stated Not stated	Not stated Not stated Not stated
Medication Delivery Devices	maxx™100	Antibiotics, intermittent medications	Electronic controlled pressure device	6.7" × 4.7" × 1.4"	10.5 oz
	maxx™250	Antibiotics, intermittent medications	Electronic controlled pressure device	5.4" × 8.6" × 1.9"	17.0 oz
River Medical	SmartDose™100	Antibiotics, intermittent medications	Chemical reaction	7.6" × 2.9" × 1.7"	5.9 oz when filled
	SmartDose™250	Antibiotics, intermittent medications	Chemical reaction	9.0" × 3.6" × 1.8"	13.9 oz when filled
Secure Medical	MedFlow II™	Antibiotics, intermittent medications	Elastomeric mechanical device	2.75" × 4.25" 2.75" × 5.5" 2.75" × 7.0"	Not stated Not stated Not stated

(From Saladow, J. [1995]. Making sense of the options. *Infusion Magazine,* April 26–27. Alexandria, VA: National Home Infusion Publishers.)

Reservoir Volumes	Flow Rates	Accuracy	Power	Battery Life	Additional Comments
100 mL	50, 100, or 200 mL/h	±15%	N/A	N/A	
105 mL	50, 100, or 200 mL/h	±15%	N/A	N/A	
275 mL	50, 100, or 250 mL/h	±15%	N/A	N/A	
				N/A	
65 mL	0.5, 2.0 mL/h	Not stated	N/A	N/A	
95 mL	0.5 mL/h	Not stated	N/A	N/A	
275 mL	1.5, 2.0, 5.0, or 10 mL/h	Not stated		N/A	
50 mL	50 mL/h	±15%	N/A	N/A	
100 mL	100 or 200 mL/h	±15%	N/A	N/A	
200 mL	175 mL/h	±15%	N/A	N/A	
50 mL	50 mL/h	±15%	N/A	N/A	The Homepump Eclipse products do not have an outer shell, making them lighter and smaller than other elastomeric infusion systems. As such, they potentially take up less storage space in both the home infusion company and the patient's home.
100 mL	100 mL/h	±15%	N/A	N/A	
200 mL	100 or 200 mL/h	±15%	N/A	N/A	
250 mL	175 mL/h	±15%	N/A	N/A	
400 mL	100 or 200 mL/h	±15%	N/A	N/A	
500 mL	100 mL/h	±15%	N/A	N/A	
65 mL	50, 100, or 200 mL/h	±15%	N/A	N/A	SideKick products are capable of delivering up to two drugs at one time.
110 mL	50, 100, or 200 mL/h	±15%	N/A	N/A	
110 mL	0.5, 1.0, 2.0, 4.0, 50, 100, or 200 mL/h	±10%	N/A	N/A	
110 mL	0.5, 1.0, 2.0, 4.0, 50, 100, or 200 mL/h	±10%	N/A	N/A	Has built-in battery for notification of fluid level and empty and near-empty alarm conditions. Battery life is 2 y.
50 mL	50 mL/h	±15%	N/A	N/A	ReadyMED products have visual infusion progress and completion indicators. They also have color-coded sets and container shells.
100 mL	100 or 200 mL/h	±15%	N/A	N/A	
250 mL	50, 100 or 167 mL/h	±15%		N/A	
100 mL	50, 100, or 200 mL/h	±15%	9V alkaline no AC power not rechargeable	5 days	Alarm features: occlusion, low battery, end of infusion, no disposable installed, open pump cover, unauthorized disposable, and pump malfunction.
250 mL	50, 100, or 200 mL/h	±15%	9V alkaline no AC power not rechargeable	5 days	Alarm features: occlusion, low battery, end of infusion, no disposable installed, open pump cover, unauthorized disposable, and pump malfunction.
110 mL	50, 100, 175, or 200 mL/h	±15%	N/A	N/A	Has a vial adaptor for mixing medications with stability limitations just prior to infusion.
265 mL	100, 175, 200 mL/h	±15%	N/A	N/A	Has a vial adaptor for mixing medications with stability limitations just prior to infusion.
100 mL	50, 100, or 200 mL/h	±15%	N/A	N/A	Sets are available with either 1.2 or a .02 μm filter.
200 mL	175 mL/h	±15%	N/A	N/A	
300 mL	100 mL/h	±15%	N/A	N/A	

TABLE 10-2
Ambulatory Electronic Infusion Pumps for the Infusion of Antibiotics

Manufacturer	Product	Size	Weight	Accuracy	Flow Rates	Volume Limits	KVO Rate	Power Sources
Abbott Laboratories	Provider® 5500	Not stated	Not stated	±3%	0.1–250 mL/h	Not stated	Not stated	AC; 2 9V alkaline batteries
Block Medical	Verifuse®	6.4" × 3.1" × 1.1"	17 oz	±6%	0.1–300 mL/h	0.1–6500 mL	0.1–0.1 mL/h	AC; 2 9V alkaline batteries; rechargeable NICAD batteries
Creative Medical Development	EZ-Flow 80-2™	6.75" × 3.5" × 1.27"	14 oz	±6%	0.6–250 mL/h	5–2000 mL	0.0–1.0 mL/h	AC; rechargeable battery pack using NICAD batteries
I-Flow	VIVUS™ 2000	7.75" × 4.5" × 1.875"	32 oz	±10%	0.1–200 mL/h per channel	Not stated	0.1–200 mL/h	AC; 5 or 10 AA batteries
	VIVUS™ 4000	7.75" × 4.5" × 1.875"	37 oz	±10%	0.1–200 mL/h per channel	Not stated	0.1–200 mL/h	AC; 5 or 10 AA batteries
Infusion Technologies	Vector™ MTI	5.6" × 3.5" × 1.4"	14.5 oz	±8%	0.1–400 mL/h	0.1–4000 mL	0.0–5.0 mL/h	AC; 2 9V batteries
MicroJect	Model 200	5" × 2" × 88"	5.8 oz	±5%	10–200 mL/h	Not stated	1 mL/h	2 AA alkaline batteries, not replaceable
Patient Solutions	MedMate™ 1100	4.4" × 3.3" × 1.4"	17 oz	Not stated	0.1–500 mL/h	0.1–9999 mL	0.1–9.9 mL/h	2 9V batteries, alkaline or lithium or optional external rechargeable

Battery Life	Recharge Time	Alarms	Proprietary Disposables	Additional Comments
Not stated	Not stated	Air-in-line, occlusion, system malfunction, and low battery	Uses proprietary IV administration sets	Programmable in mg or mL. Can infuse intermittent or continuous infusions; also can do PCA infusions.
Not stated	24 h	Door open, air-in-line, pumping complete, bar code fault, low reservoir, overvoltage, change batteries, occlusion, end of program, low batteries, bad batteries, malfunction, and pump interrupted	Uses proprietary IV administration sets. Infuses from standard IV containers	Bar code programmable, PC-based programming, and has a hand-held key pad accessory for on-site programming capability. Has a home base that allows access to equipment via modem for patient status, to change a program, or to print out a status report. In addition to antibiotics, can infuse TPN, PCA, and chemotherapy regimens.
1.5 liters minimum with full charge	Not stated	Infusion complete, source line occlusion/pump stopped, infusion line occlusion/pump stopped, low battery, and on-off switch	Uses proprietary IV administration sets with reservoir attached or with a spike that can be used with standard IV containers	Has optional KVO settings and six standard intermittent delivery cycle settings.
5–10 liters	Single-use batteries	Low and depleted battery, occlusion, stop mode (walkaway), empty reservoir, internal malfunction, motor malfunction, and open door	Uses proprietary IV administration sets, infuses from standard IV containers	Can infuse two medications, either continuously or sequentially, has remote programming and control capabilities, provides status reports via modem, and is programmed with the use of a computer. In addition to antibiotics, can infuse TPN, PCA, chemotherapy and other regimens. Can be programmed for circadian infusions.
5–10 liters	Single-use batteries	Low and depleted battery, occlusion stop mode (walkaway), empty reservoir, internal malfunction, motor malfunction, and open door	Uses proprietary IV administration sets, infuses from standard IV containers	Can infuse up to four medications, either continuously or sequentially, has remote programming and control capabilities and provides status reports via modem, and is programmed with the use of a computer. In addition to antibiotics, can infuse TPN, PCA, chemotherapy, and other regimens. Can be programmed for circadian infusions.
5000 mL	Single-use batteries	Reservoir empty, infusion finished, overpressure, check cassette, dead battery, system malfunction, air-in-line (optional), warnings on low battery, unattended, and low reservoir	Uses proprietary IV administration sets with reservoir attached or can infuse out of standard IV containers.	In addition to antibiotics, can infuse TPN, PCA, chemotherapy, epidural, and other regimens. Has custom programming options for circadian, multidose, and multivolume infusions. Has RS232 connector for remote programming capability.
15 liters	Single-use batteries	Obstruction (upstream and downstream), change driver, and malfunction	Uses proprietary IV set that allows for infusion from standard IV containers	Pump driver is disposable and is to be replaced on the conclusion of therapy or the delivery of 15 liters of fluid, whichever occurs first. Product is scheduled for release in the fourth quarter of 1995.
3000 mL at 500 mL/h	Not stated	Air-in-line, occlusion, door open, dose complete, low bag, bag end, dose due, low battery, change battery, call-back alert, program error, prime limit, and system fault	Uses proprietary IV administration sets with reservoir attached or can infuse out of standard IV containers	In addition to antibiotics, can infuse TPN, PCA, chemotherapy, and other regimens. Can infuse in either mL/h or mg.

(continued)

TABLE 10-2
Ambulatory Electronic Infusion Pumps for the Infusion of Antibiotics *(Continued)*

Manufacturer	Product	Size	Weight	Accuracy	Flow Rates	Volume Limits	KVO Rate	Power Sources
Sabratek	Sabratek 6060	4.5" × 3.75" × 2.25"	16 oz	±15%	0.1–400 mL/h	0.1–9999 mL	0.1–10 mL/h	AC; 2 9V alkaline or lithium batteries
SIMS Deltec	CADD Plus®	6.4" × 3.5" × 1.1"	15 oz	±6% nominal	0–75 mL/h	0–150 mL	0.0–10 mL/h	9V alkaline or lithium battery

PCA, patient-controlled analgesia; TPN, total parenteral nutrition.
(From Saladow, J. [1995]. Making sense of the options. *Infusion Magazine,* April, 28–29. Alexandria, VA: National Home Infusion Publishers.)

INTERMATE® INFUSION DEVICE

FIGURE 10-21   Baxter Intermate®. (Courtesy: Baxter Healthcare, Deerfield, IL)

Battery Life	Recharge Time	Alarms	Proprietary Disposables	Additional Comments
25 h at 125 mL/h	Single-use batteries	Air-in-line, door open, high rate, down occlusion, up occlusion, hold, low battery, empty battery, back-up battery, dose due, flow stop missing, low bag volume infusion complete, reprogram, remove remote PCA cord, and pump malfunction	Uses proprietary IV administration sets cassette. Can infuse out of standard IV containers or out of proprietary 150 mL reservoir set.	Has several separate delivery profiles available, each with a different delivery pattern: continuous, auto ramp, intermittent, 25 periods, and PCA. Has automatic anti-free-flow protection. Programs in either English or Spanish, mL/h or mg, and titration capabilities. Product scheduled to become available in late April 1995.
Not stated	Single use batteries	Power-up fault, pump in stop mode, low battery, depleted battery, low reservoir volume, programmed volume depleted, high pressure, and system error	Uses proprietary IV administration sets with 50 mL or 100 mL reservoir bag attached. Can also infuse out of standard IV containers with an IV spike set.	In addition to antibiotics and other intermittent therapy, can infuse continuous delivery of medications. Has a delayed start capability.

Pressure exerted by the unit is expressed in psi or mm Hg. One psi and 50 mm Hg exert the same amount of pressure.[4] The psi of an EID is important because it may affect the type of filter being used or the ability of the unit to infuse fluids through arterial lines. The psi should not exceed the pressure the filter can withstand or a rupture may occur; when the pump is used for arterial infusion, the psi must be high enough to overcome arterial pressure. Positive pressure pumps are used in most clinical settings.

Volumetric Infusion Pumps

With the volumetric pump, the unit calculates the volume delivered by measuring the volume displaced in a reservoir that is a component of the disposable administration set. The mechanism of action may be piston generated or linear.

Volumetric pumps such as Sigma International's Sigma 6000+ programmable infusion pump meet a variety of clinical needs and are cost effective, using standard IV tubing (Fig. 10-23, p. 172). Sigma's Model 8000 is a multiuse, linear peristaltic device with clinical applications for administration of large-volume parenterals, for use with syringe pumps, and for neonates, patients in need of patient-controlled analgesia, and those in the home care setting. The device incorporates a set-based anti–free-flow protection mechanism and is compatible with standard gravity IV sets supplied by Abbott, Baxter, McGaw, Braun, and several other companies (Fig. 10-24, p. 173).

The field of external EIDs includes those that are IV pole dependent yet meet a wealth of needs in the clinical setting. The Gemini PC-1, manufactured with flow- and volume-ramping capability, and the Gemini PC-2 are in Imed's product line (Fig. 10-25, p. 173). PC-1 and PC-2 do not allow free flow on infusion set removal but still allow users the option of gravity flow. Gemini PC-2 is a multichannel device, capable of simultaneously infusing from and individually monitoring two or more IV lines.

TABLE 10-3
Syringe Infusion Systems

Manufacturer	Product	Pumping Mechanism	Size	Weight	Accuracy	Flow Rates
Bard/Baxter	Mini-Infuser™ 150XL Single Speed	Syringe driver	8.5" × 4.5" × 1.6"	1 lb 2 oz	±3%	Dependent on syringe brand and size
	Mini-Infuser™ 300XL Three Speed	Syringe driver	8.5" × 4.5" × 1.6"	1 lb 2 oz	±3%	Dependent on syringe brand and size
Baxa	Dual Rate Infuser	Syringe driver	8" × 3" × 2.5"	1 lb	±3%	Normal and slow
B-D/McGaw	Infuser	Syringe driver	Not stated	2 lbs	±3%	1.5–360 mL/h
Excelsior	ESP Infusion System	Worm drive	9.2" × 4.7" × 1.7"	1.2 lbs	±3%	Normal, slow, x-slow
3M	Medifuse™	Mechanical syringe driver	13" × 2.5" × 2"	1 lb	Not stated	Dependent on syringe and set size
Medex	2001	Electronic syringe driver	7.5" × 4.5" × 3.0"	2.5 lbs	±3%	.01–378.0 mL/h
	2010	Electronic syringe driver	7.5" × 4.5" × 3.0"	2.5 lbs	±3%	.01–378.0 mL/h

McGaw's Intelligent Pump® (Fig. 10-26A, p. 174) provides volume precision of primary and secondary lines. McGaw's Profile™ 521 Plus Intelligent Pump® (Fig. 10-26B) is widely used for delivery of nutritional support and IV medications by volumetric displacement of fluid. McGaw's MicroRate® Plus Intelligent Pump® (Fig. 10-26C) is designed to meet the needs of the neonatal or pediatric patient.

Features

A wide assortment of features accompanies EIDs in today's complex health care setting. Nurses must be familiar with the literature and with the device to be used`and must take all precautions to ensure safe, efficient operation. The impact of changing

Syringes Accepted	Power	Battery Life	Recharge Time	Alarms	Proprietary Disposable	Additional Comments
5–60 mL	4 size C alkaline batteries	400 h	N/A	End of infusion, occlusion	36" and 60" microbore extension sets	Product available through Baxter Healthcare.
5–60 mL	4 size C alkaline batteries	400 h	N/A	End of infusion, occlusion	36" and 60" microbore extension sets	Product available through Baxter Healthcare.
3–35 mL	6 size AA alkaline batteries	400 h	N/A	Occlusion, end of infusion, overinfusion, low battery, end of life	None	Has built in wire hanger or optional IV pole mount.
Not stated	Battery operated	Not stated	Not stated	Occlusion, low battery, infusion complete	None	Programmable variable speed pump—time of infusion is adjustable from 10 to 60 min. Product is available through McGaw.
3–60 mL	4 size C alkaline batteries	400 h	N/A	Attention, low battery	60" Microbore tubing	Recommends use of Monoject syringes but can also use B-D syringes.
10–35 mL	Mechanical mechanism	N/A	N/A	None	55" Medifuse sets	Specific Medifuse sets determine rate of infusion.
1–60 mL	Rechargeable batteries; has AC adapter	10 h @ 5 mL/h with a 60-mL syringe	16 h maximum	Near empty, empty, volume limit, occlusion, system malfunction, low battery, depleted battery, syringe not loaded, KVO, alarm temporary delay, alarm audio volume	None	Has continuous, volume time, intermittent manual, and intermittent manual and automatic infusion modes; has a series of status alert messages.
1–60 mL	Rechargeable batteries; has AC adapter	10 h @ 5 mL/h with a 60-mL syringe	16 h maximum	Near empty, empty, volume limit, occlusion, system malfunction, low battery, depleted battery, syringe not loaded, KVO, alarm temporary delay alarm- audio volume	None	Infuses in mg/h or in mL/h; has a series of status alert messages. Has body weight, mass, continuous and volume/time infusion modes.

technology has moved us far beyond the basics of instrumentation to a field known as computer-generated technology.

Computer-Generated Technology

Now and into the future, the nursing professional is not as limited by time and space. Research, input, and data will all be computer generated. The computer will be the focal point of the IV drug delivery system. Electronic flow is now the norm rather than the exception. EIDs today are available in diverse sizes and technologies and may be found in a broad range of clinical settings. The Omni-Flow Therapist IV

Text continues of p. 174

FIGURE 10-22 LifeCare® 75 BREEZE Volumetric Controller. (Courtesy: Abbott Laboratories, North Chicago, IL)

FIGURE 10-23 Sigma International 6000+. (Courtesy: Sigma International, Medina, NY)

FIGURE 10-24 Sigma 8000 infusion pump.
(Courtesy: Sigma International, Medina, NY)

FIGURE 10-25 (**A**) Gemini PC-1. (**B**) Gemini PC-2. (Courtesy: Imed Corp., San Diego, CA)

FIGURE 10-26 McGaw devices. (**A**) McGaw 522 Intelligent Pump®. (**B**) McGaw Profile™ 521 *Plus* Intelligent Pump®. (**C**) McGaw MicroRate® *Plus* Intelligent Pump®. (Courtesy: McGaw, Inc., Irvine, CA)

Medication Management System by Abbott (Fig. 10-27) has a range of 1 to 700 mL/h, programmable in nine units of measure, with bar codes generated by the pharmacy. It is capable of infusing four medications simultaneously or intermittently (or both) from bags, bottles, or syringes.

Tapering or Ramping

These terms are used to describe the progressive increase or decrease of infusion rate.

Free Flow

Free-flow alarms may be lifesaving if the administration set has no intrinsic valves or reservoirs that require motion of the pumping mechanism to propel the solution. Many pumps incorporate free-flow alarms that are capable of detecting open flow of solution to the patient. Others have internal clamps or devices that lock into place when tubing is removed from the pump, preventing free flow of solution to the patient. Other safety features are available on a number of products.

FIGURE 10-27 Omni-Flow Therapist. (Courtesy: Abbott Laboratories, North Chicago, IL)

ECRI AND GENERAL PURPOSE INFUSION PUMPS

The Emergency Care Research Institute, now known as ECRI, is an independent nonprofit agency dedicated to improving the safety, efficacy, and cost effectiveness of health care technology, facilities, and procedures. Between January 1988 and January 1989, ECRI researchers assessed 14 general purpose infusion pumps from nine manufacturers.[3] Pumps were assessed for a variety of features. Recently, ECRI developed new criteria for evaluation of infusion pumps; the criteria are currently being reviewed by experts nationwide.

The organization is involved in developing strict evaluation criteria aimed at helping those of us in the clinical setting to deliver care with a high degree of safety and accuracy. ECRI suggests that the major issues confronting users and purchasers of general purpose infusion pumps are as follows:

- Overall performance
- Free-flow risk versus cost and conditions of acceptability
- Detecting upstream occlusion
- Detecting empty fluid containers
- Special features (including piggybacking, user-selectable occlusion alarm pressure, and pressure monitoring)

PRODUCT SELECTION AND EVALUATION

Methodology

Selection of equipment is a complex task. Hospitalized patients now receive a multitude of therapies through their intravascular systems. The type of device used to initiate flow depends on the complexity of care, the range of flow needed, pressure, the insertion site, and the delivery rate.

Needs Assessment

Product selection should be a serious consideration and should be based on needs assessment in the clinical setting. The ability to deliver a specified dose in either µg/kg/min, µg/kg/h, mg/kg/min, or mg/kg/h by entering the appropriate concentration, patient weight, bolus amount, and mass units is a feature often required in the critical care setting. Demands for features such as bolus capabilities, syringe size sensing, and delivery in body weight, mass, continuous, or volume-over-time modes have challenged today's manufacturers to produce the most advanced products ever available.

Systems

The product evaluation committee is often involved in the selection of EIDs in the clinical setting. This focus should carry into the alternative care setting as well, so that the EIDs chosen clearly meet the patients' clinical and therapeutic needs while fulfilling a real function as accessories to quality IV nursing care.

Patient Selection and Education

Patients should be carefully evaluated for their ability to comprehend and perform self-care procedures, especially when EIDs are to be used. The patient should be taught how the pump can be worn, the operating principles, care of the pump and line, technical problems, and troubleshooting techniques. Home teaching checklists addressing pump operation may be found in Chapter 24.

REFERENCES

1. Adriani, J. (1962). Venipuncture. *American Journal of Nursing, 62,* 70.
2. Boyan, C. P. (1964). Cold or warmed blood for massive transfusion. *Annals of Surgery, 160,* 282.
3. Emergency Care Research Institute. (1995). Emergency Care Research Institute Health Devices. Plymouth Meeting, PA. Draft Document: Infusion Pumps.
4. Metheny, N. M. (1996). *Fluid and electrolyte balance* (3rd ed., pp. 22–23). Philadelphia: Lippincott-Raven.
5. Revised intravenous nursing standards of practice. (1990). *Journal of Intravenous Nursing (Suppl.),* S37, S58.
6. Product Literature, Becton Dickinson Vascular Access.
7. Tarail, R. (1950). Practice of fluid therapy. *Journal of the American Medical Association, 171,* 45–49.
8. Weinstein, S. M. (1990). Math calculations for intravenous nurses. *Journal of Intravenous Nursing, 13*(4), 213–236.

BIBLIOGRAPHY

Falchuk, K. H., Peterson, L., & McNeil, B. J. (1985). Microparticulate-induced phlebitis: Its prevention by inline filtration. *New England Journal of Medicine, 312*(2), 78–82.

Frey, A. M. (1986). Taking the confusion out of multiple infusion. *Journal of the National Intravenous Therapy Association, 9*(6), 460–463.

Hadaway, L. C. (1989). Evaluation and use of advanced IV technology. Part I: Central venous access devices. *Journal of Intravenous Nursing, 12*(2), 73–82.

Quercia, R. A., Hills, S. W., Klimer, J. J., et al. (1986). Bacteriologic contamination of intravenous infusion delivery systems in an intensive care unit. *American Journal of Medicine, 80*(3), 364–368.

Ritter, H. T. M. (1990). Evaluating and selecting general-purpose infusion pumps. *Journal of Intravenous Nursing, 13*(3), 156–161.

REVIEW QUESTIONS

1. The usual infusion rate for maintenance and replacement of fluids is how many mL/m^2 body surface per minute?
   a. 2
   b. 3
   c. 4
   d. 5

2. The filter attached to a vented medication-additive IV set is what μm in size?
   a. 0.2
   b. 0.5
   c. 1.0
   d. 1.2

3. The limit to operating pressure at which an alarm is triggered on an electronic infusion device is known as what type of pressure?
   a. system
   b. needle
   c. occlusion
   d. resistance

4. The United States Pharmacopeia (USP) has established an acceptable limit of particles for single-dose infusion not to exceed how many particles per mL equal to or greater than 10.0 μm?
   a. 20
   b. 40
   c. 50
   d. 60

5. Which of the following is NOT an example of filter material?
   a. hydrophobic
   b. hydrophilic
   c. depth
   d. bubble point

6. Which of the following factors affect flow rate?
   a. height of container
   b. change in position of needle
   c. trauma to the vein
   d. temperature of solution

7. 50 mm Hg is equivalent to how many psi?
   a. 12
   b. 30
   c. 50
   d. 62

8. The rate of IV infusions should be routinely regulated by:
   a. electronic flow control
   b. manual flow control
   c. rate minders
   d. elastomerics

9. Which of the following systems was developed to reduce the incidence of needlestick injuries?
   a. needleless
   b. elastomerics
   c. Luer locks
   d. universal connection

10. Which of the following provides a guide for determining the amount of fluids and electrolytes needed?
    a. body weight
    b. height
    c. body surface area
    d. degree of hydratio

CHAPTER 11

Central Venous Catheterization

Key Terms

Axillary	Hypotension	Pressure
Basilic	Innominate	Subclavian
Central venous pressure	Insertion	Superior vena cava
Cephalic	Internal jugular	Tip placement
Complications	Preparation	Vascular
External jugular	Physiology	

Advantages of central venous catheterization include 1) placement, usually by percutaneous puncture; 2) a lower risk of infection; and 3) catheter tip placement in the superior vena cava.

The tip placement allows for rapid dilution of the infusate, thus reducing the risk of phlebitis and vein sclerosis. The tip placement also allows for monitoring central venous pressure.

VASCULAR ANATOMY

A review of the vascular system is essential in providing care to the patient with central venous access. Vessels involved include the cephalic, basilic, axillary, jugular, subclavian, and innominate veins as well as the superior vena cava (Fig. 11-1 and 11-2).

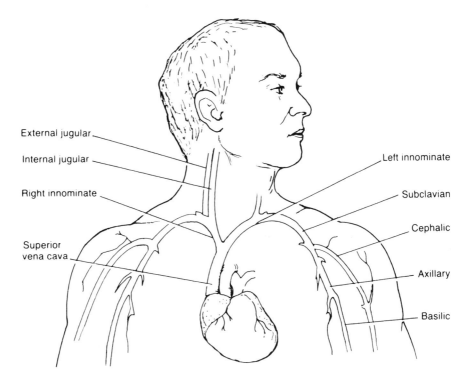

External jugular

Internal jugular

Right innominate

Superior vena cava

Left innominate

Subclavian

Cephalic

Axillary

Basilic

FIGURE 11-1 Central venous catheters are inserted through the subclavian and internal or external jugular veins.

The Cephalic Vein

The cephalic vein ascends along the outer border of the biceps muscle to the upper third of the arm. It passes in the space between the pectoralis major and deltoid muscles. It terminates in the axillary vein, with a descending curve, just below the clavicle.

The cephalic vein is occasionally connected with the external jugular or subclavian vein by a branch that passes from it upward in front of the clavicle.[3]

The Basilic Vein

The basilic vein is larger than the cephalic. It passes upward in a smooth path along the inner side of the biceps muscle and terminates in the axillary vein.[3]

The Axillary Vein

The axillary vein starts upward as a continuation of the basilic vein, increasing in size as it ascends. It receives the cephalic vein and terminates immediately beneath the clavicle, at the outer border of the first rib. At this point it becomes the subclavian vein.[3]

The External Jugular Vein

The external jugular vein is easily recognized on the side of the neck. It follows a descending inward path to join the subclavian vein above the middle of the clavicle.[3]

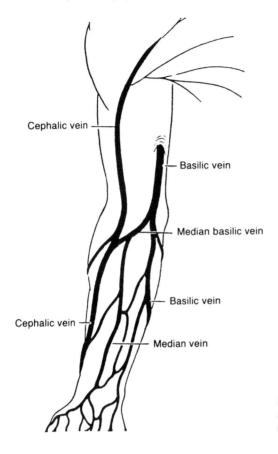

Cephalic vein

Basilic vein

Median basilic vein

Basilic vein

Cephalic vein

Median vein

FIGURE 11-2 The cephalic and basilic veins are used for peripheral insertion of central venous catheters.

The Internal Jugular Vein

The internal jugular vein descends first behind and then to the outer side of the internal and common carotid arteries. The carotid plexus is situated on the outer side of the internal carotid artery. The internal jugular vein joins the subclavian vein at the root of the neck. At the angle of junction, the left subclavian receives the thoracic duct while the right subclavian receives the right lymphatic duct.[3]

The Subclavian Vein

The subclavian vein, a continuation of the axillary, extends from the outer edge of the first rib to the inner end of the clavicle, where it unites with the internal jugular to form the innominate vein.

Valves are present in the venous system until approximately an inch before the formation of the innominate vein.[3]

The Right Innominate Vein

The right innominate vein is about an inch long. It passes almost vertically downward and joins the left innominate just below the cartilage of the first rib.[3]

The Left Innominate Vein

The left innominate vein is about 2.5 inches in length and larger than the right. It passes from left to right across the upper front chest, in a downward slant. It joins the right innominate to form the superior vena cava.[3]

The Superior Vena Cava

The superior vena cava receives all blood from the upper half of the body. It is comprised of a short trunk 2.5 to 3 inches in length. It begins below the first rib close to the sternum on the right side, descends vertically slightly to the right, and empties into the right atrium of the heart.[3]

CENTRAL VENOUS PRESSURE

Peripheral insertions of central venous catheters were first used for monitoring *central venous pressure*, which denotes the pressure in the right atrium or vena cava of the venous blood as it returns from all parts of the body. The pressure varies among individuals, usually ranging between 4 and 11 cm H_2O in the vena cava; the pressure in the right atrium is usually 0 to 4 cm H_2O.[6] The normal range has little significance because the true value lies in the change or lack of change after attempts to alter the blood volume or to improve cardiac action. Because central venous pressure relates to a fully sufficient circulation, it facilitates assessment of both the blood volume and the ability of the heart to tolerate an increased volume, thereby providing a valuable guide for fluid administration. It requires no laboratory personnel and no expensive equipment; it is simple in technique; and, once set up, it may be monitored quickly and as often as required.

Because central venous pressure relates to an adequate circulatory blood volume, it depends on[6]:

1. Blood volume
2. Status of the myocardium
3. Vascular tone

Circulatory failure may result from deficiency in any one or a combination of these essential factors.

Blood Volume

Changes in blood volume alter the tone of the blood vessels and the ability of the heart to circulate the blood. A reduced blood volume results in less pressure at the right atrium, indicated by a drop in central venous pressure; an increased blood volume produces more pressure at the atrium, with a rise in central venous pressure.[6]

In managing an inadequate circulation, one must first establish a normal blood volume. If the inadequate circulation is caused by deficiency in the blood volume, manipulation is made by administering expanders, or in the case of increased volume, phlebotomy.

If the circulation still remains insufficient, it is necessary to look at the remaining two essential components—status of the myocardium and vascular tone.

Status of the Myocardium

The myocardial status may be affected by disease, drugs, fluids, or anesthesia. Because the central venous pressure is a measure of the capacity of the myocardium as well as the blood volume, it is invaluable in monitoring the effects of anesthesia and surgery on elderly patients with arteriosclerosis or patients with myocardial insufficiency. The central venous pressure rises if the heart muscle is impaired—the pressure of the volume of blood at the heart increases because the heart muscle is no longer able to pump an adequate flow of blood out of the right atrium.[6] A high central venous pressure may suggest cardiac failure.[6] This is one of the most common causes of an elevated central venous pressure in shock.

Drugs or chemicals are administered to improve myocardial response, thus increasing cardiac output and lowering the central venous pressure.

Vascular Tone

The third essential component, the vascular tone, depends on the arterial pressure and on external and internal pressures on the veins. The arterial pressure arises from the contractile force of the left ventricle and is transmitted through the capillaries to the veins.

The external pressures on the vein result from the muscular and fascial pumping action in the extremities, the intra-abdominal pressure from straining and distention, and the intrathoracic pressure from contraction of the diaphragm and chest wall. Central venous pressure of patients on positive-pressure respirators is usually increased by 4 cm; patients on negative pressure show a decreased central venous pressure.[7]

The internal pressure on the veins is caused by the blood volume, myocardial response, and sympathomimetic amines (epinephrine, norepinephrine). By stimulating contraction of the venous wall, vasopressors decrease the capacity of the venous system and improve vascular tone.

Clinical Applications

Hypotension

The parameters used in evaluating a patient in shock consist of:

1. Blood pressure
2. Rate and quality of pulse
3. Skin temperature and color
4. Urinary output
5. Peripheral venous filling
6. Blood pH

Blood Volume

Prolonged hypovolemia may cause poor tissue perfusion with the inherent risk of renal and myocardial complication; uncorrected hypovolemia can eventually lead to shock and death. Blood volume is not necessarily reflected by the blood pressure. In cardiogenic shock, the blood volume is increased and the blood pressure is low. In septic shock, hypotension accompanies a normal blood volume.

Various methods are used to detect change in a patient's blood volume: hematocrit, change in patient's weight, and blood volume computations. Central venous pressure is a parameter used to assess blood volume. It is an important guide during the following:

1. *Surgery*, when there is a risk of overloading an anesthetized, traumatized patient who is continuously losing blood
2. *Shock*, when origin is unknown
3. *Massive fluid replacement* in open heart surgery and in critical cases, such as severely burned patients, where circulatory overload is a hazard
4. *Anuria* or *oliguria*, when questionable cause is dehydration

Total Parenteral Nutrition
Subclavian insertions were first used for administration of total parenteral nutrition. This subject is thoroughly discussed in Chapter 16.

Cancer Therapy
With the advent of tunneling techniques, antithrombogenic catheter materials, new device designs, and lowered infection rates, central venous catheters became popular for many other uses. The administration of long-term antineoplastic agents, blood or blood components, and antibiotics, as well as venous sampling, is frequently done with a central catheter device in cancer patients. See Chapters 19 and 20.

Limited Venous Access
In any hospital patient requiring a venous access whose peripheral veins cannot be cannulated, a long-term catheter may be used.

Home Intravenous Therapy
Many home patients have been taught to self-administer their continuous or intermittent medications through a central device.

CENTRAL VENOUS PRESSURE MONITORING

Central venous pressure monitoring is achieved by attaching an IV set to a three-way stopcock and to an extension tube with a radiopaque catheter of approximately 24 inches. A vertical length of infusion tubing that serves as the manometer is connected to the stopcock and attached to the IV stand against a marked centimeter tape. Central venous pressure sets are available with disposable water manometers, graduated in units. The zero mark on the tape is adjusted to the level of the patient's right atrium (Fig. 11-3). The pressure is measured at either the superior vena cava by introducing the catheter through the antecubital, jugular, or subclavian vein, or at the inferior vena cava through the femoral vein.

The superior vena cava is most commonly used. Complications have been associated with inferior vena caval catheters. Use of the femoral vein and the long duration of time the catheter is in the vein enhance the risk of thrombotic complications. A second disadvantage is the fact that abdominal distention interferes with monitoring an accurate right atrial pressure.

Central venous pressure
measurement

0 at level of right atrium

FIGURE 11-3 Central venous pressure measurement with zero point of manometer at level of right atrium. (From Metheny, N. M. [1996]. *Fluid and electrolyte balance* [3rd ed.]. Philadelphia: J. B. Lippincott.)

Equipment

With a central venous catheter in place, the following equipment is needed for monitoring central venous pressure:

IV pole

Solution as ordered

IV or transfusion tubing

Central venous manometer set

Venous pressure level (optional)

Armboard with cover

Adhesive tape

Procedure

Connecting pressure manometer to central venous catheter.

1. Wash hands thoroughly and dry.

2. Close three-way stopcock.

3. Hold and squeeze drip chamber while inserting tubing spike into upright bottle or hanging plastic bag. The use of a tubing with a Luer lock connector will aid in the prevention of a connection separation, which could result in an air embolism.

4. Release squeeze, allowing drip chamber to fill one-quarter to one-third full. Prefilling drip chamber prevents air bubbles from entering the system.

5. If the manometer is to be permanently attached to the IV pole, tape centimeter strip onto IV pole with zero point adjusted to the mid-atrial level. Patient should be in a supine position with the bed flat. Use venous pressure level for accuracy. Mid-atrial level is at a point approximately equidistant from the sternum and the back. Tape stopcock to pole at a level below patient's right atrium. Do not tape directly on the stopcock. Tape upper end of manometer taut to IV pole.

    If the manometer contains clips and will be removed for each reading, secure manometer to IV pole. When this type of manometer is used, placing a waterproof "X" on the side of the patient's chest at mid-atrial level will ensure that all readings are taken with zero point at the same level.

6. Adjust stopcock to allow solution to flow into manometer, filling it halfway.

7. Adjust stopcock to flush remainder of tubing.

8. Connect manometer system to central venous catheter.
    a. Use strict aseptic techniques while disconnecting present IV system and connecting manometer system.
    b. Be sure to use air embolism precautions when the catheter is open to air (see air embolism, under the Complications section of this chapter).
    c. Secure catheter hub–tubing connection with tape to aid in prevention of connection separation.
    d. Secure arm to covered armboard. Motion of catheter on flexion of the arm increases the potential risk of phlebitis. A kinked catheter results in unreliable readings and leads to clogging of the lumen.

Central Venous Pressure Measurement

The pressure is usually read at half-hour or hourly intervals. The patient must be quiet, not coughing or straining, and in a supine position with the zero point on the manometer at the mid-atrial level. The procedure is as follows:

1. Turn stopcock so solution flows from the container to the manometer.

2. When manometer level reaches 30 cm, turn stopcock to stop flow from the container and direct manometer flow to the patient.

3. The fluid level will drop rapidly, reaching the reading level in about 15 seconds. The central venous pressure is measured at the high point of the fluctuation.

4. Readjust the stopcock so the infusion resumes.

5. Document readings.

The catheter is presumed to be in the thoracic cavity when manometer fluid fluctuates 3 to 5 cm during breathing, and coughing and straining cause the column of water to rise. If the catheter is inserted too far and reaches the heart, higher pressure waves synchronous with the pulse will be seen.[6,8]

APPROACH TO THE PATIENT

Patient Preparation

To allay fears and to obtain patient cooperation, explain the reasons for the insertion and the procedure.

Position During Insertion

If a subclavian entry is to be used, explain to the patient that he or she will be positioned flat in bed with the head lowered and knees bent, to increase the blood supply to the vein, and that a rolled towel will be placed under the back between the shoulder blades to make it easier for the physician to enter the vein. Prior explanation will obtain patient cooperation when the uncomfortable position must be maintained.

Gowns and Masks

Explaining that the nurse and the physician will both wear gowns and masks to keep normal bacteria away from the area will allay apprehension. If the patient will be required to wear a mask, having him or her wear one before the procedure will give reassurance that a mask does not really interfere with breathing.

The Valsalva Maneuver

Practicing the Valsalva maneuver before the insertion will obtain cooperation when the patient is asked to hold the breath and "bear down" at the time the catheter is open to the air.

Becoming Acquainted With the Device

If a tunneled catheter or implanted venous access or pump device is being inserted, seeing and touching the device that will remain in their bodies is reassuring to most patients. Any limitations of activity the device will create should be thoroughly discussed. If the patient will be required to give any self-care, this should be completely explained and agreed to by the patient before insertion.

Consent Form

A patient consent form must be signed before any central venous catheter or device insertion.

Blood Studies

Preinsertion blood studies include platelet count, prothrombin time (PT), and partial thromboplastin time (PTT). Any abnormal result may require correction with vitamin K, fresh frozen plasma, or platelet concentrates before insertion is attempted.

Premedication

Depending on the type of device, insertion site, and individual patient needs, some form of sedation may be required before the procedure. This should be explained to the patient.

CENTRAL VENOUS CANNULATION _____

Any central venous catheter has its inherent risks. *If peripheral veins are obtainable and adequate for the desired treatment, a central venous catheter should not be inserted.*

Contraindications

Contraindications for any type of central venous catheter insertion may include:

1. Abnormal coagulation studies
2. Septicemia
3. Anomalies of the central venous vascular structures
4. Thrombosis of the innominate or subclavian veins or of the superior vena cava
5. Superior vena cava syndrome

Catheter Tip Placement

The preferred tip placement is usually at the junction of the superior vena cava and the right atrium. If the tip lies in the right atrium, atrial arrhythmias may occur as a result of catheter irritation. For various reasons it is not always possible to advance the catheter far enough to achieve the desired tip location. Depending on the specific purpose of the catheter, innominate or subclavian catheter tip placement may be adequate.

Infection Control

Aseptic technique will minimize the risk of infection in the patient in whom a central line is to be placed. If the patient cannot be masked during the procedure, the head should be turned away from the insertion area. The skin should be cleansed consistent with institutional policy and Centers for Disease Control and Prevention and Intravenous Nurses Society (INS) guidelines. Determine the type of catheter material before the use of acetone for defatting the skin; materials such as Silastic are often eroded by contact with acetone solutions.[5] Dress the site in the usual manner and provide catheter maintenance consistent with institutional policy.

Air Embolism Precautions

The risk of air embolism is ever present during catheter insertion because central venous pressure can be negative. Placing the patient in Trendelenburg position will increase the pressure. If possible, the patient should perform the Valsalva maneuver whenever the catheter is opened to the air.[2] If the catheter stylet has been removed, the hub should be occluded with either a syringe or the gloved finger to prevent air entry.

Patient Positioning

During a central venous catheter insertion, the patient is placed in Trendelenburg position. This not only increases central venous pressure, but it also distends the vein and facilitates entry. When the subclavian approach is used, a rolled towel is placed along the spinal cord to hyperextend the neck and elevate the clavicle. For the jugular approach, the head is turned to the opposite direction and extended. This stretches and stabilizes the vein and accentuates the muscular landmarks. During a cephalic or brachial insertion, abduction of the arm may be required to pass the catheter past the shoulder area.

INSERTION SITES

There are basically three approaches for central venous catheter insertions. The veins used for entry are the subclavian and the internal or external jugular veins for central insertion and the cephalic or basilic vein for peripheral insertion.

CENTRAL INSERTION

The subclavian vein is frequently the entry of choice. It requires the shortest length catheter because it uses the most central veins, thus creating a high blood flow around a large portion of the catheter. This results in minimal catheter irritation or obstruction. All these factors lower the risk of complications, resulting in a longer catheter life.

Subclavian Vein

A subclavian entry is a medical act; major complications can occur during or from this insertion. (See Complications section of this chapter.)

The subclavian entry may be performed by the infraclavicular or the supraclavicular approach. In both approaches, the cannula is inserted under the clavicle, aiming for the jugular notch. For the infraclavicular approach, the cannula is inserted at approximately the midpoint of the clavicle. For the supraclavicular approach, the cannula is frequently inserted at the base of the triangle formed by the sternal and clavicular heads of the sternocleidomastoid muscle.

Contraindications
Contraindications for the subclavian approach may include:

1. Radiation burns at intended insertion site
2. Fractured clavicle
3. Hyperinflated lungs
4. Malignancy at the base of the neck or apex of the lungs

Internal Jugular Vein

The insertion of central venous catheters into the internal jugular vein is usually a medical act. Many physicians select the internal jugular vein as a first choice of site for the insertion of a central venous catheter.

The constant anatomic location of the internal jugular vein makes its cannulation easier than that of the subclavian vein. The right internal jugular vein is usually chosen because it forms a straighter, shorter line to the superior vena cava. It also avoids the higher left pleura and thoracic duct. This insertion is frequently performed by first locating the vein with a small-gauge needle. After making a small skin incision to facilitate entry, a larger-gauge cannula is inserted, following the same direction as the locator needle, aiming for the ipsilateral nipple.

External Jugular Vein

The external jugular vein is observable and easily entered. Insertion complications are rare, so cannulation can be performed by specialty nurses.

The external jugular vein varies in size and its junction with the subclavian vein is acutely angulated. It contains two pairs of valves. The uppermost pair are 4 cm above the clavicle, the lower pair are located at the vein's entrance to the subclavian vein. Because of these factors, central cannulation can be difficult. Because a short cannula may be easily inserted, central cannulation may be achieved by the use of an introducer with a guidewire. Entry into the superficial vein is performed by directing the cannula toward the ipsilateral nipple.

Objections to Jugular Insertions

The main objections to any jugular cannulation are:

1. *Catheter occlusion* is a persistent problem as a result of head movement.
2. *Vein irritation* is created by the same movements. These factors result in a *shorter catheter life.*
3. It is *difficult to maintain an intact dressing* on the area.
4. The idea of having a catheter in the neck is *aesthetically and psychologically disturbing* to many patients and families.

PERIPHERALLY INSERTED CENTRAL CATHETERS

Technology has kept pace with demands for more sophisticated, long-term peripheral venous access devices. The peripherally inserted central catheter (PICC) line was the first product developed specifically for this clinical application.

Vein Selection

The *basilic vein* is usually the first choice for the peripheral insertion of a central venous catheter. It ascends obliquely in the groove between the biceps brachii and pronator teres and perforates the deep fascia slightly distal to the middle of the upper arm. With the arm held at a 90° angle, it forms the straightest, most direct route into the central venous system.

The *median cubital vein* is the second choice. Ascending on the ulnar side of the forearm, it may be divided into two vessels, one joining the basilic vein and the other the cephalic vein. This vein varies substantially, and the proper branch must be ascertained before venipuncture for PICC placement. The median antecubital basilic is preferred.

The *cephalic vein* runs proximally along the lateral side of the antecubital fossa in the groove between the brachioradialis and the biceps brachii. It becomes a deep vein at the clavipectoral fascia, ending in the axillary vein immediately caudal to the clavicle. It is much more tortuous than the basilic vein and presents a greater potential for catheter tip malposition. It is not preferred because it may also be difficult to thread.

Indications

Placement of a PICC has met with widespread acceptance in the nursing and medical communities. Indications for placement include:

1. Lack of peripheral venous access
2. Infusion of vesicant or irritant drugs
3. Infusion of hyperosmolar drugs
4. Long-term venous access
5. Infusion of antineoplastics agents, blood, or blood components
6. Patient preference
7. Clinician preference

Advantages

The PICC catheter has many advantages over the short-term peripheral catheter and the centrally placed line, including:

1. Elimination or risks associated with central venous catheter placement
2. Potential reduction of catheter sepsis
3. Ease of use
4. Preservation of the peripheral vascular system
5. Decrease in discomfort
6. Reliability

Tip Placement

Placement of a PICC may be in either the superior vena cava, providing a true central line access, and in the axillary or subclavian vein. The physical landmark used for the axillary or subclavian vein is approximately an inch distal from the head of the clavicle.

Superior Vena Cava Tip Placement

This type of placement is preferred for all antineoplastic agents, administration of vesicants, total parenteral nutrition with a final dextrose concentration in excess of 20%, and any sclerosing agents. Measurement for tip placement is from the point of insertion, along the proposed vein track to the third intercostal space.

Subclavian Tip Placement

Subclavian placement is often used for the diversity of IV therapies administered through a conventional short cannula. Measurement of tip placement is from the point of insertion, along the proposed vein track to 1 inch distal to the sternal notch.

At this point, the catheter tip should be seated in the median segment of the subclavian vein 2 to 3 cm distal to the junction of the external jugular vein.

Procedure

A physician's order is needed before placement of a PICC line. The patient should be assessed for available venous access, clinical condition, and ability to learn procedures applicable to maintenance.

1. Assemble all supplies/tray (Fig. 11-4).
2. Wash hands.
3. Place patient in a supine position with the arm to be accessed extended at 90° to the patient's trunk.
4. Place a tourniquet firmly around the mid-upper arm to access insertion site. After selecting the vein, release the tourniquet.
5. Measure the distance from the insertion site to the catheter tip termination point.
6. Open the insertion tray and establish working area.
   a. Drop sterile product onto tray.
   b. Apply first pair of gloves.
   c. Remove items from tray and place them on the sterile field.

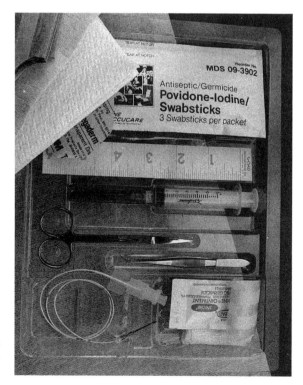

FIGURE 11-4 Per-Q-Cath tray. (Courtesy: Gesco International: San Antonio, TX)

7. Prep the site in a 3-inch concentric circle consistent with institutional guidelines and INS Standards of Practice.

8. Drape the patient's arm with the fenestrated drape provided.

9. Prepare the catheter and related items.
   a. Fill a 5-mL syringe with normal saline for injection from the previously prepped vial.
   b. Attach the injection cap to the extension set and prime.
   c. Stretch out the sterile tape measure and place the catheter beside it.
   d. If a guidewire is provided, pull it back beyond the point where trimming will be needed.
   e. Using sterile scissors, trim the catheter at a 45° angle.
   f. Advance the guidewire until it extends ¼ to ½ inch from the tip of the catheter.
   g. At the hub of the catheter, bend the guidewire at a 90° angle to prevent it from advancing beyond the end of the catheter.
   h. Pass the catheter through the introducer needle to the tip of the needle.
   i. Remove the catheter from the needle and loosely attach a syringe; pull back 2 to 3 mL to secure a flush chamber.

10. Administer lidocaine hydrochloride 1% without epinephrine intradermally (optional).

11. Reapply tourniquet.

12. Remove contaminated gloves and reglove.

13. Place a sterile 4 × 4 gauze over the tails of the tourniquet to allow release following successful cannulation.

14. Move the catheter, introducer needle and syringe, and sterile forceps to a point near the intended insertion site.

15. Stabilize the vein below the insertion site and perform venipuncture using shallow angle. Following blood return, lower the needle until it is parallel to the vein and advance the introducer needle approximately ¼ inch to ensure that the entire lumen is well within the wall of the vein.

16. Release the tourniquet, stabilize the introducer needle, and remove the syringe.

17. Remove the introducer needle.
   a. Hold catheter with forceps 1½ inch behind the introducer.
   b. Pull needle along the catheter and out of the insertion site.
   c. Stabilize the catheter at insertion site and pull needle back to the hub of the catheter.
   d. Press wings together and grasp each wing, pulling apart.

18. Advance the catheter (guidewire may remain in place for deep peripheral tip placement). If guidewire is removed, attach a syringe of normal saline to the catheter and flush gently.

19. Advance to premeasured length, remove guidewire if needed, and attach extension tubing and injection cap.

20. Check for blood return and establish ease of flushing.

21. Place a steri-strip across the wings to provide stability.

22. Cleanse site, apply skin protectant and place a folded 2 × 2 gauze above the insertion site.

23. Apply transparent dressing.

24. Heparinize catheter consistent with manufacturer's recommendations.

Alternatives to Guidewire Technique

Breakaway needle involves venipuncture made with an introducer needle. The catheter, with or without a guidewire, is threaded through the introducer. The introducer is removed from the venipuncture site, broken in half, and peeled away. The U-Wing Peelaway Needle Introducer (Fig. 11-5) is an example. The stainless steel needle introducer offers improved access to small veins and subsequent easy removal from the catheter. The T-Peel™ Peelaway Plastic Sheath introducer allows catheter threading through a plastic sheath and an integrated flashback chamber to protect the clinician and confirm placement (Fig 11-6).

Cannula technique involves use of an introducer needle to place a plastic cannula (peel-away sheath) into the vein. The catheter is then threaded through this sheath. The sheath is removed from the insertion site and peeled away from the catheter.

Assess line for evidence of redness, edema, pain, drainage, and a palpable venous cord. Postinsertion complications include:

- Bleeding (unusual after 24 hours)
- Phlebitis
- Cellulitis (tends to spread in a diffuse circular pattern into surrounding tissue)
- Catheter sepsis

FIGURE 11-5 Peelaway needle: Needle Introducer. (Courtesy: Luther Medical, Inc., Tustin, CA)

FIGURE 11-6 T-Peel™ Peelaway Plastic Sheath. (Courtesy: Luther Medical, Inc., Tustin, CA)

Postinsertion Care

A chest radiograph is always done immediately after catheter insertion to rule out pneumothorax and to document tip placement. An isotonic solution is infused until tip placement is confirmed. The site should be observed for any signs of excess bleeding or swelling. The patient's breathing should be monitored for any signs of respiratory distress. Any unexpected observation should be reported to the physician immediately. Complications associated with central line placement also apply.

PERIPHERAL PORT

The peripheral port implantable access system is designed to permit repeated access to the venous system. Consisting of a portal with a self-sealing septum, accessible by percutaneous needle puncture, and a catheter for the parenteral delivery of medications and fluids, its use is indicated when patient therapy requires repeated venous access.

Assessment

Before placement, the patient's anatomy should be accessed for evidence of prior trauma to the veins or anatomic irregularities.

Following placement, take these precautions:

1. Do not withdraw blood from or infuse medication into the arm in which the implanted system is placed without using the portal.

2. Do not attempt to measure blood pressure on this arm.

Potential Complications

Potential complications of the peripherally placed port include:

- Air embolism
- Artery or vein puncture
- Brachial plexus injury
- Cardiac arrhythmia
- Cardiac tamponade

- Cardiac puncture
- Catheter disconnection, fragmentation, embolization
- Catheter occlusion, rupture
- Drug extravasation
- Fibrin sheath formation at catheter tip
- Hematoma
- Hemothorax
- Implant rejection
- Infection
- Migration of portal/catheter
- Peripheral nerve damage
- Thoracic duct injury
- Thromboembolism
- Thrombophlebitis
- Thrombosis

Care and Maintenance

Care must be taken when administering fluid through the system because excessive pressure can be generated with all syringes. Pressure in excess of 40 psi may cause catheter rupture with possible embolization. As with any line, appropriate flushing procedures must be implemented to avoid incompatibility with heparin.

A syringe or IV administration set is attached to a 20- or 22-gauge needle, and the needle is primed. The skin is prepped and punctured directly over the septum. Advance the needle slowly through the septum until it makes contact with the bottom of the portal chamber. Do not tilt or rock the needle. Flush with an appropriate solution and administer the injection or infusate. Flush again and administer 5 mL heparinized saline to establish patency. Maintain positive pressure when withdrawing the needle to avoid reflux of blood into the catheter.

The L-CATH® for ports was designed to introduce a flexible Teflon® catheter into the septum of a subcutaneously implanted port. (Fig. 11-7). Insertion technique is described and demonstrated in Fig. 11-8.

COMPLICATIONS OF CENTRAL VENOUS CATHETERIZATION

Arterial Puncture

Arterial puncture, one of the most frequently reported complications of subclavian insertions, is usually not a major problem if it is recognized early. The puncture of an artery requires the immediate application of digital pressure for at least 5 minutes. If the patient has a coagulation abnormality, digital pressure must be maintained until all bleeding stops. If the artery puncture is not recognized and treated early, a massive hematoma resulting in tracheal compression or respiratory distress can occur.

FIGURE 11-7 L-CATH® FOR PORTS. (Courtesy: Luther Medical, Inc., Tustin, CA)

Pneumothorax

Pneumothorax, another common complication of subclavian insertion, occurs as a result of pleural puncture; the patient may experience difficult breathing or chest pain. It can be asymptomatic and discovered by radiography. A chest tube may be required to treat the symptoms.

Hemothorax

Hemothorax may result if the subclavian or adjacent veins have been traumatized or transected during the insertion. Symptoms and treatment are the same as for pneumothorax.

Hydrothorax

Hydrothorax results when the IV fluid infiltrates into the chest. The symptoms and treatment are identical to a pneumothorax.

Catheter Embolism

Catheter embolism is always a risk whenever a through-the-needle device is inserted or left in situ. During insertion, care must be taken never to withdraw the catheter back through the needle. While the through-the-needle catheter is in place, care must be taken to ensure that the needle tip is always protected with a secured tip cover. A severed catheter may require cardiac catheterization to retrieve the embolism. Breakaway needles minimize this hazard.

Air Embolism

Air embolism is always a potential danger whenever any central venous catheter is open to air. This can occur because it is always possible to have negative central venous pressure. During insertion, placing the patient in Trendelenburg position will increase central venous pressure. Placing the sterile gloved finger over the catheter hub, between catheter stylet removal and IV system connection, can prevent air from entering the catheter.

INSERTION:

1. Remove L-CATH FOR PORTS port access system from package.

2. Using sterile technique, prepare the access site.

3. Remove L-CATH FOR PORTS port access catheter from the sterile protector.

4. When using L-CATH FOR PORTS <u>with preattached extension set</u>—prime entire system with normal saline solution prior to insertion.

5. Palpate skin to find the rim of the implanted port.

6. Holding the handle at the base—firmly insert the catheter introducer through the septum perpendicular to the skin. (For side entry ports see manufacturer's access instructions). The introducer will stop when it reaches the bottom of the reservoir. **Figure 11-8A.**

7. Hold the top of the introducer and gently pull it away from patient until the catheter is free. **Figure 11-8B.**

NOTE: Do not clamp the catheter. Clamping will damage the catheter wall.

8. a. When using L-CATH FOR PORTS <u>*with*</u> preattached extension set, aspirate with syringe to confirm placement.

    b. Flush according to the port manufacturer's maintenance instructions and institutional policy and procedures.

9. a. When using L-CATH FOR PORTS <u>*without*</u> preattached extension set, attach a primed extension set with syringe partially filled with normal saline to the catheter hub. Open the slide clamp on the attached extension set and aspirate until blood completely replaces all air in the L-CATH FOR PORTS catheter. **Figure 11-8C.**

    b. Flush according to the port manufacturer's maintenance instructions and institutional policy and procedure.

NOTE: Check the priming volume of the L-CATH FOR PORTS port access catheter and add the volume of the extension set plus the volume stated by the implanted port manufacturer.

10. CLOSE THE SIDE CLAMP ON THE EXTENSION SET and remove the syringe. You mad add an injection cap or additional tubing to the extension set.

FIGURE 11-8   Insertion technique of L-CATH® FOR PORTS. (Courtesy: Luther Medical, Inc., Tustin, CA)

If the patient can cooperate, performing the Valsalva maneuver will increase central venous pressure. However, be sure that the patient takes the deep breath and bears down *before* the disconnection. Performing the disconnection while the patient is inhaling can *increase* the risk of air embolism. During tubing changes, the same precautions are necessary to prevent air embolism. Using junction securement devices can reduce the risk of tubing separations resulting in air embolism.[2,4]

Air embolism precautions should be taken during catheter removal. The Valsalva maneuver should also be performed at this time. Positioning the patient flat in bed and, immediately on catheter removal, placing a sterile sponge with antimicrobial ointment directly over the puncture site will prevent air from entering the system. This dressing should be left intact for 24 to 48 hours to allow time for tissue healing.

Signs and symptoms of air embolism can include chest pain, dyspnea, hypoxia, apnea, tachycardia, hypotension, or a precordial murmur. Immediate treatment includes placing the patient in a supine position on the left side with the feet elevated. This position is used in an attempt to trap the air in the right atrium, where it can be aspirated with an intracardiac needle.

Catheter-Related Infection

Catheter-related infection is a serious complication of central venous catheterization, occurring at the exit site, tunnel, or port pocket. The majority of steps taken in maintenance of the IV system and site are performed to prevent IV-related sepsis.

Whenever a patient with a central venous catheter has an unexpected fever spike, IV-related sepsis must be suspected. The insertion site should be carefully inspected for any signs of infection. A blood culture drawn through the catheter may be ordered. To rule out all sources of contamination, all tubings and containers should be changed immediately and sent promptly to bacteriology for culturing. A complete "fever work-up" must be done to rule out any other obvious source of infection. If the fever remains and no other possible source can be established, catheter removal may be necessary.

Some practitioners perform a catheter exchange with a guidewire. If the blood culture is positive or the semiquantitative culture of the catheter tip yields 15 or more colonies, the new catheter is removed and the patient is considered to have catheter sepsis. If both cultures are negative, then the catheter can be used despite the fever. If septic shock, shaking chills, recent positive blood cultures for *Staphylococcus* or *Candida*, or local infection of the catheter entry site is present, the catheter must be removed immediately.[9] In situ treatment of catheter-related sepsis with a combination of systemic antibiotics and local thrombolytic agents has been reported. Antibiotic lock technique has also been used (see Chapters 8 and 10).[10]

Of primary importance in the prevention of IV-related infection is maintaining strict aseptic technique during insertion, admixture, any line manipulations, and aseptically performing recommended site dressing and tubing changes.

Deep-Vein Thrombosis

Deep-vein thrombosis is not as common with the new catheter materials. The addition of 1000 U heparin per liter of infusate has been recommended as a preventive measure.[9] Thrombosis may be present without any symptoms. Arm and neck pain may suggest the diagnosis. A venogram may be necessary to establish the diagnosis.

Signs and symptoms of pulmonary embolism in a patient with a central venous catheter strongly suggest deep-vein thrombosis. Treatment consists of thrombolytic therapy with streptokinase or urokinase.[9]

Thrombus Catheter Occlusion

Thrombus catheter occlusion used to be a frequent cause for catheter removal. A fibrin sheath forms, originating at the intimal injury, either where the catheter enters the vessel or where the catheter tip touches the intima. By 1 to 7 days, an unorganized, unendothelialized fibrin sleeve is apparent on venography.[11] This may result in only a withdrawal occlusion. In this case, it is impossible to withdraw a blood sample, but there is no difficulty with infusion. If there is little or no infusion flow, the patency of the catheter can be restored with the use of a thrombolytic agent. Small-dose vials are available for the declotting procedure.

Preparing the Solution

Urokinase 5000 IU is packaged in a two-chamber vial. The following steps are used to prepare the solution:

1. Remove protective cap and turn plunger–stopper a quarter turn, press to force diluent into lower chamber.
2. Roll and tilt to dissolve; avoid shaking solution.
3. Sterilize stopper top with alcohol.
4. Insert needle through the center of stopper until tip is barely visible. Invert vial and withdraw dose.

Declotting the Catheter

An aliquot of solution equal in volume to the luminal volume of the catheter is used for each injection. Catheter declotting, with urokinase, may be achieved by the following steps, wearing gloves[1]:

1. Using air embolism precautions, aseptically disconnect the IV tubing at the catheter hub and attach an empty 10-mL syringe.
2. Gently attempt to aspirate blood. If aspiration is not possible, remove the syringe.
3. Attach a 1-mL tuberculin syringe filled with prepared urokinase.
4. Slowly and gently inject amount equal to volume of catheter.
5. Remove syringe and connect empty 5-mL syringe.
6. Wait at least 5 minutes before attempting to aspirate drug and residual clot.
7. Repeat aspiration attempts every 5 minutes.
8. If the catheter cannot be opened within 30 minutes, cap the catheter and allow drug to remain for 30 to 60 minutes.
9. A second urokinase injection may be required and may be repeated as long as systemic thrombolysis is not induced.
10. When patency is restored, aspirate 4 to 5 mL blood to ensure removal of all drug and clot residual.

11. Remove blood-filled syringe and connect 10-mL syringe with 0.9% sodium chloride and gently flush to ensure patency.

12. Remove syringe and aseptically reconnect sterile IV tubing to catheter hub.

Care and Maintenance

Risks and complications associated with central venous catheterization may be reduced when a team of qualified nursing specialists assumes responsibility for assisting with insertions, maintaining lines, and providing ongoing IV care. Astute nursing assessment and a comprehensive understanding of the vascular access device in place may avert complications such as dislodgment, migration, pinch-off syndrome, and skin eros ion.

Electronic Infusion Devices

Electronic instrumentation should be used to maintain flow accuracy and catheter patency. The diversity of electronic infusion devices today ensures availability for patients with central venous access devices.

When a positive-pressure instrument is used, the pressure must not exceed that which is recommended for the type of catheter or electronic infusion device in use.

Catheter Clamps

Smooth-jaw clamps are used when tunneled silicone catheters are placed to prevent damage to the catheter material. Ideally, the clamp is applied to the distal two-thirds portion of the external catheter. If clamp damage should occur, catheter repair is easily facilitated in this area. Clamp sites should be alternated to prevent a weakened area on the catheter itself. Second-generation Silastic catheters use integral, soft-jaw clamps.

Catheter Repair

A sterile repair kit, specific to the individual type of catheter, should be readily available. Repairing the external portion of a tunneled catheter is a sterile procedure requiring surgical gloves, mask, and cap. It may be performed by the following steps.

Equipment

Sterile repair kit containing 1) replacement silicone rubber segment with Luer lock connector; 2) silicone rubber splice sleeve; 3) splice segment; 4) Luer lock cap; 5) tube of medical adhesive; and 6) blunt 18-gauge needle.

Sterile drapes, gloves	Guarded hemostat
3-mL syringe	Tongue blade
4 × 4 inch sterile sponges	Povidone-iodine solution
Small beaker for alcohol	Alcohol
Scalpel blades	Heparin flush
Iris scissors	Tape

Procedure

1. Surgically prep catheter and create sterile field. Put on gloves.
2. Clean powder from gloves with 4 × 4 inch sponge and alcohol.
3. Load adhesive into syringe barrel, then insert plunger and attach blunted needle.
4. If catheter is not clamped, clamp with guarded hemostat near chest wall.
5. Cut off the existing damaged catheter 15 to 20 cm from chest wall.
6. Insert splice segment into lumen of catheter (lubricate with alcohol if necessary but be sure all alcohol is removed or evaporated before proceeding).
7. Trim repair segment to desired length and slip onto the splice segment protruding from the implanted catheter. Do not remove the larger splice sleeve loose mounted on the repair segment.
8. Inject adhesive on the outside of the tubing in the area of the splice segment and slide the larger splice sleeve over the area of the splice segment. Inject adhesive underneath each end of splice sleeve. Roll between fingers to extrude excess adhesive and wipe excess adhesive away.
9. A sterile field is no longer required. Splint the repaired joint by taping the area to a tongue blade.
10. Remove clamp and *gently* flush with heparin. Excessive pressure may rupture joint.

The catheter may be used for infusion after a few hours. The splint may be removed after 48 hours, when the joint will have achieved full mechanical strength.

Some manufacturers provide catheter repair kits that may be used to repair most catheters (Fig. 11-9).

FIGURE 11-9 Universal catheter repair kit. (Courtesy: GISH Biomedical Inc., Santa Ana, CA) The Hemed™ catheter repair kit consists of a catheter repair assembly, boot dilator, and locking sleeve.

0.2-μm Air-Eliminating Filter

Taping a Luer lock air-eliminating filter directly to the catheter hub will reduce the risk of connection separation and air infusion that could result in a fatal embolism. If a separation occurs distal to the filter, this device will prevent air infusion and an inadvertent bleed. The 0.2-μm filter can also prevent any particulate matter, fungi, bacteria, and endotoxins from entering the system through the filter.

Intravenous Containers and Admixtures

All recommendations for peripheral containers or admixtures should be strictly adhered to for central catheter usage. To prevent risks of contamination, all manipulation for admixture and container changes must be performed with strict adherence to aseptic technique.

Tubing Changes

All tubings should be aseptically changed according to INS Standards of Practice.[4] It is extremely important to remember that there is always the possibility of negative pressure with a central catheter. Therefore, the risk of an air embolism is always present when the catheter is open to the air. If the patient cannot perform the Valsalva maneuver, consider using an extension tubing with a clamp that can be closed during the tubing change. Many practitioners use this system especially for critically ill patients. Care must be taken to maintain the sterility of the extension tubing during each IV tubing change. The extension tubing is changed at least weekly.

Between changes of components the system should be maintained as a closed system. All entries into the system should be made through injection ports that have been disinfected immediately before use.

Looping the tubing and taping it to the chest wall will prevent any related stress to the connection or insertion site when the tubing is pulled or inadvertently stretched. All connections should use junction securement devices or Luer locking connections, consistent with INS Standards of Practice.[4]

REFERENCES

1. Bjeletich, J. (1987). Declotting central venous catheters with urokinase in the home by nurse clinicians. *Journal of the National Intravenous Therapy Association, 10*(6), 428–430.
2. Coppa, G. F., Gouge, T. H., et al. (1981). Air embolism: A lethal but preventable complication of subclavian vein catheterization. *Journal of Parenteral and Enteral Nutrition, 5,* 166–168.
3. Gray, H. (1977). *Anatomy, descriptive and surgical* (Rev. American ed. from the 15th English ed.). New York: Crown.
4. *Revised intravenous nursing standards of practice.* (1990). *Journal of Intravenous Nursing* (Suppl.), S45–48, S40.
5. Maki, D. G., & Band, J. D. (1981). A comparative study of polyantibiotic and iodophor oint-

ments in prevention of vascular-catheter-related infection. *American Journal of Medicine, 70,* 739–744.
6. Metheny, N. M. (1996). *Fluid and electrolyte balance* (3rd ed., pp. 25–26). Philadelphia: J. B. Lippincott.
7. Hudak C., Gallo B., & Benz J. (1990). *Critical care nursing.* (5th ed., p. 123). Philadelphia: J. B. Lippincott.
8. Ryan, G. M., & Howland, W. S. (1966). An evaluation of central venous pressure monitoring. *Anesthesia and Analgesia, 45,* 754–759.
9. Ryan, J. A., Jr., & Gough, J. A. (1984). Complications of central venous catheterization for total parenteral nutrition. *Journal of the National Intravenous Therapy Association, 7*(1), 29–35.

10. Schuman, E. S., Winters V., Gross, G. F., & Hayes, J. F. (1985). Management of Hickman catheter sepsis. *American Journal of Surgery, 149,* 627.

11. Fischer, J. E. (1991). *Total parenteral nutrition* (2nd ed., pp. 36–37). Boston: Little, Brown.

BIBLIOGRAPHY

Bradham, G. B., & Walsh, N. (1965). Silastic for intravenous intubation. *Journal of S.L. Medical Association, 61,* 165.

Brendel, V. (1983). Current concepts in the care of central line catheters. *Journal of the National Intravenous Therapy Association, 6,* 272–274.

Camp-Sorrell, D. (1990). Advanced central venous access. *Journal of Intravenous Nursing, 6,* 361–365.

Gilligan, J. E., Phillips, P. J., et al. (1979). Streptokinase and blocked central venous catheter. *Lancet, 2,* 1189.

Hoshal, V. L. Jr., Ause, R. G., et al. (1971). Fibrin sleeve formation on indwelling subclavian central venous catheters. *Archives of Surgery, 102,* 353–358.

Hurtubise, M. R., Bottino, J. C., & Lawson, M. (1980). Restoring patency of occluded central venous catheters. *Archives of Surgery, 115,* 212–213.

Lindblad, B. (1982). Thromboembolic complications and central venous catheters [Letter]. *Lancet, 2,* 936.

Maki, D. G., Weise, C. E., & Sarafin, H. W. (1977). A semiquantitative culture method for identifying intravenous-catheter-related infection. *New England Journal of Medicine, 296,* 1305–1309.

Mansell, C. W. (1983). Peripherally inserted central venous catheterization by I.V. nurses: Establishing a precedent. *Journal of the National Intravenous Therapy Association, 6,* 355–356.

Nursing Photobook. (1980). *Managing I.V. therapy.* Horsham, PA: Intermed Communications, Inc.

Ostrow, L. S. (1981). Air embolism and central venous lines. *American Journal of Nursing, 81,* 2036.

Peters, W. R., Bush, W. H., et al. (1973). The development of fibrin sheath on indwelling venous catheters. *Surgery, Gynecology and Obstetrics, 137,* 43–47.

Rubin, R. N. (1983). Local installation of small doses of streptokinase for treatment of thrombotic occlusions of long-term access catheters. *Journal of Clinical Oncology, 1,* 572.

Sriram, K., Kaminski, M. V., et al. (1982). A safe technique of central venous catheterization. *Journal of Parenteral and Enteral Nutrition, 6,* 245–248.

Stephens, W., & Lawler, W. (1982). Thrombus formation and central venous catheters. *Lancet, 2,* 664.

REVIEW QUESTIONS

1. The ideal tip location for a central venous catheter is which of the following?
   a. junction of superior vena cava and right atrium
   b. junction of inferior vena cava and right atrium
   c. in the right atrium
   d. in the internal jugular

2. When measuring central venous pressure, zero point on the manometer is adjusted to the level of:
   a. patient's heart
   b. right atrium
   c. left lung
   d. sternum

3. The vein of choice for insertion of a PICC is:
   a. basilic
   b. axillary
   c. median carpal
   d. innominate

4. The Valsalva maneuver is used to minimize the risk of:
   a. serratia
   b. air embolism
   c. septic shock
   d. speed shock

5. Clinical parameters used to evaluate a patient in shock include all of the following EXCEPT:
   a. blood pressure
   b. rate/quality of pulse
   c. temperature
   d. urinary output

6. Measurement of central venous pressure is an important guide during all of the following EXCEPT:
   a. surgery
   b. shock
   c. anuria
   d. polyuria

7. Alternatives to guidewire insertion technique for the PICC catheter include which of the following?
   a. laser
   b. breakaway needle
   c. cannula technique
   d. fluoro

8. All connections should use all of the following systems EXCEPT:
   a. taping
   b. junction securement
   c. Luer locking
   d. slide clamps

9. Repair of an external tunneled catheter is what type of procedure?
   a. clean
   b. sanitary
   c. sterile
   d. nonsterile

10. Main objections to jugular cannulation include all of the following EXCEPT:
    a. catheter occlusion
    b. vein irritation
    c. difficulty in assessing sterility
    d. difficulty in maintaining dressin

CHAPTER 12

Advanced Vascular Access

Key Terms

Bonded	Implanted	Tunneled
Catheter materials	Intraosseous	Ventricular reservoir
Design	Specialty	

Vascular access has become a highly complex area of nursing specialization. With newer and more advanced therapies available to patients with diverse clinical needs, the infusion therapy nursing specialist must remain cognizant of changes in this exciting field. Manufacturers have kept pace with demands for more sophisticated products specific to various therapeutic modalities. In all clinical settings, a working knowledge of advanced vascular access is an essential part of IV nursing care.

DEVICES

Central venous catheterization is an integral component of the care of critically ill patients, allowing hemodynamic monitoring as well as administration of fluids, blood products, medications, and nutritional solutions. Central venous catheterization is now also an integral component of the care of patients in alternative settings, freeing the patient for months or a lifetime of nutritional support and related therapies.

Central venous access devices include tunneled lines, implanted ports, pumps, and reservoirs, and a diversity of central venous catheter products including single-, double-, and triple-lumen catheters with and without J wires, with and without introducer needles, and with and without peel-away sheaths. Each product is aimed at simplifying infusion therapy in a safe, efficient manner.

CATHETER MATERIALS

The ideal material for a central venous catheter would inhibit thrombus formation, be biocompatible, easily insertable, and be radiopaque (Table 12-1).

Deep-Vein Thrombosis

Deep-vein thrombosis from central venous catheters has many contributing factors. Any foreign material in the bloodstream becomes coated with a protein and fibrin deposit. Internal coagulation is activated, causing platelet activation, and platelets adhere to the catheter. Damage to endothelial cells at the puncture site enhances platelet activation. Patients requiring central venous catheters often have activated coagulation systems because of trauma or severe disease, both of which also promote the development of central venous catheter thrombosis. Thrombosis may be limited to a fibrin sheath formation or may be severe enough to cause vein occlusion. It may have no clinical significance or it may result in a fatal pulmonary embolism.[16]

Biocompatibility

Biocompatibility or bioinertness indicates that the tissues of the body do not react to the materials as a foreign substance. Silicone is the most bioinert material currently in use in the manufacturing process.

The majority of central venous catheters are made of polyvinylchloride (PVC), Teflon (™DuPont), polyurethane, or silicone.

Polyvinylchloride
Polyvinylchloride was the first catheter material. High incidences of thrombosis have been associated with this material.[10] Today, most central venous catheters are made of less thrombogenic materials.

Teflon
Teflon catheters are easily inserted because they are relatively stiff. However, they are reported to have a high incidence of thrombus formation.[11]

Polyurethane
Polyurethane is only moderately firm, so it is not as easily inserted. Thrombus formation is reported to be less than with Teflon. Hydromer-coated polyurethane catheters reportedly have a low incidence of thrombus formation.[2]

Silicone
Silicone catheters are very soft, much like a wet noodle, so they require special mechanisms for insertion. They are reported to have the lowest incidence of thrombus formation.

Radiopaque Catheters
Radiopaque catheters are available in all materials. This property is required to affirm catheter tip placement after insertion.

TABLE 12-1
Catheter Materials

PVC/Teflon

- Stiff
- Causes damage to the tunica intima
- Increased risk of platelet aggregation and subsequent thrombus formation
- Limited to subclavian or jugular insertion due to lack of flexibility

Polyurethane

- Rigid during insertion but softens at body temperature
- Less thrombogenicity
- Can be used at all sites

Silicone Elastomer/Silastic

- Very flexible
- Minimal thrombus formation
- Biocompatible
- Good for long-term use
- Dramatic fibrin sheath formation when particulate matter is present; rinse gloves and catheter before insertion

Elastomeric Hydrogel

- Available in peripheral lines; central lines in production
- Combines stretchable polymer with hydrophilic substance (water absorbing and similar to extended-wear contact lenses)
- Rinse with normal saline; easier to insert

BONDED CATHETERS

The most frequent life-threatening complication of central venous catheters is septicemia. Most related septicemias derive from invasion of the catheter wound by organisms from the patient's cutaneous microflora. Studies involving a triple-lumen polyurethane central venous catheter in which the entire catheter is impregnated with silver sulfadiazine and chlorhexidine proved favorable. It is believed that use of such a bonded catheter may substantially reduce the incidence of catheter-related infection, can extend the time that such lines may safely remain in place, and is cost efficient.[11] Known as Vita Cuff®, the product is available as a stand-alone to be used with Arrow's single-, double-, and triple-lumen catheters, percutaneous sheath introducers, and hemodialysis catheters[12] (Fig. 12-1).

The cuff is composed of two concentric layers of materials: an inner silicone sleeve that secures the cuff in place around a catheter, and an outer collagen matrix. The collagen matrix is made from purified type I bovine tendon collagen. Silver ions are chelated to the collagen matrix. Silver possesses a broad antimicrobial spectrum and has been used extensively in topical antimicrobial preparations in burn patients.

FIGURE 12-1 Vita Cuff® is composed of two concentric layers of material; used with Arrow's triple-lumen catheter. (Courtesy: Arrow International, Inc., Reading, PA)

The cuff, with introducer attached, is placed around a catheter before catheter insertion. The catheter is inserted percutaneously to the desired level. Then, the cuff is placed subcutaneously with the introducer, which is then separated from the cuff. After insertion, subcutaneous tissue grows into the collagenous matrix, anchoring the catheter and creating a barrier against invasion by extrinsic organisms. Significant antimicrobial activity associated with the Arrow catheter has been demonstrated using zone of inhibition bioassays against the following organisms:

- *Escherichia coli*
- *Pseudomonas aeruginosa*
- *Staphylococcus epidermidis*
- *Klebsiella pneumoniae*
- *Candida albicans*

Another bonding technique uses surfactant and antibiotics. A trial study[9] yielded a sevenfold reduction in the incidence of infection when catheters coated with penicillins and cephalosporins were used.

CATHETER DESIGNS

The design of the device is frequently related to the properties of the catheter material. The design also dictates insertion methods.

Through-the-Needle Catheter

The through-the-needle catheter (TNC) is often made of polyurethane or PVC.

Device Components

The unit consists of a stainless steel needle attached to a plastic sheath containing a catheter with or without a stylet and needle tip cover.

Insertion Technique

The venipuncture is performed with the stainless steel needle. The catheter is advanced through the needle. The needle is drawn back over the catheter and its tip protected with a cover.

Device Features

Because of its stiffness, the catheter is easy to insert a short distance into the vein. When attempting to thread a long catheter, difficulty may be encountered because of the stiffness. If this occurs, the stylet (if present) can be partially withdrawn to soften the catheter. A smooth insertion requires a vein without sharp twists or curves. The TNC is always a single-lumen catheter. If not used according to manufacturer's instructions, this device has a high risk of catheter embolism. During insertion the catheter must never be drawn back through the needle. The sharp needle can easily sever the catheter with a resultant embolism. Because the sharp needle must remain over the catheter, there is always the risk of catheter severance if manufacturer's instructions as to needle point protection are not followed. The TNC is a *short-term* inpatient central venous catheter. It was not designed for long-term or home care usage.

Catheter With Removable Introducer

Catheters with removable introducers are frequently made of polyurethane.

Device Components

The unit consists of an introducer catheter or syringe and needle and a catheter with stylet.

Insertion Technique

The venipuncture is performed with the needle and syringe. The syringe is removed and the catheter threaded through the needle. The needle is withdrawn from the vein and removed from the catheter by splitting the needle into two parts (Fig. 12-2).

Device Features

A catheter with a removable introducer is a single-lumen catheter with a fairly easy method of insertion. Because the device is usually made of polyurethane, it is softer than Teflon and easier to thread through twists and curves. Removal of any sharp needle eliminates the risk of catheter embolism. Because thrombus formation can be a problem with polyurethane, this may not be the catheter of choice for long-term therapy. However, minimal thrombus formation has been reported with hydromer-coated polyurethane and long-term usage.

Catheter With Introducer and Guidewire

A catheter with an introducer and guidewire allows for the insertion of a multiple-lumen silicone catheter.

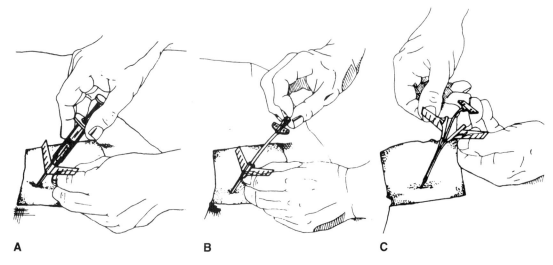

FIGURE 12-2 Insertion technique for catheter with removable introducer. (**A**) Venipuncture is performed with the introducer needle and syringe. (**B**) The syringe is removed and the catheter threaded through the needle. (**C**) The needle is withdrawn from the vein and removed from the catheter by splitting into two parts. (Courtesy: Luther Medical Products, Inc., Santa Ana, CA)

Introducer Needle
Appropriate gauge and length

**Straight and Curved Safe-T-J®
Double Flexible Tip Wire Guide**
Appropriate length, Teflon coated stainless steel

Catheter
Radiopaque polyurethane

FIGURE 12-3 (**A**) Components of a catheter with introducer and guidewire. (Courtesy: Cook Critical Care, Bloomington, IN) (**B**) Groshong OTG catheter (Courtesy: Davol, Inc., Subsidiary CR Bard Inc., Salt Lake City, UT)

Device Components

The unit consists of a syringe and needle or an over-the-needle catheter (ONC), long central catheter, and a guidewire (Fig. 12-3).

Insertion Technique

The venipuncture is performed with the syringe and needle or ONC. The syringe or stylet is removed. The guidewire is threaded through the short catheter or needle, and the short catheter or needle is withdrawn. The puncture site may be enlarged with a no. 11 scalpel blade. The long catheter is threaded over the guidewire (Fig. 12-4), and the guidewire withdrawn, leaving the long catheter in the vein.

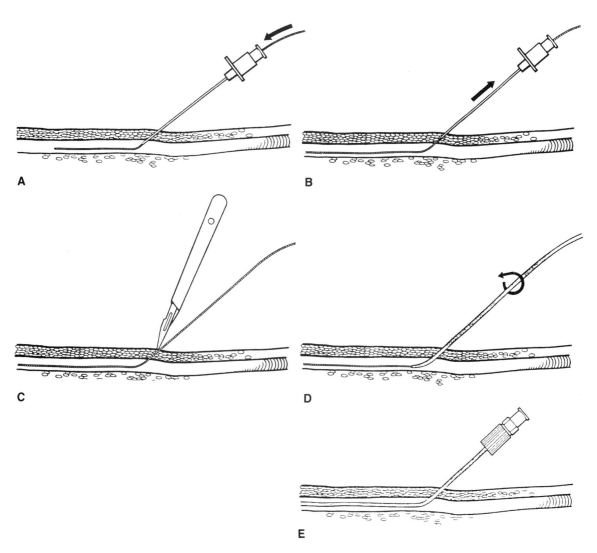

FIGURE 12-4 Insertion technique for catheter with introducer and guidewire. (**A**) The guidewire is threaded through the inserted needle. (**B**) The needle is withdrawn from the vein. (**C**) The puncture site may be enlargd with a no. 11 scalpel blade. (**D**) The catheter is threaded over the guidewire. (**E**) The guidewire is withdrawn, leaving the catheter in the vein. (Courtesy: Cook Critical Care, Bloomington, IN)

Device Features

The silicone catheter has the lowest reports of thrombus formation. The design allows for multiple-lumen catheter placement. It requires a fairly complex method of insertion with a large amount of "in-and-out" manipulation in the vein. The silicone catheter is an excellent *long-term* central catheter for both inpatient and home care use.

Tunneled Catheters

The indwelling tunneled catheter is made of polymeric silicone.

Device Components

This single- or double-lumen catheter contains a Dacron cuff. The external end has a "ring" with a threaded Luer lock adapter covered with a Luer lock cap. An integral clamp may be present (Fig. 12-5). One version of this catheter has a closed tip and a lateral two-way valve. The valve opens outward for infusion and inward for blood sample drawing. This model does not require heparin flush to maintain catheter patency.

Insertion Technique

The insertion may be performed by cutdown or percutaneous puncture. This is performed under fluoroscopy, usually in a minor surgery operating room.

The catheter is placed by locating the subclavian vein, forming a tunnel from the vein to an area between the sternum and the nipple, pulling the catheter through the tunnel, inserting it into the vein, and threading it until the tip is in the superior vena cava (Fig. 12-6).

Device Features

Fibrous tissue forms around the Dacron cuff. The cuff and tunnel anchor the catheter and help prevent infection. Because the material is polymeric silicone, this catheter has reports of a low incidence of thrombus formation. It is a perfect central venous catheter for home IV therapy. This catheter is also inserted for long-term inpatient use.

FIGURE 12-5   Dual-lumen Hickman catheter. (Courtesy: Davol, Inc., Subsidiary CR Bard Inc., Salt Lake City, UT)

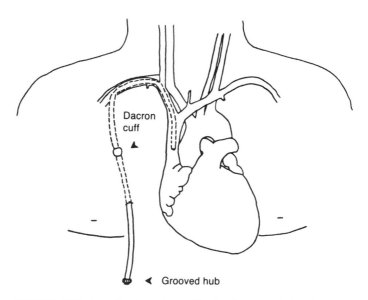

FIGURE 12-6 Insertion technique of indwelling tunneled catheter. A funnel is formed from the vein to an area between the sternum and the nipple. The catheter tip is placed in the superior vena cava.

Implanted Ports and Other Venous Access Devices

Totally implanted devices for repeated venous access eliminate the need for frequent venipunctures.

Device Components

The unit consists of a silicone catheter attached to a reservoir with a self-sealing septum. At the present time, four manufacturers make this device (Figs. 12-7 through 12-10). Units are available with single or double lumens. Special noncoring needles are required to access these devices.

Insertion Technique

The unit is surgically placed under local or general anesthesia. The insertion technique is similar to that used for implanted tunneled catheters. The catheter is placed in the subclavian vein and threaded into the vein until the tip lies in the superior vena cava. This position is confirmed by fluoroscopy. A pocket is made for the reservoir. The reservoir is sutured in the pocket. Because the center of the port will be punctured repeatedly, when the pocket is closed the suture line is lateral, medial, superior, or inferior to the port septum (Fig. 12-11).

Device Features

This device has reports of a low incidence of thrombus formation from the silicone catheter. When not in use, the only care required is a monthly heparin flush. The fact that this is totally implanted, leaving no catheter exiting from the chest, makes it a favorite device with many patients. It is an "artificial vein" perfect for any patient receiving *long-term periodic* infusion therapy in the home or in the hospital.

FIGURE 12-7 PORT-A-CATH® Implantable Peritoneal Access System (Property of SIMS Deltec, St. Paul, MN)

FIGURE 12-8 PORT-A-CATH® Venous Access System with PolyFlow™ catheter. (Property of SIMS Deltec, St. Paul, MN)

FIGURE 12-9   PORT-A-CATH® Implantable Dual-Lumen Venous Access System (Property of SIMS Deltec, St. Paul, MN)

SPECIALTY DEVICES

Totally Implanted Pump

Totally implanted pumps are designed for continuous, low-volume, long-term ambulatory therapy. They may be used for arterial or venous infusion and tissue perfusion.

Device Components

The device consists of two chambers separated by flexible metal bellows. One chamber is the drug reservoir; the other contains the charging fluid in a completely sealed

FIGURE 12-10   SidePort (Courtesy: Norfolk Medical, Skokie, IL)

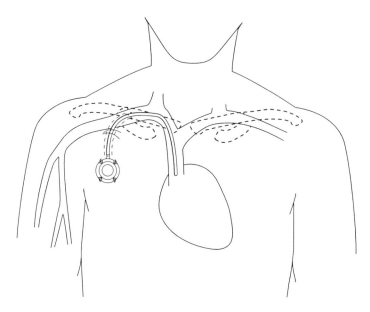

FIGURE 12-11   Placement of the PORT-A-CATH® Venous Access System with PolyFlow™ catheter. (Property of SIMS Deltec, St. Paul, MN)

compartment. The vapor pressure of the charging fluid exerts a constant pressure on the bellows, forcing the drug out of the reservoir through an outlet filter and flow restrictor into a silicone catheter (Fig. 12-12). When the pump is refilled, the increasing pressure within the drug chamber exerts a pressure on the charging fluid, causing the fluid vapor to condense to its liquid state, thereby storing energy for the next pumping cycle.

Various models are available. The basic device has one catheter. One model also has a direct access port that bypasses the reservoir for administering bolus injections. Another model has double catheters, which can be used to administer a drug to more than one site.

Insertion Technique

The pump is implanted in the operating room under fluoroscopy. To activate the charging fluid, the pump must be heated for 30 minutes at 30° to 40°C before implantation. This is done with a heating pad. The insertion technique is the same as that for the implanted venous access. The pocket is frequently located below the umbilicus on the abdomen.

Device Features

Several factors will influence the pump flow rate. If the catheter site is arterial and *arterial blood pressure increases significantly*, the flow rate can decrease by as much as 15%. *Hypotension* can increase the rate by as much as 6%. When the patient moves from one *altitude* to another, the rate can increase by as much as 38%. *Fever* can increase flow rate by as much as 13%. The *amount of drug in the reservoir* will affect the flow rate. The pump flow rate is established with the reservoir half full. At full volume the rate will be approximately 3% faster and at low volume 3% slower than the mean flow rate.[7]

The silicone catheter results in a low incidence of thrombus formation. This is an excellent method for *continuous long-term administration* of *low-volume* narcotics or chemotherapeutic agents to cancer patients. Because there are no external parts, it requires no care between port refills.

Contraindications

Contraindications for the implanted pump include:

1. All but very small volumes of drugs
2. A body size not large enough for the size and weight of the pump
3. Patients with severe emotional, psychiatric, or neurologic disturbances
4. Patients who travel extensively or frequently and experience altitudinal changes[7]

Aids for Preventing Catheter Clotting

While the nurse injects the heparin flush, the clamp is applied before the syringe is completely empty. The syringe and needle are removed while pressure is applied on the plunger. This prevents reflux of blood into the lumen, which could result in catheter clotting.

When the catheter is not in use, taping the hub to the chest wall above heart level will minimize blood pressure at the catheter tip.

FIGURE 12-12   Components of the implanted pump. Infusaid™. (Courtesy: Intermedics Infusaid, Inc., Norwood, MA)

Discontinuing Infusion

When an infusion is completed, an injection cap and heparin flush are used to maintain catheter patency. A normal saline flush is given before the heparin to rinse the IV fluid from the catheter. If the catheter is of a material that cannot be clamped without possible damage and there is no extension tubing that can be clamped, the patient must perform the Valsalva maneuver at any time the catheter is open to the air.

The following steps may be used to discontinue the infusion, connect an injection cap, and flush with normal saline and heparin.

Equipment

Smooth blade catheter clamp (1)   Povidone-iodine swab (3)

Luer lock injection cap (1)   Alcohol sponge (1)

10 mL syringe (1)   Sterile 2 × 2 inch sponge (1)

22 gauge × 1 inch needle (1)   Tape

Sodium chloride 0.9% 10 mL (1)   Sterile gloves one pair (optional)

Prefilled syringe with heparin flush (1)

Procedure

1. Wash hands thoroughly and dry.
2. Aseptically open all sterile supplies.
3. Prepare air-purged 10 mL 0.9% sodium chloride syringe with a 22-gauge × 1-inch needle.
4. Prepare air-purged heparin flush.
5. Shut infusion off and clamp catheter.
6. Remove old tape from catheter filter–IV tubing connection.
7. Cleanse connection with povidone-iodine swab for 30 seconds.
8. Place connection on sterile 2 × 2 inch sponge and allow to dry.
9. Put on gloves, they may be used at this time. Pick up connection by holding catheter hub with the sterile sponge.
10. Aseptically disconnect and discard infusion tubing.
11. Aseptically connect and lock injection cap.
12. Remove clamp.
13. Cleanse rubber end of injection cap with povidone-iodine for 30 seconds. Allow to dry.
14. *Carefully* insert needle of syringe with normal saline flush into center of injection cap. Do not exert force. If an obstruction is felt, realign needle angle.
15. Inject normal saline flush.
16. While still holding catheter hub, remove empty syringe. Recleanse injection cap end with povidone-iodine for 30 seconds; allow to dry.
17. *Carefully* insert needle of heparin flush. Do not force insertion. If an obstruction is felt, realign needle angle.

18. Inject heparin flush. Before the syringe is completely empty, close catheter clamp.
19. Remove syringe and needle, applying pressure on plunger during withdrawal.
20. Remove clamp.
21. Secure injection cap to catheter with a strip of tape.
22. Tape catheter hub on the chest wall above heart level.

Routine Flushing

Routine flushing is required to maintain patency of unused catheters. If the catheter has more than one lumen, remember to flush each unused lumen. Either heparin or saline may be used.

The following steps may be used to perform heparin flush without changing the intermittent injection cap.

Equipment

Smooth-blade catheter clamp (1)

Prefilled syringe with heparin dosage (1) (Fig. 12-13)

Povidone-iodine swab (1)

Tape

Procedure

1. Wash hands thoroughly and dry.
2. Prepare air-purged heparin flush.
3. Remove tape holding end of catheter to chest wall.
4. Cleanse rubber end of injection cap with povidone-iodine for 30 seconds. Allow to dry.
5. While stabilizing the catheter hub, carefully insert needle of heparin flush syringe into center of cap. If an obstruction is felt, do not apply force but realign needle angle.
6. Gently inject heparin flush. Clamp the catheter before the syringe is completely empty.
7. Apply pressure on plunger while removing syringe and needle.
8. Remove clamp.
9. Tape catheter hub on chest wall above heart level.

Changing Intermittent Injection Cap

The injection cap must be changed at routine intervals. If the catheter is flushed every other day, cap changing may be coordinated with each third flushing (every 6 days). Using an intermittent injection cap that has a very small amount of dead space eliminates the need to preflush the cap. This minimizes the risk of touch contamination.

FIGURE 12-13 Wyeth's Tubex Injector, loaded for instillation of saline or heparin in lock. (Courtesy: Wyeth-Ayerst Laboratories, Philadelphia, PA)

If the catheter contains more than one lumen, remember to change the caps on all unused lumens. If the catheter is made of a material that cannot be clamped without catheter damage, be sure that the patient is flat in bed and performs the Valsalva maneuver at any time the catheter is open to the air.

The following steps may be used to change the intermittent injection cap at the time of heparin flushing.

Equipment

Smooth-blade catheter clamp (1)

Prefilled syringe with heparin dosage (1)

Luer lock intermittent injection cap (1)

Sterile 2 × 2 inch sponge (1)

Povidone-iodine swabs (2)

Tape

Procedure

1. Wash hands thoroughly and dry.

2. Aseptically prepare sterile supplies. Put on gloves.

3. Prepare air-purged heparin flush.

4. Remove tape holding catheter to chest wall. Remove tape securing cap to catheter.

5. Cleanse cap–catheter connection point with povidone-iodine for 30 seconds. Place on sterile sponge and allow to dry.

6. Close clamp.

7. Pick up catheter hub protected by sterile sponge. Be careful not to touch the cleansed connection.

8. *Carefully* unlock, remove, and discard old cap.

9. Holding the new cap by the rubber injection end, connect and lock to catheter.

10. Secure connection with a strip of tape.

11. Remove clamp.

12. Cleanse rubber end of injection cap with povidone-iodine for 30 seconds. Allow to dry.

13. *Carefully* insert needle of heparin flush into center of rubber end. Do not force insertion. If an obstruction is felt, realign needle angle.

14. Gently inject heparin. Before the syringe is completely empty, close clamp.

15. Apply pressure on plunger while withdrawing syringe and needle.

16. Remove clamp.

17. Tape catheter hub on the chest wall above heart level.

Venous Sampling

Many central venous catheters are placed on patients without available peripheral veins or to minimize peripheral venipunctures. Therefore, drawing blood specimens through central catheters is common practice. Three basic methods are used with tunneled and nontunneled catheters: 1) drawing specimens from a continuous infusion line maintaining the closed system; 2) drawing specimens from a continuous infusion line by opening the system; and 3) drawing specimens from a catheter with an in-place intermittent injection cap.

If the system does not have the possibility of catheter clamping, the patient must be placed flat in bed and perform the Valsalva maneuver whenever the catheter is open to the air. If this is not done, air embolism is always possible.

Prothrombin Time and Partial Thromboplastin Time Tests and Heparin
Any blood specimen drawn through a central catheter that has been flushed with heparin or that has heparin as a solution additive should not be used for prothrombin time or partial thromboplastin time testing. Heparin adheres to the catheter and can result in falsely elevated values for these tests.

Patient Identification
Before drawing any blood specimens the patient must be accurately identified. This should be done by the patient's hospital identification band. Asking the patient to state his or her name may supplement but should never be substituted for some form of written identification on the patient.

Labeling Specimen Tubes
Before drawing the blood specimen, all tubes should be labeled with the patient's full name, room number, hospital identification number, and the initials of the person

drawing the blood. This is done to prevent mislabeling, which can result in inadequate or inappropriate treatment.

Drawing Blood Specimens From Continuous Infusion Line Maintaining a Closed System

This procedure requires an injection port between the filter and the catheter. It may be performed by using the following equipment and procedure.

Equipment

Vacuum tube holder (1)

Multiple draw needle: 22 gauge × 1 inch (1)

Appropriate number and type vacuum tube(s) for tests

0.9% sodium chloride 10 mL (2)

10-mL syringe (2)

Needles: 22 gauge × 1 inch (2)

Povidone-iodine swab (3)

Alcohol sponge (1)

Procedure

1. Put on gloves. Strict aseptic technique must be used throughout the entire procedure.
2. Prepare two air-purged 10 mL 0.9% sodium chloride syringes with 22-gauge × 1-inch needles.
3. Prepare vacuum tube holder, needle, and tube. Do not fully insert tube into needle because vacuum will be lost.
4. Shut off infusion for 1 minute before drawing blood specimens to prevent blood contamination with infusion fluid. This is especially important when total parenteral nutrition is infusing.
5. Close clamp distal to injection port (Fig. 12-14A).
6. Cleanse injection port with povidone-iodine for 30 seconds. Allow to dry.
7. Hold injection port while performing all entries and withdrawals. Aseptically insert needle of first normal saline flush directly into center of port. Gently inject solution to flush extension tubing (if used) and catheter of infusate (Fig. 12-14B).
8. Withdraw syringe full (10 mL) of blood and fluid mixture. Remove and discard syringe and needle.
9. Recleanse injection port with povidone-iodine for 30 seconds. Allow to dry.
10. Aseptically insert needle of vacuum tube unit into center of injection port.
11. Fully insert tube into needle. Allow tube to fill with blood (Fig. 12-14C).
12. Remove tube. Continue to insert, allow to fill, and remove required tube(s) for blood specimen(s). Be sure to mix, by gentle rotation, all specimens drawn in tubes with an anticoagulant.
13. Remove holder, tube, and needle.

FIGURE 12-14 Procedure for drawing blood specimens from continuous infusion line maintaining a closed system. (**A**) The clamp distal to the injection port is closed. (**B**) Normal saline is injected to clear system of infusate. (**C**) Allow vacuum tube to fill with blood.

14. Recleanse injection port with povidone-iodine for 30 seconds. Allow to dry.

15. Aseptically, insert needle of second syringe with 0.9% sodium chloride into center of injection port. Gently flush to rinse blood cells from the catheter.

16. Open clamp and regulate infusion drip rate.

Drawing Blood Specimens From Continuous Infusion Line by Opening the System

This procedure requires a catheter that can be clamped because the catheter will be opened to the air several times. An extension tubing that contains a clamp may be aseptically Luer locked and taped to the catheter hub as a substitute. Extreme care must be taken to maintain sterility when the extension tubing is used for this purpose. This procedure should be performed in correlation with the tubing change to avoid reconnecting a used tubing after the blood specimens are drawn.

The following equipment and steps may be used to perform the venous sampling.

Equipment

Catheter clamp or in-site extension tubing with clamp (1)

Appropriate number and type vacuum tubes for tests

Syringe large enough to hold required amount of blood (1)

10-mL syringes (2)

Needles: 20 gauge × 1 inch (3)

FIGURE 12-14   *(Continued)*

0.9% sodium chloride 10 mL (2)

Povidone-iodine swab (1)

Alcohol sponge (1)

Sterile 2 × 2 inch sponge (1)

Appropriate infusion tubing (1)

Luer lock 0.2-μm air-eliminating filter (1)

Procedure

1. Put on gloves. Strict aseptic technique must be maintained throughout the entire procedure.

2. Prepare fresh IV system, flush tubing and filter.

3. Prepare two air-purged syringes of 10 mL 0.9% sodium chloride.

4. Shut infusion off for 1 minute. Close clamp.

5. Remove old tape at catheter–tubing or filter connection.

6. Cleanse connection for 30 seconds with povidone-iodine swab. Place on sterile sponge to dry.

7. Pick up connection by protecting catheter hub with sterile sponge.

8. Disconnect and discard infusion system.

9. Continue to hold hub with sterile sponge during all connection and disconnection manipulations. Connect first air-purged syringe of 0.9% sodium chloride.

10. Open clamp. Gently inject flush to rinse catheter, and extension tubing, if used.

11. Withdraw 10 mL blood and fluid mixture. Close clamp.

12. Disconnect and discard syringe.

13. Connect large syringe, open clamp, and withdraw required amount of blood for all ordered tests.

14. Close clamp. Disconnect syringe filled with blood. A second person may be required to add needle and fill specimen tube(s). Be sure to mix by gentle rotation all tubes with an anticoagulant.

15. Connect second air-purged syringe with 0.9% sodium chloride. Open clamp and inject flush to rinse blood from catheter.

16. Close clamp, remove syringe. Connect, lock, and tape Luer lock connection of IV tubing or filter to catheter. Open clamp. Reestablish infusion flow rate.

17. Tape tubing to chest wall to prevent relayed stress to the connection if the tubing is pulled or stretched.

Drawing Blood Specimens From Catheters With Injection Cap in Place

This procedure is frequently performed, especially with multiple-lumen catheters. The most proximal lumen is usually reserved for this purpose. By using the distal lumen(s) for infusions, the fluid is downstream from the site where the blood will be drawn. This decreases the risk of blood contamination with the infusate if the solution cannot be turned off or can be turned off only for a very short period of time.

When inserting needles into an intermittent injection cap, force should never be applied. If an obstruction is felt, realigning the angle of the needle will facilitate entry.

Blood may be drawn from a central catheter with an injection cap in place by using the following equipment and steps.

Equipment

Vacuum tube holder (1)

Multiple-sample needle: 22 gauge × 1 inch (1)

Appropriate number and type vacuum tubes for tests

0.9% sodium chloride 10 mL (2)

10-mL syringes (2)

Needles: 22 gauge × 1 inch (2)

Prefilled syringe with heparin dosage (1)

Povidone-iodine swabs (4)

Alcohol swab (1)

Tape

Procedure

1. Put on gloves. Aseptic technique must be maintained throughout the entire procedure.

2. Prepare two air-purged 10-mL 0.9% sodium chloride flushes. Prepare air-purged heparin flush.

3. Prepare vacuum tube holder and needle with first tube. Do not fully insert tube into needle because vacuum will be lost.

4. Cleanse rubber end of injection cap with povidone-iodine for 30 seconds. Allow to dry.

5. Hold catheter hub without touching end of injection cap during all needle entries and withdrawals. Insert needle of first air-purged syringe with normal saline flush into center of rubber cap.

6. Inject flush to rinse heparin from catheter.

7. Withdraw 10 mL blood and solution mixture. Remove and discard needle and syringe.

8. Recleanse rubber end of injection cap with povidone-iodine for 30 seconds. Allow to dry.

9. Insert needle of vacuum tube unit into center of injection cap. Fully insert tube into needle. Allow tube to fill with blood. Remove tube.

10. Insert, allow to fill, and remove required specimen tubes. Be sure to mix by gentle rotation all tubes with an anticoagulant.

11. Recleanse rubber end of injection cap with povidone-iodine for 30 seconds. Allow to dry.

12. Insert needle of second syringe with normal saline flush into center of injection cap.

13. Inject flush to rinse blood from catheter. Remove syringe and needle.

14. Recleanse rubber end of injection port with povidone-iodine for 30 seconds. Allow to dry.

15. Insert needle of heparin flush into center of injection cap.

16. Gently inject heparin. Before the syringe is completely empty, clamp tubing. Apply pressure on plunger while withdrawing needle and syringe.

17. Remove clamp and tape catheter hub on chest wall above heart level.

18. Remove gloves and wash hands.

TUNNELED CATHETERS

Originally available as a Broviac catheter and later modified with a larger diameter by Hickman and associates, today's tunneled right atrial catheter is made of silicone and is available in a single-, double-, and triple-lumen configuration (Fig. 12-15). Many tunneled lines feature an integral catheter clamp and a reinforced segment of catheter to reduce the risk of silicone fatigue after repeated clamping.

Insertion is performed as a surgical procedure, through a cutdown in which the vein is isolated and the catheter is inserted. After locating the catheter tip in the central vein, the remaining portion is threaded or tunneled into the subcutaneous tissue 3 to 5 cm to an exit site outside the skin. Typical exit sites are below the nipple, in the abdomen, or in the groin. A Dacron cuff is an integral part of the tunneled line and extends from the exit site. Granulation tissue forms around the cuff in 10 to 14 days, preventing migration of microorganisms into the catheter pathway.

When a dual-lumen catheter is used, the lumens should be labeled to indicate the purpose and function of each port.

Manufacturers have continued to provide more advanced product options. In addition to the Hickman and Broviac catheters and their multiple-lumen styles, the Groshong catheter (Davol) offers an alternative. The Groshong catheter is distinguished by the construction of a rounded, blunt catheter tip that incorporates a three-way valve. A three-position pressure-sensitive valve (Fig. 12-16) that remains closed at normal vena caval pressure restricts either entrainment of air into the venous system or backflow of blood from the catheter. Application of a vacuum with a syringe allows the valve to open inward for blood aspiration. Positive pressure into the catheter by the infusion forces the valve to open outward. Advantages of this type of catheter include:

- Decreased risk of bleeding or air emboli
- Elimination of catheter clamping
- Elimination of the use of heparin in the catheter
- Reduction of flushing between use

FIGURE 12-15   Dual-lumen Hickman catheters. (Courtesy: Davol, Inc., Subsidiary CR Bard Inc., Salt Lake City, UT)

FIGURE 12-16   Groshong valve. (Courtesy: Davol, Inc., Subsidiary CR Bard Inc., Salt Lake City, UT)

For the valve to function properly, catheter tip position is critical. The tip must be situated in the midsuperior part of the vena cava.[13] If the tip is in the right atrium, thrombus formation around the tip could result, followed by malfunction and loss of valve competence. Occasional use of a fibrinolytic agent may restore valve function. Clamping and flushing with heparin similar to the procedure followed with non-valved catheters may be needed.

The Hemed central venous catheter (GISH Biomedical, Inc.) is a long-term tunneled catheter composed of biocompatible silicone and available in single- and dual-lumen configurations. A locking clip holds the dilator and sheath together as a unit during surgical insertion. GISH Biomedical also manufactures a CathCap Catheter System in which a prefilled povidone-iodine cap immerses and bathes the hub while the cap serves as a barrier against airborne, waterborne, and touch-contamination microorganisms.

IMPLANTED PORTS

Implanted ports are designed to permit repeated access to the vascular system. In general, the portal consists of one or two self-sealing silicone septa, accessible by percutaneous needle puncture, and a single- or dual-lumen catheter. For the patient in need of long-term vascular access, the implanted port system is ideal. As with any central venous access system, potential complications exist, including:

* Air embolism
* Artery or vein puncture

- Arteriovenous fistula
- Brachial plexus injury
- Cardiac arrhythmia
- Cardiac puncture
- Cardiac tamponade
- Catheter disconnection/fragmentation/embolization
- Catheter occlusion
- Catheter rupture
- Drug extravasation
- Erosion of portal/catheter through skin and/or blood vessel
- Fibrin sheath formation
- Hematoma
- Hemothorax
- Implant rejection
- Infection/sepsis
- Migration of portal/catheter
- Pneumothorax
- Thoracic duct injury
- Thromboembolism
- Thrombosis

The implanted port may be used for arterial access or implanted into the epidural space, peritoneum, pericardia, or pleural cavity (Fig. 12-17). Vascular access ports may be side entry or top entry. In a side-entry port, the needle is inserted almost

FIGURE 12-17 Accessing the PORT-A-CATH® Venous Access System. (Property of SIMS Deltec, St. Paul, MN)

parallel to the reservoir. In a top-entry port, the needle is inserted perpendicular to the reservoir. Only noncoring needles should be used to access the port. A noncoring needle has an angled or deflected point that slices the septum on entry. When removed, the septum reseals itself. Noncoring needles are available in straight and 90° angle configurations, with or without extension sets. Some clinicians recommend the use of an ONC for continuous access to an implanted port. A winged noncoring needle, such as the Gripper™ by SIMS Deltec, is also helpful and relatively easy to stabilize (Fig. 12-18).

Sterile Technique

Because this device is placed for long-term usage, extreme care must be taken to maintain sterile technique while performing any manipulations.

Needles

To prevent septum damage, only noncoring needles may be used for cannulation of the device. Straight needles are used for heparin flush, bolus injection, or blood drawing. Needles bent to a 90° angle are used for continuous or frequent intermittent infusions. The bent needle may also be used for heparin flush, bolus injection, or blood drawing. Noncoring needles are also available with a permanently attached extension tubing and clamp.

Needles are available, with metal or plastic hubs, in gauges 24 to 19, and in lengths from 0.5 inch to 2.5 inches. The needle length required will depend on how superficial or deep the septum is implanted. The gauge will depend on the type and rate of infusate to be given. Packed red cells may require a 19-gauge needle, whereas a 24-gauge needle may be adequate for flushing.

The needle must be held securely against the needle stop during all procedures to avoid injecting the drug into the subcutaneous tissue. Do not use an angular motion or

FIGURE 12-18 PORT-A-CATH® Gripper™ Needle. Access of implanted ports is facilitated by the use of a needle with gripping device. (Property of SIMS Deltec, St. Paul, MN)

twist the needle once in the septum. This action will cut the septum and create a drug leakage path. If the heparin flush is given without an extension tubing, 3 mL heparin (100 U/mL) is used. If an extension tubing is used, 5 mL heparin may be required.

Access of the side port is similar (Fig. 12-19).

Heparin Flush

Implanted catheters require heparin flushing after each use and monthly when not in use. This is almost universally done with 3 to 5 mL of 100 U/mL heparin.

The heparin flush may be performed by the following steps:

Equipment

Sterile noncoring needle (1)

Sterile syringe with 3 mL heparin flush (100 U/mL)

Sterile gloves (1 pair)

Sterile towel (1)

Sterile fenestrated drape (optional)

Povidone-iodine swabs (3)

Procedure

1. Identify septum by palpating the outer perimeter of the port. Confirm septum location.
2. Wash hands thoroughly and dry.
3. Aseptically prepare sterile supplies on opened sterile towel.
4. Put on sterile gloves. Observing sterile technique, perform *three* separate skin preps with povidone-iodine. Start at center of septum and work outward toward the periphery of the port.

FIGURE 12-19 Access side port. (Courtesy: Norfolk Medical, Skokie, IL)

5. Place fenestrated drape over prepped area (optional). The availability of a sterile field at the insertion site will decrease risk of touch contamination during the procedure.

6. Attach syringe with heparin flush to noncoring needle and eliminate air from syringe and needle. A straight or 90° angled needle may be used for heparin flush.

7. *While stabilizing the port*, using a *perpendicular angle*, insert needle into septum until the needle stop is felt.

8. Inject flush no faster than 5 mL/min.

9. Withdraw needle while *maintaining stability of the port*.

10. Examine the site closely for any signs of infiltration or leakage. Apply sterile dressing if necessary.

Connecting Implanted Catheter to Continuous Infusion System

When a continuous infusion is to be started, the device is cannulated with an extension tubing connected between the needle and the infusion tubing. If frequent intermittent infusions are given, the needle and extension tubing are left in place and the extension tubing covered with an intermittent injection cap. This prevents the need for frequent septum punctures.

Equipment

Electronic infusion device (optional)

Appropriate infusion tubing

Luer lock air-eliminating 0.22-μm filter (1)

Luer lock extension tubing with clamp or stopcock (1)

Admixture or infusion solution

Noncoring 90° angled needle

Sterile towel (1)

Sterile fenestrated drape (optional)

Sterile 10-mL syringe with 0.9% sodium chloride

Sterile strip of tape (1)

Povidone-iodine swabs (3)

Povidone-iodine ointment (optional)

Sterile gloves (1 pair)

Sterile 2 × 2 inch sponges (2)

Sterile transparent tape dressing (1)

Procedure

1. Identify septum by palpating the outer perimeter of the port. Confirm septum location.

2. Wash hands thoroughly and dry.

3. Prepare solution container, tubing, and filter. Flush system. If infusion pump is used, be sure psi is less than 15 to prevent possibility of catheter rupture.

4. Aseptically prepare all sterile supplies on opened sterile towel.

5. Put on sterile gloves. Using sterile technique perform *three* separate site preps with povidone-iodine. Start at the center of the septum and work outward beyond the periphery of the port.

6. Place fenestrated drape over prepped area (optional).

7. Attach 10-mL syringe with 0.9% sodium chloride to extension tubing.

8. Firmly lock noncoring 90° angle needle to extension tubing.

9. Flush extension tubing and needle with the 0.9% sodium chloride. Close stopcock or clamp.

10. *While stabilizing the port*, using a perpendicular angle, insert needle into septum until the needle stop is felt. Digital pressure on top of the needle at the bend point will facilitate septum entry.

11. Open stopcock or clamp, stabilize port, and inject normal saline to affirm needle placement. Carefully observe site for any signs of infiltration. If desired, a small amount of blood may be withdrawn to affirm septum entry.

12. Close stopcock or clamp and remove syringe.

13. Securely connect and lock prepared infusion system to the extension tubing. The use of Luer locks and taping connections will reduce the risk of separation.

14. Open stopcock or clamp and start the infusion.

15. If the needle does not lie flush with the skin, place a sterile sponge under needle or needle hub.

16. If povidone-iodine ointment is to be used, apply to insertion site. The use of an ointment at this access point may create increased risk of needle movement with resultant dislodgment and can prevent direct observation of the insertion site.

17. Placing a strip of sterile tape over the needle at the insertion site can help prevent needle dislodgment.

18. Using aseptic technique, apply sterile transparent tape dressing over the site and a portion of the extension tubing. Using clear sterile tape allows for site inspection without removing the dressing.

19. Loop the tubing and tape on the skin to prevent stress at the needle site if the tubing is stretched or pulled.

Discontinuing Infusion

A continuous infusion may be discontinued by the following steps:

1. Shut infusion off. Close clamp on extension tubing or turn stopcock off.

2. Aseptically disconnect IV tubing from stopcock or extension tubing.

3. Aseptically connect air-purged syringe with 10 mL 0.9% sodium chloride. Open clamp or stopcock. Inject sodium chloride to flush system. Close clamp or stopcock.

4. Remove empty syringe. Connect air-purged syringe with 5 mL (100 U/mL) heparin. Open clamp or stopcock. Inject heparin flush.

5. Stabilize the needle while removing the clear tape and any sponges.

6. Remove the needle while *maintaining* stability.

7. Examine injection site for any signs of swelling or fluid seepage.

8. Apply a sterile dressing if necessary.

Administering a Bolus Injection

A bolus injection may be given by the following steps:

Equipment

Sterile noncoring needle (1)

Sterile extension tubing with clamp or two-way stopcock (1)

Sterile syringes 10 mL (2)

Sterile syringe 5 mL (1)

Sterile syringe appropriate size for drug (1)

Sterile needles: 22 gauge × 1 inch (4)

Sodium chloride 0.9% 20 mL

Heparin flush 5 mL (100 U/mL)

Drug to be injected

Sterile gloves (1 pair)

Sterile towel (1)

Sterile fenestrated drape (optional)

Povidone-iodine swabs (3)

Alcohol sponge (1)

Procedure

1. Identify septum by palpating the outer perimeter of the port. Confirm septum location.

2. Wash hands thoroughly and dry.

3. Open sterile towel and aseptically prepare all sterile supplies.

4. Put on sterile gloves. Observing sterile technique perform *three* separate skin preps with povidone-iodine. Start at center of septum and work outward toward the periphery of the port.

5. Place fenestrated drape over prepped area (optional). The availability of a sterile field at the needle insertion site will decrease risk of touch contamination during the procedure.

6. Using sterile technique, prepare two air-purged syringes with 10 mL normal saline, one air-purged syringe with 5 mL heparin flush, and an air-purged syringe with drug to be injected.

7. Connect extension tubing or stopcock to first syringe with 0.9% sodium chloride and noncoring needle. Flush the system. Close clamp or turn stopcock off.

8. While stabilizing port, using a perpendicular angle insert needle into septum until needle stop is felt. Open clamp or turn stopcock on. Inject sodium chloride. To prevent needle dislodgment during any injection, the needle should be stabilized either digitally or with a 90° angle needle by the use of a sterile strip of tape.

9. Turn stopcock off or clamp extension tubing, disconnect empty syringe, and connect air-purged syringe with drug. Turn stopcock on or open tubing clamp, inject drug at recommended rate but no faster than 5 mL/min.

10. Turn stopcock off or clamp extension tubing, disconnect empty syringe, and connect second air-purged 10-mL syringe of 0.9% sodium chloride. Turn stopcock on or open tubing clamp, inject flush.

11. Turn stopcock off or clamp extension tubing, disconnect empty syringe, and connect air-purged syringe with heparin flush. Turn stopcock on or open tubing clamp, and inject heparin flush.

12. Remove needle while *maintaining stability of the port.*

13. Examine site closely for any signs of infiltration or leakage. Apply sterile dressing if necessary.

Venous Sampling

Blood samples may be drawn as a separate procedure, at the time of a bolus injection, or during continuous infusion. To draw a blood sample as a separate procedure or at the time of a bolus injection:

1. Follow all steps including the first flush with 0.9% sodium chloride given for a bolus injection (steps 1 through 7).

2. Using the empty syringe, draw back 10 mL blood and saline mixture. Close stopcock or clamp and remove and discard syringe with blood.

3. Attach fresh sterile syringe, open stopcock or clamp, and withdraw required amount of blood for ordered specimen. Close stopcock or clamp and remove syringe.

4. Immediately attach second syringe with 10 mL 0.9% sodium chloride. Open stopcock or clamp and flush device. Close stopcock or clamp.

5. If bolus injection is to be given, proceed with bolus procedure after first 0.9% sodium chloride flush (steps 8 through 11).

6. If the catheter will not be used, perform heparin flush by the following steps.
   a. Remove empty syringe and connect air-purged heparin syringe.
   b. Inject flush at 5 mL/min.
   c. Remove needle while *maintaining positive pressure* (Fig. 12-20). Inspect

FIGURE 12-20   Withdraw needle while maintaining positive pressure.

site closely for any signs of infiltration or leakage. Sterile dressing may be applied to site if necessary.

Drawing Blood Samples During Continuous Infusion

1. Shut off infusion.
2. Close clamp on extension tubing.
3. Aseptically disconnect system at extension tubing–IV system connection. Blood samples should be drawn in coordination with tubing and filter changes. This prevents unnecessary manipulation of the system and prevents the risk of contamination that is present if the same tubing is reconnected.
4. Aseptically connect air-purged syringe with 10 mL 0.9% sodium chloride. Open clamp. Inject normal saline to flush infusate from septum and catheter.
5. Using empty syringe, withdraw 10 mL blood and saline mixture. Close clamp.
6. Aseptically remove and discard syringe with blood and connect empty syringe. Make sure the syringe is large enough to collect all blood required for specimens.
7. Open clamp and withdraw required amount of blood. Close clamp.
8. Aseptically remove syringe with blood, attach air-purged syringe with 10 mL sodium chloride.
9. Open clamp and inject to flush blood from the catheter and septum.

10. Close clamp. Remove syringe. Reconnect sterile IV system and lock and tape connections.

11. Reestablish flow rate.

Tubing and Dressing Changes

Tubing and filter down to the extension tubing should be changed consistent with institutional guidelines and Intravenous Nursing Society (INS) standards.

MRI® Port

The MRI® Port, designed by Davol (Cranston, RI), is designed to eliminate interference caused by metal ports during magnetic resonance imaging or computerized tomography.

IMPLANTED PUMPS

The implanted pump provides long-term venous or arterial access, a safe means of treatment for those with chronic diseases, direct infusion that can be targeted at a tumor or organ, a decreased infection rate, and enhanced patient mobility.

Criteria for use of implanted pumps include the following:

- Histologically proven primary or metastatic hepatic cancer
- Absence of extrahepatic disease or malignant ascites
- Measurable hepatic disease
- Satisfactory condition for major surgery
- Absence of acute infection/prolonged fever

Insertion is performed during laparotomy in which the infusion catheter is threaded through a gastric artery to a common hepatic artery. The catheter is then sutured in place and the feeding arteries are ligated. A pump pocket is prepared, and the pump is sutured to the underlying fascia. An infusate is injected into the pump reservoir and remains in place for 4 to 6 postoperative days. Then, the pump is emptied and filled with an initial dose of chemotherapy.

Patient Identification Card

When the pump is implanted, the surgeon should fill out the Patient Registration and Implantation Record. The manufacturer will issue the patient a wallet-sized identification card containing information pertinent to the implanted pump. The physician should fill in the space provided for any medical emergency instructions. This card should be carried by the patient at all times.

Postimplantation Care

Patients should be monitored carefully after implantation to confirm proper pump performance, wound healing, and favorable response to therapy. The pump should not be used for the administration of drugs for several days after implantation to allow for adequate wound healing.[7]

Patient Instructions

The patient should be instructed to[7]:

1. Avoid traumatic physical activity to prevent tissue damage around the implant site.
2. Avoid long hot baths, saunas, and other activities that increase body temperature and result in increased drug flow.
3. Consult the physician during febrile illness to assess the effects of increased drug flow.
4. Consult the physician before air travel or change of residence to another geographic location. Adjustments in drug dosage may be required to compensate for an anticipated change in drug flow.
5. Avoid deep sea or scuba diving.
6. Report any unusual symptoms or complications relating to the specific drug therapy or the device.
7. Return at the prescribed time for pump refill.

Pump Refill Procedure

The pump will require refills at specific intervals of time. The intervals will depend on the volume of the reservoir and the rate of administration.

The pump may be refilled by the following steps[7]:

Equipment

Sterile fenestrated drape (1)

Sterile towel (1)

50-mL syringe with drug solution (1)

Sterile empty 50-mL syringe (1)

Sterile noncoring needle (1)

Sterile extension tubing with clamp (1)

Sterile gloves (1 pair)

Sterile 2 × 2 inch sponge (1)

Povidone-iodine swabs (3)

Heating pad (1)

Procedure

1. Warm 50-mL syringe with drug solution to 15° to 35°C with the heating pad.
2. Identify the outer perimeter of the pump by palpating the pump pocket. Locate pump septum.
3. Wash hands thoroughly and dry.
4. Using sterile technique, place all sterile items on opened sterile towel.
5. Put on sterile gloves.

6. Disinfect pump site with povidone-iodine. Use *three* separate preps. Start at the center of the pump and work outward beyond the periphery of the pump.

7. Place fenestrated drape over prepped pump site. Sterile template may be aligned over septum.

8. *Securely* connect *barrel* of empty 5-mL syringe and extension tubing to the noncoring needle. Close clamp.

9. Using a perpendicular angle, insert needle into center of septum.

10. Open clamp. Lower syringe barrel to below patient level and allow pump to empty (see Figure 12-21A).

11. Close clamp. Record returned volume, adding 1 mL for amount of drug remaining in extension tubing. Disconnect and discard syringe barrel.

12. *Securely* attach air-purged syringe with drug solution to extension tubing. Open clamp.

13. Using both hands, inject 5 mL of solution into pump. Release pressure and allow drug to return to syringe. This test confirms proper needle placement. Continue to inject and check needle placement at 5-mL increments until syringe is emptied (see Figure 12-21B).

14. Pull needle out quickly and apply digital pressure with sterile sponge. If necessary, apply a sterile adhesive bandage.

Important Considerations

Never attempt to aspirate fluid from the pump. This will cause blood to be drawn back into the catheter, resulting in occlusion. If no fluid is returned into the syringe barrel, either the septum has not been penetrated or the pump is completely empty of

A   **B**

FIGURE 12-21 Pump refill procedure. (**A**) The syringe barrel is lowered to allow the pump to empty. (**B**) Using both hands, 5 mL is injected into the pump. (Courtesy: Intermedics Infusaid, Inc., Norwood, MA)

infusate. To test for septum penetration, remove the syringe barrel and connect 5-mL syringe with normal saline. Inject the solution and release the plunger to allow the fluid to return to the syringe. If the fluid does not return, again attempt to locate and penetrate the septum, using 5 mL normal saline to test penetration. If you are not successful, the physician should be notified because pump failure may have occurred. Accurate fill and refill records are essential to ensure that the pump is refilled at the required intervals; these records also document appropriate pump functioning.

Bolus Injection Through the Side Port

A bolus injection may be given through the side port of the implanted pump by the following steps[7]:

Equipment

Sterile 5-mL syringes (2)

Sterile syringe appropriate size for drug to be injected (1)

Sterile needles 22 gauge × 1 inch (3)

Noncoring needle (1)

Stopcock or extension tubing with clamp (1)

0.9% sodium chloride 10 mL (1)

Drug to be injected (1)

Sterile towel (1)

Sterile fenestrated drape (1)

Sterile gloves (1 pair)

Alcohol sponge (1)

Povidone-iodine swabs (3)

Procedure

1. Identify the outer perimeter of the pump by palpating the pump pocket. Locate the *side port* septum.
2. Wash hands thoroughly and dry.
3. Using sterile technique, place all sterile items on opened sterile towel.
4. Put on sterile gloves.
5. Disinfect side port septum with povidone-iodine. Use *three* separate preps. Start at the center of the side port and work outward beyond the periphery of the port.
6. Place fenestrated drape over prepped area.
7. Using sterile technique, prepare two syringes with 5 mL 0.9% sodium chloride. Prepare drug to be injected in separate syringe.
8. Connect first normal saline syringe to stopcock or extension tubing and noncoring needle. Secure all connections. Flush system with solution. Close clamp or stopcock.

9. While stabilizing port, insert noncoring needle into *side port* septum at a perpendicular angle.

10. Open stopcock or clamp. Inject saline to flush catheter and confirm needle placement. Close stopcock or clamp.

11. Disconnect and discard syringe. Connect syringe with drug. Open stopcock or clamp. Inject drug at manufacturer's recommended rate, but do not exceed 10 mL/min. Close stopcock or clamp. Disconnect and discard syringe.

12. Connect second syringe with normal saline flush. Open stopcock or clamp. Flush catheter. Close clamp.

13. Stabilize port while gently withdrawing needle.

14. Carefully check area for any signs of infiltration or leakage. A sterile dressing may be applied if necessary.

INTRAOSSEOUS ACCESS

When factors such as venous collapse in shock, anatomic scarcity of veins, and thrombosis of venous sites preclude the ability to establish peripheral venous access, intraosseous (IO) infusion should be considered. First used in patients in 1934, this technique has endured for nearly 60 years and has recently gained acceptance and interest as a viable alternative to peripheral or central venous access.

Historical Background

Use of the bone marrow for infusion of IV fluids was first proposed by Drinker of Harvard in 1922.[4] During the 1940s, Tocantins and O'Neill became the best known advocates of IO infusions.[20] Principal indications for IO infusion were:

- Pediatric emergencies
- Adults with mutilated skin
- Transportation of uncooperative patients
- Shock

Commonly administered fluids were colloids, crystalline solutions, plasma, blood products, antibiotics, epinephrine, morphine, and glucose. Interest in IO infusions dwindled between 1950 and 1970 because of the development of disposable IV needles and catheters. Since 1976, interest in this route of administration has grown dramatically.

Indications

Indications for the use of IO infusions include anaphylaxis, burns, cardiac arrest, coma, dehydration, drowning, respiratory arrest, septic shock, hypovolemia, diabetic acidosis, status epilepticus, status asthmaticus, sudden infant death syndrome (SIDS), and trauma. Standard protocol calls for the establishment of an IO line in children if percutaneous peripheral venous access cannot be established within 60 to 120 seconds.[1,3] It may be the route of choice in event of cardiac arrest or hypotension.[15]

Anatomy

Bones are vascular structures with dynamic circulation capable of accepting large volumes of fluid and rapidly transporting fluids or drugs to the central circulation.[17] Long bones consist of a shaft called the diaphysis with a very dense cortex, the epiphysis (or the rounded ends of the bone), and the metaphysis (the transitional zone). The epiphysis and the metaphysis have a much thinner cortex and contain cancellous, or spongy, bone. The iliac crest is comprised of a thin cortex and is filled with cancellous bone. The hollow core of the shaft of long bones and the spaces within the cancellous bone are referred to as the medullary space and contain the marrow.

The marrow cavity has been appropriately called the noncollapsible vein.[14,19] The intramedullary space is an integral part of the vascular system and is made up of a vastly interconnected network of venous sinusoids, analogous to a sponge.[18] The marrow is supplied by nutrient arteries that penetrate the cortex of the bone.

Technique

Many sites have been used for IO infusions, including the sternum, the tibia (Fig. 12-22), the femur, and the iliac crest. In children under the age of 5, the site of choice is the flat anterior medial surface of the proximal tibia just below the tibial tubercle or the distal tibia, followed by the distal femur.[5] In adults, the iliac crest is the bone of choice.

FIGURE 12-22 Possible insertion sites of percutaneous intraosseous infusion device in the lower extremities. (Reproduced with permission of *Journal of Emergency Nursing*)

Strict asepsis is essential and the skin preparation should be consistent with INS Standards of Practice. Local anesthesia may be used for conscious patients.

A sturdy needle with a stylet, such as a standard bone marrow needle, is used. The IO needle is quickly advanced through the skin to the bony cortex. With firm pressure and a rotary motion, the needle is further advanced into the marrow cavity. Insertion resistance decreases as the needle penetrates the cortex, also known as the "trap door effect." The stylet is removed and the correct position is verified by observing the needle standing without support and the ability to aspirate blood and marrow contents. Once these criteria are fulfilled, a continuous infusion can begin.[6] If, however, an attempt is unsuccessful, further attempts must be undertaken in other bones because if IO infusion were established in the same bone, the infused fluid would leak from the original abandoned hole in the cortex.[5,17,18]

Intraosseous Access Needles

The standards throughout the industry for IO access have been the Kormed/Jamshidi bone marrow biopsy needle, the Osgood needle, and the Cook IO infusion needle; these products come in several sizes and with various tips.

The Osteoport, an improved IO access needle, was developed by Von Hoff and his colleagues and was patented as the intramedullary catheter (Fig. 12-23). To decrease the complications of insertion, threads were added to the needle so that the IO needle could be precisely placed within the marrow. To decrease the rate of leakage, a cone was added to provide a tight seal between the bone and the Osteoport. To decrease the rate of osteomyelitis and cellulitis, the Osteoport was made implantable so that there would not be a direct conduit from outside the body into the bone marrow. To increase comfort to the patient, the Osteoport has a low profile and does not require a stiff needle protruding through the skin. For repeated use, the patient will not require repeated bone punctures.[5,21]

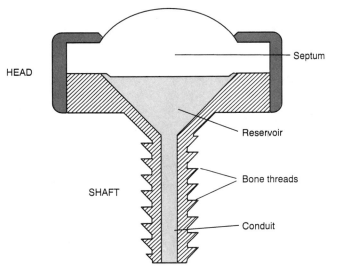

FIGURE 12-23 Osteoport.

The Osteoport is made of medical implant-grade titanium. Thread size and shape are identical to commonly accepted orthopedic devices. The Silastic membrane is made of medically implantable-grade Silastic, commonly used in IV catheters and implanted ports.

Primary indications for the Osteoport are patients who require access to the vascular system but have exhausted all other reasonable IV sites. The recommended duration of implant is less than 30 days.[21]

The Osteoport consists of a 1-inch titanium or stainless steel needle with a self-sealing cap. The hollow device, which resembles a partially threaded bolt (see Figure 12-24), is implanted in a large bone of the hip or leg. Once the incision is closed, the device is ready for use. The implant may be performed under local or general anesthesia.

FIGURE 12-24   Intraosseous infusion via Osteoport.

To initiate the flow of fluids, a needle attached to the IV tubing is inserted through the skin into the Osteoport's cap. The physician will be able to locate the device by feeling it under the skin (Fig. 12-24 A&B.)

Because it is implanted in bone, the device offers numerous advantages:

- Fluids are rapidly absorbed by the blood from the marrow cavity.
- Clotting and lung puncture problems are eliminated.
- The risk of infection is reduced.

VENTRICULAR RESERVOIRS

The ventricular implanted reservoir is used to provide access directly into the cerebrospinal fluid (CSF) without performing a spinal tap, to measure CSF pressure, to obtain CSF specimens, and to instill medication.[8] Implanted surgically, it is positioned in the right frontal region, into the lateral ventricle, sutured to the pericranium, and covered with a skin flap (see Chapter 19).

Major complications include:

- Infection, characterized by tenderness, redness, drainage, fever, neck stiffness, and headache with or without vomiting
- Reservoir malfunction in which the catheter is obstructed from the distal subarachnoid blockage of CSF, causing inability to aspirate or inject the port and slow refilling of the reservoir after manual expression of fluid
- Displacement or migration of the catheter, assessed by slow or absent refilling of the reservoir after manual expression of fluid and confirmed by computed tomography and change in neurologic status

The following procedure applies to accessing and administering medications through the ventricular reservoir:

1. Explain procedure to patient/family.
2. Gather supplies.
3. Obtain vital signs.
4. Place patient in comfortable position; Trendelenburg's is recommended to facilitate gravitational force for specimen collection.
5. Wash hands.
6. Put on gloves and mask.
7. Open packages using aseptic technique; use a sterile field.
8. Scalp hair over the port may be clipped to facilitate access.
9. Swab area vigorously with povidone-iodine in a concentric circle, covering an area 2 inches in diameter.
10. Repeat skin preparation; allow to air dry.
11. Remove and discard gloves.
12. Apply new sterile gloves.
13. Attach syringe to a 23- or 25-gauge winged infusion set.

14. Using nondominant hand, palpate and stabilize reservoir port (this hand is no longer sterile).

15. Puncture the reservoir obliquely with a 23- or 25-gauge needle.

16. Withdraw 3 mL CSF and detach syringe; place on sterile field.

17. Attach syringe with medication to access needle.

18. Administer medication as ordered over 5 minutes. Monitor patient during administration and immediately thereafter for presence of nausea/vomiting, headache/dizziness.

19. Detach medication syringe and attach syringe with 3 mL reserved CSF.

20. Flush reservoir with CSF.

21. Maintain positive pressure on syringe and withdraw access needle.

22. Apply gentle pressure over the site with sterile gauze.

23. Instruct patient to remain in supine position without a pillow under his head for 30 minutes following this procedure.

24. Discard biohazardous waste consistent with institutional policy.

25. Document in appropriate area of clinical record.

TROUBLESHOOTING/APPLICABLE STANDARDS

Catheter Withdrawal Occlusion

The inability to withdraw blood through a central venous catheter even though infusion creates no difficulties is frequently encountered. It has been postulated that the formation of a fibrin sheath over the catheter tip allows infusion but inhibits blood withdrawal.[11] Having the patient cough or move into various positions may be helpful. Sometimes the problem will be intermittent; after an hour's wait, blood specimens can be obtained without difficulty. At other times and in some patients, it may continue to be impossible to withdraw blood through the central venous catheter. Flushing the catheter with normal saline before blood withdrawal appears to be helpful.

CATHETER DECLOTTING

Clots develop when thrombin, an enzyme made from prothrombin, converts fibrinogen to fibrin, a collagen. The fibrin forms the clot. Activated plasminogen forms plasmin, an enzyme that dissolves the clot and keeps fibrinogen from reforming fibrin; this process is known as *fibrinolysis.*

Within the lumen of a right atrial catheter, clot or fibrin sheath occludes the line, and fibrinolytic agents are often used to restore patency. Urokinase dissolves clots by stimulating the conversion of plasminogen to plasmin, triggering fibrinolysis. When urokinase is used as directed for IV catheter clearance, therapeutic serum levels are not observed, because only minute amounts of the drug enter the bloodstream.

To declot catheters using a fibrinolytic agent, perform the following procedure:

1. Connect a 10-mL syringe to the catheter. Put on gloves.

2. Gently attempt to aspirate blood from the catheter.

3. If occlusion is present and cannot be aspirated, attach a 5-mL syringe filled with urokinase in a concentration equal to the volume of the catheter:
   • 11 Fr Hickman = 0.8–0.9 mL
   • 6 Fr = 0.5–0.7 mL
   • Port-A-Cath = 1.3 mL

4. Slowly and gently inject the drug into the lumen of the catheter.

5. Cap the catheter and wait 10 minutes.

6. Attempt to aspirate drug and residual clot with a 10-mL syringe. If unsuccessful, reattempt every 10 minutes.

7. After 30 minutes, wait 30 additional minutes before trying again.

8. If unsuccessful, draw the urokinase from the catheter, clamp it, and remove the syringe.

9. Place a sterile, Luer lock cap on the catheter and unclamp it.

10. Wait 1 hour and repeat procedure.

Studies report success in restoring patency to an occluded implantable port using a 10-mL syringe with 0.2 mL to 1 mL of 0.1 N concentration hydrochloric acid solution left to dwell for 1 to 2 hours.[10]

CATHETER REPAIR

Tunneled Catheter Repair

Although conventional methods of catheter repair using adhesives have been available for some time, emergency, temporary repair may be accomplished as follows:

1. Clamp the catheter between the chest wall and the tear.
2. Clean the torn area with povidone-iodine solution.
3. Using sterile scissors, cut off the damaged portion.
4. Insert a blunt-end needle (14 or 16 gauge) into the distal end of the catheter.
5. Insert an injection cap in the hub of the needle and heparinize the catheter.
6. Secure the needle and catheter with silk suture material.
7. Release the clamp.
8. Determine patency by flushing with saline solution.

Permanent repair may be needed and is accomplished by splicing a new section of catheter with an end connector to the remainder of the line. GISH Biomedical also provides a nonadhesive repair kit. Developed specifically to be used with GISH Biomedical's central catheter line, the kit may also be used for other tunneled and central venous catheters. Key components of the kit are featured in Figure 12-25.

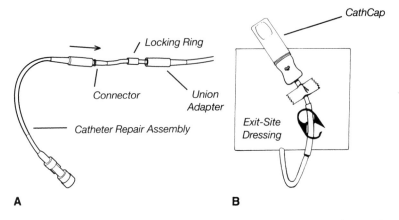

FIGURE 12-25 Hemed™ central venous access catheter nonadhesive repair kit. (Courtesy: GISH Biomedical, Inc., Santa Ana, CA). (**A**) The union adapter and locking ring are unique to the GISH repair kit. (**B**) Repaired catheter with exit-site dressing in place.

Clinicians have indicated that several items, not included in the repair kits, but recommended during the repair of Hemed™ Catheters are as follows:

Isopropyl alcohol swab

Povidone-iodine 4 × 4 gauze

Padded/jawless clamp heparin flush

Surgical gloves sterile drapes

Syringe aseptic garments (ie, mask)

The padded clamp is placed between the damaged area and the body exit site, at least 2½ inches from the damaged area, to facilitate repair. Using the GISH method:

1. Cleanse and drape the body exit site area. Using sterile technique, carefully cut off the damaged portion of the catheter, allowing at least 2½ inches between the cut end and the clamp to permit catheter repair. Discard the damaged tubing and the old Luer.

2. The union adapter slides onto the remaining tubing, tapered end first; ½ inch of tubing should extend beyond the tabbed union adapter.

3. Grasp the adapter tab with one hand and the union adapter and silicone tubing with the other hand. The adapter tab is removed with a slight twist while pulling.

4. The locking ring easily slides over the extended catheter tubing.

5. Remove the end cap and carefully insert the straight end of the guidewire through the Luer fitting on the catheter repair assembly, consistent with GISH recommendations for the use of its products, specifically as they apply to the use of the guidewire assembly.

6. Slip the catheter tubing onto the connector of the catheter repair assembly. The tubing should be positioned approximately two-thirds up the connector.

7. The GISH locking ring is advanced onto the connector until it is against the flange. The locking ring will pull the catheter tubing up over the flange.

8. The union adapter is then advanced over the locking ring and the flange and adjusted for a tight fit.

9. Grasp the tubing on both sides of the repair site and pull gently to remove any kinks in the tubing under the union adapter.

10. The manufacturer warns the clinician to aspirate the repaired catheter before use to remove any air.

Regardless of the type of repair product used, the clinician must be familiar with the manufacturer's recommendations for use. A working knowledge of the intricacies of the catheter itself and repair methodologies will ensure safe practice and return a damaged catheter to patency.

CATHETER SITE CARE

A regular, standardized site inspection, disinfection, and dressing change should minimize catheter-related sepsis. Catheter site care and dressing change should be performed consistent with institutional policy and dressing material. If the dressing becomes wet, soiled, or loose, it should be changed immediately. Aseptic technique must be maintained during the procedure.

Nontunneled Catheter

Many variations are acceptable for performing site care and changing central venous catheter dressings. However, they are all based on the same principles. On a routine basis, the old dressing must be removed; both site and catheter carefully inspected, cleaned, and disinfected; an antimicrobial ointment applied; and an occlusive dressing secured. The person performing the care thoroughly washes the hands and wears sterile gloves and a mask. If the patient cannot be masked, the face should be turned away from the dressing site.

Equipment

The use of a prepackaged dressing kit will ensure the immediate availability of all required supplies. It will also help to ensure that all persons performing the care are using a standard procedure.

Procedure

1. Prepare a clean table for a work area.

2. Prepare the patient in a comfortable position on the bed.

3. Put on the mask, wash hands thoroughly, and dry. Put on gloves.

4. Carefully, remove old dressing. Removing the tape from the outside edges inward toward the center will prevent stress at the insertion site. The site should be carefully inspected for any signs of discharge or leakage. The catheter should be inspected to ensure that the sutures are intact, that the length of the external portion has not increased, that any needle protective cover is in place and locked, and that the catheter and hub are intact.

If the hands should become contaminated during the dressing removal, they must be rewashed. If the procedure is performed with two pairs of gloves, the first pair is worn to remove the old dressing.

5. Open kit. The overlay will provide a sterile field.

6. Put on the sterile gloves.

7. The site and the portion of the catheter close to the site should be cleansed of all debris. Polyurethane and silicone catheters should not come in contact with 100% acetone, which could weaken the material and cause leakage. Concentrated acetone may also cause skin irritation, which can increase the risk of infection. Some practitioners use a combination of dilute acetone and alcohol for cleansing purposes. The cleansing is performed in a circular fashion, starting at the center and working outward. The cleansing agent must be allowed to dry before the disinfection is started.

8. Disinfection may be done with 1% or 2% tincture of iodine followed by a complete removal with alcohol or with povidone-iodine solution. Povidone-iodine must not be removed with alcohol. The skin prep is applied in the circular method as described for cleansing. The nurse must not forget to disinfect the portion of the catheter that is close to the insertion site. Allow the agent to dry.

9. Apply antimicrobial ointment sparingly directly to the insertion site. Povidone-iodine is recommended for central catheter sites.

10. Placing a sterile 2×2 inch sponge directly over the ointment will ensure that the ointment stays at the site. A sterile sponge may be placed under the catheter and hub for patient comfort.

11. If the tape causes skin damage, tincture of benzoin may be used to protect the exposed skin. Be sure that it dries before applying the tape.

12. An adhesive cover is applied to maintain an occlusive dressing. Several types are available. Foam adhesive bandage or transparent tape is frequently used. The sterile tape is placed directly over the site with the catheter exiting from the bottom of the tape. This position is important to prevent stress at the catheter hub–tubing connection when the patient moves. Be sure this connection is outside the tape to facilitate tubing changes.

13. The catheter hub–tubing connection is inspected to be sure that it is locked and taped. The tubing is looped and taped to the chest wall to prevent stress at the connection or insertion site when the tubing is pulled or stretched.

14. The dressing change label is signed, dated, and applied to the dressing (Fig. 12-26A).

15. Transparent dressings may be used (Figure 12-26B).

Tunneled Catheters

The dressing change procedure may be modified for the tunneled catheter. If the patient is immunosuppressed or if site healing is not complete, the same care given to the nontunneled catheter may be used for this catheter. If the patient is not immunosuppressed and site healing is complete, site care may be limited to daily inspection and cleansing with soap and water while bathing.

FIGURE 12-26 (**A**) Connections are taped and the site is labeled. (**B**) Transparent dressings may also be used. (Courtesy: Acme United Corp., Fairfield, CT)

Totally Implanted Devices

Totally implanted devices do not require any site care because the entire device is under the skin.

CATHETER MAINTENANCE

Heparin Flush

After using the catheter and at routine intervals, flushing with heparin solution will maintain catheter patency. For tunneled or nontunneled catheters, the frequency and heparin strength vary considerably among institutions. The volume of heparin needs to be only slightly more than the volume of the catheter—2.5 to 5 mL should be sufficient. Many practitioners have found that every-other-day flushes maintain catheter patency. The strength of heparin may depend on the condition of the patient, usually 10–100 U/mL.

Prefilled Heparin Flush Syringe

Using a prefilled heparin syringe reduces the risk of touch contamination during preparation and ensures administration of the correct dosage of heparin. Saline flush may also be used.

Gauge and Length of Needles

Whenever injections are made into injection ports or intermittent injection caps, using a short needle prevents the risk of accidental puncture of the tubing or catheter. Small-gauge needles prevent large holes in the cap or injection port, which can result in fluid leakage or an entry point for air or bacteria.

STANDARDS OF PRACTICE

Quality central venous care mandates the development of policies and procedures based on INS Standards of Practice and the Oncology Nursing Society (ONS) Recommendations for Nursing Practice for venous catheters. A clinical practicum and evaluation tool should be developed to ensure safe practice by those professionals responsible for accessing and maintaining long-term venous access.

RECOMMENDATIONS FOR NURSING PRACTICE

(Source: Oncology Nursing Society, reprinted with permission.) See also Box 12-1.

    I. Venous catheters

        The nursing care of patients with venous catheters is complex, and numerous controversial issues surround the care of these catheters. While much research is in progress, current study results have not conclusively resolved these practice issues.

        The recommendations in this document are consistent with the literature cited to date and are deemed reasonable in the absence of definitive studies. Healthcare professionals who work with venous catheters should study new information as it becomes available.

      A. Policies

        1. The registered professional nurse is designated as qualified to care for patients with short-term or long-term venous catheters after adequate educational preparation according to the individual care setting's policies and procedures.

        2. After adequate educational preparation, the registered professional nurse should demonstrate knowledge and skills in the following areas:

          a) Patient preparation for catheter placement

          b) Immediate post-procedural care of the patient,

Text continues on p. 256

Box 12-1
Long-Term Catheter Practicum

LONG-TERM VENOUS CATHETERS

Part I—Clinical Practicum Evaluation

As part of the nurse's evaluation, the preceptor will verify the nurse's performance of basic skills with a long-term venous catheter by indicating whether the nurse completes the following steps.

SKILL	MET	NOT MET
A. Patient Preparation		
1. Performs preplacement assessment of patient		
2. Explains procedure to patient and/or significant others		
3. Performs preplacement preparation		
4. Performs postoperative assessment of patient and catheter		
5. Confirms position of catheter prior to initiating treatment		
B. Assessing the Long-Term Venous Catheter		
1. Organizes catheter care to minimize entry into system		
2. Maintains strict aseptic technique		
3. Never leaves catheter open to air		
4. Uses only smoothed edged clamps or latex- or plastic-covered clamps		
5. Protects catheter prior to clamping		
6. Tapes catheter securely to patient's body		
7. Washes hands		
8. Prepares appropriate equipment		
9. Applies gloves		
10. Accesses catheter		
C. Blood Drawing		
1. Follows procedures for accessing system		
2. Removes at least 5 mL blood/solution and discards		
3. Clamps catheter at appropriate times		
4. Withdraws desired amount of blood		
5. Flushes catheter with 10 mL normal saline		
6. Using alcohol swab, removes any blood from catheter hub		
7. Heparinizes catheter or connects an appropriate solution		

(continued)

Box 12-1
Long-Term Catheter Practicum *(Continued)*

SKILL	MET	NOT MET
D. Maintaining Patency		
1. Heparinizes catheter with correct dose of heparin at appropriate frequency		
E. Injection Cap Change		
1. Washes hands		
2. Prepares appropriate equipment		
3. Applies gloves		
4. Cleanses catheter		
5. Changes injection cap with appropriate frequency		
F. Exit Site Care		
1. Washes hands		
2. Prepares appropriate equipment		
3. Carefully removes old dressing		
4. Inspects exit site		
5. Applies sterile gloves		
6. Cleanses exit site		
7. Applies appropriate dressing		
G. Damaged Catheter		
1. Clamps catheter proximal to severance		
2. Obtains repair kit and follows direction to repair catheter		
H. Occlusion		
1. Diagnoses occlusion		
2. Obtains physician order to instill urokinase		
3. Verifies catheter placement prior to beginning procedure		
4. Checks patient's platelet count prior to beginning procedure		
5. Accesses long-term venous catheter		
6. Prepares urokinase		
7. Instills urokinase		
8. Aspirates catheter		
I. Documentation/Patient Education		
1. Documents all procedures		
2. Teaches patient or significant others short-term venous catheter care		

(continued)

Box 12-1
Long-Term Catheter Practicum (Continued)

Part II—Clinical Practicum Evaluation

The nurse performs the following activities at a satisfactory level. If there has not been an opportunity to carry out a particular activity, indicate N/A (not applicable) in the space provided. Under "Comment" give examples of how the nurse met each objective or performed each activity.

BEHAVIOR   MET   NOT MET

1. Participates in interdisciplinary planning related to insertion and care of the patient's long-term venous catheter (eg, physician, social service, home care)
   Comment:

2. Anticipates complications associated with long-term venous catheters and takes action to prevent/minimize complications
   Comment:

3. Involves patient or significant others in care planning and establishes interventions specific to the individual needs of the patient
   Comment:

4. Instructs patient or significant others how to care for the long-term venous catheter including:
   a. care of the exit site
   b. flushing the catheter and heparinization
   c. changing the injection cap
   d. possible complications
   Comment:

5. Demonstrates knowledge of the principles of infection control related to long-term venous catheters
   Comment:

6. Demonstrates knowledge and skill in the assessment and management, and follow-up care of the extravasation of chemotherapy
   Comment:

(continued)

Box 12-1
Long-Term Catheter Practicum *(Continued)*

BEHAVIOR   MET   NOT MET

7. Demonstrates knowledge of the assessment and management of a damaged long-term venous catheter
Comment:

_____

8. Demonstrates knowledge of the assessment and management of an occluded long-term venous catheter
Comment:

_____

9. Demonstrates knowledge of the assessment and management of a migrated long-term venous catheter
Comment:

_____

10. Demonstrates knowledge of the assessment and management of a thrombosed long-term venous catheter
Comment:

_____

11. Demonstrates knowledge of the assessment and management of a long-term, venous catheter that has lost blood return
Comment:

_____

(Reproduced with permission of Oncology Nursing Society.)

c) Methods of accessing short-term and long-term venous catheters
d) Methods of maintaining patency of short-term and long-term venous catheters
e) Care of the exit site
f) Recognition of complications associated with short-and long-term venous catheters
g) Management of a severed or damaged catheter
h) Management of an occluded catheter
i) Management of a migrated catheter
j) Management of a thrombosed catheter
k) Management of catheter where there is no blood return
l) Management of chemotherapy extravasation (see *ONS Cancer Chemotherapy Guidelines*, Module V—*Recommendations for the Management of Extravasation and Anaphylaxis*, 1988.)

m) Documentation procedures

n) Policies and procedures on patient education

3. A mechanism for annually evaluating the registered professional nurse's knowledge and skill in caring for patients with short-term or long-term venous catheters should be established by the administrative authorities of the institution.

4. Ongoing participation in continuing education on venous catheter care is recommended to maintain a current knowledge base.

5. Only registered professional nurses or physicians with specialized training should care for patients with short-term or long-term venous catheters.

6. Personnel who insert short- or long-term venous catheters should be familiar with the specific equipment used as well as the proper selection of insertion site and catheter type, size, and length.

7. Proper aseptic technique must be used in caring for short-term and long-term venous catheters.

8. Patients with short-term and long-term venous catheters should be cared for within the framework of the nursing process and taught self-care management of the device.

9. Patients should be informed of the therapeutic benefits and risks of a short-term or long-term venous catheter in the degree of detail they desire.

10. The individual care setting should have written policies and procedures on:

   a) Short-term and long-term venous catheter placement

   b) Infection control practices for short-term and long-term venous catheters

   c) Short-term and long-term venous catheter care

   d) Declotting the long-term venous catheter

   e) Management of a damaged long-term venous catheter

   f) Management of a migrated catheter

   g) Extravasation of chemotherapy

B. Outcomes

1. Only adequately prepared registered professional nurses who are skilled in caring for patients with short-term or long-term venous catheters will assume responsibility for the care of the device to insure quality patient care and maintain the highest standards of patient and personnel safety.

2. The patient will verbalize the consequences of the treatment decision to have a short-term or long-term venous catheter.

3. The sterility of the short-term or long-term venous catheter system will be maintained.

4. The patient and/or significant other will be able to manage the short-term or long-term venous catheter.

C. Procedures

(Review product information supplied by the manufacturer to become familiar with the specifics of the catheter before using.)

    1. Short-term venous catheters

        a) Patient preparation and short-term venous catheter placement

            (1) Perform a pre-placement assessment of the patient to determine if a short-term venous catheter is appropriate, including any or all of the following characteristics:

                (a) Short-term treatment with chemotherapy (45–60 days)

                (b) Short-term infusions of vesicant chemotherapy

                (c) Single bolus injections of chemotherapy

                (d) Brief life expectancy

                (e) Frequent venous access requirements

                (f) Limited venous access availability

                (g) Patient's desire for venous catheter

                (h) Total parenteral nutrition

                (i) Pain management

                (j) Hydration

                (k) Antibiotic therapy

                (l) Other supportive therapies

REFERENCES

1. American Academy of Pediatrics and American College of Emergency Physicians. (1989). *Advanced pediatric life support*, pp. 3, 10–11, 39, 76–77, 123.
2. Brendel, V. (1984). Catheters utilized in delivering total parenteral nutrition. *Journal of the National Intravenous Therapy Association, 7*(6), 488–490.
3. Brunette, D. D., & Fischer, R. (1988). Intravascular access in pediatric cardiac arrest. *American Journal of Emergency Medicine, 6*(6), 577–579.
4. Drinker, C. K., Drinker, K. R., & Lund, C. C. (1922). The circulation in the mammalian bone marrow. *American Journal of Physiology, 62*(1).
5. Fuentes-Afflick, E. (1990). Use and management of intraosseous infusions. Presentation to the Bay Area Vascular Access Nurses (BAVAN) Fourth Annual Conference. March 12, 1990, San Francisco, CA.
6. Ho, M. T., & Saunders, C. E. (1990). *Current emergency diagnosis and treatment* (3rd ed.). Norwalk, CT: Appleton & Lange.
7. Intermedics Infusaid Corp. (1983). *Implantable drug delivery system—Physician's manual.* Norwood, MA: Author.
8. *Revised intravenous nursing standards of practice.* (1990). Journal of Intravenous Nursing (Suppl.), S73.
9. Kamal, G. D., Pfaller, M. A., & Rempe, L. E. (1991). Reduced intravascular catheter infection by antibiotic bonding. *Journal of the American Medical Association, 265,* 2364–2368.
10. Kupensky, D. T. (1995). Use of hydrochloric acid to restore patency in an occluded implantable port. *Journal of Intravenous Nursing, 18*(4), 198–201.
11. McIntyre, P. B., Laidlow, J. M., et al. (1982). Thromboembolic complications and central venous catheters [Letter]. *Lancet, 2,* 936.
12. Product literature. (1990). Arrow Corp. VitaCuff® Technical Report. Arrow-Howes Multilumen catheter with antiseptic surface and VitaCuff.
13. Product literature. (1991). Davol Inc., subsidiary of C. R. Bard, Inc., PO Box 8500, Cranston, RI. Groshong three-way valve.
14. Rosen, P., Baker, F. J., II, Barkin, R. M., Braen, G. R., Dailey, R. H., & Lewvy, R. C. (1988). *Emergency medicine concepts and clinical practice* (Vol. 1). St. Louis: C. V. Mosby.
15. Rosetti, V. A., Thompson, B. M., Miller, J., Mateer, J. R., & Aprahamian, C. (1985). Intraosseous infusion: An alternative route of pediatric intravascular access. *Annals of Emergency Medicine, 14,* 885–888.
16. Ryan, J. A., Jr., & Gough, J. A. (1984). Complications of central venous catheterization for total parenteral nutrition: The role of the nurse. *Journal of the National Intravenous Therapy Association, 7*(1) 29–35.
17. Spivey, W. H. (1991). Clinical procedure in emergency medicine. In J. Roberts & J. Hedges (Eds.), *Intraosseous infusion* (Chap. 24). Philadelphia: W. B. Saunders.
18. Spivey, W. H. (1987). Intraosseous infusions. *Journal of Pediatrics, 3*(5), 639–643.

19. Standards for CPR and ECC. (1986). Part V: Pediatric advanced life support. *Journal of the American Medical Association, 255*(21), 2961–2969.
20. Tocantins, L. M., O'Neill, J. F., & Price, A. H. (1941). Infusions of blood and other fluids via the bone marrow: Application in pediatrics. *Journal of the American Medical Association, 117,* 1229–1234.

BIBLIOGRAPHY

Esparza, D. M., & Weyland, J. B. (1982). Nursing care for the patient with an Ommaya reservoir. *Oncology Nursing Forum, 9*(4), 17–20.

Handy, C. M. (1989). Vascular access devices. *Journal of Intravenous Nursing, 12*(1S), S12–S14.

Manley, L. (1989). Intraosseous infusion: A lifesaving technique that should be used more widely. *Journal of Intravenous Nursing, 12*(6), 367–368.

Newton, R., DeYoung, J. L., & Levin, H. J. (1985). Volumes of implantable vascular access devices and heparin flush requirements. *Journal of the National Intravenous Therapy Association, 8*(2), 137–140.

Scharping, S., Hirschman, M. L. (1994). Venous access devices study: Identification of the number of patients with venous access device lines. *Journal of Intravenous Nursing, 17*(6), 277–281.

Winter, V. (1984). Implantable vascular access devices. *Oncology Nursing Forum, 11,* 25–30.

REVIEW QUESTIONS

1. Central venous access devices include all of the following EXCEPT:
   a. tunneled line
   b. implanted port
   c. tunneled port
   d. reservoir

2. The majority of central venous catheters are made of which of the following materials?
   a. polyvinylchloride
   b. silicone
   c. Teflon
   d. polystyrene

3. The collagen matrix in a bonded catheter is made of what type of material?
   a. purified type I bovine tendon collagen
   b. human collagen
   c. purified type II bovine artery
   d. animal artery

4. The blunt catheter tip with three-way valve is a feature of what type of catheter?
   a. Groshong
   b. Hickman
   c. Broviac
   d. peripherally inserted central catheter

5. Complications associated with the implanted port include all of the following EXCEPT:
   a. speed shock
   b. cardiac tamponade
   c. catheter occlusion
   d. fibrin sheath formation

6. The implanted port may be implanted into all of the following sites EXCEPT:
   a. peritoneum
   b. epidural space
   c. pleural cavity
   d. right atrium

7. Catheter declotting may be performed with the instillation of:
   a. urokinase
   b. saline
   c. 10-U heparin flush
   d. lidocaine

8. IO access has routinely been performed with all of the following EXCEPT:
   a. bone marrow biopsy needle
   b. laser device
   c. Osgood needle
   d. IO port

9. Principal indications for IO infusion include all of the following EXCEPT:
   a. pediatric emergencies
   b. adults with mutilated skin
   c. cancer
   d. shock

10. Major complications with the implanted reservoir include all of the following EXCEPT:
    a. infection
    b. malfunction
    c. displacement
    d. air embolis

CHAPTER 13

Intra-arterial Therapy

Key Terms

Arterial	Buffers	Parameters
Arterial blood gas	Femoral	Pressure monitoring
Arrhythmias	Hydrogen	Radial
Base excess	Nitrogen	Volume
Bicarbonate		

Through technical advancement of blood analyzers, it is now possible to obtain measurements of blood levels and pressures of carbon dioxide and oxygen as well as bicarbonate blood levels. Because arterial blood supplies all body tissues, medical practitioners recognized the advantages gained for diagnosis and assessment of treatment if this blood analysis were performed on arterial rather than venous blood. Placement of indwelling arterial catheters to allow for multiple drawings of arterial blood specimens and continuous arterial pressure monitoring is an almost routine IV nursing practice.

PURPOSE

An arterial puncture may be performed with a syringe and needle for a one-time sample of arterial blood for arterial blood gas (ABG) measurement or by insertion of an indwelling catheter to obtain serial or daily ABG samples and constant arterial pressure monitoring.

Arterial Access

The *radial artery* is usually the site of first choice because 1) it is superficial and easiest to enter; 2) its location at the wrist makes it easy to stabilize for a quick entry; 3) if thrombosis should occur, the ulnar artery will, by collateral circulation, supply blood to the entire hand (shown by Allen's test); and 4) it is easy to apply a postpuncture pressure dressing at this site.

Second and third site choices vary according to institution and personal preferences.

The *ulnar artery* is usually much deeper and more difficult to stabilize than the radial artery, so, although it may be larger, it is usually not the first choice as an entry site. Most authors will agree that if the radial artery has been entered, the ulnar artery of the same arm should not be used.

The *brachial artery* at the antecubital fossa frequently lies deep, close to nerves and tendons, and is difficult to stabilize. If thrombosis should occur in the brachial artery, blood supply to the forearm and hand may be compromised (Fig. 13-1).

The *femoral artery* located midway between the anterior superior spine of the ilium and the symphysis pubis (Fig. 13-2) is the largest accessible artery and is easily palpated, stabilized, and entered. However, digital pressure is required for postpuncture pressure. If postpuncture thrombosis should occur in the femoral artery, a limb- or life-threatening condition may result.

ONE-TIME ARTERIAL BLOOD GAS SAMPLING

Patient Preparation

Steps for patient preparation for ABG sampling include:

1. The physician's order should include the fraction of inspired oxygen (FIO_2) or room air fraction of oxygen (21% O_2), and the patient should be at this steady state continuously for 15 to 20 minutes before the blood sample is drawn.

2. Unless a postexercise sample is ordered, the patient should be at rest for this period of time.

3. The patient's position can result in varied ABG measurements. Having the patient in a supine position may result in more difficult breathing than would sitting upright. The most comfortable position for the patient should be used for all blood sampling procedures.

4. The procedure must be fully explained to the patient because anxiety and fear can cause hyperventilation and alteration of the blood values.

5. The person performing the arterial puncture should be competent because undue trauma will cause pain, often leading to hyperventilation by the patient and resulting in alteration of the blood values.

Equipment

The laboratory requisition form should have all identifying patient information plus the oxygen status of the patient, time of day (for serial drawings), and, if the patient is on a respirator, all pertinent settings. In some institutions, the patient's tempera-

Biceps muscle

Brachial artery

Brachioradialis
muscle

Pronator teres
muscle

Palmaris longus
muscle

Flexor carpi
ulnaris muscle

Flexor carpi
radialis muscle

Radial artery

Ulnar artery

FIGURE 13-1 Anatomic location of
radial, ulnar, and brachial arteries.

ture and hemoglobin count are also required. Follow recommended institutional
policy.

Blood samples can be drawn with existing equipment or a prepackaged kit may
be used.

Needed supplies are:

- Gloves
- Airtight syringe (2–10 mL)
- Appropriate size needles (2)
  - For radial or brachial artery: 25 gauge × ⅝ inch or 22 gauge × 1 inch
  - For femoral artery: 22 gauge × 1½ inch or 20 gauge × 1½ inch
- Sodium heparin 1 mL (1000 USP U/mL)

Deep femoral artery

Rectus femoris muscle

Vastus medialis muscle

Patella

Femoral artery

Gracilis mucle

Sartorius musle

FIGURE 13-2 Anatomic location of the femoral artery.

- Alcohol swab
- Iodophor prep
- Sterile 2 × 2 inch sponge
- Rubber stopper or syringe cap
- Labeled container with ice (paper cup or emesis basin)
- 1-inch adhesive tape

To heparinize the syringe, attach a needle other than the one to be used for puncture to the syringe, cleanse top of heparin vial or neck of ampule with alcohol swab, and open ampule. Withdraw 1 mL heparin into the syringe, draw plunger back and forth several times to coat plunger with heparin, and rotate plunger to eliminate dry spots. To eliminate any air bubbles, hold the syringe with the needle upright and gently tap sides of syringe, or turn syringe with needle pointed downward and *slowly* invert syringe upright. Discard needle used for heparinization, and place and *secure tightly* needle selected for arterial puncture. With syringe in inverted position, push plunger up and expel all excess heparin. *The only heparin remaining should be in the dead space of the needle and on the walls of the syringe.* Excess heparin or air bubbles will alter the resultant ABG values.

Use of an ABG kit is inexpensive and the kit contains, except for ice and tape, all equipment needed to perform a one-time arterial puncture. If the kit contains a heparinized prefilled syringe, remove syringe cap, place and secure appropriate size needle, wet inner walls of syringe with heparin, and expel excess heparin with the same method used for a syringe that is not prefilled. Most ABG kits contain a plastic bag for the iced blood sample.

Note: An ABG blood sample that has not been immediately placed in ice can have faulty results because red blood cells will continue to metabolize oxygen and give off carbon dioxide.

Procedure

Radial Puncture

As with any invasive procedure, begin by putting on gloves. Check the site for a palpable pulse and take precautions to monitor the condition of skin, surrounding tissues, and any previous arterial puncture marks. Perform Allen's test to ensure the adequacy of collateral circulation (Fig. 13-3).

A rolled towel may be placed under the wrist, causing hyperextension of the hand to stretch and stabilize the artery. The skin is prepped with iodophor, wiping with the circular method and allowing at least a 30-second contact time with the intended puncture site. Gloves should be worn.

A local anesthetic is not always necessary for an arterial puncture with a needle. With it, the chances for a quick, successful entry are less, and the anesthetic does not help the discomfort of arterial entry. However, if a difficult entry is anticipated or multiple attempts are necessary, a local anesthetic injected at the intended entry site may eliminate skin discomfort.

To perform the radial puncture, palpate the artery and align two or three fingertips along the direction the artery follows. Hold syringe no higher than a 30° angle with the needle pointed directly toward the artery. With one smooth step, quickly en-

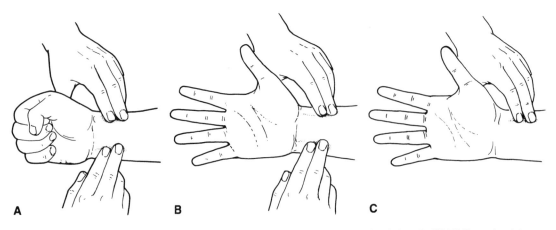

FIGURE 13-3 Performing Allen's test: (**A**): Starting point. (**B**) Lower patient's hand. (**C**) While maintaining pressure.

ter skin and artery. Artery pressure will usually cause the blood to spontaneously pulsate back into the syringe. If blood pressure is low or the syringe not free flowing, it may be necessary to withdraw *gently* on the plunger.

The plunger should be withdrawn 1 to 2 mL before the stick. This accomplishes two purposes: 1) if the sample is indeed arterial and not venous, the patient's pressure will cause a brisk and often pulsatile reflux of blood into the syringe (unless the patient is severely hypotensive); and 2) this prevents complications such as arterial spasm and blood hemolysis.

The blood return will stop when the level of the automatic shutoff is reached. If a shutoff feature is not available, 1 to 2 mL blood is sufficient for the blood gas analyzer.

The 2 × 2 inch sterile sponge is folded to form a pressure point and, immediately after the quick withdrawal of the needle and syringe, is applied with digital pressure to the puncture site. Taking precautions not to encircle the entire wrist, the pressure dressing is firmly secured with tape.

If a syringe cap is to be used, remove the needle from the syringe and attach the cap quickly and securely. If a rubber stopper is to be used, stick the needle tip into the center of the stopper. Roll the syringe back and forth between the hands for 5 to 10 seconds to ensure mixing of the blood and heparin. The unit is then placed in the iced container and taken immediately for analysis. A small amount of cold water added to the ice provides for even, cold distribution and facilitates placement of the sample so that all the blood in the barrel is in contact with iced water.

Femoral Puncture

The femoral artery is usually easily palpated with the patient in the supine position. If the patient is very obese, assistance may be needed to hold the abdomen away or the patient's buttocks may be placed on an inverted bedpan. If the abdomen is pendulous, you may tape it up and away to provide easier access and maintain sterility.

Wearing gloves, prepping of patient's skin, and finger prepping are done in the same manner as for a radial artery puncture.

The following two different techniques may be used for a femoral arterial puncture:

1. The artery is located and "fixed" between two fingers, allowing pulsation to be felt on both fingers but at the same time allowing enough room between them for the needle entry. The syringe and needle are held almost straight down. When the puncture is made in this manner, care must be taken not to pierce through the other wall of the artery.

2. The entry may be performed with the same techniques used for a radial artery puncture. Two or three fingertips are placed along the direction of the femoral artery, and the syringe and needle are held no higher than a 30° angle. This method must be used for femoral artery catheter placement and, if used for a one-time needle and syringe sample, there is less chance of artery perforation.

Regardless of the method used, when pulsation is strong, it will be relayed up through the needle and syringe as the needle touches and penetrates the artery. The walls of the femoral artery are usually thick and resistant to puncture, so feeling pulsations can be a good guide to needle tip placement. When the artery is entered, the blood will usually pulsate back into and fill the syringe without any traction being applied on the plunger.

Box 13-1
Post-Procedure Patient Interventions

- Determine if the oxygen status of the patient has been altered *only* for the blood sampling.
- If so, resume presampling status as soon as the blood specimen is drawn.
- Maintain pressure dressing long enough—usually 5 min—to prevent excessive seepage of blood into the tissue.

  Note: The pressure dressing must not be so restrictive as to cause blanching or severe restriction of venous blood in the hand.
- Remove pressure dressing when bleeding has stopped.

  Note: If the patient is receiving anticoagulation therapy, apply digital pressure. Digital pressure is also preferable to the use of a C clamp at the femoral site because significant occult bleeding into the retroperitoneal space can occur rapidly and might result in unnecessary blood loss and discomfort for the patient.

When the needle and syringe are removed, digital pressure is needed because a pressure dressing with tape is difficult to maintain in the femoral artery area.

Maintain pressure for at least 10 minutes, and 20 minutes or longer in an anticoagulated patient. It is helpful to remember to release pressure slowly. A sudden release often causes undue pressure against the arterial wall and the patient will begin bleeding.

The care of the blood sample is the same as that outlined for a radial artery puncture.

Postprocedure patient care and nursing responsibilities are described in Box 13-1.

INDWELLING ARTERIAL CATHETER

Serial or Daily Arterial Blood Gas Sample Drawing

Frequently, serial or daily ABG sample drawing is necessary. To avoid multiple punctures, it may be advisable to place an indwelling catheter to obtain the blood samples.

The *radial artery* is usually the site of first choice because it is the easiest to enter, easiest to maintain with intact sterile dressings, and allows the patient the greatest freedom of movement. It is imperative that Allen's test be performed before placing any indwelling catheter in the radial artery because the long-term placement with decreased blood flow will increase the risk of thrombosis.

The *brachial artery* is rarely used because the catheters easily become fractured or bent, thus increasing the chance of embolization. The brachial artery also provides inaccurate readings.

The *femoral artery* may be a favorable site because it can accommodate a catheter of substantial diameter to achieve consistent monitoring and sampling of blood. Care must be taken at all times not to leave the patient in bed at a 30° angle or less. Frequent pedal pulse checks for strength of pulsatile flow and color of limb should be maintained and documented. The patient should have a shave prep before the procedure, and a sterile occlusive dressing may then be maintained intact.

Note: If the catheter is to be maintained for a substantial period of time, it is probably more prudent to suture it in place. This is also true with arterial lines to be maintained in the radial artery.

When inserting any indwelling arterial catheter, extra precautions must be taken to wash hands thoroughly. Skin prepping in this instance may include an acetone defatting as well as a complete iodophor prep. In some institutions, sterile gloves are mandatory for this procedure and should always be used where probing is anticipated.

A local anesthetic may be injected at the insertion site, especially if an 18-gauge or larger catheter is being used. It is preferable that only experienced personnel perform this procedure; a successful entry with the first attempt is highly desirable because the availability of suitable arteries is limited.

Catheter Insertion and Sample Drawing

Catheter with Obturator

When using a catheter with obturator, follow the procedure outlined below.

1. Wearing gloves, insert catheter at a 30° angle, using the same techniques as those used to perform venipuncture of a superficial vein without a tourniquet.

2. As the catheter tip touches and enters the artery, pulsation can be felt up through the catheter. The artery walls are thicker and more resistant to entry than vein walls, making this procedure painful if not done quickly and expertly.

3. When the artery is fully entered, blood will pulsate back into the stylet; the catheter is then fully advanced.

4. To maintain a sterile field while removing the stylet and placing the obturator, an iodophor swab or sterile 2 × 2 inch sponge may be placed under the catheter hub.

5. To facilitate the stylet–obturator change, the arterial blood flow may be temporarily shut off, either by digital pressure at the catheter tip or by adequate placement of a tourniquet proximal to the insertion site.

6. After the obturator is removed from its protective shield, the stylet is removed from the catheter, the obturator is inserted and locked by twisting in place, and arterial pressure is released.

7. Label the arterial entry, and include the date and time of insertion and the initials of the person performing the procedure on the dressing.

8. Document the procedure stating the date, time, type, and gauge catheter used, insertion site, any patient reactions, name of person performing procedure, and pertinent data regarding distal extremity, including color, pulse, warmth.

Arterial Blood Gas Sample. When an ABG sample is needed:

1. Wearing gloves, prepare heparinized syringe without needle.
2. Apply digital or tourniquet arterial pressure.
3. Place iodophor swab or sterile 2 × 2 inch sponge under catheter hub.
4. Remove obturator.
5. Connect heparinized syringe to catheter hub.
6. Release arterial pressure.
7. Allow syringe to fill with required amount of blood.
8. Reapply arterial pressure.
9. Remove syringe from catheter.
10. Insert and lock new sterile obturator.
11. Release arterial pressure.
12. Cap syringe and treat sample as for a one-time puncture for ABG specimen.

Intermittent Catheter (Heparin Lock)

When using a heparin lock, observe the following method:

1. Wearing gloves, insert catheter using same techniques used for catheter with obturator.
2. Pressure to stop arterial blood flow is not needed because there is no stylet–obturator change.
3. Flush catheter with dilute heparin solution.
4. Dressing, documentation at site, and charting are the same as for catheter with obturator.

Arterial Blood Gas Sample. When an ABG sample is needed:

1. Wearing gloves, prepare:
   a. Heparinized syringe with 1 inch × 22-gauge needle for the blood sample
   b. Plain syringe with 1 inch × 22 gauge-needle for withdrawal of dilute heparin in heparin lock
   c. Syringe and needle with dilute heparin solution for flushing the catheter after drawing the ABG sample
2. Cleanse injection site of catheter with antiseptic.
3. Securely anchor catheter hub with free hand to prevent excessive pressure at insertion site and insert needle with plain syringe.
4. Withdraw and discard approximately 0.5 mL blood with dilute heparin from catheter.
5. Recleanse injection port and insert needle in syringe heparinized for ABG sample.
6. Allow syringe to fill with enough blood for sample. Remove syringe with needle.
7. Recleanse injection port and, still maintaining secure anchorage of catheter

---

Box 13-2
Postarterial Care

1. Observe the site for thrombosis of the artery, hematoma formation, perforation of artery, and catheter kinking or dislodgment.
2. Check the hand for adequate blood supply by noting color and temperature.
3. Maintain secure, clean, and intact dressings.
4. Avoid undue stress at insertion site by using the unaffected arm for blood pressure monitoring and venipunctures.

---

hub, insert needle of syringe with dilute heparin and flush catheter. Remove syringe and needle.

8. Treat blood sample in the same manner as for one-time puncture for ABG specimen.

Note: When entering any intermittent catheter with a needle, *extreme care must be taken to use a needle short enough that the needle tip cannot pass beyond the catheter hub* into the catheter itself. If the needle tip does enter the catheter, the catheter can be pierced and broken off by the needle tip with a resultant catheter embolus. The needle gauge must be small enough to allow postpuncture closure of the entry site, otherwise leakage of blood and risk of contamination are increased.

Postarterial Care

Close site monitoring is required after placement of any type of indwelling arterial catheter (Box 13-2).

CONSTANT ARTERIAL PRESSURE MONITORING _____

Placement of Catheter

Constant arterial pressure monitoring requires placement of an indwelling arterial catheter. This procedure allows for:

1. Continuous systolic, diastolic, and mean arterial pressure readings
2. An assessment of the cardiovascular effects of vasopressor/vasodilator drugs during the treatment of shock
3. Simultaneous drawing of arterial blood for ABG measurements

A cardiac monitor with a module for measuring arterial pressure is required. The monitor is connected by cable and a transducer to a special IV setup (Fig. 13-4). The IV system consists of a 500-mL bag of normal saline solution that has been heparinized (usually 500–2000 U/500 mL) to inhibit catheter clotting and thrombus formation at the catheter tip. *Klebsiella, Enterobacter,* and *Serratia* species and *Pseudomonas cepacia* show rapid growth within 24 hours with 5% dextrose in water. The bag is connected to an IV tubing and placed inside a pressure infusor bag

To patient

Pressure
infuser bag

Pressure tubing

Three-way stopcock

Continuous flush device

Transducer

To monitor

FIGURE 13-4   System for constant arterial pressure monitoring.

with a gauge and inflation bulb, the same one used to pump blood transfusions. Some institutions prefer microdrip tubings, but air bubbles are more persistent with this size drip. Other hospitals prefer macrodrip tubings; this size drip allows a larger volume of fluid to be infused.

The IV tubing is connected by a high-pressure extension tubing, a continuous flush attachment, and three-way stopcocks to a transducer dome. Most of these systems deliver 3 to 5 mL solution. The entire system is flushed. *All connections must be secured and all air bubbles eliminated.* The transducer is covered with the dome and secured on a plate attached to an IV pole at the level of the patient's right atrium. Each manufacturer provides detailed instructions for this setup, which should be read and carefully followed.

Any indwelling catheter may be used for this procedure and the insertion is the same as that shown for serial or daily ABG sample drawing. The catheter is connected to the primed IV tubing by placing an iodophor swab or sterile 2 × 2 inch sponge under the catheter hub, applying digital or tourniquet arterial pressure distal to the site, removing the stylet, connecting and securing the tubing adapter, and releasing arterial pressure. The pressure infusor bag is inflated to 300 mm Hg to automatically deliver a designated volume, depending on the drip size, of fluid per hour.

A sterile dressing is applied to the insertion site and taped securely. The site is labeled to clearly denote arterial access, date, time, type and gauge of catheter, and initials of person performing the insertion. A short handboard may be required to limit wrist motion. If restraints are necessary, they should be applied around the handboard, not the patient's wrist, because this could cause arterial pressure interference and increase the risk of catheter kinking or dislodgment.

Aftercare

Aftercare of the insertion site is the same as that for an indwelling catheter placed for serial or daily ABG drawing.

Arterial Blood Gas Sample

When an ABG sample is needed, a sampling port provides an easy arterial access.

Another method is to attach a three-way stopcock connection as close as possible to the site. Cap the sampling site with a heparin lock (intermittent infusion cap). Remove the cap when sampling and attach appropriate syringe. Turn the stopcock off to pressure or to the sampling site. Gently withdraw the sample and handle consistent with institutional policy. Flush the port and turn the stopcock back to pressure.

Malfunctions and Complications

Malfunctions

Common malfunctions occurring in arterial pressure lines are listed in Table 13-1.

TABLE 13-1
Malfunctions Occurring in Arterial Pressure Monitoring

Malfunction	Intervention
1. Air bubbles may cause distorted wave patterns.	1. Eliminate air from system in setup; avoid entry of air in manipulation.
2. Near-exsanguination has been reported.	2. Secure all connections.
3. "Damped" pressure tracing (almost flat) may occur if tip lies against artery wall.	3. Secure catheter hub; ensure use of intact dressings.
4. Catheter clotting can occur if pressure is <300 mm Hg.	4. Check pressure bag to ensure that it is maintained.
5. Abnormally high or low reading may occur if height of transducer is zero reference point or is the type placed with a plate on an IV pole.	5. Identify type of system used on the control switch of patient's bed.

1. Observe the site for thrombosis of the artery, hematoma formation, perforation of artery, and catheter kinking or dislodgment.

2. Check the hand for adequate blood supply by noting color and temperature.

3. Maintain secure, clean, and intact dressings.

4. Avoid undue stress at insertion site by using the unaffected arm for blood pressure monitoring and venipunctures.

Complications

Certain complications are related to arterial pressure lines.

1. The incidence of thromboses, hematomas, pseudoaneurysms, and prolonged arterial spasms may be reduced by the clinician's exercising expertise during catheter insertion and by careful monitoring of insertion sites.

2. Infection is a serious threat. Arterial pressure monitoring has been related to as high as 13% of reported outbreaks of nosocomial bacteremia. Incidences of contaminated transducers, transducer domes, and flush solutions have all been well documented. Sterilizing the transducer after each use, using disposable domes, and changing the entire monitoring system except for the catheter every 2 days reduce infection rates. As with any invasive procedure, thorough handwashing before insertion and maintaining of aseptic techniques during setup of the entire system, during insertion, and during all manipulations of the line are mandatory.

SWAN-GANZ CATHETERS

Although the insertion sites for Swan-Ganz catheters are veins, they are included in arterial access because they enter the pulmonary artery and measure arterial pressures. Central venous pressure lines give assessment only of right heart pressure. Swan-Ganz catheters, however, give assessment of both right and left heart pressures so they are frequently used for diagnosis and management of treatment in heart failure resulting from myocardial infarction and cardiogenic shock. In the treatment of cardiogenic shock, the Swan-Ganz catheter not only serves as a guide for IV therapy administration, a site for this administration, and evaluation of any therapeutic drugs given but also provides information regarding the cause of shock.

Basic Swan-Ganz catheters have double or triple lumens. Catheters are approximately 110 cm in length and come in sizes 5 Fr, 6 Fr, 7 Fr, and 7.5 Fr. Each has a balloon tip that is inflated with 0.8 to 1.5 mL air, depending on the size and manufacturer. A double-lumen catheter contains a larger port, which is connected to an IV system and monitor to measure pulmonary artery wedge pressure (PAWP), and a smaller port, with a two-way stopcock for inflation and deflation of the balloon. Triple-lumen catheters contain a third proximal port, which is connected to another IV system and may be used to monitor right atrial pressure.

The *IV system* contains a heparinized bag, pressure infusor bag, pressure tubings with stopcocks, and transducer with cable connected to a monitor. This equipment is the same as that used for arterial monitoring except that for Swan-Ganz catheters the lines may be coded in blue to differentiate them from arterial lines, which may be coded in red.

Insertion

The Swan-Ganz catheter may be inserted either percutaneously or by cutdown in any accessible vein large enough to allow passage of the catheter. As the catheter is threaded and the tip passes the superior vena cava, inflation of the balloon will allow normal blood flow to assist catheter advancement. The tip enters the right atrium and passes through the tricuspid valve, entering the right ventricle. It then passes through the pulmonic valve into the pulmonary artery. Use of a cardiac monitor is essential during this insertion because the pattern shows definite changes with each advancement, thus providing a guide for tip location, and simultaneously allowing for patient monitoring throughout the procedure. The catheter tip placement must be confirmed by radiography.

Pulmonary capillary wedge pressure (PCWP), which reflects left heart pressure, is measured intermittently by inflating the balloon to its recommended level (Fig. 13-5). Care should be taken not to overinflate or to inflate too frequently. Typically, one would inflate every 4 hours, with the pressure maintained no longer than 1 to 2 minutes.

Complications

Possible complications include:

1. Cardiac arrhythmias may occur during insertion. Lidocaine hydrochloride and defibrillation equipment must be readily available. Serious arrhythmias during insertion are rare.

FIGURE 13-5 Pulmonary capillary wedge pressure.

2. Catheter knotting may occur with the 5 Fr catheter when it is advanced too far for the chamber whose pressure is being registered.

3. Balloon rupture is possible in a patient without intracardiac shunting of blood.

4. Pulmonary damage may result from pulmonary artery blood flow obstruction caused by peripheral migration of the catheter to a wedged position. This is avoidable with constant monitoring and by following recommendations regarding balloon inflation.

5. Infection is always a threat. The use of disposable equipment has minimized the occurrence of infection. Strict adherence to aseptic technique is mandatory.

PARAMETERS

The purposes of arterial blood gas interpretation are to cope with respiratory imbalances, specifically, to diagnose, regulate oxygen therapy, and assess all other therapy—and metabolic imbalances—in particular, to diagnose and assess the effectiveness of the therapy.

To interpret ABG values, it is necessary to understand the physiologic, chemical, and physical processes that influence each parameter.

pH

pH is the parameter that refers to the degree of acidity or alkalinity of the blood. It is not an absolute measurement but shows an approximation of hydrogen ion concentration. The pH scale is as follows (numbers are inversely related to the degree of acidity): 1) the range compatible with life is roughly 6.8 to 7.8; and 2) the normal range lies between 7.35 and 7.45. A pH increase represents a decrease in acidity and a pH decrease represents an increase in acidity; a pH decrease of 0.3 shows a doubling of hydrogen concentration. Blood pH 7.10 has twice the hydrogen concentration of blood pH 7.40.

Blood pH is directly proportional to the ratio of carbonic acid to bicarbonate (HCO_3^-). When there is 1 part carbonic acid to 20 parts bicarbonate, the resultant pH is 7.35 to 7.45. If only carbonic acid increases or only bicarbonate decreases, the ratio becomes closer (1:5–16) and acidosis results. Conversely, when only carbonic acid decreases or only bicarbonate increases, the ratio widens (1:25–50) and alkalosis results.

Carbonic acid or bicarbonate changes themselves produce no toxic effects; it is the ratio alteration and resultant pH change that interfere severely with enzyme activity.

Hydrogen

Cell metabolism produces hydrogen, which combines with bicarbonate to form carbonic acid. This breaks down into water, which is excreted by the kidneys, and carbon dioxide, which is excreted by the lungs.

Because waste products of metabolism are mainly acidic, humans are by nature acid-producing animals. The body generates and processes 15,000 to 20,000 mEq hydrogen daily. The majority (99.8%) is nonfixed or volatile acid, which means it can change into gaseous form. The remainder (0.2%) is fixed or nonvolatile.

Body processing of hydrogen is accomplished without any appreciable change in blood concentration by elimination of volatile acid as carbon dioxide by the lungs, by excretion and reabsorption of fixed acid and bicarbonate by the kidneys, and by chemical buffering.

Buffers

A *buffer* is a solute that resists pH change when acids or bases are added. The buffer base consists of bicarbonate and all nonbicarbonate buffers. The bicarbonate buffer system cannot buffer volatile acids but does buffer approximately 75% of all the fixed acid generated by the body. The nonbicarbonate buffer system consists primarily of proteins, hemoglobin, and phosphate. It buffers volatile, nonfixed, acids.

Bicarbonate

The primary metabolic parameter bicarbonate may be reported as carbon dioxide content, carbon dioxide combining power, carbon dioxide, or standard bicarbonate, any of which refers to the same factor. Bicarbonate is measured by concentration and reported as mEq/L. It is universally related to the quantity of fixed acid *excess* and therefore is more a controlled than a controlling factor.

Sources of fixed acids are: 1) organic and inorganic dietary acids; 2) lactic acid as a by-product of cell metabolism without oxygen; and 3) keto acids as by-products of cell metabolism without glucose or insulin.

The normal excretion rate of fixed acid by the kidneys is 50 mEq each day. However, the excretion and reabsorption of both hydrogen and bicarbonate can be greatly increased or decreased by body demands.

The normal bicarbonate range is 24 ± 3 mEq/L. The minimal stated as being compatible with life is 1 mEq/L, the maximal is 48 mEq/L.

Base Excess

The parameter base excess (BE) is the sum total in concentration of all the buffer anions (bicarbonate and nonbicarbonate) in a sample of whole blood, equilibrated with a normal P_{CO_2} (40 mm Hg). As base excess is equilibrated with a normal P_{CO_2}, it is not affected by primary respiratory imbalances.

Normal base excess is 48 ± 3 mm/L but is reported as plus or minus zero, with zero representing 48 mm/L. In metabolic acidosis, base excess is minus; in metabolic alkalosis, base excess is plus.

Physics of Gas

So far we have discussed parameters that are measured by concentration. The two respiratory parameters measured by pressure (intensity) warrant a brief review of the physics of gas.

Gas has *volume*, which refers to the space the gas occupies and is measured in centimeters (cc). Gas has *pressure*, which is measured mathematically as force per unit area by noting height to which force can support a column of mercury, and is expressed in millimeters of mercury (mm Hg). Gas has *temperature*, which is generated by gas molecules in constant motion and is measured in degrees centigrade (°C) or Fahrenheit (°F).

Dalton's law regarding the behavior of gas in a mixture, as applied to oxygen in the atmosphere (room air), tells us the following:

1. The total pressure of the gas mixture equals the sum of the partial pressures of each gas, or total pressure of atmosphere (P_{atm}) = partial pressure oxygen (Po_2) + partial pressure nitrogen (PN_2) + partial pressure carbon dioxide (Pco_2).

2. Each gas acts independently, as if it alone occupied the total space.

3. Each gas contribution to the total pressure depends solely on the percentage of the total gas it occupies. The contribution of oxygen to the total atmospheric pressure is 21%. (Other variables not discussed here can exist.)

4. The partial pressure of each gas depends on the number of molecules existing in the fixed space. At high elevations, because the number of oxygen molecules is decreased, Po_2 will be decreased.

5. Each gas is unaffected by any changes in other gas molecules. The Po_2 will not increase or decrease because Pco_2 is increased or decreased.

Partial Pressure Carbon Dioxide

The Pco_2 value reflects the adequacy of alveolar ventilation. It is the primary respiratory parameter.

Carbon dioxide is eliminated by the lungs at the same rate formed by the tissues and at the same time maintains constant blood levels.

Arterial Pco_2 is inversely related to the level of ventilation. With hypoventilation, carbon dioxide is retained and the Pco_2 elevates; with hyperventilation, carbon dioxide is blown off and the Pco_2 decreases.

The Pco_2 normal range is 40 ± 4 mm Hg. The minimal value stated as compatible with life is 9 mm Hg, with the maximal value 158 mm Hg.

Partial Pressure Oxygen

The Po_2 value is also an intensity factor, measured in mm Hg. It tells how fast and for how long oxygen will pass from blood into tissue. The Po_2 is usually not a direct influence in acid–base balance.

Normal Po_2 values are oxygen and age dependent. When the FIO_2 is 21% (room air) and the patient is 60 years of age or less, the Po_2 should be at least 80 mm Hg. With each 10-year advance in age, the normal Po_2 will decrease by 10 mm Hg. If the Po_2 is 50 mm Hg or below in a patient less than 60 years of age, respiratory failure is present. A Po_2 between 50 and 75 mm Hg reflects moderate hypoxemia.

Hypoxemia

Hypoxemia is insufficient oxygenation of the blood and can be measured directly by the Po_2. Hypoxia is insufficient oxygenation of the tissues; it cannot be directly measured but is presumed if the partial pressure oxygen, venous blood (P_vO_2) is 30 mm Hg or below. To avoid hypoxia when hypoxemia is present, either the cardiovascular system must increase the rate of tissue perfusion or the hemoglobin content must be elevated.[2]

Shunting is frequently a cause of hypoxemia. *Shunting* is any impediment in the blood transport system that results in blood not coming in contact with oxygen. This can be seen in vascular lung tumors, a right-to-left intracardiac shunt, or capillary shunting where pulmonary capillary blood comes in contact with totally unventilated alveoli (dead space).

Oxygen Saturation

Oxygen saturation (O_2 Sat) is the parameter that tells the amount of oxygen taken up by hemoglobin when fully saturated. It is a quantity factor and is measured in percentage. It may also be called $Po_2\%$.

The normal adult values are 96% to 97% under age 65 years and 95% to 96% in older patients. Oxygen saturation:

1. Depends on Po_2. When the pressure exceeds a certain value, the amount of oxygen taken in no longer increases.

2. Is altered by pH. If Po_2 remains constant, O_2 Sat will decrease when the pH decreases and increase when the pH increases.

3. Is altered by temperature. If the Po_2 is constant, O_2 Sat will decrease when the temperature increases and increase when the temperature decreases.

This tells us that hyperthermia causes metabolic acidosis and hypothermia causes metabolic alkalosis. In hypothermia, the oxygen need is decreased, but the oxygen is bound so tightly to the hemoglobin that the ability to deliver it is greatly decreased. Inhalation of carbon dioxide may be used to cause acidosis and release the bound oxygen.

Chemoreceptors

Chemoreceptors located peripherally in aortic and carotid bodies and centrally in the brain play a role in body responsive changes to abnormal Pco_2 and Po_2 values. Chemoreceptors signal the brain to stimulate or depress ventilation, according to body needs. The response to an elevated Pco_2 is greater than a decreased Po_2 because Pco_2 elevation is a danger signal of respiratory failure. At high altitudes where oxygen supply is lowered, oxygen need is greater than Pco_2 constancy; the chemoreceptors stimulate hyperventilation to obtain more oxygen, but this hyperventilation results in a decreased Pco_2.

Arterial Blood Gas Normal Values (at sea level)[1]

pH: 7.35–7.45

Pco_2: 36–44 mm Hg

Po_2: 80–95 mm Hg

O_2 Sat: 95%–96%

Hco_3^-: 22–26 mEq/L

BE: ± 3

PRIMARY ACID–BASE IMBALANCES

Metabolic Acidosis

Metabolic acidosis is a process resulting from an excess of fixed acids or a primary bicarbonate deficit.

The primary causes are:

1. Increased production of fixed acids
   a. Keto acids, as seen in diabetic acidosis or starvation, where glucose and insulin are unavailable for cell metabolism
   b. Lactic acid, as seen in cardiopulmonary failure when oxygen is unavailable for cell metabolism
2. Failure of kidneys to excrete fixed acid
3. Primary bicarbonate deficit
   a. Severe diarrhea
   b. Bowel or biliary fistula

This is a metabolic imbalance because bicarbonate is the parameter primarily affected. Acidosis is present because the carbon dioxide level has not changed, but the decrease in bicarbonate has caused the ratio to go closer than 1 part acid to 20 parts base. It can be between 1:16 and 1:5, depending on the degree of bicarbonate deficit. Because pH is dependent on the acid–base ratio, and this ratio has now narrowed, acidosis is present. Base excess is minus because there is not enough bicarbonate to buffer the fixed acid.

Arterial Blood Gas Values in Metabolic Acidosis

pH: <7.35

HCO_3^-: <22 mEq/L

PCO_2: normal (40±4 mm Hg)

BE: <−3

If the metabolic acidosis is of renal origin, the kidneys cannot respond. If it is of nonrenal origin, the kidneys will increase the excretion of hydrogen and increase the reabsorption of bicarbonate. This response is slow, but, once started, can be maintained for weeks or months.

The chemoreceptors are sensitive to the increase in hydrogen and will stimulate compensatory hyperventilation to blow off carbon dioxide, decreasing the PCO_2 less than 40 mm Hg to obtain an acid–base ratio closer to normal (1:20) needed for a normal pH. This compensatory respiratory response is prompt and predictable—it will occur within minutes but becomes less effective with time. The limit of compensatory hyperventilation is when the PCO_2 reaches 12 mm Hg.

After the kidneys and lungs have responded, bicarbonate will increase to a level closer to normal, PCO_2 will decrease, and the acid–base ratio will come closer to 1:20 with a resultant pH closer to normal. Compensation thus occurs.

With bicarbonate administration, the bicarbonate level will revert to normal, and the lungs will stop hyperventilating. Therefore, PCO_2 will revert to normal, resulting in a 1:20 acid–base ratio and allowing a normal pH (7.35–7.45). Correction thereby is achieved.

Metabolic Alkalosis

Metabolic alkalosis results from a decrease in body content of fixed acids or a primary bicarbonate excess. The primary causes are:

1. Excessive loss of fixed acids by
   a. Prolonged vomiting
   b. Gastric suctioning
   c. Potassium deficit

2. Primary bicarbonate excess by
   a. Excessive administration of sodium bicarbonate or sodium citrate
   b. Chloride deficit, where bicarbonate increases to maintain cation–anion balance
   c. Sodium deficit, with bicarbonate excretion dependent on sodium

This is a metabolic imbalance because the primary parameter affected is bicarbonate. Alkalosis is present because the acid–base ratio has widened to 1 part acid to 25 to 50 parts base. This ratio results in a pH elevation; because there is an excess of bicarbonate, the base excess is plus.

Arterial Blood Gas Values in Metabolic Alkalosis

pH: >7.45

HCO_3^-: >26 mEq/L

PCO_2: normal (40± 4 mm Hg)

BE: > + 3

Whether the kidneys respond to metabolic alkalosis depends on several factors. An increase in bicarbonate causes the excretion of bicarbonate to increase, provided there is no deficit of chloride or potassium. If a chloride depletion is present, bicarbonate will be reabsorbed as the accompanying anion for sodium. Because a bicarbonate increase is usually accompanied by an increase in sodium, a decrease in chloride, and a potassium deficit, bicarbonate is not excreted but reabsorbed.

Compensatory respiratory response to metabolic alkalosis is variable. The degree of hypoventilation that occurs depends on the causative factors. Regardless of the cause, hypoventilation as a compensatory response will rarely be sufficient to bring the PCO_2 above 55 mm Hg because an elevated PCO_2 will cause the chemoreceptors to stimulate breathing to prevent respiratory failure.

When the lungs and kidneys do respond, some compensation will occur—bicarbonate will decrease, PCO_2 will increase, and the acid–base ratio will come closer to 1:20; thus the pH will decrease to a level closer to normal.

Correction occurs with the administration of solutions containing chloride and potassium.

In the assessment and treatment of respiratory imbalances, ABG measurements are an absolute clinical necessity because ventilation is reflected in PCO_2 and oxygenation in Po_2. Furthermore, acute respiratory failure may occur with slight changes in pulse, blood pressure, or alertness until cardiopulmonary collapse occurs.

Respiratory Acidosis

Respiratory acidosis is always caused by carbon dioxide retention from hypoventilation. This is rarely seen without hypoxemia (Po_2 < 60 mm Hg). The causes of hypoventilation include:

1. Anesthesia, narcotics
2. Central nervous system (CNS) disease such as polio, spinal cord lesions
3. Severe hypokalemia
4. Intrathoracic collection of blood, fluid, or air
5. Pulmonary diseases
    a. Restrictive (congestive heart failure, tumors, atelectasis)
    b. Obstructive (bronchitis, emphysema, asthma, or foreign body)

This process is respiratory because the Pco_2 is the primary parameter involved. Nonfixed, volatile, acid (Pco_2) is in excess but the base (bicarbonate) is normal. The acid–base ratio is closer than 1:20; it is between 1:5 and 1:20, resulting in acidosis.

Arterial Blood Gas Values in Respiratory Acidosis

pH: <7.35

Pco_2: >44 mm Hg

Hco_3^-: normal (24 ± 2 mEq/L)

Because the lungs are always the primary cause of respiratory acidosis, they cannot play any role in compensation. Renal compensation is always slow in onset but effective once started: generation and reabsorption of bicarbonate will increase, excretion of hydrogen will increase, and the excretion of chloride will increase, resulting in a chloride deficit.

With renal response, bicarbonate will elevate above normal, and Pco_2 will remain unchanged. The acid ratio will be closer to 1:20, allowing for some compensation, with a pH closer to normal.

Correction of respiratory acidosis is possible only by correction of the pulmonary cause. Chloride solutions are usually given to treat the chloride deficit.

Respiratory Alkalosis

Respiratory alkalosis is always caused by a carbon dioxide deficit due to hyperventilation. Factors causing hyperventilation include:

1. Chemoreceptor response to hypoxemia. The chemoreceptors sense the decrease in oxygen and send a message to the brain to stimulate ventilation. This hyperventilation results in carbon dioxide being blown off, thus decreasing Pco_2. This is normal at high altitudes.

2. Respiratory response to metabolic acidosis. This response can persist for several hours or days after the metabolic acidosis is corrected because of higher levels of hydrogen excess in cerebrospinal fluid and the fact that chemoreceptors are more responsive to cerebrospinal fluid than to blood.

3. CNS malfunctions (trauma, infection, brain lesions)

4. Anxiety, pain, fever, shock

5. Anemia, carbon monoxide poisoning

6. Epinephrine, salicylates, and progesterone

7. Improper mechanical ventilation. Any patient with chronic obstructive pulmonary disease who is overcorrected by mechanical ventilation so that the Pco_2 decreases faster than 10 mm Hg/h will have respiratory alkalosis.

This hyperventilation process is respiratory because Pco_2 is the primary parameter affected. Alkalosis is present because carbon dioxide is decreased and the bicarbonate value is normal, resulting in an acid–base ratio between 1:25 and 1:50. This ratio results in a pH above 7.45.

Arterial Blood Gas Values in Respiratory Alkalosis

pH: >7.45

Pco_2: <36 mm Hg

Hco_3^-: normal (24 ± 2 mEq/L)

Because the lungs are the primary cause of respiratory alkalosis, they cannot respond for compensation. Renal response occurs after several hours or days. The kidneys will decrease excretion of hydrogen and increase excretion of bicarbonate. The urine cannot become more alkaline than pH 7.0. This renal response will create some *compensation*. The bicarbonate value will decrease below 24 mEq/L. The acid–base ratio will come closer to 1:20, allowing the pH to come closer to normal.

Respiratory alkalosis can be corrected by administering chloride solutions to replace the bicarbonate ion load. However, the buffering capacity of the plasma has been compromised as a result of the alkalosis and any additional insult to the balance will be poorly tolerated.

MIXED ACID–BASE IMBALANCES

In the hospital setting, two or more primary imbalances may coexist in the same patient. The following combinations sometimes occur:

1. Metabolic acidosis and metabolic alkalosis appear in a patient with diabetic acidosis who is vomiting.

2. Metabolic acidosis and respiratory acidosis occur in a patient with severe pulmonary edema, followed by cardiogenic shock.

3. Metabolic acidosis and respiratory alkalosis are seen in a patient with both kidney and liver failure.

4. Respiratory acidosis and metabolic alkalosis appear in a patient with chronic respiratory insufficiency who is on a salt-poor diet and taking diuretics.

5. Respiratory alkalosis and metabolic alkalosis are usually seen as a result of mechanical overventilation.

Respiratory acidosis and respiratory alkalosis cannot coexist because a person cannot hypoventilate and hyperventilate at the same time.

REFERENCES

1. Metheny, N. M. (1996). *Fluid and electrolyte balance. Nursing considerations* (3rd ed., pp. 169–174). Philadelphia: Lippincott-Raven.
2. Ryabov, G. (1995, November 30). Hypoxia: incidence, identification, and interventions. Lecture. Mount Sinai Hospital Medical Center/Finch University of Health Sciences.

BIBLIOGRAPHY

Bennett, J. V., & Brachman, P. S. (1986). *Hospital infections* (2nd ed., pp. 572–575). Boston: Little, Brown.

Covey, M., McLane, C., Smith, N., et al. (1988). Infection related to intravascular pressure monitoring: Effects of flush and tubing changes. *American Journal of Infection Control, 16*(5), 206–213.

REVIEW QUESTIONS

1. Before insertion of an indwelling catheter in the radial arterial, the following test should be done:
   a. Abbott's
   b. Allen's
   c. Demer's
   d. Swan's

2. The ABG parameter that reflects ventilation is:
   a. bicarbonate
   b. P_{O_2}
   c. pH
   d. P_{CO_2}

3. The primary metabolic parameter in ABGs is:
   a. bicarbonate
   b. P_{CO_2}
   c. base excess
   d. P_{O_2}

4. The physician's order for ABG sampling should include:
   a. postexercise or at rest
   b. FIO_2

   c. outside air
   d. room air

5. In a patient receiving anticoagulants, the drawing of an ABG sample should include:
   a. personal observation
   b. chest pressure
   c. digital pressure
   d. avoid use of heparin

6. Two methods used ONLY for drawing ABG samples include:
   a. syringe and needle
   b. catheter with heparin lock
   c. needle with heparin lock
   d. peripherally inserted central catheter

7. At the onset of metabolic acidosis, what parameters will be decreased:
   a. pH
   b. bicarbonate
   c. base excess
   d. P_{O_2}

8. At the onset of respiratory acidosis, which of the following will be increased?
   a. P_{CO_2}
   b. P_{O_2}
   c. positive end-expiratory pressure
   d. pulmonary artery wedge pressure

9. Strong traction on the plunger of the syringe to withdraw ABG samples faster may increase the chance of:
   a. air contamination
   b. blood hemolysis

   c. arterial spasm
   d. venous spasm

10. Blood pH is directly proportional to the ratio of:
    a. carbonic acid to bicarbonate
    b. carbonic acid to P_{CO_2}
    c. bicarbonate to carbonic acid
    d. P_{CO_2} to carbonic acid

PART IV

Application of Intravenous Therapy for Homeostasis

CHAPTER 14

Fluid and Electrolyte Balance

Key Terms

Acidosis	Deficit	Ionization
Alkalosis	Glycosuria	Insensible loss
Balance	Homeostasis	Metabolic
Base excess	Hypokalemia	Pituitary
Biologic	Hyperkalemia	Physiology

OVERVIEW OF PHYSIOLOGY

Over the past 30 years our knowledge of fluid and electrolyte balance has increased to the extent that we now recognize an imbalance as a threat to life. With this increased knowledge has come an increase in the nurse's responsibility in parenteral therapy. Not only is accurate recording of the patient's intake and output important, but so too is the ability to recognize symptoms of imbalance; prompt recognition of an imbalance may indicate adjustment in therapy that may be crucial to the patient's safety.

Today electrolyte therapy is used extensively. At least 80% of all fluids administered contain some electrolytes. Electrolyte therapy is often a lifesaving procedure; its safe and successful administration is essential. Knowledge of the fundamentals of fluid and electrolyte metabolism contributes to safe electrolyte therapy. This knowledge alerts the nurse to the necessity for accurate fluid and electrolyte administration, the potential dangers of electrolyte therapy, and a change in the patient's condition that could alter the therapy prescribed.

Abnormalities of body fluid and electrolyte metabolism present certain therapeutic problems. When the mechanisms normally regulating fluid volume, electrolyte composition, and osmolality are impaired, therapy becomes complicated. An understanding of these metabolic abnormalities enables the nurse to understand the problems involved. Such problems exist in patients with renal insufficiency, adrenal insufficiency, adrenal hyperactivity, and other kinds of impaired organ function. For example, correction of a severe potassium deficit resulting from vomiting and diarrhea presents a problem in the dehydrated patient. Potassium replacement is imperative. However, potassium administered to patients with renal insufficiency results in potassium toxicity; the kidneys are unable to excrete electrolytes. The adverse effects of excess potassium on the heart muscle are arrhythmia and heart block. The nurse must recognize the importance of both hydrating the patient before potassium can be administered safely and watching for diminished diuresis that could necessitate a change in therapy. Once antidiuresis occurs, the potassium infusion must be interrupted and the physician notified.

Therapeutic problems also exist in patients with impaired liver function. Gastric replacement is necessary when excessive loss of gastric fluid has occurred. Most deficits caused by gastric suction, unless severe, are treated with 0.9% sodium chloride in 5% dextrose in water or 0.33% sodium chloride in 5% dextrose in water. However, severe loss may call for gastric replacement solutions containing ammonium chloride, which can be potentially dangerous when administered to patients with impaired liver function. Ammonium chloride administered to a patient with severe liver damage may result in ammonia intoxication because of the liver's inability to convert ammonia to hydrogen ion and urea.

These examples illustrate how knowledge of fluid and electrolyte metabolism contributes to safe, successful therapy in the critically ill patient.

FLUID CONTENT OF THE BODY

The total body water content of an individual varies with age, weight, and sex. The amount of water depends on the amount of body fat. Body fat is essentially water free; the greater the fat content, the less is the water content.

In the typical adult patient, approximately 60% of weight consists of fluid (water and electrolytes; Fig. 14-1). After age 40, mean values for total body fluid in per-

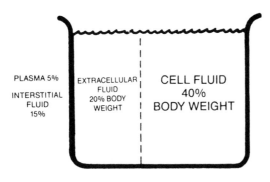

PLASMA 5%

INTERSTITIAL FLUID 15%

EXTRACELLULAR FLUID 20% BODY WEIGHT

CELL FLUID 40% BODY WEIGHT

FIGURE 14-1 Total body fluid is 60% of body weight. (From Metheny, N.M. [1996]. *Fluid and electrolyte balance* [3rd ed. p. 4]. Philadelphia: J. B. Lippincott.)

centage of body weight decrease for both men and women; the sex differentiation, however, remains. After 60 years of age, the percentage may decrease to 52% in men and 46% in women. With aging, lean body mass decreases in favor of fat. Infants have a high body fluid content, approximately 70% to 80% of their body weight.[4]

Compartments

The total body fluid is functionally divided into two main compartments: the intracellular and the extracellular compartments. The intracellular compartment consists of the fluid inside the cells and comprises about two-thirds of the body fluid, or 40% of the body weight. The extracellular compartment consists of the fluid outside the body cells—the plasma representing 5% of the body weight and the interstitial fluid (fluid in tissues) representing 15% of the body weight. Figure 14-2 is a schematic representation of compartments.[6]

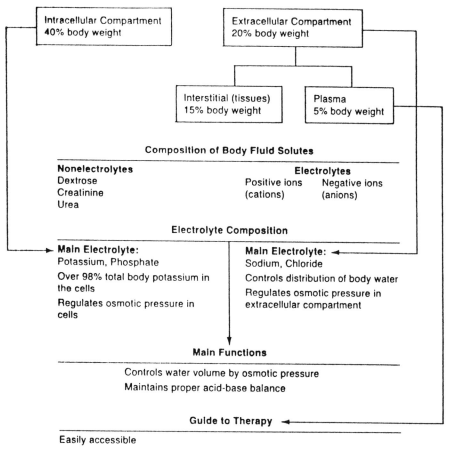

FIGURE 14-2 Total body water composition.

In newborn infants the proportion is approximately three-fifths intracellular and two-fifths extracellular. This ratio changes and reaches the adult level by the time the infant is about 30 months old.

There is one additional compartment, the transcellular compartment. The transcellular fluid is the product of cellular metabolism and consists of secretions such as gastrointestinal secretions and urine. Analysis of the secretions may assist the physician in tracing lost electrolytes and prescribing proper fluid and electrolyte replacement. Excessive fluid and electrolyte loss must be replaced to maintain fluid and electrolyte balance in the two main compartments. The amount of body water loss is easily computed by weighing the patient and noting loss of weight: 1 L body water is equivalent to 1 kg, or 2.2 lb, of body weight. Up to 5% weight loss in a child or adult may signify moderate fluid volume deficit—more than 5% may indicate severe fluid volume deficit.[5] Weight changes are also valuable as indicators of body water gains—acute weight gain may indicate water excess.

COMPOSITION OF BODY FLUID

The body fluid contains two types of solutes (dissolved substances): the electrolytes and the nonelectrolytes, as shown in Figure 14-2. The *nonelectrolytes* are molecules that do not break into particles in solution but remain intact. They consist of dextrose, urea, and creatinine.

Electrolytes are molecules that break into electrically charged particles called ions. The ion carrying a positive charge is called a cation, the ion with a negative charge, an anion. Potassium chloride is an electrolyte that, dissolved in water, yields potassium cations and chloride anions. Chemical balance is always maintained; the total number of positive charges equals the total number of negative charges. The quantity of charges and their concentration is expressed as milliequivalents (mEq) per liter of fluid. Because the number of negative charges must equal the number of positive charges for chemical balance, the milliequivalents of cations must equal the milliequivalents of anions[1] (see Tables 14-1 and 14-2 later in this chapter for an example).

Electrolyte Composition

Each fluid compartment has its own electrolyte composition (see Figure 14-2). The extracellular compartment (plasma and interstitial fluid) contains a high concentration of sodium, chloride, and bicarbonate and a low concentration of potassium. The composition of the intracellular fluid is quite different; the concentrations of potassium, magnesium, and phosphate are high, whereas the sodium and chloride concentrations are relatively low.

Electrolyte composition of the intracellular fluid is in part related to electrolyte composition of the plasma and interstitial fluids. Disturbances in the extracellular fluid are reflected in the patient's symptoms. These facts, combined with the accessibility of plasma, make the analysis of plasma a valuable guide to therapy. Occasionally, however, the electrolyte determination of plasma may be misleading. For example, concentration of potassium in plasma may be high while there is a body deficit. This surplus is due to the shift of potassium from intracellular to extracellular fluid in the process of large potassium losses through the kidneys. Determination of plasma sodium may also present a false picture. In the case of an edematous cardiac patient, the plasma concentration may be low despite excess body sodium because total body sodium is equal to the sum of the products of volume times concentration in the various compartments.

Electrolytes serve two main purposes: to act in controlling body water volume by osmotic pressure and to maintain the proper acid–base balance of the body.

Osmolality

Osmolality is the total solute concentration and reflects the relative water and total solute concentration because it is expressed per liter of serum. The osmotic pressure is determined by the number of solutes in solution. If the extracellular fluid contains a relatively large number of dissolved particles and the intracellular fluid contains a small amount of dissolved particles, the osmotic pressure would cause water to pass from the less concentrated fluid to the more concentrated. Therefore, fluid from the intracellular compartment would pass into the extracellular compartment until the concentration became equal.

The unit of osmotic pressure is the osmole and the values are expressed in milliosmoles (mOsm). Normal blood plasma has an osmolality of about 290 mOsm/kg water. The determination of serum osmolality is sometimes used to detect dehydration or overhydration. Because sodium chloride is the principal solute in the extracellular fluid, the osmolality reading usually parallels the sodium reading or is close to two times the serum sodium plus 10. Therefore, measurement of sodium concentration also indicates the water needs of the body. At times the osmolality reading may falsely indicate dehydration. Because the osmolality is the total solute concentration, nonelectrolytes are included in the reading. An elevated level of blood urea can therefore increase the osmolality without exerting osmotic pressure. A determination of blood urea nitrogen may supply a correction to the osmolality reading in cases of increased serum urea.

Units of Measure

Concentrations of solutes may be expressed in several ways in addition to mEq/L; for example, milligrams per deciliter (mg/dL) or millimoles per liter (mmol/L). Each of these units of measure may be used in a clinical setting. A *milliequivalent* of an ion is its atomic weight expressed in milligrams divided by the valence. This is the measure most often used for expressing small concentrations of electrolytes in body fluids because it emphasizes the principles that ions combine milliequivalent for milliequivalent. *Milligrams per 100 mL (deciliter)* expresses the weight of the solute per unit volume. In those countries in which the *Système Internationale (SI)* is used, electrolyte content in body fluids is expressed in *millimoles*. One *mole* (mol) of a substance is defined as the molecular (or atomic) weight of that substance in grams. For example, a mole of sodium is equivalent to 23 g (the atomic weight of sodium is 23). A *millimole* is one-thousandth of a mole, or the molecular or atomic weight expressed in milligrams. Therefore, a *millimole* of sodium equals 23 mg.

Sometimes it is necessary to convert from millimoles per liter to milliequivalents per liter. The following formula applies: mEq/L = mmol/L × valence (Fig. 14-3).[5]

For a univalent ion like sodium, 1 mmol equals 1 mEq

For a divalent ion like calcium, 1 mmol equals 2 mEq

FIGURE 14-3 Millimoles versus milliequivalents for univalent and divalent ions. (From Metheny, N. M. [1996]. *Fluid and electrolyte balance* [3rd ed., p. 7]. Philadelphia: Lippincott-Raven.

Acid–Alkaline (Base) Balance

The alkalinity or acidity of a solution depends on the degree of hydrogen ion concentration. An increase in the hydrogen ions results in a more acid solution; a decrease results in a more alkaline solution. Acidity is expressed by the symbol pH, which refers to the amount of hydrogen ion concentration. A solution having a pH of 7 is regarded as neutral.

The extracellular fluid has a pH ranging from 7.35 to 7.45 and is slightly alkaline. When the pH of the blood is higher than 7.45, an alkaline condition exists; when lower than 7.35, an acid condition exists.

The biologic fluids, both extracellular and intracellular, contain a buffer system that maintains the proper acid–base balance. This buffer system consists of fluid with salts of a weak acid or weak base. A base or hydroxide neutralizes the effect of an acid. These weak acids and bases maintain pH values by soaking up surplus ions or releasing them; acids yield hydrogen ions, bases accept hydrogen ions.

The carbonic acid–sodium bicarbonate system is the most important buffer system in the extracellular compartment. The normal ratio is 1 part of carbonic acid to 20 parts of base bicarbonate, which represents 1.2 mEq carbonic acid to 24 mEq base bicarbonate.[5]

Acid–Base Imbalance

Acid–base imbalances are normally the result of an excess or a deficit in either base bicarbonate or carbonic acid. Deviations of pH from 7.35 to 7.45 are combated by the buffer system and by the respiratory and renal regulatory mechanisms. Two types of disturbance can affect the acid–base balance: respiratory and metabolic. A diagrammatic presentation of the following information is found in Figure 14-4.

Respiratory Disturbances

Respiratory disturbances affect the carbonic side of the balance by increasing or decreasing carbonic acid; when carbon dioxide unites with extracellular fluid, carbonic acid is produced.

Respiratory alkalosis is caused when excess carbon dioxide is exhaled during rapid or deep breathing. Carbonic acid is depleted because of the carbon dioxide loss. Respiratory alkalosis may occur as the result of emotional disturbances, such as anxiety and hysteria, and also from lack of oxygen or from fever.[5,6]

Symptoms are convulsions, tetany, and unconsciousness. Laboratory determination is a urinary pH above 7 and a plasma bicarbonate concentration less than 24 mEq/L.[5] The body attempts to restore the ratio to normal by depressing the bicarbonate so as to compensate for the deficit in the carbonic acid.

Respiratory acidosis occurs when exhalation of carbon dioxide is depressed; the excess retention of carbon dioxide increases the carbonic acid. It may occur in conditions that interfere with normal breathing, such as emphysema, asthma, and pneumonia.[5,6]

Symptoms are weakness, disorientation, depressed breathing, and coma. Urinary pH is below 6, and plasma bicarbonate concentration is above 24 mEq/L. The bicarbonate increase is due to the body's attempt to restore the carbonic acid–bicarbonate ratio.[5,6]

Metabolic Disturbances

Metabolic disturbances affect the bicarbonate side of the balance. Kidney function controls the bicarbonate concentration by regulating the amount of cations (hydrogen, ammonium, and potassium) in exchange for sodium ions to combine with the reabsorbed bicarbonate in the distal tubular lumen. As hydrogen ions are excreted, bicarbonate is generated, maintaining the proper acid–base balance of the blood. Ammonia excretion is increased in response to a high acidity; bicarbonate replaces the ammonia.

Metabolic alkalosis is a condition associated with excess bicarbonate. This condition occurs when chloride is lost. Chloride and bicarbonate are both anions, which must equal the total number of cations. When the chloride anions are lost, the deficit must be made up by an equal number of anions to maintain electrolyte equilibrium; bicarbonate increases in compensation and alkalosis occurs.

Metabolic alkalosis is also associated with decreased levels of intracellular potassium. Potassium escapes from the cell into the extracellular fluid and is lost through the transcellular fluid. When body potassium is lost, the shift of the sodium and hydrogen ions from the extracellular fluid causes alkalosis, while the increase of hydrogen ions in the intracellular fluid causes acidosis of the cells.

Muscular hyperactivity, tetany, and depressed respiration are symptoms of metabolic alkalosis. The muscular hyperactivity and the tetany are symptoms of the deficit in ionized calcium that exists in alkalosis. Laboratory determinations are urinary pH above 7, plasma pH above 7.45, and bicarbonate level above 24 mEq/L.[5]

Treatment consists of the administration of solutions containing chloride to replace bicarbonate ions. Excess of bicarbonate ions is accompanied by potassium deficiency, so potassium must also be replaced.

Metabolic acidosis is a condition associated with a deficit in the bicarbonate concentration. This occurs when 1) excessive amounts of ketone acids accumulate, as in uncontrolled diabetes or starvation; 2) inorganic acids like phosphate and sulfate accumulate, as in renal disease; and 3) excessive losses of bicarbonate occur from gastrointestinal drainage or diarrhea. Acidosis may occur also from IV administration of excessive amounts of sodium chloride or ammonium chloride, causing chloride ions to flood the extracellular fluid.

Stupor, shortness of breath, weakness, and unconsciousness are the symptoms of metabolic acidosis, and laboratory determinations of metabolic acidosis are a urinary pH below 6, plasma pH below 7.35, and plasma bicarbonate concentration below 24 mEq/L.[5]

Treatment and clinical management consist of increasing the bicarbonate level. Solutions of sodium lactate are often used, but because lactate ion must be oxidized to carbon dioxide before it can affect the acid–base balance, it is advisable to use

RESULT OF TWO DISTURBANCES

Respiration

Controls carbonic acid concentration by
regulating amount of CO_2 through action of the
lungs

Respiratory Alkalosis

Deficit of CO_2 ⟶ **Deficit** ← Body compensates

			Excretes bicarb. ions (urine alkaline)
Occurs in:	Symptoms:	Treatment:	Retains H ions
Hyperventilation	Convulsions	Correct pulmonary problem	
Fever	Tetany	Low CO_2 concentration in inspired air	
Lack of oxygen	Unconsciousness		

Carbonic Acid
H_2CO_3

normal ratio:
1 to 20

Retention of CO_2 ⟶ **Excess** ← Body compensates

			Excretes H ions (urine acid)
Occurs in:	Symptoms:	Treatment:	Conserves base bicarbonate
Pneumonia	Disorientation	Correct pulmonary problem	
Asthma	Respiratory embarrassment		
Emphysema	Weakness — coma		

Respiratory Acidosis

FIGURE 14-4 Acid-base imbalances as a result of respiratory or metabolic disturbances.

sodium bicarbonate solutions, which are effective even when the patient is suffering
from oxygen lack.

HOMEOSTATIC MECHANISMS

The body contains regulating mechanisms that maintain the constancy of body fluid
volume, electrolyte composition, and osmolality. These mechanisms consist of the
renocardiovascular, endocrine (adrenal, pituitary, and parathyroid), and respiratory
systems. The kidneys, skin, and lungs are the main regulating agents.[4-6]

The *kidney* plays a major role in fluid and electrolyte balance. To function adequately, the kidney depends on its own soundness as well as on the coordination of
all the regulating organs. The distal renal tubules in the kidney are important in regu-

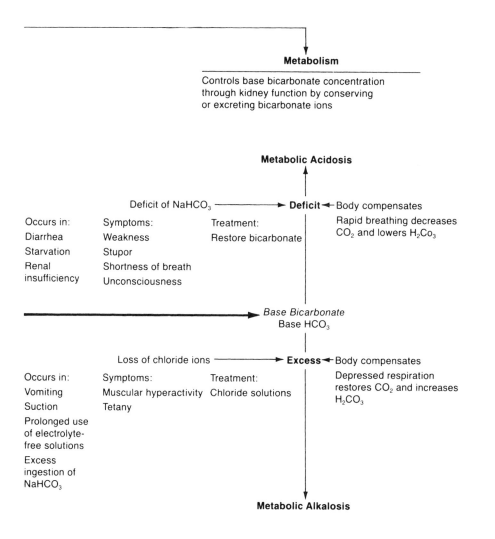

Metabolism

Controls base bicarbonate concentration
through kidney function by conserving
or excreting bicarbonate ions

Metabolic Acidosis

Deficit of $NaHCO_3$ ⟶ **Deficit** ◄ Body compensates

Rapid breathing decreases
CO_2 and lowers H_2Co_3

Occurs in:	Symptoms:	Treatment:
Diarrhea	Weakness	Restore bicarbonate
Starvation	Stupor	
Renal insufficiency	Shortness of breath	
	Unconsciousness	

Base Bicarbonate
Base HCO_3

Loss of chloride ions ⟶ **Excess** ◄ Body compensates

Depressed respiration
restores CO_2 and increases
H_2CO_3

Occurs in:	Symptoms:	Treatment:
Vomiting	Muscular hyperactivity	Chloride solutions
Suction	Tetany	
Prolonged use of electrolyte-free solutions		
Excess ingestion of $NaHCO_3$		

Metabolic Alkalosis

lating the body fluid. They selectively retain or reject electrolytes and other substances to maintain normal osmolality and blood volume; sodium is retained and potassium is excreted.[1]

The kidneys also play an important part in acid–base regulation. The distal tubule has the ability to form ammonia and exchange hydrogen ion (in form of ammonia) for bicarbonate to maintain the carbonic acid–bicarbonate ratio.

The *lungs* and the *skin* play an important role in fluid balance—the skin in loss of fluid through insensible perspiration and the lungs in loss of fluid by expiration. It has been noted that normal intake of 2500 mL from all sources will deliver a loss of about 1000 mL in breath and perspiration, 1400 mL in urine, and 100 mL in feces.[2]

The *renocardiovascular system* maintains fluid balance by regulating the amount and composition of urine. Plasma must reach the kidneys in sufficient volume to permit regulation of water and electrolyte balance. Renal disease, cardiac failure, shock, postoperative stress, and alarm impair this regulating mechanism.

The *adrenal glands* influence the retention or excretion of sodium, potassium, and water. These glands secrete aldosterone, a hormone that increases the reabsorption of sodium from the renal tubules in exchange for potassium, thus maintaining normal sodium concentration.[5] Any stress, such as surgery, increases the secretion of aldosterone, thus increasing the reabsorption of sodium bicarbonate. Adrenal hyperactivity also increases the secretions of the hormone and causes excess sodium retention. Excess loss of sodium occurs with adrenal insufficiency.

The *pituitary gland* is another important organ in the control of fluid and electrolyte balance. The posterior lobe of the pituitary releases antidiuretic hormone (ADH), which inhibits diuresis by increasing water reabsorption in the distal tubule. Increased concentration of sodium in the extracellular fluid stimulates the pituitary to release ADH. This hormone increases the reabsorption of water to dilute the sodium to the normal level of concentration. Increased body fluid osmolality, decreased body fluid volume, stress, and shock are conditions that increase ADH secretion. Increased body fluid volume, decreased osmolality, and alcohol inhibit ADH secretion.[4,5]

The *parathyroid glands*, pea-sized glands embedded in the corners of the thyroid gland, regulate calcium and phosphate balance by means of parathyroid hormone (PTH). When calcium level is low, PTH secretion is stimulated. When calcium concentration is too high, PTH secretion is depressed so that almost no bone reabsorption occurs.

The *pulmonary system* regulates acid–base balance by controlling the concentration of carbonic acid through exhalation or retention of carbon dioxide.

ELECTROLYTES OF BIOLOGIC FLUIDS

Electrolyte content of the intracellular fluid differs from that of extracellular fluid. Because specialized techniques are required to measure electrolyte concentration in the intracellular fluid, it is customary to measure the electrolytes in the extracellular fluid, chiefly plasma. Plasma electrolyte concentrations may be used to assess and manage patients with a diversity of electrolyte imbalances. Although some tests are performed on serum, the terms serum electrolytes and plasma electrolytes are used interchangeably. Table 14-1 lists the electrolytes in intracellular fluid and Table 14-2 lists those in plasma.

Potassium

Potassium is one of the most important electrolytes in the body. An excess or deficiency of potassium can cause serious impairment of body function and even result in death.

Potassium is the main electrolyte in the intracellular compartment, which houses more than 98% of the body's total potassium. The healthy cell requires a high potassium concentration for cellular activity. When the cell dies, there is an exchange of potassium into the extracellular fluid with a transfer of sodium into the cell. This process also occurs to some degree when cellular metabolism is impaired, as in catabolism (breaking down) of cells from a crushing injury.

Serum concentration of potassium is 3.5 to 5.0 mEq/L.[4] In the cell, the normal concentration is 115 to 150 mEq/L fluid. Variations from either of these levels can

TABLE 14-1
Approximation of Major Electrolyte Content in Intracellular Fluid

Electrolytes		Electrolytes	
Cations	mEq/L	Anions	mEq/L
Potassium (K+)	150	Phosphates	
Magnesium (Mg²⁺)	40	Sulfates	150
Sodium (Na+)	10	Bicarbonate (HCO₃⁻)	10
Total cations	200	Proteinate	40
		Total anions	200

(From Metheny, N. M. [1996]. *Fluid and electrolyte balance* [3rd ed., p. 5]. Philadelphia: Lippincott-Raven.)

produce critical effects. When a repeated potassium level is above 5.6 mEq/L, a potassium excess is indicated; renal impairment will usually be shown by renal function studies. High serum concentrations have an adverse effect on the heart muscle and may cause cardiac arrhythmias; elevation to two to three times the normal level may result in cardiac arrest. The electrocardiogram (ECG) may detect signs of potassium excess with peaked and elevated T waves; P waves later disappear, and finally, "biphasic deflections [result] from fusion of the QRS complex, RST segment, and the T waves."[5] *Hypokalemia* is the term that expresses serum potassium level below normal; *hyperkalemia* denotes a serum potassium level above normal.[6]

TABLE 14-2
Plasma Electrolytes

Electrolytes		Electrolytes	
Cations	mEq/L	Anions	mEq/L
Sodium (Na+)	142	Chloride (Cl⁻)	103
Potassium (K+)	5	Bicarbonate (HCO₃⁻)	26
Calcium (Ca²⁺)	5	Phosphate (HPO₄²⁻)	2
Magnesium (Mg²⁺)	2	Sulfate (SO₄²⁻)	1
Total cations	154	Organic acids	5
		Proteinate	17
		Total anions	154

(From Metheny, N. M. [1996]. *Fluid and electrolyte balance* [3rd ed., p. 5]. Philadelphia: Lippincott-Raven.)

Hypokalemia

Hypokalemia, or a serum potassium level less than 4 mEq/L, may result when any one of the following conditions occurs: 1) total body potassium is below normal; 2) concentration of potassium in cells is below normal; or 3) concentration of potassium in serum is below normal.[3,7]

These conditions are often caused by variations in the intake or output of potassium. A decreased intake of potassium from prolonged fluid therapy (lacking potassium replacement) may result in hypokalemia. It also may occur during a "starvation diet" because the kidneys do not normally conserve potassium. An increased loss of potassium usually results from polyuria, vomiting, gastric suction (prolonged), diarrhea, and steroid therapy.[3,6]

These conditions of potassium deficiency may be unrelated to intake and output. They can be caused by a sudden shift of potassium from extracellular fluid to intracellular fluid, such as that occurring from anabolism (building up of cells), healing processes, or the use of insulin and glucose in the treatment of diabetic acidosis.[3] The shifts resulting from anabolism and healing processes are not usually of severe consequence unless accompanied by intervening factors. In the treatment of diabetic acidosis, the potassium shift may occur suddenly with grave consequences. When cells are anabolized, potassium shifts into the cells. During the use of glucose in the treatment of diabetic acidosis, the glucose in the cells is quickly metabolized into glycogen for storage, causing a sudden shift of potassium from the extracellular fluid to the intracellular fluid.[3,7] This process results in hypokalemia.

The signs and symptoms of hypokalemia are malaise, skeletal and smooth muscle atony, apathy, muscular cramps, and postural hypotension. Treatment consists of administration of potassium orally or parenterally.

Hyperkalemia

Hyperkalemia may result from renal failure with potassium retention or from excessive or rapid administration of potassium in fluid therapy. It may also occur in conditions unrelated to retention or excessive intake. A sudden shift of potassium from intracellular to extracellular fluid results when catabolism of cells occurs, as in a crushing injury; potassium shifts from cells to plasma.

The signs and symptoms of hyperkalemia are similar to those of hypokalemia. In addition to the signs already listed, the patient may experience tingling or numbness in the extremities, and the heart rate may be slow. A serum potassium level greater than 5.5 mEq/L confirms the diagnosis.[6,7]

Treatment consists of stopping the potassium intake. Dialysis may be necessary for a long-term renal problem. If the cause is a shift of potassium from cells to plasma, glucose and insulin therapy may be used.

Sodium

Sodium is the main electrolyte in the extracellular fluid; its normal concentration is 135 to 145 mEq/L plasma. The main role of sodium is to control the distribution of water throughout the body and to maintain a normal fluid balance. Alterations in sodium concentration markedly influence the fluid volume: the loss of sodium is accompanied by water loss and dehydration; the gain of sodium, by fluid retention.

The body, by regulating the urinary output, normally maintains a constant fluid volume and isotonicity of the plasma. The urinary output is controlled by ADH, secreted by the pituitary gland. If a hypotonic concentration results from a low sodium concentration, the fluid is drawn from the plasma into the cells. The body attempts to correct this process; the pituitary inhibits ADH and diuresis results, with a loss of extracellular fluid. This loss of fluid increases sodium concentration to a normal level.

If a hypertonic concentration results from increased concentration of extracellular sodium, fluid is drawn from the cells. Again the body reacts, and the pituitary is stimulated to secrete ADH. This causes a retention of fluid that dilutes sodium to normal concentrations.

Therefore, increased sodium concentration stimulates the production of ADH, with retention of water, thus diluting sodium to the normal level; a decrease in sodium concentration inhibits the production of ADH, resulting in a loss of water, which raises the concentration of sodium to the normal level.

In the kidneys, sodium is reabsorbed in exchange for potassium. Therefore, with an increase in sodium there is loss of potassium; with a loss of sodium there is an increase in potassium.

A *sodium deficit* may be present when plasma sodium concentration falls below 135 mEq/L. It is caused by excessive sweating combined with a large intake of water by mouth (salt is lost and fluid increased, thus reducing sodium concentration), excessive infusion of nonelectrolyte fluids, gastrointestinal suction plus water by mouth, and adrenal insufficiency, which causes large loss of electrolytes.

The symptoms of a sodium deficit are apprehension, abdominal cramps, diarrhea, and convulsions.

Dehydration results from loss of sodium and leads to peripheral circulatory failure. When sodium and water are lost from the plasma, the body attempts to replace them by a transfer of sodium and water from the interstitial fluid. Eventually the water will be drawn from the cells and circulation will fail; plasma volume will not be sustained.

Sodium excess may be present when the plasma sodium rises above 145 mEq/L. Its causes are excessive infusions of saline, diarrhea, insufficient water intake, diabetes mellitus, and tracheobronchitis (excess loss of water from lungs because of rapid breathing).

The symptoms of sodium excess are dry, sticky mucous membranes, oliguria, excitement, and convulsions.

Calcium

Calcium is an electrolyte constituent of the plasma present in a concentration of about 4.6 to 5.1 mg/dL ionized calcium.[4] Total calcium range is 8.9 to 10.3 mg/dL. Calcium serves several purposes. It plays an important role in formation and function of bones and teeth. As ionized calcium, it is involved in normal clotting of the blood and regulation of neuromuscular irritability.

The parathyroid glands control calcium metabolism. By acting on the kidneys and bones, PTH regulates the concentration of ionized calcium in the extracellular fluid. Impairment of this regulatory mechanism alters the calcium concentration. Hyperparathyroidism causes an elevation in the serum calcium level and a decrease in the serum phosphate level.

Calcium deficit may occur in patients with diarrhea or with problems in gastrointestinal absorption, in extensive infections of the subcutaneous tissue, and in burns.[5] This deficiency can result in muscle tremors and cramps, in excessive irritability, and even in convulsions.

Calcium ionization is influenced by pH; it is decreased in alkalosis and increased in acidosis. With no loss of calcium, a patient in alkalosis may develop symptoms of calcium deficit: muscle cramps, tetany, and convulsions. This is due to the decreased ionization of calcium caused by the elevated pH.

A patient in acidosis may have a calcium deficit with no symptoms because the acid pH has caused an increased ionization of available calcium. Symptoms of calcium deficit may appear if acidosis is converted to alkalosis.

It is estimated that 98% of patients with *hypercalcemia*, or calcium excess, have one of the following three conditions: malignancy, hyperparathyroidism, or thiazide diuretic use.[4] Characteristics include muscular weakness, tiredness, lethargy, constipation, anorexia, polyuria, polydipsia, shortened QT interval on the ECG, and a serum calcium concentration greater than 10.5 mg/dL.

Other Electrolytes

The primary role of *magnesium* is in enzyme activity, contributing to the metabolism of both carbohydrates and proteins. Its serum concentration is 1.3 to 2.1 mEq/L. A *magnesium deficit* is a common imbalance in critically ill patients. Deficits may also occur in less acutely ill patients, such as those experiencing withdrawal from alcohol and those receiving parenteral or enteral nutrition after a period of starvation. Neuromuscular irritability, disorientation, and mood changes are indicative of hypomagnesemia. *Hypermagnesemia* is generally uncommon, but it may be seen in patients with advanced renal failure. Magnesium is excreted by the kidneys; therefore, diminished renal function results in abnormal renal magnesium retention.[4,5]

Chloride, the chief anion of the extracellular fluid, has a plasma concentration of 97 to 110 mEq/L. A deficiency of chloride leads to a deficiency of potassium, and vice versa. There is also a loss of chloride with a loss of sodium, but because this loss can be compensated for by an increase in bicarbonate, the proportion will differ.[1]

Phosphate is the chief anion of the intracellular fluid; its normal level in plasma is 1.7 to 2.3 mEq/L.*

OBJECTIVES OF FLUID AND ELECTROLYTE THERAPY _____

Parenteral therapy has three main objectives: 1) to maintain daily body fluid requirements; 2) to restore previous body fluid losses; and 3) to replace present body fluid losses.

---

*Convert to mg/dL by multiplying by 1.2

Maintenance

Maintenance therapy consists of providing all the nutrient needs of the patient: water, electrolytes, dextrose, vitamins, and protein. Of these needs, water is the most important. The body may survive for a prolonged period without vitamins, dextrose, and protein, but without water, dehydration and death occur.

Water

Water is needed by the body to replace the insensible loss that occurs with evaporation from the skin and evaporated moisture from the expired air. An average adult loses from 500 to 1000 mL water per 24 hours through insensible loss. The skin loss varies with the temperature and humidity.

Water is essential for kidney function; the amount needed depends on the amount of waste products to be excreted as well as the concentrating ability of the kidneys. Protein and salt increase the need for water.

An individual's fluid requirements are based on age, height, weight, and amount of body fat. Because fat is water free, a large amount of body fat contains a relatively low amount of water; as body fat increases, water decreases in inverse proportion to body weight.[2,6] The normal fluid and electrolyte requirements based on body surface area are more constant than when expressed in terms of body weight. Many of the essential physiologic processes such as heat loss, blood volume, organ size, and respiration have a direct relationship to the body surface area.[2,6] The fluid and electrolyte requirements are also proportionate to surface area, regardless of the patient's age.[2] These requirements are based on square meters of body surface area and are calculated for a 24-hour period. Nomograms are available for determining surface area (see Chapter 10).

Balanced electrolyte solutions are available for maintenance. The average requirements of fluid and electrolytes are estimated for a healthy person and applied to a patient. The balanced solutions contain electrolytes in proportion to the daily needs of the patient, but not in excess of the body's tolerance, as long as adequate kidney function exists. When a patient's water needs are provided by these maintenance solutions, the daily needs of sodium and potassium are also met. For maintenance, 1500 mL/m^2 body surface area is administered over a 24-hour period.[3,5]

Glucose

Because it is converted into glycogen by the liver, hence improving hepatic function, glucose has an important role in maintenance. By supplying necessary calories for energy, it spares body protein and minimizes the development of ketosis caused by the oxidation of fat stores for essential energy in the absence of added glucose.

The basic daily caloric requirement of a 70-kg adult at rest is about 1600 calories. However, the administration of 100 g glucose a day is helpful in minimizing the ketosis of starvation[3]; 100 g is contained in 2 L 5% dextrose in water or 1 L 10% dextrose in water.[8]

Protein

Protein is another nutrient important to maintenance therapy. Although a patient may be adequately maintained on glucose, water, vitamins, and electrolytes for a limited time, protein may be required to replace normal protein losses over an extended period. It is necessary for cellular repair, wound healing, and synthesis of vitamins and some enzymes. The usual daily protein requirement for a healthy adult is 1 g/kg body weight.[2] Protein is available as amino acids; taken orally, it is broken down into amino acids before being absorbed into the blood.

Vitamins

Vitamins, although not nutrients in the true sense of the word, are necessary for the utilization of other nutrients. Vitamin C and the various B complex vitamins are the most frequently used in parenteral therapy. Because these vitamins are water soluble, they are not retained by the body but lost through urinary excretion. Because of this loss, larger amounts are required parenterally to ensure adequate maintenance than may be required when administered orally. Vitamin B complex vitamins play an important role in the metabolism of carbohydrates and in maintaining gastrointestinal function. Vitamin C promotes wound healing and is frequently used for the surgical patient. Vitamins A and D are fat-soluble vitamins, better retained by the body and not generally required by the patient on maintenance therapy.

Restoration of Previous Losses

Restoration of previous losses is essential when past maintenance has not been met—when the output has exceeded the intake. Severe dehydration may occur from failure to replace these losses. Therapy consists of replacing losses from previous deficits in addition to providing fluid and electrolytes for daily maintenance. Kidney status must be considered before electrolyte replacement and maintenance can be initiated; urinary suppression may result from decreased fluid volume or renal impairment. A hydrating solution such as 5% dextrose in 0.2% (34.2 mEq) sodium chloride is administered. Urinary flow will be restored if the retention is functional. The patient must be rehydrated rapidly to establish an adequate urinary output. Only after kidney function is proved adequate can large electrolyte losses be replaced. Potassium chloride must be used with considerable caution and is considered potentially dangerous if administered when renal function is impaired. A buildup of potassium, caused by the kidney's inability to excrete salts, can prove hazardous; arrhythmia and heart block can result from the effect of excess potassium on the heart muscle.

Replacement of Present Losses

Replacement of present losses of fluid and electrolytes is also an essential component of maintenance therapy. Accurate measurement of all intake and output is a significant means of calculating fluid loss. Fluid loss may be estimated by determining loss of body weight; 1 L body water equals 1 kg, or 2.2 lb, body weight. An osmolality determination may indicate the water needs of the body. If necessary, a corrective blood urea nitrogen determination may be done in conjunction with the osmolality.

The type of replacement depends on the type of fluid being lost. A choice of appropriate replacement solutions is available. Excessive loss of gastric fluid must be replaced by solutions resembling the fluid lost, such as gastric replacement solutions. Excessive loss of intestinal fluid must be replaced by an intestinal replacement fluid. Examples of conditions that may result from current losses are alkalosis and acidosis. Table 14-3 describes identification of these conditions.

TABLE 14-3
Differentiation of Alkalosis/Acidosis

Cause		Physiology	Symptoms	Intervention
Alkalosis	Loss NaCl/KCl gastric fluid	Concentration of bicarbonate	Slow shallow respiration, pallor	Replacement fluids
		Gastric ions; anions must equal cations.		
		Ammonia is converted into urea and hydrogen ion. If liver fails to convert ammonia to urea, ammonia retention and toxicity result.	Sweating, tetany, coma	
Acidosis	Excess fluid is alkaline.	Intestinal secretions contain excessive bicarbonate ions; with loss, chloride ion	Shortness of breath; rapid breathing;	Administer base salts; ie, sodium lactate or sodium

ELECTROLYTE AND FLUID DISTURBANCES— PATIENT-SPECIFIC APPROACHES

The Surgical Patient

A knowledge of the endocrine response to stress helps the nurse better understand the imbalances and problems associated with them. It also contributes to safe and successful parenteral therapy. The nurse knows what to expect, is alert to the possible dangers of imbalances, and recognizes early symptoms.

Neuroendocrine Response

The neuroendocrine response stimulated by many anesthetic agents is further heightened by surgical stress. Apprehension, pain, and duration and severity of trauma give rise to surgical stress and contribute to an increased endocrine response during the first 2 to 5 days after surgery.

The stress reaction is normal and is nature's way of protecting the body from hypotension resulting from trauma and shock. Correction is often unnecessary and may, in fact, be harmful.

The two major endocrine homeostatic controls affected by stress are the pituitary gland and the adrenal gland (Figure 14-5). The posterior pituitary controls quantitative secretions of ADH. The anterior pituitary controls secretions of corticotropin, which stimulates the adrenal gland to increase mineralocorticoid secretions (aldosterone) and glucocorticoid secretions (hydrocortisone).[2] The adrenal medulla secretes vasopressors (epinephrine and norepinephrine) to help maintain the blood pressure.

A direct physiologic effect occurs when stress increases the secretions of these various hormones. When the posterior pituitary increases ADH secretions, antidiuresis is effected, thus helping maintain blood volume. When the anterior pituitary increases corticotropin secretions, the adrenal gland is stimulated to increase aldo-

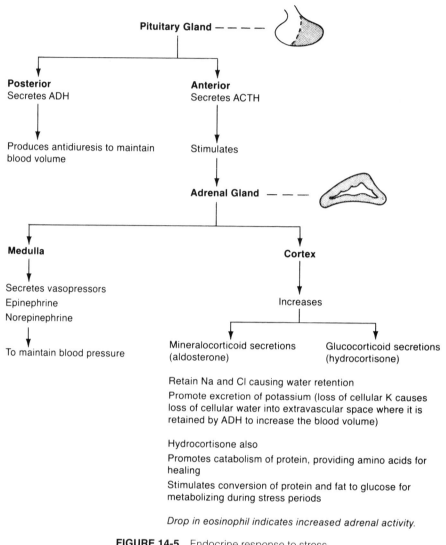

FIGURE 14-5 Endocrine response to stress.

sterone and hydrocortisone secretion. These two adrenal hormones help maintain blood volume by causing the retention of sodium ions and chloride anions, thereby causing water retention, and promoting the excretion of potassium (loss of cellular potassium ions causes loss of cellular water into extracellular space, where it is retained by ADH to maintain blood volume).[2]

Hydrocortisone also promotes the catabolism of protein to provide necessary amino acids for healing and stimulates the conversion of protein and fat to glucose for metabolism during the stress period. This metabolic activity may elevate the blood sugar level, a finding that may mistakenly suggest diabetes mellitus. A drop in the eosinophil count and an elevated level of serum 17-hydroxycorticosteroid hormones indicate increased adrenal activity.[2]

Fluid Needs

Accurate records of intake and output measurements are important for assessing fluid requirements and preventing serious fluid imbalances during the early postoperative period. The daily requirement of 1500 to 2000 mL varies with the patient's needs. Caution must be taken not to overhydrate the patient—the intake should be adequate but should not exceed the fluid losses.

We have seen how the adrenocortical secretions, increased by trauma and stress of surgery, cause some water and sodium retention. This retention may be severe enough to give a false picture of oliguria. Excessive quantities of nonelectrolyte solutions (such as 5% dextrose in water) administered at a time when antidiuresis is occurring may cause a serious fluid imbalance, hyponatremia.

Hyponatremia. In hyponatremia, the serum sodium concentration is less than normal. Water-yielding solutions, infused in excess of the body's tolerance, expand the extracellular compartment, lowering the electrolyte concentration. By osmosis, water invades the cells, with a resulting excess accumulation of intracellular fluid. Usually there is no edema because edema is the result of an excess accumulation of fluid in the extracellular compartment.[2,7,8]

Symptoms of water excess include confusion, hallucinations, delirium, weight gain, hyperventilation, muscular weakness, twitching, and convulsions. If these occur during the early postoperative stages, the nurse should suspect water excess. This is of particular concern in the young and the elderly. Serious consequences, even death, can result.

Restricting the fluid intake may correct mild water excess, but for more severe cases, the administration of high concentrations of sodium chloride may be indicated. The electrolyte concentration of the plasma, increased by the concentrated saline, causes an increase in the osmotic pressure, drawing fluid from the cells for excretion by the kidneys.

Often parenteral therapy during the stress period consists of administering conservative amounts of 5% dextrose in water. Because some sodium retention results from the endocrine response to stress, caution is taken to avoid administration of excessive quantities of saline at a time when there is an interference in the elimination of salt. During this early period, the physician frequently gives 5% dextrose in quarter- or half-strength saline to avoid sodium excess.

Hypernatremia. In hypernatremia, the serum sodium concentration is higher than normal. This excess can cause expanded extracellular fluid volume or edema and possible disruption of cellular function (in potassium-depleted patients the sodium may replace the intracellular potassium).

Symptoms of sodium excess include flushed skin, elevation in temperature, dry and sticky mucous membranes, thirst, and a decreased or absent urinary output. Treatment consists of reducing the salt and water intake and promoting diuresis to eliminate the excess of salt and water from the plasma.

Nutrients

Carbohydrates. Carbohydrates provide an indispensable source of calories for the postoperative patient unable to receive oral sustenance. When carbohydrates are inadequate, the body will use its own fat to supply calories; the by-products are ketone bodies. These acid bodies neutralize bicarbonate and produce metabolic acidosis. The only by-products excreted in the metabolism of carbohydrates are water and carbon dioxide.

By providing calories for essential energy, carbohydrates also reduce catabolism of protein. During the stress response, the renal excretion of nitrogen (from the catabolism of protein) exceeds the intake. By reducing the protein breakdown, glucose helps prevent a negative nitrogen balance.

Carbohydrates do not provide adequate calories for the patient receiving prolonged therapy. One liter of 5% dextrose in water provides 170 calories. Many liters, a volume too great for most patients to tolerate, would be required to provide a patient with 1600 calories. Greater concentrations of glucose, 20% and 50%, may be administered to provide calories for patients unable to tolerate large volumes of fluid (eg, patients with renal insufficiency). The concentrated solutions must be administered slowly for glucose utilization to occur. Rapid administration results in diuresis; the concentrated glucose acts as a diuretic, drawing interstitial fluid into the plasma for excretion by the kidneys.

Alcohol.   Alcohol solutions may be administered to the postoperative patient for nutritional and physiologic benefits. Nutritionally, the alcohol supplements calories provided by the glucose, 1 g ethyl alcohol yielding 6 to 8 calories.[6] Because alcohol is quickly and completely metabolized, it provides calories for essential energy, sparing fat and protein. Metabolized in preference to glucose, alcohol allows the infused glucose to be stored as glycogen.

Physiologically, alcohol produces a sedative effect, reducing pain; 200 to 300 mL of a 5% solution per hour produces sedation without intoxication in the average adult.[6] Alcohol also inhibits the secretion of ADH, promoting water excretion.

Solutions containing alcohol, particularly hypertonic solutions, can cause phlebitis. These solutions, if allowed to infiltrate, may cause tissue necrosis. The cannula should be carefully inserted within the lumen of the vessel and inspected frequently to detect any infiltration.

Protein.   Patients who receive parenteral fluid therapy for a prolonged time require protein for cellular repair, wound healing, and growth. Stress states accompanying surgical procedures and trauma frequently result in protein deficiency.

During the stress period, increased secretions of glucocorticoids from the adrenal cortex cause protein breakdown and the conversion of protein and fat to glucose for energy. More urinary nitrogen is lost than normal. When nitrogen loss exceeds intake, the patient is said to be in a *negative balance*. This response to stress is normal. However, protein losses must be counteracted; preservation of body cell mass is essential. A depleted body cell mass can be restored only by hyperalimentation. Approximately 1 g/kg body weight is required by a healthy adult to replace normal protein loss.[6]

Because of the high ammonia level, extreme caution is required if administered to patients with hepatic insufficiency or emaciation. Organ-specific formulas have been developed for the patient with renal or hepatic disease.

Supplemental medications added to the solution may result in incompatibilities. Always check with the pharmacist before adding any medication to solutions.

Solutions, once opened, must be used immediately. Storing a partially used container of solution in the refrigerator for future use provides a culture medium for the growth of bacteria. No solutions that are cloudy or that contain precipitate should be used.

Fat Emulsions.   Fat emulsions provide a source of calories and essential fatty acids for metabolic processes. They provide a high caloric yield, 9 kcal/g as compared with 4 kcal/g from carbohydrates.

Potassium.   Once the stress period is past, adrenal activity decreases and diuresis begins. At this time, usually after the second to the fifth postoperative day, potassium is given daily to prevent a deficit; potassium is not conserved by the body but is lost in the urine. Electrolyte maintenance fluids may be used or potassium may be added to parenteral solutions. When potassium is added to parenteral fluids, the container, bag, or bottle should be thoroughly shaken to mix and dilute the potassium. Potassium should *never* be added to a hanging container while the infusion is running; such action could result in a bolus injection of the drug. Rapid injection, which increases the drug concentration in the plasma, can result in trauma to the vessel wall and even in cardiac arrest. Potassium should never be given by IV push or bolus administration.

The status of the kidneys must be considered. If kidney function is inadequate, the patient must be rehydrated. During this infusion, the nurse must watch for diminished diuresis and notify the physician if antidiuresis occurs.

Usually 40 mEq/L is sufficient to replace normal potassium loss. It is usually infused over an 8-hour period. Premixed potassium replacement solutions are available in a variety of strengths.

In extreme cases of hypokalemia, when the serum potassium concentration is less than 2.0 mEq/L, it may be necessary to infuse potassium at a much faster rate, not faster than 40 mEq/h. When the serum K concentration reaches 2.5 mEq/L and ECG manifestations of hypokalemia diminish, the rate should be decreased to no more than 10 mEq/h, using a solution that contains no more than 30 mEq/L.[4] Continuous ECG monitoring is required when high doses of potassium are infused. The solution containing potassium should be conspicuously labeled and must never be used when positive pressure is indicated—rapid infusion may result in cardiac arrest.

Potassium is irritating to the vein and may cause a great deal of pain, especially if infused into a vein where a previous venipuncture has been performed. Slowing the rate may decrease the pain.

Vitamins.   Vitamins B complex and C are usually added to parenteral solutions if, after 2 or 3 days, the patient is unable to take fluids orally. Vitamin C is important in promoting healing in the surgical patient, and vitamin B complex aids carbohydrate metabolism.

Nursing Diagnoses
Nursing diagnoses for the postsurgical patient should address relevant fluid and electrolyte disturbances. Table 14-4 lists some possible nursing diagnoses for this patient.

The Burned Patient

The body mechanisms that regulate fluid and electrolyte balance are altered when severe burns occur. The changes during the first 48 hours must be recognized and dealt with. Fluid and electrolyte therapy sufficient to replace losses and maintain a status

TABLE 14-4
Examples of Nursing Diagnoses for a New Postoperative Patient After Abdominal Surgery

Nursing Diagnosis	Etiologic Factors	Defining Characteristics
FVD related to actual fluid loss and third-space fluid shift during surgical procedure	Vomiting after reaction to anesthesia GI suction Third-space fluid shift at surgical site	Postural tachycardia Postural hypotension initially; later, low BP in all positions Decreased skin turgor Decreased capillary refill time Oliguria (<30 mL/h in adult) Weight change depends on cause (decreased if actual fluid loss, as in GI suction; usually increased if fluid loss is due to third-space shift, provided parenteral fluids are given in an attempt to correct hypovolemia)
Altered tissue perfusion (renal) related to hypotension during surgical procedure	Hypotensive effects of anesthesia Hypovolemia due to direct or indirect loss of fluid Hypovolemia due to inadequate parenteral fluid replacement	Oliguria or polyuria in presence of elevated serum creatinine
Alteration in sodium balance (hyponatremia) related to excessive ADH activity	Major surgery with its premedication, anesthesia, decreased blood volume, and postoperative pain results in increased ADH release (causing water retention with sodium dilution)	Serum sodium < 135 mEq/L May be asymptomatic if Na > 120 mEq/L Lethargy, confusion, nausea, vomiting, anorexia, abdominal cramps, muscular twitching
Alteration in acid–base balance (metabolic alkalosis) related to vomiting or gastric suction	Vomiting after reaction to anesthesia Gastric suction, particularly if patient is allowed to ingest ice chips freely	Tingling of fingers, toes, and circumoral region, due to decreased calcium ionization pH > 7.45, bicarbonate above normal, chloride below normal
Altered nutrition (less than body requirements) related to negative nitrogen balance arter surgical stress, and inadequate caloric intake	Catabolic response to stress of surgery Inability to tolerate oral feedings during first few postoperative days due to decreased GI motility, anorexia, nausea, and general discomfort Failure of health care providers to administer sufficient calories via the parenteral route	Weight loss of approximately ¼ to ½ lb/d in adult (provided fluids are not abnormally retained) Perhaps a decrease in serum albumin, transferrin, and retinol binding protein levels (although delivery of a large volume of blood products or the long half-life of certain secretory proteins can interfere with correct interpretation)

ADH, antidiuretic hormone; BP, blood pressure; FVD, fluid volume deficit; GI, gastrointestinal
(From Metheny, N. M. [1996]. *Fluid and electrolyte balance* [3rd ed., p. 252]. Philadelphia: Lippincott-Raven.)

quo increase the patient's chances of survival. Awareness of these physiologic changes contributes to intelligent therapy and aids in the patient's recovery.

Fluid and Electrolyte Changes

Intravascular to Interstitial Fluid Shift.   The shift from intravascular to interstitial fluid, followed by shock, begins immediately after the burn. This fluid shift represents the water, electrolytes, and protein lost through the damaged capillaries, resulting in edema and a marked reduction in plasma volume. The severity of the shift depends on the degree and extent of the burn. In an adult with a 50% burn, the edema may exceed the total plasma volume of the patient. Parenteral fluids must be given immediately to replace the fluid loss and combat shock.

Dehydration.   In the early phases of fluid shift from plasma to tissues, water and electrolytes are lost in larger quantities than is the protein (protein, because of its larger molecular size, does not readily pass through the capillary walls). The osmotic pressure, increased by the higher protein concentration of the plasma, draws fluid from the undamaged tissues and generalized tissue dehydration occurs.

A much more significant fluid loss occurs as exudate from the burned area, water in the form of vapor at the burned area, and blood lost through the damaged capillaries. These losses further contribute to dehydration and hypovolemia.

Decreased Urinary Output.   Decreased urinary output occurs when the lowered blood volume causes a diminished renal blood flow. Increased endocrine secretions further contribute to the decreased urinary output; adrenocortical secretions cause sodium and water absorption; ADH causes increased water reabsorption by the kidneys.

In deep burns free hemoglobin, released by destruction of red blood cells, may produce renal damage.

Potassium Excess.   In the early postburn period, when excessive amounts of potassium build up in the extracellular fluid, potassium excess occurs; cell destruction releases potassium and decreased renal flow obstructs normal excretion of potassium. Plasma potassium concentrations may rise to a dangerously high level. Because of the tendency to plasma potassium excess and the uncertainty of the extent of renal impairment in the burned patient, administration of potassium is contraindicated.

Sodium Deficit.   When plasma is lost in edema and exudate, sodium, the chief electrolyte of the extracellular fluid, is lost with the plasma, and sodium deficit occurs. Further loss may occur as sodium moves into the cells to replace lost potassium.

Metabolic Acidosis.   Acidosis develops within a few hours due to accumulation of fixed acids released from injured tissues.[2]

Fluid Needs

When moderate or severe burns occur, immediate fluid therapy is necessary to combat hypovolemic shock and prevent renal depression. A large-gauge indwelling venous catheter is inserted to ensure venous access during this critical period. Because the measurement of venous pressure is an important guide against overinfusion, a central venous pressure line may be placed.

Solutions such as lactated Ringer's, a balanced salt solution, is often used. It supplies salt and water and helps correct the metabolic acidosis associated with burns.

Hypertonic crystalloid solutions were introduced to decrease the fluid volume needed to correct burn shock and to minimize formation of edema. If used, they are prescribed during the first 24 hours of fluid therapy.[2] In general, they are prescribed after the first 24 hours of fluid therapy. Albumin is also frequently used. Nonprotein colloids, including dextran and hetastarch, have molecular size and increased oncotic pressure to help maintain blood volume and cardiac output by pulling water from the interstitial space of nonburned tissue. Blood is generally not administered unless sufficient loss of blood has occurred from an associated injury. A nonelectrolyte solution, such as 5% dextrose in water, may be used to replace insensible water loss.

During the initial 24 hours, caution must be taken to avoid overzealous administration of water. During the early phase, water contributes little to the maintenance of normal cardiovascular function. Later, when fluid shifts back into the plasma, excess parenteral fluid can cause overburdened circulation and pulmonary edema. If smoke and heat damage have impaired lung function, the threat of pulmonary edema is further increased. Only enough fluid to maintain blood volume and urinary output is administered.

The shift from interstitial fluid to plasma begins on the second to third day after the burn and accounts for the large reduction in parenteral fluids. An increase in the urinary output should alert the nurse to the edema mobilization occurring and the need to decrease fluid therapy.

The "rule of nines" has been commonly used to estimate burned area (Table 14-5). The body's surface area is divided into areas equal to 9% or multiples of 9%. The portion of these areas that have sustained second- or third-degree burns is determined. The total represents the percentage of total body surface area burned. This method may be inaccurate in children, and hence, other charts are available for accurately determining percentage of body surface area burned.

Formulas

Fluid requirements for the first 24 hours range from 2 to 4 mL/kg body weight per percent of body surface area burned. Several factors must be considered, including age of the patient, size and depth of the burn, type of fluid, and complication factors such as inhalation injury, electrical burns, or multiple trauma.[2] Numerous formulas

---

TABLE 14-5
"Rule of Nines" for Estimating Burned Body Area in Adults

Part of Body	Percentage of Body
Head and neck	9
Anterior trunk	18
Each arm	9
Posterior trunk	18
Genitalia	1
Each leg	18

have been developed for this purpose (Table 14-6), but an ideal rate of infusion is one that maintains perfusion, as reflected by a urinary output of 0.5 mL/kg body weight per hour in the adult patient.

Assessment

Ongoing assessment of the patient is needed to allow tailoring of fluid replacement to individual needs. Monitoring parameters include urine volume, sensorium, vital signs, and central venous pressure.

TABLE 14-6
Formulas for Fluid Replacement/Resuscitation

	First 24 Hours			Second 24 Hours		
	Electrolyte	Colloid	Glucose in Water	Electrolyte	Colloid	Glucose in Water
Burn budget of F. D. Moore	1000–4000 mL Lactated Ringer's solution and 1200 mL 0.5% saline	7.5% of body weight	1500–5000 mL	1000–4000 mL Lactated Ringer's solution and 1200 mL 0.5% saline	2.5% of body weight	1500–5000 mL
Evans	Normal saline 1 mL/kg/% burn	1.0 mL/kg/% burn	2000 mL	One-half of first 24-h requirement	One-half of first 24-h requirement	2000 mL
Brooke	Lactated Ringer's solution, 1.5 mL/kg/% burn	0.5 mL/kg/% burn	2000 mL	One-half to three-quarters of first 24-h requirement	One-half to three-quarters of first 24-h requirement	2000 mL
Parkland	Lactated Ringer's solution, 4 mL/kg/% burn				20%–60% of calculated plasma volume	
Hypertonic sodium solution	Volume to maintain urine output at 30 mL/h (fluid contains 250 mEq Na/L)			One-third of salt solution orally, up to 3500 mL limit		
Modified Brooke	Lactated Ringer's solution, 2 mL/kg/% burn				0.3–0.5 mL/kg/% burn	Goal: maintain adequate urinary output
Burnett Burn Center	Isotonic or hypertonic alkaline sodium solution/% burn/kg			D_5 ¼ NS maintenance	Colloid 0.5 mL/% burn/kg	D_5W (% burn) (TBSAm³)

TBSA, total body surface area

(Hudak, C., Gallo, B., & Benz, J. [1990]. *Critical care nursing* [5th ed., p. 766]. Philadelphia: J. B. Lippincott with permission.)

Urine output is the best indicator of adequate fluid resuscitation. Adult output should be 30 to 50 mL/h. Lack of urine output or a substantial decrease in volume may be attributed to inadequate fluid replacement, gastric dilation, or renal failure. Daily weights are a helpful tool for monitoring the burned patient. A weight gain of 15% to 20% may indicate fluid retention.

Adequacy of tissue perfusion is measured by assessing the patient's sensorium. Sensorium should remain normal with appropriate fluid replacement unless other factors, such as head injury, are present.

Vital signs should be monitored hourly in the burned patient. Blood pressure should remain at near normal values with consideration given to the patient's baseline pressure. Temperature may be elevated and tachycardia may be present. Rate and character of respirations should be evaluated. Peripheral pulses and capillary refill times should be monitored. Vasoconstriction of unburned skin is a compensatory response to help preserve normal blood flow in the hours immediately after a severe burn. Hence, unburned skin may be cool to the touch and appear pale at first.

Central venous and arterial pressure monitoring may be used to evaluate the effects of fluid replacement. Inadequate fluid replacement is evidenced by decreased urinary output, thirst, restlessness and disorientation, hypotension, and increased pulse rate. Circulatory overload may be indicated by elevated central venous pressure reading (15–20 cm), shortness of breath, and moist crackles.[2]

Diabetic Acidosis

Diabetic acidosis is an endocrine disorder causing complex fluid and electrolyte disturbances. It occurs when a lack of insulin prevents the metabolism of glucose, and essential calories are provided instead by the catabolism of fat and protein. Acidosis results from the accumulation of acid by-products. Knowledge of the physiologic changes in diabetic acidosis aids the nurse in early detection of imbalances and in an understanding of the treatment involved.

Physiologic Changes

Lack of insulin prevents cellular metabolism of glucose and its conversion into glycogen. Glucose accumulates in the bloodstream (*hyperglycemia*). When the blood sugar rises above 180 mg/100 mL, glucose spills over into the urine (*glycosuria*). The kidneys require 10 to 20 mL water to excrete 1 g glucose; water excretion increases (*polyuria*).

The body's fat and protein are used to provide necessary calories for energy. Ketone bodies, metabolic by-products, reduce plasma bicarbonate, and acidosis occurs.

Fluid and Electrolyte Disturbances

Dehydration.   Dehydration results from excessive fluid and electrolyte losses. Cellular fluid deficit occurs when water is drawn from the cells by the hyperosmolality of the blood. Extracellular deficit occurs when 1) glycosuria increases the urinary output; 2) ketone bodies increase the load on the kidneys and the water to excrete them; 3) vomiting causes loss of fluid and electrolytes; 4) oral intake is reduced because of the patient's condition; and 5) hyperventilation is induced by the acidotic state.

Decreased Kidney Function. Dehydration lowers the blood volume, decreasing renal blood flow, and the kidneys produce less of the ammonia needed to maintain acid–base balance. Severe dehydration may lower the blood volume enough to cause circulatory shock and oliguria.

Ketosis. Ketosis is the excessive production of ketone bodies in the bloodstream. Ketone bodies are the end products of oxidation of fatty acids. Ketosis occurs when a lack of insulin results in excessive fatty acids being converted by the liver to ketones and the decreased utilization of ketones by the peripheral tissues. Electrolytes and ketone bodies, retained in high serum concentration, increase the acidosis; the increase in the number of hydrogen ions, from the retention of ketone bodies, may drop the blood pH to 7.25 and lower. The bicarbonate anions decrease to compensate for the increase in ketone anions and may drop the bicarbonate level to 12 mEq/L or less.[5]

Hyperglycemic Hyperosmolar Nonketotic Coma. Hyperglycemic hyperosmolar nonketotic (HHNK) coma is a syndrome that may develop in the middle-aged or elderly type II diabetic patient. This condition is often associated with the stress of cardiovascular disease, infection, or pharmacologic treatment with steroids or diuretics. It is also precipitated by too-rapid infusion of parenteral nutrition solution. Blood sugars may reach 4000 mg/dL but without the ketosis of diabetic ketoacidosis.[2] Fluid volume deficit is profound and may lead to death. Underlying factors contributing to development of diabetic ketoacidosis or HHNK coma are found in Table 14-7.

Signs and Symptoms of Diabetic Acidosis

The nurse should be familiar with the signs and symptoms that characterize diabetic acidosis. By recognizing impending diabetic acidosis, early treatment may be initiated and complications prevented.

1. *Hyperglycemia* occurs when a lack of insulin prevents glucose metabolism; glucose accumulates in the bloodstream.

2. *Glycosuria* occurs when the accumulation of glucose exceeds the renal tolerance and spills over into the urine.

3. *Polyuria.* Osmotic diuresis occurs when the heavy load of nonmetabolized glucose and the metabolic end products increase the osmolality of the blood, and the increased renal solute load requires more fluid for excretion.

4. *Thirst* is prompted by cellular dehydration arising from the osmotic effect produced by hyperglycemia.

5. *Weakness* and *tiredness* come from the inability of the body to use glucose and from a potassium deficit.

6. *Flushed face* results from the acid condition.

7. *Rapid deep breathing* is the body's defense against acidosis; expiration of large amounts of carbon dioxide reduces carbonic acid and increases the pH of the blood.

8. *Acetone breath* results from an increased accumulation of acetone bodies.

9. *Nausea* and *vomiting* are caused by distention from atony of gastric muscles.

TABLE 14-7
Factors Contributing to Development of DKA or HHNC in Susceptible Persons

DKA	HHNC
Infections, illness	Chronic renal disease
Physiologic stresses (*eg,* trauma, surgery, myocardial infarction, dehydration, pregnancy)	Chronic cardiovascular disease
	Acute illness, infection
	Surgery, burns, trauma
Psychological/emotional stress	Hyperalimentation, tube feedings
Omission/reduction of insulin	Peritoneal dialysis
Failure of insulin delivery system (pump)	Mannitol therapy
	Pharmacologic agents
Excess alcohol intake	Chlorpromazine
	Cimetidine
	Diazoxide
	Diuretics (thiazide, thiazide-related, and loop diuretics)
	Glucocorticoids and immunosuppressive agents
	L-asparaginase
	Phenytoin
	Propranolol

DKA, diabetic ketoacidosis; HHNK, hyperglycemic hyperosmolar nonketotic coma

(From Metheny, N. M. [1996]. *Fluid and electrolyte balance* [3rd ed., p. 325]. Philadelphia: Lippincott-Raven.)

---

10. *Weight loss* accompanies an excess loss of fluid (1 L body water equals 2.2 lb, or 1 kg, body weight) and a lack of glucose metabolism.

11. *Low blood pressure* results from a severe fluid deficit.

12. *Oliguria* follows the decreased renal blood flow that results from a severe deficit in fluid volume.

Parenteral Therapy

Insulin is given to metabolize the excess glucose and combat diabetic acidosis. Because absorption is quickest by the bloodstream, insulin is administered IV. When given subcutaneously or intramuscularly, the slower rate of absorption of insulin may be further decreased by peripheral vascular collapse in the presence of shock. The dose of insulin, when administered by continuous infusion, is usually 4 to 8 U/h.[3] Many types of infusion pumps are available to ensure accurate and continuous administration of medications.

Parenteral fluids are administered to increase the blood volume and restore kidney function. Early treatment of the hypotonic patient usually consists of the administration of sodium chloride (0.9% NaCl) to replace sodium and chloride losses and to expand the blood volume. Later, hypotonic fluids with sodium chloride may be used. Bicarbonate replacement may be necessary when severe acidosis is present.

Potassium administration is contraindicated in the early treatment of diabetic acidosis. During the later stages (10–24 hours after treatment), the plasma potassium level falls; improved renal function increases potassium excretion and, in anabolic states, as the glucose is converted into glycogen, a sudden shift of potassium from extracellular fluid to intracellular fluid further lowers the plasma potassium level. If the patient is hydrated, potassium should be administered when the plasma potassium concentration falls.

A severe potassium deficit may occur if symptoms are not recognized and early treatment begun. Symptoms include weak grip, irregular pulse, weak picking at the bedclothes, shallow respiration, and abdominal distention.

REFERENCES

1. Baxter Healthcare. (1996). *Clinical guide to infusion therapy. Water and electrolytes.* Publisher pending. Edited by Sharon Weinstein.
2. Burgess, R. E. (1965). Fluid and electrolytes. *American Journal of Nursing, 65*, 90–95.
3. Crowell, C. W., & Staff of Educational Design, Inc. New York. (1967). Potassium imbalance. *American Journal of Nursing, 67*, 343.
4. Dunagan, W., & Ridner, M. (1989). Manual of medical therapeutics (26th ed.). Boston: Little, Brown.
5. Metheny, N. M. (1996). *Fluid and electrolyte balance* (3rd ed., pp. 10, 56–58, 182, 223, 308, 311, 289–316). Philadelphia: Lippincott-Raven.
6. Metheny, N. M., & Snively, W. D., Jr. (1985). *Nurses' handbook of fluid balance* (4th ed., pp. 18, 19, 91, 147–154, 161, 185–192, 293–297). Philadelphia: J. B. Lippincott.
7. Terry, J. (1994). The major electrolytes: Sodium, potassium, and chloride. *Journal of Intravenous Nursing, 17*(5), 240–243.
8. Terry, J., et al. (1995). *Intravenous therapy: Clinical principles and practice* (pp. 111–115). St. Louis: Mosby and the Intravenous Nurses Association.

BIBLIOGRAPHY

Corbett, J. V. (1992). *Laboratory tests and diagnostic procedures with nursing diagnosis* (3rd ed., pp. 109–110, 229). Norwalk, CT: Appleton and Lange.

Smeltzer, S. C., & Bare, B. G. (1992). *Brunner and Suddarth's textbook of medical-surgical nursing* (7th ed., p. 125). Philadelphia: J. B. Lippincott.

REVIEW QUESTIONS

1. Nonelectrolytes found in body fluid include which of the following:
   a. dextrose
   b. urea
   c. creatinine
   d. bicarbonate

2. Osmolality of normal blood plasma is:
   a. 210 mOsm/kg water
   b. 230 mOsm/kg water
   c. 270 mOsm/kg water
   d. 290 mOsm/kg water

3. Which of the following controls distribution of water throughout the body?
   a. sodium
   b. potassium
   c. calcium
   d. phosphorus

4. Objectives of infusion therapy include which of the following?
   a. maintain daily requirements
   b. restore previous losses
   c. replace present losses
   d. restore future losses

5. Which electrolyte is considered potentially dangerous if administered to the patient with impaired renal function?
   a. sodium
   b. potassium
   c. phosphate
   d. calcium

6. One liter of body water equals how much body weight?
   a. 1 kg
   b. 2 kg
   c. 3 kg
   d. 4 kg

7. Blood volume is maintained by which of the following hormones?
   a. aldosterone
   b. cortisone
   c. hydrocortisone
   d. norepinephrine

8. Immediately after severe burns, what fluid shift occurs?
   a. interstitial to intravascular
   b. intravascular to interstitial
   c. plasma to tissues
   d. tissues to plasma

9. Rapid administration of 20% or 50% glucose promotes:
   a. diuresis
   b. dehydration
   c. hydration
   d. emesis

10. What fluid shift occurs on the second to third day after a burn?
    a. interstitial to intravascular
    b. intravascular to interstitial
    c. plasma to tissue
    d. tissue to plasma

CHAPTER 15

Principles of Parenteral Fluid Administration

Key Terms

Acidifying	Hydrating	Hypotonic
Alkalyzing	Hypodermoclysis	Isotonic
Contraction	Hyperinsulinism	Turgor
Dehydration	Hypertonic	Water intoxication
Expansion		

PARENTERAL FLUIDS

A knowledge of parenteral fluids is essential in the delivery of infusion therapy; rapid critical changes in fluid and electrolyte balance may be caused by infusates, affecting patient outcomes.

Until the 1930s, IV fluids consisted of dextrose and saline; little was known about electrolyte therapy. Today, with more than 200 types of commercially prepared fluids available and with the great increase in their use, fluid and electrolyte disturbances are more common. With the increased administration of fluids in alternative care settings, nurses must know the chemical composition and the physical effects of the infusions they administer.

Nurses have a legal and professional responsibility to know the normal amount and both the desired and untoward effects of any IV infusion they administer. The type of fluid, the amount, and the rate of flow are determined only after the physician has carefully assessed the patient's clinical condition. Attention to detail and a comprehensive assessment of a patient's fluid and electrolyte status will ensure positive IV patient outcomes.

Definition of Intravenous Infusion

Today, methods of infusion have changed dramatically, and small-volume parenterals may be administered as a secondary infusate or in a volume-controlled reservoir for electronic drug delivery.

An infusion is usually regarded as an amount of fluid in excess of 100 mL designated for parenteral infusion because the volume must be administered over a long period of time. However, when medications are administered by "piggyback" small-volume parenterals (50–100 mL), a shorter period (usually 30–60 minutes) may be required, whereas volumes of 150 to 200 mL may require more than an hour. Today, methodologies have changed consistent with clinical needs of patients, and alternate delivery systems are readily available (see Chapter 10).

Intravenous fluids are mistakenly referred to as *IV solutions*. The term *solution* is defined in the United States Pharmacopeia (USP) as a liquid preparation that contains one or more soluble chemical substances usually dissolved in water. Solutions are distinguished from injections, for example, because they are not intended for administration by infusion or injection.[11] They may vary widely in methods of preparation. The USP refers to parenteral fluids as injections, and methods of preparation must follow standards for injection.

Official Requirements of Intravenous Fluids

Intravenous injections must meet the tests, standards, and all specifications of the USP applicable to injections. This includes quantitative and qualitative assays of infusions, including tests for pyrogens and sterility.

Particulate Matter

Each container must be carefully examined to detect cracks and the fluid examined for cloudiness or presence of particles. The final responsibility falls on the pharmacist and the nurse who administers the fluid. Tests to detect the presence of particulate matter and standards for an acceptable limit of particles have been established by the USP. A large-volume injection for single-dose infusion meets the requirements of the test if it contains not more than 50 particles per milliliter that are equal to or larger than 10.0 μm and not more than 5 particles per milliliter that are equal to or larger than 25.0 μm in effective linear dimension.[10]

pH

The pH indicates hydrogen ion concentration or free acid activity in solution.[7] All IV fluids must meet the pH requirements set forth by the USP. Most of these requirements call for a solution that is slightly acid, usually ranging in pH from 3.5 to 6.2.

Dextrose requires a slightly acid pH to yield a stable solution. Heat sterilization, used for all commercial solutions, contributes to the acidity.

It is important to know the pH of the commonly used IV fluids because it may affect the stability of an added drug and cause the drug to deteriorate. The acidity of dextrose solutions has been criticized for its corrosive effect on veins.

Tonicity

Parenteral fluids are classified according to the tonicity of the fluid in relation to the normal blood plasma. The osmolality of blood plasma is 290 mOsm/L. Fluid that approximates 290 mOsm/L is considered isotonic. IV fluids with an osmolality significantly higher than 290 mOsm (+ 50 mOsm) are considered hypertonic, whereas those with an osmolality significantly lower than 290 mOsm (– 50 mOsm) are hypotonic.[2] Parenteral fluids generally range from approximately one-half isotonic (0.45% sodium chloride) to 5 to 10 times isotonic (25%–50% dextrose).

The tonicity of the fluid when infused into the circulation has a direct physical effect on the patient. It affects fluid and electrolyte metabolism and may result in disastrous clinical disturbances. Hypertonic fluids increase the osmotic pressure of the blood plasma, drawing fluid from the cells; excessive infusions of such fluid can cause cellular dehydration. Hypotonic fluids lower the osmotic pressure, causing fluid to invade the cells; when such fluid is infused beyond the patient's tolerance for water, water intoxication results. Isotonic fluids cause increased extracellular fluid volume, which can result in circulatory overload. By knowing the osmolality of the infusion and the physical effect it produces, the nurse is alerted to the potential fluid and electrolyte imbalances.

The choice of veins used for an infusion is affected by the tonicity of the fluid; hyperosmolar fluids must be infused through veins with a large blood volume to dilute the fluid and prevent trauma to the vessel.

The tonicity of the fluid affects the rate at which it can be infused; hypertonic dextrose infused rapidly may result in diuresis and dehydration.

Because of the direct and effective role osmolality plays in IV therapy, it is helpful for the nurse involved in the administration of IV fluids to be familiar with the terminology and subsequent calculations.

The osmotic pressure is proportional to the total number of particles in the fluid. The milliosmole is the unit that measures the particles or the osmotic pressure. By converting milliequivalents to milliosmoles, an approximate osmolality may be determined. A quick method for approximating the tonicity of IV injections follows.[13]

Fluids Containing Univalent Electrolytes

Each milliequivalent is approximately equal to a milliosmole because univalent electrolytes, when ionized, carry one charge per particle. Normal saline injection (0.9% sodium chloride) contains 154 mEq sodium and 154 mEq chloride per liter, making a total of 308 mEq/L, or approximately 308 mOsm/L.

Fluids Containing Divalent Electrolytes

Because each particle carries two charges when ionized, the milliequivalents per liter or the number of electrical charges per liter when divided by the charge per ion (2) will give the approximate number of particles or milliosmoles per liter. As an example, when 20 mEq magnesium sulfate is introduced into a liter of fluid, each particle ionized will carry two charges. By dividing 20 mEq or 20 charges by 2, an approximate 10 particles or 10 mOsm/L is reached for each component, or 20 mOsm/L total.

The osmolality of electrolytes in solution may be accurately computed but involves the use of the atomic weight and the concentration of the given electrolytes in milligrams per liter. The methods for accurately computing the osmolality of an electrolyte in solution follow.[10]

Osmolality of a Given Electrolyte in Solution

Formula:

$$\frac{\text{milligrams of electrolyte/L}}{(\text{Atomic weight})(\text{valance})} = \text{milliosmoles/L}$$

Example: 35 mg K/L

$$\frac{39}{39 \times 1} = 1 \text{ mOsm/L}$$

Example: 40 mg K/L

$$\frac{40}{40 \times 2} = \frac{1}{2} \text{ mOsm/L}$$

DEXTROSE IN WATER

When glucose occurs as a part of parenteral injections, it is usually referred to as *dextrose*, a designation by USP for glucose of requisite purity. Dextrose is available in concentrations of 2.5%, 5%, 10%, 20%, and 50% in water. To determine the osmolality or the caloric value of a dextrose solution, it is necessary to know the total number of grams or milligrams per liter. Because 1 mL water weighs 1 g, and 1 mL is 1% of 100 mL, milliliters, grams, and percentages can be used interchangeably when calculating solution strength. Thus, 5% dextrose in water equals 5 g dextrose in 100 mL equals 50 g dextrose in 1 L.

Calories

Hexoses (glucose or dextrose and fructose) do not yield 4 calories[15] per gram as do dietary carbohydrates (eg, starches). Each gram of hydrous or anhydrous dextrose provides about 3.4 or 3.85 calories, respectively. One liter of 5% glucose solution yields 170 calories; 1 liter of 10% glucose yields 340 calories[1] (see page 332).

Tonicity of 5% Dextrose in Water

Dextrose 5% in water is considered an isotonic solution because its tonicity approximates that of normal blood plasma, 290 mOsm/L. Because dextrose is a nonelectrolyte and the total number of particles in solution does not depend on ionization, the osmolality of dextrose solutions is determined differently from that of electrolyte solutions. One millimole (one formula weight in milligrams) of dextrose represents 1 mOsm (unit of osmotic pressure). One millimole of monohydrated glucose is 198 mg, and 1 liter of 5% dextrose in water contains 50,000 mg. Thus:

$$\frac{50,000 \text{ mg}}{198} = 252 \text{ mOsm/L}$$

pH

The USP requirement for pH of dextrose solutions is 3.5 to 6.5. This broad pH range may at times contribute to an incompatibility in one bottle of dextrose and not in another when an additive is involved (see Chapter 16).[12]

Metabolic Effects of Dextrose[13]

1. Dextrose provides calories for essential energy.
2. Because glucose is converted into glycogen by synthesis in the liver, it improves hepatic function.
3. It spares body protein (prevents unnecessary breakdown of protein tissue).
4. It prevents ketosis or excretion of organic acid, which frequently occurs when fat is burned by the body without an adequate supply of glucose.
5. When deposited intracellularly in the liver as glycogen, dextrose causes a shift of potassium from the extracellular to the intracellular fluid compartment. This effect is used in the treatment of hyperkalemia by infusing dextrose and insulin.

Indications for Use

Dehydration
Dextrose 2.5% in water and dextrose 5% in water provide immediate hydration to the dehydrated patient and often are used for hydrating the medical and surgical patient. Dextrose 5% in water is considered isotonic only in the bottle; once infused into the vascular system, the dextrose is rapidly metabolized, leaving the water. The water decreases the osmotic pressure of the blood plasma and invades the cells, providing immediately available water to dehydrated tissues.

Hypernatremia
If the patient is not in circulatory difficulty with extracellular expansion, 5% dextrose may be administered to decrease the concentration of sodium.

Vehicle for Administration of Drugs
Many of the drugs for IV use are added to infusions of 5% dextrose in water.

Nutrition
Concentrations of 20% and 50% dextrose in conjunction with electrolytes provide long-term nutrition. Insulin is frequently added to prevent overtaxing of the islet tissue of the pancreas.

Hyperkalemia
Infusions of dextrose in high concentration with insulin cause anabolism (build-up of body cells), which results in a shift of potassium from the extracellular to the intracellular compartment, thereby lowering the serum potassium concentration.

Dangers

Hypokalemia
Because the kidneys do not store potassium, prolonged fluid therapy with electrolyte-free fluids may result in hypokalemia. When cells are anabolized by the metabolism of glucose, a shift of potassium from extracellular to intracellular fluid may occur, resulting in hypokalemia.

Dehydration

Osmotic diuresis occurs when dextrose is infused at a rate faster than the patient's ability to metabolize it. A heavy load of nonmetabolized glucose increases the osmolality of the blood and acts as a diuretic; the increased solute load requires more fluid for excretion. A normal, healthy individual with a urinary specific gravity of 1.029 to 1.032 requires 15 mL water to excrete 1 g solute, whereas individuals with poor kidney function or low concentrating ability of the kidneys require much more water to excrete the same amount of solute.[8,14]

Hyperinsulinism

This condition may occur from a rapid infusion of hypertonic carbohydrate solutes. In response to a rise in blood sugar, extra insulin pours from the beta islet cells of the pancreas in its attempt to metabolize the infused carbohydrate. Termination of the infusion may leave excess insulin in the body, resulting in symptoms such as nervousness, sweating, and weakness caused by the severe hypoglycemia that may be induced. Frequently, after infusion of hypertonic dextrose, a small amount of isotonic dextrose is administered to cover the excess insulin.[8]

Water Intoxication

This imbalance results from an increase in the volume of the extracellular fluid from water alone. Prolonged infusions of isotonic or hypotonic dextrose in water may cause water intoxication. This condition is compounded by stress, which leads to inappropriate release of antidiuretic hormone (ADH) and fluid retention. The average adult can metabolize water at a rate of about 35 to 40 mL/kg/d, and the kidney can safely metabolize only about 2500 to 3000 mL/d in an average patient receiving IV therapy.[6] Under stress, the patient's ability to metabolize water is decreased.

Administration

Isotonic dextrose may be administered through a peripheral vein. Hyperosmolar fluids such as 50% dextrose in water should be infused into the superior vena cava through central venous access. Hypertonic dextrose administered through a peripheral vein with small blood volume may traumatize the vein and cause thrombophlebitis; infiltration can result in necrosis of the tissues.

Sodium-free dextrose injections should not be administered by hypodermoclysis. Dextrose solutions, by attracting body electrolytes in the pooled area of infusions, may cause peripheral circulatory collapse and anuria in sodium-depleted patients.

Electrolyte-free dextrose injections should not be used in conjunction with blood infusions. Dextrose mixed with blood causes hemolysis of the red blood cells.

The amount of water required for hydration depends on the condition and the needs of the patient. The average adult patient requires 1500 to 2500 mL water each day. In patients with prolonged fever, the water requirement depends on the degree of temperature elevation. The 24-hour fluid requirement for a temperature between 101°F and 103°F increases by at least 500 mL; the requirement for a prolonged temperature above 103°F increases by at least 1000 mL.[4]

The rate of administration depends on the patient's condition and the purpose of therapy. When the infusion is used to supply calories, the rate must be slow enough to allow complete metabolism of the glucose (0.5 g/kg/h in normal adults). The maximum rate should generally not exceed 0.8 g/kg/h.[1] When the infusion is used to produce diuresis, the rate must be fast enough to prevent complete metabolism of the dextrose, thereby increasing the osmolality of the extracellular fluid.

ISOTONIC SODIUM CHLORIDE INFUSIONS

Sodium Chloride Injection (0.9%), USP (normal saline), contains 308 mOsm/L (sodium, 154 mEq/L; chloride, 154 mEq/L); has a pH between 4.5 and 7.0; and is usually supplied in volumes of 1000, 500, 250, and 100 mL. The term *normal* or *physiologic* is misleading because the chloride in normal saline is 154 mEq/L, compared to the normal plasma chloride value of 103 mEq/L, whereas the sodium is 154 mEq/L, or about 9% higher than the normal plasma value of 140 mEq/L. Because the other electrolytes present in plasma are lacking in normal saline, the isotonicity of the solution depends on the sodium and chloride ions, resulting in a higher concentration of these ions.[1]

Indications for Use

1. Extracellular fluid replacement when chloride loss has been relatively greater than or equal to sodium loss.

2. Treatment of metabolic alkalosis in the presence of fluid loss; the increase in chloride ions provided by the infusion causes a compensatory decrease in the number of bicarbonate ions.

3. Sodium depletion. When there is an extracellular fluid volume deficit accompanying the sodium deficit, an isotonic solution of sodium chloride is used to correct the deficit.[8]

4. Initiation and termination of blood transfusions. When 0.9% sodium chloride is used to precede a blood transfusion, the hemolysis of red blood cells, which occurs with dextrose in water, is avoided.

Dangers

Sodium chloride (0.9%) provides more sodium and chloride than the patient needs. Marked electrolyte imbalances have resulted from the almost exclusive use of normal saline. Untoward effects are described below.

Hypernatremia

An adult's dietary requirement for sodium is about 90 to 250 mEq/d, with a minimum requirement of 15 mEq and a maximum tolerance of 400 mEq.[3] When 3 L 0.9% sodium chloride or 5% dextrose in 0.9% sodium chloride is administered, the patient receives 462 mEq sodium (154 mEq/L × 3), a level that exceeds normal tolerance. Such an infusion at a time when sodium retention is occurring, as during stress, can result in hypernatremia.

The danger of hypernatremia is increased in the elderly, in patients with severe dehydration, and in patients with chronic glomerulonephritis; these patients require more water to excrete the salt than do patients with normal renal function. Isotonic saline does not provide water but requires most of its volume for the excretion of salt.

Acidosis
One liter of 0.9% sodium chloride contains one-third more chloride than is present in the extracellular fluid. When infused in large quantities, the excess chloride ions cause a loss of bicarbonate ions and result in acidosis.

Hypokalemia
Infusion of saline increases potassium excretion and at the same time expands the volume of extracellular fluid, further decreasing the concentration of the extracellular potassium ion.

Circulatory Overload
Continuous infusions of isotonic fluids expand the extracellular compartment and lead to circulatory overload.

Requirements

In an average adult, the daily requirements of sodium chloride are met by infusing 1 L of 0.9% sodium chloride or 1 to 2 L of 4.5% sodium chloride, but the dosage depends on the patient's age, weight, clinical condition, and fluid, electrolyte, and acid–base balance.[1]

ISOTONIC SALINE WITH DEXTROSE

Dextrose 5% in 0.9% Sodium Chloride

Dextrose 5% in 0.9% sodium chloride contains 252 mOsm dextrose (chloride, 154 mEq/L; sodium, 154 mEq/L); has a pH of 3.5 to 6.0; and is available in volumes of 1000, 500, 250, and 150 mL.

When normal saline is infused, the addition of 100 g dextrose prevents both the formation of ketone bodies and the increased demand for water the ketone bodies impose for renal excretion. The dextrose prevents catabolism and, consequently, loss of potassium and intracellular water.

Indications for Use
1. Temporary treatment of circulatory insufficiency and shock caused by hypovolemia in the immediate absence of a plasma expander.
2. Early treatment along with plasma or albumin for replacement of loss caused by burn.
3. Early treatment of acute adrenocortical insufficiency.

Dangers
The hazards are the same as those for normal saline (see preceding section).

Dextrose 10% in 0.9% Sodium Chloride

Dextrose 10% in 0.9% sodium chloride contains 504 mOsm/L dextrose (sodium, 154 mEq/L; chloride, 154 mEq/L), has a pH of 3.5 to 6.0, and is usually supplied in volumes of 1000 and 500 mL.

Indications for Use
This fluid is used as a nutrient and an electrolyte (sodium and chloride) replenisher.

Dangers
Hypernatremia, acidosis, and circulatory overload may result when normal saline is administered in excess of the patient's tolerance.

Administration
Dextrose 10% in 0.9% sodium chloride, because of its hypertonicity, must be administered IV, preferably through a vein of large diameter to dilute the fluid and reduce the risk of trauma to the vessel. Close observation and precautions are necessary to prevent infiltration and damage to the tissues.

HYPERTONIC SODIUM CHLORIDE INFUSIONS

These infusions include 3% sodium chloride (sodium, 513 mEq/L; chloride, 513 mEq/L) and 5% sodium chloride (sodium, 850 mEq/L; chloride, 850 mEq/L).

Indications for Use

Severe Dilutional Hyponatremia (Water Intoxication)
Hypertonic sodium chloride, on infusion, increases the osmotic pressure of the extracellular fluid, drawing water from the cells for excretion by the kidneys.

Severe Sodium Depletion
Infusions of hypertonic saline replenish sodium stores. An estimate of the sodium deficit can be made by taking the difference between the normal sodium concentration and the patient's current sodium concentration and multiplying it by 60% of the body weight in kilograms; sodium depletion is based on total body water and not on extracellular fluid.[9]

Administration

Hypertonic sodium chloride injection must be administered with great caution to prevent pulmonary edema. Frequent reevaluation of the clinical and electrolyte picture during administration is advised. A 3% or 5% solution of sodium chloride is used to correct the deficit if the fluid volume is normal or excessive; the amount of sodium administered depends on the sodium deficit in the plasma.[8]

Hypertonic saline solutions should be infused slowly (such as 200 mL over a minimum of 4 hours),[8] and the patient should be observed constantly. The fluid must

---

TABLE 15-1
Summary of Important Nursing Considerations in Administration of Hypertonic Saline Solutions (3% and 5% NaCl)

1. Check the serum sodium level before administering these solutions and frequently thereafter.

2. Be aware that these solutions are dangerous and should be used only in critical situations in which the serum sodium is very low (such as <110 mEq/L) and neurologic symptoms are present.

3. Administer these solutions only in intensive care settings where the patient can be closely monitored. Watch for signs of pulmonary edema and worsening of neurologic signs. Use with great caution in patients with congestive heart failure or renal failure.

4. Be aware that only small volumes are needed (such as 5 mL or 6 mL/kg body weight of 5% NaCl) to elevate the serum sodium level by 10 mEq/L. For example, elevating the serum sodium level of a 70-kg patient from 110 to 120 mEq/L would require approximately 350 to 420 mL.

5. The serum sodium should not be raised more rapidly than 2 mEq/L/h unless the clinical state of the patient indicates the need for more rapid treatment.

6. Use an electronic infusion device to administer the fluid; maintain close vigilance on the device as none is foolproof.

7. Be aware that the aim of therapy is not to elevate the serum sodium level to normal quickly; rather, it is to elevate it only enough to alleviate neurologic signs. It has been recommended that the serum concentration be raised no higher than 125 mEq/L with hypertonic saline.

8. Be aware that the physician may prescribe flurosemide to promote water loss and prevent pulmonary edema. Urine should be saved as renal sodium and potassium losses may need to be measured to allow for replacement.

(From Metheny, N. M. [1996]. *Fluid and electrolyte balance* [3rd ed., p. 75]. Philadelphia: Lippincott-Raven.)

---

be infused by vein, with great care taken to prevent infiltration and trauma to the tissues. Table 15-1 summarizes the important nursing considerations in the administration of hypertonic saline.

HYPOTONIC SODIUM CHLORIDE IN WATER

One-half hypotonic saline (0.45% saline containing sodium, 77 mEq/L, and chloride, 77 mEq/L) is used as an electrolyte replenisher. When there is a question regarding the amount of saline required, hypotonic saline is preferred over isotonic saline. In general, 0.45% sodium chloride is preferable to 0.9% sodium chloride.

HYDRATING FLUIDS

Because solutions consisting of dextrose with hypotonic saline provide more water than is required for excretion of salt, they are useful as hydrating fluids. These solutions include 2.5% dextrose in 0.45% saline (dextrose, 126 mOsm/L, with sodium, 77 mEq/L, and chloride, 77 mEq/L), 5% dextrose in 0.45% saline (dextrose, 252 mOsm/L, with sodium, 77 mEq/L, and chloride, 77 mEq/L), and 5% dextrose in 0.2% saline (dextrose, 252 mOsm/L, with sodium, 34.2 mEq/L, and chloride, 34.2 mEq/L).

Indications for Use

1. Commonly called *initial hydrating solutions*, hypotonic saline dextrose infusions are used to assess the status of the kidneys before electrolyte replacement and maintenance are initiated.

2. Hydration of medical and surgical patients.

3. Promotion of diuresis in dehydrated patients.

Administration

To assess the status of the kidneys, the fluid is administered at the rate of 8 mL/m^2 body surface area (BSA) per minute for 45 minutes. The restoration of urinary flow shows that the kidneys have begun to function; the hydrating fluid may be replaced by more specifically needed electrolytes. If after 45 minutes the urinary flow is not restored, the rate of infusion is reduced to 2 mL/m^2 BSA per minute for another hour. If this does not produce diuresis, renal impairment is assumed.[8]

Initial hydrating fluids must be used cautiously in edematous patients with cardiac, renal, or hepatic disease. Once good renal function is obtained, appropriate electrolytes should be administered to prevent hypokalemia.

HYPOTONIC MULTIPLE-ELECTROLYTE FLUIDS

Hypotonic multiple-electrolyte fluids are patterned after the type devised by Butler. Butler, with his coworkers at the Massachusetts General Hospital, was the first to emphasize that basic water and electrolyte requirements are proportionate to the BSA. Butler-type fluids are one-third to one-half as concentrated as plasma. They provide fluid to meet the patient's fluid volume requirement and in so doing provide cellular and extracellular electrolytes in quantities balanced between the minimal needs and the maximal tolerance of the patient. These fluids, because of their hypotonicity, provide water for urinary and metabolic needs and take advantage of the body's homeostatic mechanisms to retain the electrolytes and reject those not needed, thus maintaining water and electrolyte balance.[8]

Hypotonic fluids should contain 5% dextrose for its protein-sparing and antiketogenic effect.[5] The dextrose will increase the tonicity of the fluid in the container, but once infused the dextrose will be metabolized, leaving the water and salt. Whether the patient has received too much or too little water depends on the tonicity of the electrolyte and not the osmotic effect of dextrose.

A balanced solution of hypotonic electrolytes is ideal for routine maintenance. There are several modifications of the Butler-type fluids. Those containing 75 mEq total cation per liter are used for older infants, children, and adults.

Administration

A useful formula for maintenance water requirements, based on studies by Crawford, Butler, and Talbot, is: maintenance water equals 1600 mL/m^2 BSA per day.[5] For obese or edematous patients, this should be calculated on ideal weight rather than actual weight. The water requirement must be patterned after the condition of the patient.

When infection, trauma involving the brain, or stress lead to inappropriate release of ADH, maintenance requirements are less. Excessive fluid losses through urine, stool, expired air, and so forth require increased water. The rate of infusion is usually 3 mL/m^2 BSA per minute.

Dangers

Hyperkalemia
When renal function is impaired, IV potassium should be used cautiously. The nurse should be alert for signs of hyperkalemia. If such signs develop, the physician should be notified and the fluid replaced by more appropriate electrolytes.

Water Intoxication
The patient's tolerance limits for water can be exceeded. Care should be exercised in maintaining the prescribed flow rate and in ensuring that the patient receives the prescribed volume of fluid. Water intoxication is more likely to occur when inappropriate release of ADH, in response to stress, causes water retention. These patients should be carefully watched to detect any early signs of an imbalance, so that a change in therapy can be initiated before the condition becomes precarious. Weighing the patient is the best way to monitor the status of water balance. Daily weights are extremely important in following the state of hydration in extremely ill patients.

ISOTONIC MULTIPLE-ELECTROLYTE FLUIDS

Many types of commercial replacement fluids are available. When severe vomiting, diarrhea, or diuresis results in a heavy loss of water and electrolytes, replacement therapy is necessary. Balanced fluids of isotonic electrolytes having an ionic composition similar to plasma are used.

Administration

Rapid initial replacement is seldom necessary. However, if impaired circulation and renal function of a severely dehydrated patient become evident and it is necessary to restore the patient's blood pressure quickly, 30 mL/kg of an isotonic fluid may be provided in the first hour or two.[5] Fluid overload must be prevented. Central venous pressure monitoring is especially helpful in the elderly patient and in patients with renal or cardiovascular disorders.

Extracellular replacement can generally be assumed to be complete after 48 hours of replacement therapy unless proved otherwise by clinical or laboratory evidence. To continue replacement fluids after deficits have been corrected may result in sodium excess leading to pulmonary edema or heart failure.[5] Patients receiving replacement therapy should be observed closely to detect any signs of circulatory overload.

Gastric replacement fluids provide the usual electrolytes lost by vomiting or gastric suction. They contain ammonium ions, which are metabolized in the liver to hydrogen ions and urea, replacing the hydrogen ion lost in gastric juices. They are useful in metabolic alkalosis caused by excessive ingestion of sodium bicarbonate. The usual adult dose is 500 to 2000 mL, and the rate should be consistent with the patient's clinical condition but not exceed 500 mL/h.

Gastric replacement fluids are contraindicated in the presence of hepatic insufficiency or renal failure. They require the same precautions as any fluid containing potassium and should be avoided in patients with renal damage or Addison's disease. Also, the low pH causes incompatibilities with many additives.

Lactated Ringer's injection is considered safe in certain conditions. Because the electrolyte concentration closely resembles that of the extracellular fluid, it may be used to replace fluid loss from burns and fluid lost as bile and diarrhea. Lactated Ringer's injection has been useful in mild acidosis, the lactate ion being metabolized in the liver to bicarbonate.

Dangers

Three liters contain about 390 mEq sodium, which can quickly elevate the sodium level in a patient who is not deficient.[3] Lactated Ringer's injection is contraindicated in severe metabolic acidosis or alkalosis and in liver disease or anoxic states that influence lactate metabolism.

ALKALIZING FLUIDS

When anesthesia or disorders such as dehydration, shock, liver disease, starvation, and diabetes cause retention of chlorides, ketone bodies, or organic salts, or when excessive bicarbonate is lost, metabolic acidosis occurs. Treatment consists of infusion with an appropriate alkalizing fluid. These fluids include one-sixth molar isotonic sodium lactate (1.9%, with sodium, 167 mEq/L, and lactate ions, 167 mEq/L, and a pH of 6.0–7.3), one-sixth molar Sodium Bicarbonate Injection, USP (1.5%, with sodium, 178 mEq/L, and bicarbonate, 178 mEq/L, and a pH of 7.0–8.0), and hypertonic sodium bicarbonate injection (7.5% or 5%).

One-Sixth Molar Sodium Lactate

The lactate ion must be oxidized in the body to carbon dioxide before it can effect acid–base balance; the complete conversion of sodium lactate to bicarbonate requires about 1 to 2 hours.[1] Because oxidation is necessary to increase the bicarbonate concentration, sodium lactate is not used for patients suffering from oxygen lack, as in shock or congenital heart disease with persistent cyanosis. It is also contraindicated in liver disease because the lactate ions are improperly metabolized.

One-sixth molar sodium lactate is used when acidosis results from a sodium deficiency in such disorders as vomiting, starvation, uncontrolled diabetes mellitus, acute infections, and renal failure.[1]

The usual dose is 1 L of a one-sixth molar solution, but the dosage depends on the patient's condition and the serum sodium level. One-sixth molar infusion may be administered by venoclysis or hypodermoclysis and usually at a rate not greater than 300 mL/h.[1] The patient should be observed closely for any evidence of alkalosis.

Sodium Bicarbonate

Sodium Bicarbonate Injection, USP (1.5%, with sodium, 178 mEq/L, and bicarbonate, 178 mEq/L), is an isotonic solution that provides bicarbonate ions in conditions in which excess depletion has occurred. It is used for severe hyperpnea early in the treatment of severe acidosis until the signs of dyspnea and hyperpnea are relieved. The bicarbonate ion is released in the form of carbon dioxide through the lungs, leaving an excess of sodium cation behind to exert its electrolyte effect.[1] Recommendations and practice related to pharmacologic management of cardiopulmonary resuscitation suggest a cautious use of sodium bicarbonate to manage acidosis.[8]

The usual dose is 500 mL in a 1.5% solution. The dosage depends on the patient's weight, condition, and carbon dioxide content. If the isotonic infusion is not available, it may be made by adding two 50-mL ampules containing 3.75 g each of sodium bicarbonate to 400 mL hypotonic saline. The fluid should be infused slowly intravenously. Rapid injection may induce cellular acidity and death. The patient should be watched for signs of hypocalcemic tetany, and calcium supplement should be administered if required; calcium does not ionize well in an alkaline medium. Extravasation of hypertonic sodium bicarbonate injections must be avoided.[1] Bicarbonate therapy should cease when the pH reaches 7.2.[9]

ACIDIFYING INFUSIONS

Normal saline (0.9% Sodium Chloride Injection, USP) is not usually listed among the acidifying infusions. However, because metabolic alkalosis is a condition associated with excess bicarbonate and loss of chloride, isotonic saline provides conservative treatment. When the chloride ions are infused, the bicarbonate decreases in compensation and the alkalosis is relieved.

Ammonium chloride, the usual acidifying agent, is available as isotonic 0.9% ammonium chloride injection (ammonium, 167 mEq/L; chloride, 167 mEq/L) and hypertonic 2.14% ammonium chloride injection (ammonium, 400 mEq/L; chloride, 400 mEq/L). The pH range is 4.0 to 6.0. Both concentrations are supplied in 1-liter bottles.

Indications for Use

Ammonium chloride is used as an acidifying infusion in severe metabolic alkalosis caused by loss of gastric secretions, pyloric stenosis, or other causes. The ammonium ion is converted by the liver to hydrogen ion and to ammonia, which is excreted as urea.

Administration

The 2.14% ammonium chloride is usually used in the treatment of the adult patient; 0.9% ammonium chloride is used for children.[8]

The dosage depends on the condition of the patient and on an accurate chemical picture, including plasma carbon dioxide–combining power. Ammonium chloride must be infused at a very slow rate to enable the liver to metabolize the ammonium ion, not to exceed 5 m/L minute in adults.[1] Rapid injection can result in toxic effects, causing irregular breathing, bradycardia, and twitching.[1]

Precautions

Because its acidifying effect depends on the liver for conversion, ammonium chloride must not be administered to patients with severe hepatic disease or renal failure. It is contraindicated in any condition with a high ammonium level.

Contents of selected solutions and comments are found in Table 15-2.

EVALUATION OF WATER AND ELECTROLYTE BALANCE

A rational approach is necessary if the patient is to receive safe and successful IV therapy. In the past, emphasis was placed on the technical responsibility of the nurse in maintaining the infusion and in maintaining patent venous access. With the increase in the use of IV therapy, clinical disturbances in fluid and electrolyte metabolism are more common. Changes can occur quickly and in the absence of the physician. Today the nurse's responsibility consists of monitoring the fluid and electrolyte status of the patient as well as the progress of the infusion. Greater emphasis must be placed on the causes and effects of fluid and electrolyte abnormalities so that these imbalances may be anticipated and recognized before they become disastrous. The nurse should be familiar with the parameters used in evaluating fluid and electrolyte imbalances and in supplying fluid and electrolyte requirements.

Central Venous Pressure

Central venous pressure monitoring provides a simple, accurate, and valuable guide in detecting changes in blood volume and in assessing fluid requirements. It is particularly valuable in assessing the ability of the heart to tolerate the infusion. Many erroneous conclusions are drawn from false values recorded when the line is not properly responsive to right atrial pressures.

A normal venous pressure indicates an adequate circulatory blood volume.

An elevated venous pressure may mean an increase in circulatory volume and right heart pressure, with the possibility of circulatory overload. It may also indicate other problems such as a pulmonary embolus, myocardial infarction, or lack of digitalis. Determination of the hematocrit value will supplement clinical information.[6]

A low venous pressure, too low to measure, indicates that the patient has probably lost fluid or blood. One must not overlook the fact that fluid loss can result from drug-induced vasodilation[8] or improper administration of IV fluids. If rapid infusion of dextrose exceeds the patient's tolerance, massive diuresis with dehydration and diminished circulatory volume may occur. The decreased venous blood return into the right atrium is reflected by a decrease in the central venous pressure.

Pulse

The pulse quality and rate provide valuable clinical information for assessing fluid and electrolyte changes in the patient. A high pulse pressure, bounding and not easily obliterated by pressure, indicates a high cardiac output caused by circulatory overload. A regular pulse, easily obliterated by pressure, indicates low cardiac output resulting from a lowered blood volume. A bounding, easily obliterated pressure signifies a drop in blood pressure with a wide pulse pressure, indicative of impending

TABLE 15-2
Contents of Selected Water and Electrolyte Solutions With Comments About Their Use

Solution	Comments
5% dextrose in water (D$_5$W): No electrolytes 50 g of dextrose	Supplies approximately 170 cal/L and free water to aid in renal excretion of solutes Should not be used in excessive volumes in patients with increased ADH activity or to replace fluids in hypovolemic patients
0.9% NaCl (isotonic saline): Na$^+$ 154 mEq/L Cl$^-$ 154 mEq/L	Isotonic fluid commonly used to expand the extracellular fluid in presence of hypovolemia Because of relatively high chloride content, it can be used to treat mild metabolic alkalosis
0.45% NaCl (1/2-strength saline): Na$^+$ 77 mEq/L Cl$^-$ 77 mEq/L	A hypotonic solution that provides Na$^+$, Cl$^-$, and free water Na$^+$ and Cl$^-$ provided in fluid allows kidneys to select and retain needed amounts Free water desirable as aid to kidneys in elimination of solutes
0.33% NaCl (1/3-strength saline): Na$^+$ 56 mEq/L Cl$^-$ 56 mEq/L	A hypotonic solution that provides Na$^+$, Cl$^-$, and free water Often used to treat hypernatremia (because this solution contains a small amount of Na$^+$, it dilutes the plasma sodium while not allowing it to drop too rapidly.)
3% NaCl: Na$^+$ 513 mEq/L Cl$^-$ 513 mEq/L	Grossly hypertonic solutions used only to treat severe hyponatremia See Table 15-1 for summary of important nursing considerations in administration
5% NaCl: Na$^+$ 855 mEq/L Cl$^-$ 855 mEq/L	Dangerous solutions
Lactated Ringer's solution: Na$^+$ 130 mEq/L K$^+$ 4 mEq/L Ca^{++} 3 mEq/L Cl$^-$ 109 mEq/L Lactate (metabolized to bicarbonate) 28 mEq/L	A roughly isotonic solution that contains multiple electrolytes in approximately the same concentrations as found in plasma (Note that this solution is lacking in Mg and PO$_4$.) Used in the treatment of hypovolemia, burns, and fluid lost as bile or diarrhea Useful in treating mild metabolic acidosis

(continued)

circulatory collapse. As the patient's condition deteriorates, the pulse will become rapid, weak, thready, and easily obliterated, signifying circulatory collapse.

Hand Veins

Examination of the hand veins provides a means of evaluating the plasma volume. The hand veins will usually empty in 3 to 5 seconds when the hand is elevated and will fill in the same length of time when the hand is lowered to a dependent position. Peripheral vein filling takes longer than 3 to 5 seconds in patients with sodium depletion and extracellular dehydration.[8] Slow emptying of the hand veins indicates overhydration and an excessive blood volume; slow filling indicates a low blood volume and often precedes hypotension. Hand veins that become engorged and clearly visible

TABLE 15-2 *(Continued)*

Solution	Comments
Sodium lactate solution, ⅙ M: Na+ 167 mEq/L Cl- 167 mEq/L	A roughly isotonic solution used to correct severe metabolic acidosis (lactate is metabolized to bicarbonate in 1–2 h by the liver.) Not used in patients with liver disease (lactate cannot be converted to bicarbonate in such individuals); also, not used in patients with oxygen lack (unable to adequately convert lactate to bicarbonate)
Sodium bicarbonate, 5%: Na+ 595 mEq/L Cl- 595 mEq/L	A very hypertonic solution used to correct severe metabolic acidosis Should be cautiously administered at a slow rate, under careful volume control Should be administered only with extreme caution to salt-retaining patients (eg, those with cardiac, renal, or liver damage)
Ammonium chloride, 2.14%:	Acidifying solution used to correct severe metabolic alkalosis Due to high ammonium content, must be administered cautiously to patients with compromised hepatic function
Potassium chloride, 0.15% K+ 20 mEq/L Cl- 20 mEq/L	Premixed potassium chloride solution
Potassium chloride, 0.30% K+ 40 mEq/L Cl- 40 mEq/L	Premixed potassium chloride solution

ADH, antidiuretic hormone

(From Metheny, N. M. [1996]. *Fluid and electrolyte balance* [3rd ed., p. 183]. Philadelphia: Lippincott-Raven.)

indicate an increase in the plasma volume secondary to an interstitial-to-vascular fluid shift or an increase in extracellular fluid volume.[8]

Neck Veins

Changes in fluid volume are reflected by changes in neck vein filling, provided the patient is not in heart failure. In the supine position, the patient's external jugular veins fill to the anterior border of the sternocleidomastoid muscle. Flat neck veins in the supine position indicate a decreased plasma volume.[8]

Weight

A sudden gain or loss in weight is a significant sign of a change in the fluid volume. A change in the volume of body fluid can be computed by weighing the patient daily at the same time of day, on the same scales, with the same amount of clothing. A loss or gain of 1 kg body weight reflects a loss or gain of 1 liter body fluid. A rapid 2% loss of total body weight (TBW) indicates mild fluid volume deficit (FVD), and a rapid loss of 8% or more represents severe FVD. Conversely, weight gain occurs when total fluid intake exceeds total fluid output. A rapid 2% gain of; TBW indicates mild fluid volume excess (FVE); a 5% gain represents a moderate FVE; and 8% or greater indicates a severe FVE.[8]

Thirst

Thirst is an important symptom denoting a deficit in body fluid or, more specifically, cellular dehydration. This type of dehydration occurs when the extracellular fluid becomes hypertonic, either as a result of water deprivation or the infusion of hypertonic saline. The increase in osmotic pressure causes fluid to be drawn from the cells, resulting in cellular dehydration, the stimulus to thirst.

Normally, thirst governs the need for water but, in certain conditions, the lack of thirst may accompany dehydration. This is especially true in the aged, in whom thirst is not urgent. These patients may lose their thirst and as a result become severely dehydrated before the condition is recognized.

In the severely burned patient, the great thirst experienced may lead to ingestion of excess water and to a serious sodium deficit.

Intake and Output

Water intake and output should be carefully measured and recorded. Hourly urine output measurements may be particularly important. A urine output of 200 mL/h indicates that too much water is being infused too rapidly. By regulating the urine output between 30 and 50 mL/h, the patient receives at least enough fluid for the kidneys to work efficiently.[6]

A decreased urinary output accompanies a decreased blood volume; changes in the arterial pressure and pressure in the glomeruli result in the oliguria or anuria of profound shock. The increase in urinary output accompanying an increase in blood volume is primarily caused by changes in arterial pressure and pressure in the glomeruli.[8] Output should include urine, vomitus, diarrhea, drainage from fistulas, and drainage from suction apparatus.[8]

Skin Turgor

Observing changes in skin turgor (elasticity) and texture is helpful in assessing the state of water balance. To test skin turgor, pinch the skin over the sternum, inner aspect of the thigh, or forehead in the adult or the medial aspects of the thigh or abdomen[8] in the child, and then release it; in the normal individual, the pinched skin will return to its original position. Skin that remains in a raised position for several seconds indicates a deficit in fluid volume.

Tongue Turgor

A dry, leathery tongue may indicate a fluid volume deficit or mouth breathing. To differentiate between the two, the mucous membrane may be checked for moisture by running the finger between the gums and the cheek; dryness indicates a fluid volume deficit.

Normally, the tongue has one longitudinal furrow. In the patient with fluid volume deficit, additional longitudinal furrows are present and the tongue is smaller because of the fluid loss. Not significantly affected by age, the tongue is a good parameter to measure in all age groups.

Edema

Edema reflects an increase in the extracellular fluid volume outside the circulating intravascular compartment. It depends on an imbalance or a disturbance in the exchange of water and electrolytes between the patient and the environment or the exchange of water and electrolytes between the compartments of the body. The fluid and electrolyte exchange between the body compartments may be affected by an alteration in the circulatory system, the lymphatic system, or the concentration of albumin in the serum; water and electrolytes escape from the circulation faster than they enter, and edema ensues. Edema may be generalized, as in congestive failure; localized, as with ascites; or peripheral.

By detecting edema early, a clinical imbalance may be corrected before the patient's condition deteriorates. Early peripheral edema may be detected by fingerprinting, a procedure in which the finger is rolled over the bony prominence of the sternum or tibia. As edema increases, pitting edema will occur and may be detected by pressure of the fingers on the subcutaneous tissue.

In generalized edema, such as that seen in cardiac failure, total extracellular water volume as well as interstitial edema increase. Symptoms such as venous engorgement, restlessness, dyspnea, cyanosis, and pulmonary rales indicate generalized edema.

Laboratory Values

Laboratory values, when used to supplement clinical observations, aid in forming diagnostic and therapeutic guidelines.

Electrolyte studies (serum sodium, potassium, chloride, bicarbonate, and pH) performed daily are important in assessing the fluid and electrolyte status of the patient receiving IV fluids. In patients with massive electrolyte losses, such studies may be required two or three times a day.

Blood cell count and *hematocrit* determinations are helpful in detecting hemoconcentration or hemodilution; hemoconcentration reflects a diminished plasma volume caused by dehydration, and hemodilution, an increased volume from overtreatment with water.

Measurement of *serum protein with the albumin/globulin ratio* helps in detecting a change in fluid volume; large quantities of parenteral fluid rapidly administered dilute and decrease the serum protein concentration. This determination is helpful when used to supplement clinical observation—otherwise it may be misleading and interpreted as showing actual depletion. A decrease in serum protein reduces the osmotic pressure of the extracellular compartment, causing some edema and loss of plasma volume.

Blood urea nitrogen should be measured frequently to evaluate kidney function, an important parameter in treating fluid and electrolyte imbalances.

CLINICAL DISTURBANCES OF WATER AND ELECTROLYTE METABOLISM

Most of the common clinical disturbances in water and electrolyte balance result from changes in the volume of total body water or in one or more of the fluid compartments of the body. Clinical disturbances in water and electrolyte metabolism have been classified into six types: isotonic, hypertonic, and hypotonic expansion and isotonic, hypertonic, and hypotonic contraction. These are discussed in the following pages and are summarized in Tables 15-3 and 15-4.

Isotonic Expansion

Isotonic expansion (circulatory overload) occurs when fluids of the same tonicity as plasma are infused into the vascular circulation. Because solutions isotonic to plasma do not affect the osmolality, water does not flow from the extracellular to the intracellular compartment. The extracellular compartment expands in proportion to the fluid infused and is the only compartment affected. The increase in the volume of fluid dilutes the concentration of hemoglobin and lowers the hematocrit and total protein levels, but the serum sodium level remains the same.

Isotonic expansion is a critical complication of IV therapy. Patients who receive isotonic fluids around the clock are prime targets and should be observed closely for early signs of circulatory overload. Sodium chloride (0.9%) or solutions containing balanced isotonic multiple electrolytes are used for preexisting or continuing fluid and electrolyte losses and are not the ideal fluids for maintenance therapy. The electrolyte isotonicity of these solutions causes expansion of the extracellular compartment and does not provide the extra water that balanced hypotonic solutions provide for the kidney to retain or secrete as needed.[3]

The early postoperative or posttrauma patient is susceptible to this critical complication. The increased endocrine response to stress during the first 2 to 5 days after surgery results in retention of sodium chloride and water.[8] When a patient under stress is receiving isotonic infusions, the nurse must anticipate and watch for signs of circulatory overload.

Elderly patients receiving isotonic fluids must be carefully monitored because they have a lower tolerance to fluids and electrolytes. Because they are also likely to have some degree of cardiac and renal impairment, the ability of the kidneys to eliminate fluid is likely to be diminished. The status of these patients can change quickly.

In the patient who has had a craniotomy, large-volume isotonic infusions can increase the intracranial pressure and prove detrimental.

Patients who are potential candidates for isotonic expansion must be watched carefully and turned frequently to prevent fluid from settling in the lungs. Pulmonary edema can result from the cardiac and pulmonary side effects of IV therapy. The apices of the lungs, which are high, will tend to be fairly dry, but the bases of the

TABLE 15-3
Comparison of Three Types of Dehydration (Contraction)

	Isotonic	Hypertonic	Hypotonic
Cause	Loss of blood or isotonic fluid	Excess loss of water or insufficient intake	Loss of salt
Effect on fluid compartments	ECF volume ↓	ICF and ECF volume ↓	ICF volume ↑ ECF volume ↓
Clinical signs			
Weight	↓	↓	↓
Rate of H_2O excretion	↓	↓	↑
Rate of Na excretion	↓	↓	↓
Thirst	—	Early sign, due to cellular dehydration	—
Pulse rate	Regular, easily obliterated by pressure	Regular and normal in early stages	Increased, weak and thready, easily obliterated by pressure
Hand vein filling time (normal = 3–5 sec)	May ↑ —	May be normal	Normal to ↑
Behavior		Irritability, restlessness, possibly confusion	Possibly vomiting and cramps
Signs in late stages	Developing shock with pulse weak and thready	Skin turgor diminished; dry, furrowed tongue; death, possibly due to rise of osmotic pressure	Skin turgor may be diminished; thready pulse; possibly confusion and apathy; death from peripheral circulatory failure
Laboratory values			
Hematocrit	↑	↑	↑
Hemoglobin	↑	↑	↑
Total protein and albumin globulin ratio	↑	↑	↑
Sodium concentration	—	↑	↓

ECF, extracellular fluid; ICF, intracellular fluid

lungs, posteriorly and inferiorly, can be fairly wet.[6] As a result, hypostatic pneumonia secondary to gravity may develop.

Manifestations

The nurse who monitors IV infusions must be familiar with the early clinical manifestations that accompany isotonic expansion to recognize and prevent its development; mild pulmonary edema progressing to severe pulmonary edema is a late stage that must be prevented. Early clinical manifestations include: 1) weight gain; 2) increased

TABLE 15-4
Comparison of Three Types of Fluid Expansion

	Isotonic	Hypertonic	Hypotonic
Cause	in Infusion of excess quantities of isotonic fluids	Infusion of excess quantities of hypertonic saline	Increased intake or infusion of water in excess of patient's tolerance
Effects on fluid compartments	ECF volume ↑	ECF volume ↑ ICF volume ↓	ECF and ICF volume ↑
Clinical signs			
Weight	↑	↑ depending on amount infused	↑
Rate of H_2O excretion	↑	↓	↑
Rate of Na excretion	↑	↑	↑
Thirst	—	Present	—
Pulse rate	Bounding, not easily obliterated by pressure	Full, bounding (significant)	May be regular and not easily obliterated by pressure
Hand vein emptying time (normal = 3–5 sec)	↑	↑	↑
Edema	May be present	Early, tibial edema; later, pitting edema; diminished skin turgor	Tibial edema with finger printing
Signs of intracranial pressure	—	—	Irritability, headache, confusion
Signs in late stages	Hoarseness, pulmonary edema, cyanosis, coughing, dyspnea	Water rales, pulmonary edema	Pulmonary edema
Other signs	—	Hoarseness (a frequent early sign)	Cramping of exercised muscles
Laboratory values			
Hematocrit	↓	↓	↓
Hemoglobin	↓	↓	↓
Total protein and albumin globulin ratio	↓	↓	↓
Sodium concentration	—	↑	↓

ECF, extracellular fluid; ICF, intracelluar fluid

fluid intake over output; 3) a high pulse pressure, bounding and not easily obliterated, showing signs of high cardiac output; 4) increase in central venous pressure; 5) peripheral hand vein emptying time longer than normal 3 to 5 seconds when the hand is elevated from a dependent position; 6) peripheral edema, depending on the extent of fluid expansion; and 7) hoarseness. If IV therapy is allowed to continue, isotonic expansion becomes more apparent and dangerous, with easily recognized signs: cyanosis, dyspnea, coughing, and neck vein engorgement.

Laboratory characteristics include a drop in the hematocrit value and reduced concentrations of hemoglobin and total protein.

Treatment

Treatment for circulatory overload when detected early is relatively simple and consists of withholding all fluids until excess water and electrolytes have been eliminated by the body. After the condition is rectified, hypotonic maintenance fluids will provide the patient with fluid and a minimum daily requirement of electrolytes. The hypotonicity of the fluid allows the kidneys to maintain the needed amount and selectively retain or excrete the excess.

Isotonic Contraction

Isotonic contraction occurs when there is loss of fluid and electrolytes isotonic to the extracellular fluid, such as whole blood or large volumes of fluid from diarrhea or vomiting. The extracellular compartment contracts. Because the fluid lost is isotonic, the osmolality of the extracellular compartment remains unchanged and no movement of water occurs between the compartments; only the extracellular volume is affected.

Manifestations

Because of the loss of fluid, the hematocrit level and the concentrations of hemoglobin and total protein are increased. The serum sodium concentration does not change.

Clinical manifestations are: 1) weight loss; 2) negative fluid balance (a decrease in urinary output but a greater output than total fluid intake); 3) pulse regular in rate, easily obliterated by pressure, and, as the patient's condition deteriorates, weak and thready; and 4) possible increase in peripheral hand filling time above the normal 3 to 5 seconds when the hand is moved from an elevated to a dependent position.

Treatment

Treatment consists of replacing the fluid loss with isotonic solutions containing balanced electrolytes.

Hypertonic Expansion

Hypertonic expansion occurs when the volume of body water is increased by the IV infusion of hypertonic saline. Sodium chloride 3% or 5% is used to replace a massive sodium loss or to remove excess accumulation of body fluids, but, if it is rapidly infused, hypertonic expansion can result. The saline increases the osmotic pressure of the extracellular compartment, causing water to be drawn from the intracellular compartment until both compartments are isosmotic. The volume of the extracellular compartment increases and that of the intracellular compartment decreases. The osmolality of the extracellular fluid is higher than before the infusion but lower than the high level after the infusion because of the increased extracellular fluid volume.[1]

Caution must be used in the IV administration of hypertonic saline. Circulatory overload with hypernatremia can occur. An understanding of the reason for the infusion, the condition of the patient, the proper rate of administration, and the signs and symptoms of hypertonic expansion provides a basis for sound IV practice.

Manifestations

Clinical manifestations include a gain in body weight dependent on the volume infused. A small volume (500 mL) will not contribute to a significant weight gain.[13] An increased sodium load results in a decreased rate of water excretion; however, the abrupt increase in plasma volume may cause an increase in the rate of water excretion as the body attempts to excrete the excess salt and water. The degree of thirst will depend on the hypertonicity of the plasma and consequently the amount of cellular dehydration. Peripheral hand vein emptying time may be increased beyond the normal 5 seconds when the hand is elevated but depends on the degree of expansion of the extracellular compartment. A bounding pulse is significant in detecting hypertonic expansion. The serum sodium concentration is increased. The hematocrit level and the concentrations of hemoglobin and total serum protein are decreased as a result of the expanded fluid volume in the extracellular compartment.

Treatment

Treatment consists of stopping the infusion to allow the kidneys to eliminate the overload of salt and water. If no cardiovascular side effects are noted, 5% dextrose in water may be infused slowly to reduce the tonicity of the extracellular fluid and replace body water.

Hypertonic Contraction

Hypertonic contraction (hypertonic dehydration) occurs when water is lost without a corresponding loss of salt. This condition occurs in patients who are unable to take sufficient fluid for a prolonged period or in patients with excess insensible water loss through the lungs and skin.

In the elderly, hypertonic dehydration is a common clinical disturbance; they frequently have a decrease in the thirst stimuli in response to hypertonicity of body fluids, and adequate intake of fluid is not met. In the unconscious or incontinent patient, frequency and excess urination may go undetected or may be recognized as a sign of good renal function. A loss of tubular ability to concentrate urine in the aged will result in a large urinary volume when an increased solute load is presented to the patient.[8] Elderly patients also have a diminished response to ADH. Large amounts of dilute urine may be lost, resulting in hypertonic dehydration.

To prevent fluid imbalance, the nurse must recognize that individuals differ widely in the water they require; patients whose kidneys do not concentrate well require more water than those whose kidneys concentrate well. The daily fluid requirement must be met.

In hypertonic contraction, the loss of water from the extracellular compartment results in an increase in the osmolality, causing water to flow from the cells to the extracellular compartment. Dehydration occurs as water leaves the cellular compartment to replace the plasma volume. Both compartments, the intracellular and the extracellular, are affected by the water loss; there is a decrease in volume and an increase in osmolality in both compartments. In contrast, in isotonic contraction only the extracellular compartment is affected and the contraction is more serious.

Because signs of hypertonic contraction are not obvious in the early stages, the nurse must anticipate such an imbalance and be alert to any changes.

Manifestations

Clinically, thirst is an early and reliable sign of hypertonic contraction but may be absent in the elderly, complicating early recognition of this imbalance. Weight loss occurs. Negative fluid balance (output greater than intake) is present. Hourly output measurements show a decrease in the rate of excretion of water. The pulse has a normal quality and is regular in the early stages of hypertonic contraction. The hand vein filling time may be within the normal limits; cellular fluid has partly replenished the plasma. Irritability, restlessness, and possibly confusion may be present. Skin turgor diminishes and is a sign of dehydration in the later stages. A dry mouth with a furrowed tongue indicates dehydration.

Laboratory studies show an increase in serum sodium concentration, hematocrit level, hemoglobin concentration, and total serum protein concentration.

Treatment

Treatment consists of hydrating the patient by administering a balanced hypotonic solution such as the Butler-type solutions; 2400 mL/m² BSA per day for moderate preexisting deficit and 3000 mL/m² BSA per day for severe preexisting deficit.[8] The usual rate for IV administration is 3 mL/m² BSA. A therapeutic test for functional renal depression may be necessary before infusing water and electrolytes for maintenance.

Hypotonic Expansion

Hypotonic expansion (water intoxication, dilutional hyponatremia) occurs when the increase in the volume of body fluids is caused by water alone. Water expands the extracellular compartment, causing a decrease in the concentration. Water then diffuses into the cells until both compartments are isosmotic. Both the extracellular and the intracellular compartments are affected; the volume is increased and the concentration is decreased. The serum sodium concentration and the hematocrit, hemoglobin, and total serum protein levels are reduced.

Hypotonic expansion occurs in patients who are receiving large quantities of electrolyte-free water to replace excessive fluid and electrolytes lost from gastric suction, vomiting, diarrhea, or diuresis, or insensibly through the skin.

Patients receiving continuous infusion of 5% dextrose in water are particularly susceptible to water intoxication. This solution contains 252 mOsm dextrose per liter, making it an isotonic solution in the container. Once introduced into the circulation, the dextrose is quickly metabolized, leaving the water free to dilute and expand the extracellular compartment. With the decreased osmolality of the extracellular fluid, water diffuses into the cells and hypotonic expansion occurs.

The patient's tolerance to water can be exceeded by infusion of excess amounts of hypotonic fluids. The kidneys of the normal adult can metabolize water in amounts of 35 to 45 mL/kg/d, but the kidneys of the average patient can metabolize only 2500 to 3000 mL/d; above these volumes, abnormal accumulation of water occurs.[6]

Hypotonic expansion is more likely to occur during the early postoperative period, when retention of water is being affected by the response to stress, particularly in the elderly patient, in whom the response to stress is compounded by impairment in renal function. Small amounts of adjusted hypotonic saline (sodium, 90 mEq/L; chloride, 60 mEq/L; and lactate, 30 mEq/L) may be used in the early postoperative management of the aged.

Manifestations

When acute onset of behavioral changes, such as confusion, apathy, and disorientation, occurs in the elderly patient postoperatively, overhydration should be suspected. Central nervous system disturbances such as weakness, muscle twitching, and convulsions are seen, as are headaches, nausea, and vomiting.

Fluid intake is increased over fluid output. Weight gain is always present. Blood pressure usually is normal but may be elevated. Peripheral hand veins are usually full, and hand emptying time is increased beyond the normal 5 seconds when the hand is elevated from a dependent position. The pulse may be regular and not easily obliterated when pressure is applied.

Treatment

Treatment consists of withholding all fluids until the excess water is excreted. In severe hyponatremia, it may be necessary to administer small quantities of hypertonic saline to increase the osmotic pressure and the flow of water from the cells to the extracellular compartment for excretion by the kidneys. Hypertonic saline must be used cautiously and must not be administered to patients with congestive heart failure.

Hypotonic Contraction

Hypotonic contraction (hypotonic dehydration) occurs when fluids containing relatively more salt than water are lost from the body. This loss results in a decrease in the effective osmolality of the extracellular compartment. Water is drawn into the cells until osmotic equilibrium is established. Because of the invasion of water, the intracellular compartment is expanded and the extracellular compartment is contracted.

This imbalance may result from the loss of salt from any one of several sources: urine of patients receiving diuretics, fistula drainage, severe burns, vomitus, and sweat. The elderly are affected by the loss of small quantities of sodium.

Manifestations

Clinical manifestations include 1) weight loss; 2) negative fluid balance; 3) pulse rate increased, weak or thready, and easily obliterated; 4) increased hand filling time; and 5) decreased skin turgor.

Laboratory studies show a decrease in serum sodium concentration and an increase in hematocrit, hemoglobin, and total serum protein levels.

Treatment

Treatment of hypotonic contraction consists of replacing the fluids and electrolytes that have been lost. Because other electrolytes are usually lost along with the sodium loss, a balanced electrolyte solution may be administered.

REFERENCES

1. American Society of Hospital Pharmacists. (1995). Bethesda, MD: American Hospital Formulary Service, 1486, 1490, 1514–1517, 1527–1529.
2. Burgess, R. E. (1965). Fluid and electrolytes. *American Journal of Nursing, 65,* 90.
3. Burns, W. (1972). Indications for IV therapy. In Health Care Worldwide. *Proceedings of Clinical Seminar* (pp. 7, 8, 12), San Francisco, 1968. North Chicago, IL: Abbott Laboratories.
4. Condon, R., & Nyhus, L. (Eds.). (1975). *Manual of surgical therapeutics* (3rd ed., p. 203). Boston: Little, Brown.
5. Drug and Therapeutic Information, Inc. (1970). Parenteral water and electrolyte solutions. *Medical Letter on Drugs and Therapeutics, 12*(19), 77.
6. Dudrick, S. J. (1971). Rational IV therapy. *American Journal of Hospital Pharmacy, 28,* 83–85.
7. Lebowitz, M. H., MaSuda, J. V., & Beckerman, J. H. (1971). The pH and acidity of intravenous infusion solutions. *Journal of the American Medical Association, 215,* 1937.
8. Metheny, N. M. (1996). *Fluid and electrolyte balance* (3rd ed., pp. 12–29, 169, 174, 273). Philadelphia: Lippincott-Raven.
9. Dunagan, W., & Ridner, M. (1989). *Manual of medical therapeutics* (26th ed., pp. 2, 65). Boston: Little, Brown.
10. Stoklosa, M. J. (1974). *Pharmaceutical calculations* (6th ed., pp. 236, 237). Philadelphia: Lea & Febiger.
11. United States Pharmacopeia. (1980). (20th ed., pp. 803, 1027). Easton, PA: Mack Publishing.
12. Vanatta, J., & Fogelman, M. (1988). *Moyer's fluid balance: A clinical manual* (4th ed., p. 45). Chicago: Year Book Medical Publishers.
13. Voda, A. M. (1970). Body water dynamics. *American Journal of Nursing, 70,* 2597, 2598, 2600–2601.
14. Weisberg, H. F. (1969). Parenteral fluid therapy in adults. In H. F. Conn (Ed.). *Current therapy* (p. 414). Philadelphia: W. B. Saunders.
15. Weisberg, H. F. (1964). Pitfalls in fluid and electrolyte therapy. *Journal of St. Barnabas Medical Center, 2,* 106.

REVIEW QUESTIONS

1. Fluids with the same tonicity as plasma are known as:
   a. isotonic
   b. hypotonic
   c. hypertonic
   d. base fluids

2. How many grams of dextrose are in 250 mL 20% dextrose in water?
   a. 25
   b. 50
   c. 75
   d. 100

3. How much water can the kidney safely metabolize in the average patient receiving IV therapy?
   a. 1500-1999 mL daily
   b. 2000-2499 mL daily
   c. 2500-2999 mL daily
   d. 3000-3500 mL daily

4. Hydrating fluids are used to:
   a. assess status of kidneys
   b. hydrate medical and surgical patients
   c. promote diuresis in dehydrated patients
   d. assess status of liver

5. What type of fluids are indicated when a retention of chlorides, ketone bodies, or organic salts occurs as in shock, liver disease, and starvation?
   a. alkalinizing fluids
   b. acetic fluids
   c. isotonic fluids
   d. hypertonic fluids

6. What fluid imbalance may result from continuous infusion of 5% dextrose in water?
   a. water intoxication
   b. dehydration
   c. hypertonic expansion
   d. peripheral edema

7. Loss of fluid and electrolytes of the same tonicity as plasma through vomiting, diarrhea, or loss of whole blood may result in:
   a. hypertonic contraction
   b. isotonic contraction
   c. hypotonic expansion
   d. hypertonic expansion

8. Which of the following sites is best used to assess skin turgor in the adult patient?
   a. skin over forehead or sternum
   b. skin over medial aspect of thigh
   c. skin over lateral aspect of thigh
   d. skin over abdomen

9. Which of the following parameters provide valuable information concerning fluid and electrolyte status?
   a. central venous pressure
   b. peripheral veins
   c. quality and rate of pulse
   d. laboratory values

10. Dextrose and hypotonic saline are considered hydrating fluids because:
    a. they provide more water than is required for excretion of salt
    b. the water they provide equals that needed for excretion of salt
    c. they minimize retention of salt
    d. they maximize retention of potassium in the cell

C HAPTER 16

Parenteral Nutrition

Key Terms

Admixture	Nutrition	Total nutrient
Drug–nutrient	assessment	admixture
interaction	Nutrition screening	Transitional
feeding		
Enteral nutrition	Nutrition support	Vascular access
Malnutrition	Parenteral nutrition	device
Nutrient		

HISTORY

Development of hyperalimentation began in the early 1960s in the Harrison Department of Surgical Research at the University of Pennsylvania. Dr. Stanley Dudrick devised a central venous system of feeding that resulted in the normal weight gain and growth of beagle puppies who were fed only by vein.[22] His animal experiments quickly led to human applications; he successfully hyperalimented a severely ill infant who was unable to sustain herself with any type of gastrointestinal feeding due to small-bowel atresia.[81]

Further applications followed in the adult population. The term "parenteral hyperalimentation" was coined by Dr. Jonathan E. Rhoads and Dr. Dudrick and defined as "the intravenous administration of nitrogen, calories, and other nutrients sufficient to achieve tissue synthesis and anabolism in patients with normal or excessive nutritional needs."[22] These accomplishments led the way for further research and application as other clinicians and researchers realized its potential.

Hyperalimentation soon became a recognized specialty and nutrition support teams were formed. JoAnne Grant was the first nurse hired exclusively for work with this new form of nutrition support at the University of Pennsylvania in 1967.[32] In

1976, a multidisciplinary group of professionals (physicians, nurses, dietitians, and pharmacists) was organized and the American Society for Parenteral and Enteral Nutrition (ASPEN) held its first Clinical Congress in Chicago.

The 1980s saw hyperalimentation evolve as a science and become more commonly known as total parenteral nutrition (TPN) or parenteral nutrition (PN). Disease-specific formulas were developed to address the particular needs of patients with renal, cardiac, or hepatic disease and became commercially available. The rehabilitation of patients surviving catastrophic illnesses by maintenance on home PN (HPN) led to the formation of support groups such as LifeLine and the Oley Foundation. Nutrition support research continued at a fast pace.

From this modest beginning, PN has evolved into a sophisticated field of therapeutic intervention that has its own multidisciplinary specialists and a large body of established knowledge. The role of amino acids such as arginine and glutamine; the indications for medium-, short-, or long-chain triglycerides, and structured lipids; the implications of antioxidants, growth hormone, and cytokines are some of the areas of ongoing research.

The 1990s, with the changing health care environment and emergence of managed care, have brought additional changes and challenges to the area of nutrition support. There is more of a focus on home care and home nutritional support, while, at the same time, more stringent restrictions on reimbursement for home nutritional support are being drafted. Nutrition support teams are also moving into the outpatient setting or being eliminated.

INDICATIONS

Indications for PN are diverse and depend on the patient's clinical status, severity of current illness, degree of catabolism, presence of complications and other diagnoses, and length of time the patient will be without gastrointestinal function and adequate oral intake.[48] Guidelines for the use of parenteral and enteral nutrition in hospitalized patients have been published by ASPEN and are widely used.[2] Georgetown University also published a report on the evaluation of PN, known as the "Georgetown Report."[23]

Although the need for PN is clear in patients with a nonfunctional gastrointestinal tract who are expected to eat in 7 to 10 days, the expense and risk of complications associated with such treatment mandates careful consideration of its use in others. The standard rule is still appropriate—when the gut works, use it! The enteral route is preferred whenever possible because it is more physiologic—it maintains the integrity and function of the gastrointestinal system. It is also less expensive, less invasive, and easier to manage, with generally fewer complications.

Some general guidelines for the use of PN, developed at a community hospital with a nutrition support team, are outlined in Table 16-1.

NUTRITIONAL ASSESSMENT

A nutritional assessment should be included in the overall assessment of patients, particularly on admission to the hospital and periodically throughout their hospital stay.

Many hospitals have established formal nutritional screening programs for all hospital admissions, to identify patients most at risk or already malnourished. Mod-

TABLE 16-1
Guidelines for Parenteral Nutrition (PN) Support[2,68]

Criteria

Nonfunctioning gastrointestinal tract:

- Cannot be used safely and effectively
- Use is undesirable or contraindicated for prolonged period
- Unable to tolerate adequate nutrition orally

Guidelines

1. Normally nourished patients unable to eat for 7–10 days generally *do not* require PN
2. PN should be promptly initiated as soon as it is determined that enteral starvation will persist for 7–10 days or more, even if normally nourished.
3. Moderately malnourished patients who require intensive medical or major surgical intervention should be started on PN immediately.
4. Markedly hypercatabolic patients (burns, sepsis, trauma) should be started on PN immediately, even if well nourished.
5. Severely malnourished patients should begin PN immediately.
6. Acute metabolic derangements should be corrected *before* PN is initiated (should be hemodynamically stable).
7. Examples of situations in which PN may be useful:
   - Acute pancreatitis
   - Enterocutaneous fistulas
   - Intractable vomiting, diarrhea
   - Hyperemesis gravidarum
   - Intensive cancer chemotherapy, radiation therapy
   - Inflammatory bowel disease
   - Short-bowel syndrome

Contraindications

1. Patients who have a functional and usable gastrointestinal tract capable of absorption of adequate nutrients.
2. The anticipated need for PN is less than 5 days.
3. When aggressive nutrition support is not desired by the patient or legal guardian, in accordance with hospital policy and existing law.
4. Prognosis does not warrant aggressive nutrition support—should not be used when malnutrition is due to rapidly progressive disease not amenable to curative or palliative therapy (not used to sustain the hopelessly ill; may only prolong suffering).
5. PN should not be used during periods of acute hemodynamic instability.
6. PN should not be used during surgical operations, unless it is a short procedure under local anesthesia.
7. When the risks of PN are judged to exceed the potential benefit.

(Courtesy of West Jersey Hospital Nutrition Support Committee, Voorhees, NJ)

erate to severe malnutrition has been reported in up to 50% of hospitalized patients.[69] Inadequate nutrition has been found to increase complications, especially infection, decrease the ability to heal wounds, prolong length of stay, and contribute to
anorexia and weakness.

Suggested goals of nutritional assessment include:

1. To identify nutritional status and deficiencies that adversely affect health

2. To obtain specific information to assist in planning and delivery of nutrition
   support

3. To evaluate the efficacy of nutrition support and to modify the patient's care
   plan as needed to obtain the desired result[27]

Three major types of malnutrition have been identified, characterized by pathogenesis and specific clinical findings:

1. Marasmus (calorie)—a gradual wasting of body fat and muscle, with intact
   visceral protein stores. This patient is emaciated; marasmus is often associated with chronic illness and starvation.

2. Kwashiorkor (protein) or hypoalbuminemia—loss of visceral protein stores in
   the presence of adequate fat and muscle. It is usually associated with poor
   protein intake in the presence of adequate calories and in acute situations
   with increased stress.

3. Mixed marasmus and hypoalbuminemia—a combination of both fat loss and
   muscle wasting with depleted visceral protein stores.[15]

In hospitalized patients, another clinical state has recently been recognized—
acute hypoalbuminemia.[34] This is commonly seen with acute stress and hypermetab-
olism. Rapid and marked decreases in serum albumin occur, often characterized by
edema or generalized anasarca. The acute fall is caused by redistribution of albumin
into extravascular compartments, external losses, and, to a lesser extent, by alterations in protein synthesis to meet demands for acute phase proteins and increased
albumin degradation.

Early nutritional intervention is recommended to avoid additional complications
of malnutrition. Although not due to malnutrition, acute hypoalbuminemia is associated with increased morbidity and mortality.

Effective in 1995, the Joint Commission on the Accreditation of Healthcare
Organizations (JCAHO) standards for both hospital and home care mandate nutritional assessment as part of the specific nutrition care standards, emphasizing
an interdisciplinary approach. An algorithm for nutritional screening is found in Figure 16-1. Primary care, outpatient management, and the new standards have moved
the role of nutritional assessment into the physician's office and home care as well.
A nutritional assessment traditionally begins with a complete history that includes
a diet history, anthropometric measurements, physical assessment, and complete medical history, including drug–nutrient interactions, and biochemical evaluation.

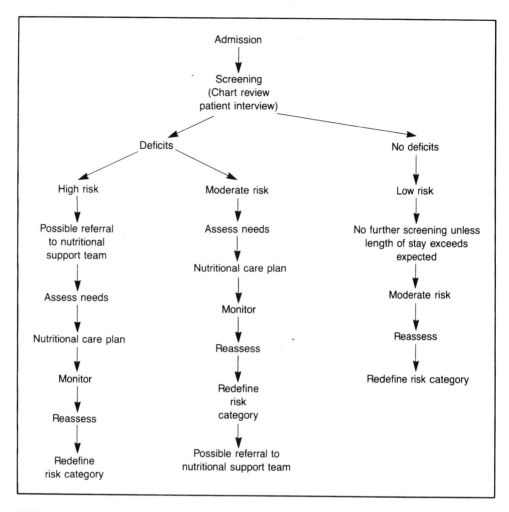

FIGURE 16-1   Nutritional screening. [Courtesy: Grant, DeHoog. Nutritional Assessment and Support, 1991.)

Patient History

The patient's usual and current dietary intake is helpful in identifying the adequacy of nutrient intake and possible nutritional deficiencies. Dietary factors that may alter intake include food allergies, aversions, and intolerances; fad diets; diet modifications (low sodium, low cholesterol, low fat); poor dentition or ill-fitting dentures; chewing or swallowing difficulties; oral sores; alterations in taste and smell; breathing difficulties; and inability to prepare food or feed oneself.[16,33] The medical history should include any acute or chronic diseases that may have an impact on nutrient intake or utilization and conditions that increase metabolic needs or fluid and electrolyte losses. Certain drugs, such as analgesics, antacids, anticonvulsants, antibiotics, diuretics, laxatives, antineoplastic drugs, or oral contraceptives, alter dietary intake or nutrient utilization.[33]

Social factors that can influence nutrient intake include religion, ethnic background, income, education, psychologic or physical disabilities, and alcohol and substance abuse.

Physical Assessment

A thorough physical assessment by an experienced clinician can detect signs and symptoms that may indicate nutritional deficiencies. These include but are not limited to changes in hair, eyes, skin, nails, and all organ systems (Table 16-2).

Anthropometrics

Anthropometric measurements consist of simple, noninvasive, inexpensive techniques for obtaining body measurements used to evaluate a patient's nutritional status. The patient's actual height and weight should be obtained and used as a baseline. The weight should be measured periodically thereafter—using the same scale and same amount of clothing, and at the same time of day.[16,69] In assessing body weight, the current weight is compared to usual body weight (UBW) and ideal body weight (IBW). Standard reference tables such as the 1983 Metropolitan Life Insurance tables, based on sex, height, and body frame size, can be used to determine IBW. Body frame size can be determined by measuring wrist circumference just distal to the styloid process (Table 16-3). Weight loss has been directly correlated to morbidity and weight loss of 35% to 40% is usually not compatible with life.[65,69] Current weight as

---

TABLE 16-2
Physical Assessment for Nutritional Deficiencies

I. Hair changes associated with protein–calorie malnution
   A. Lackluster
   B. Thinness, sparseness
   C. Pigmentation changes
   D. Easy pluckability (inspect comb, pillow, and bed for hair)

II. Lip changes
   A. Angular stomatitis
      1. Associated with deficiencies of one or more B vitamins
      2. Cracks, redness at corners of mouth
      3. May result in scars when healed
   B. Cheilosis
      1. Associated with riboflavin and niacin deficiency
      2. Vertical cracks in lips

III. Tongue changes
   A. Most changes associated with deficiencies of one or more B vitamins
   B. May change color (eg, become purplish red or beefy red)
   C. Fissures
   D. May be painful and hypersensitive, with burning
   E. Atrophy of taste buds; tongue may appear smooth and pale

IV. Skin changes
   A. Consider general characteristics of skin (dryness and flakiness may be associated with deficiency of vitamin A, essential fatty acids)
   B. Petechiae
      1. Hemorrhagic spots on skin at pressure points
      2. May occur in presence of liver disease or during anticoagulation
      3. Associated with deficiencies of vitamins C and K

Adapted from Curtas, S. (1988). Nutritional assessment. In C. Caldwell-Kennedy & P. Guenter (Eds). *Nutritional support nursing: Core curriculum.* Silver Spring, MD: American Society for Parenteral and Enteral Nutrition.

TABLE 16-3
Determination of Body Frame Size[31]

	Males	*Females*
Small	r >10.4 cm	r >11.0 cm
Medium	r = 9.6–10.4 cm	r = 10.1–11.0 cm
Large	r = <9.6 cm	r = <10.1 cm

$$r = \frac{\text{Height (cm)}}{\text{Wrist circum (cm)}}$$

a percentage of UBW is usually the most accurate determinate of weight loss and can be calculated as follows:

$$\% \text{ usual weight} = \frac{\text{actual weight}}{\text{usual weight}} \times 100$$

Percent IBW may also be used and can be determined by the above formula substituting IBW for UBW. It is generally not as accurate. A normally thin person, with stable weight, may be incorrectly identified as malnourished if the weight is less than IBW; obese patients with significant recent weight loss may be overlooked if they are still above IBW[33] (Table 16-4).

Fluid status should be considered when evaluating weight—significant edema or ascites may contribute significant fluid weight.[16]

TABLE 16-4
Evaluation of Weight Change

Loss	*Significant Weight Loss*	*Severe Weight Loss*
1 wk	1–2%	>2%
1 mo	5%	>5%
3 mo	7.5%	>7.5%
6 mo	10%	>10%

*Values charted are for percent weight change:

$$\text{Percent Weight Change} = \frac{(\text{Usual weight} - \text{Actual weight})}{(\text{Usual weight})} \times 100$$

Blackburn, G.J., Bistrian, B.R., Maini, B.S., Schlamm, B.A., & Smith, M.F. (1977). Nutritional and metabolic assessment of the hospitalized patient. *Journal of Parenteral and Enteral Nutrition.* 1(1), p. 7.

Other anthropometric measurements include triceps skinfold, which estimates subcutaneous fat stores, and midarm muscle circumference, which estimates somatic protein stores (skeletal muscle mass). These indices are not as widely used any more because of questions concerning their validity. Reproducibility of these measurements requires strict adherence to protocol and may vary widely in the same individual by different examiners.[48] A more detailed discussion can be found in other references.[16,26,33,69]

Biochemical Assessment

A variety of biochemical tests are used to assess nutritional status, with a broad range of cost and sensitivity. The most commonly used, and most readily available, are visceral proteins and tests to evaluate immune function.

Visceral Proteins

Depletion of visceral proteins is characteristic of protein malnutrition, which occurs acutely in the hospitalized patient (hypoalbuminemia). An estimate of visceral protein status can be obtained from measurements of specific serum transport proteins that are synthesized in the liver. These include albumin, transferrin, thyroxine-binding prealbumin, and retinol-binding protein (Table 16-5). Although the long half-life of albumin makes it less valuable in monitoring acute changes in nutritional status, it is still regarded as the best single test for predicting outcome in hospitalized patients.[49] It is recommended that serum albumin measurements be included in the initial chemical profile when screening for malnutrition.[71,77] Prealbumin, with a shorter half-life, seems to be a more sensitive and specific indicator to monitor the effectiveness of nutritional support.[71,77,78] It is more expensive and may not be available in smaller hospitals. The changes in the levels of these proteins should be evaluated together because they reflect different processes in the body.[69] Consideration should also be given to assessment for nonnutritional factors that may affect these visceral proteins as well. Even though these current tests are useful, new nutritional markers are needed that better identify malnourished patients and precisely monitor the effectiveness of nutritional intervention on nutritional status. Other proteins are being investigated to determine their efficacy.

Immune Function

Alterations in the immune system may be influenced by stress, specific disease states, and malnutrition. The total lymphocyte count (TLC) is indicative of a patient's ability to fight infection and to maintain host integrity, and is known to fall with malnutrition. The TLC can be derived from a complete blood count with differential as follows:

$$\mathrm{TLC} = \frac{\mathrm{percent\ lymphocytes} \times \mathrm{white\ blood\ cells}}{100}$$

Values between 1200 and 2000/mm^3 are associated with mild depletion, values of 800 to 1200/mm^3 are associated with moderate depletion, and counts less than 800/mm^3 are associated with severe depletion.[33]

Cell-mediated immunity is most frequently evaluated with delayed cutaneous hypersensitivity skin tests. The responses to interdermal injection of three or more

TABLE 16-5
Visceral Proteins[15,25,31,70]

Visceral Protein	Half-life	Normal Range	Causes of Decrease	Causes of Increase
Albumin Maintains plasma oncotic pressure Carrier protein (zinc, calcium, magnesium, fatty acids)	18–21 d	Normal: >3.5 g/dL Mild depletion: 2.8–3.5 g/dL Mod. depletion: 2.1–2.7 g/dL Severe depletion: <2.1 g/dL Reflects *chronic,* not acute change	Metabolic stress Infection, Inflammation Liver disease ↑ losses (wounds, burns, fistulas) Inadequate protein intake Fluid imbalance (ascites, edema, overhydration) Malabsorptive states	Dehydration may falsely ↑ levels Salt-poor albumin infusion
Transferrin Carrier protein for iron	8–10 d	Normal: >200 mg/dL Mild depletion: 150–200 mg/dL Mod. depletion: 100–150 mg/dL Severe depletion: <100 mg/dL	Chronic infection Inflammatory state Acute catabolic states ↑ iron stores Liver damage Overhydration	Pregnancy Hepatitis Iron deficiency anemia Dehydration Chronic blood loss
Thyroxine-binding prealbumin (Transthyretin) Carrier protein for retinol-binding protein Transport protein for thyroxine	2–3 d	Normal: >20 mg/dL Mild depletion: 10–15 mg/dL Mod. depletion: 5–10 mg/dL Severe depletion: <5 mg/dL Sensitive to acute changes in protein status Limited use in situation in which there is a sudden demand for protein synthesis	Infection Acute catabolic states Postsurgery (5–10 mg/dL drop first week) Liver disease Altered energy and protein balance Hyperthyroid	Chronic renal failure Corticosteroids
Retinol-binding protein Transport retinol (alcohol of vitamin A)	10–18 h	Normal: 3–5 mEq/dL Reflects acute change	Vitamin A deficiency Acute catabolic states Postsurgery Liver disease Hyperthyroid	Renal disease

common recall antigens are assessed at 24 and 48 hours. Plastic, disposable multitest applicators are available, including tetanus toxoid, diphtheria toxoid, streptococcus, Old tuberculin, candida, trichophyton, proteus, and a glucerin-negative control. Interpretation of results and methods for measuring the results are not standardized. Results are classified as anergic if there is no response to any of the antigens, relatively anergic if only one response occurs, and normal or reactive if there is a response to two or more antigens. These results must be weighed with other findings in the nutritional assessment because nonnutritional factors such as infection, sepsis, cancer, liver disease, renal failure, immunosuppressive diseases, and immunosuppressive drugs may also affect immunocompetence.[79]

Nitrogen Balance

A 24-hour urine specimen for urine urea nitrogen (UUN) is obtained to determine nitrogen balance and is an objective method of evaluating the efficacy of the patient's nutritional regimen. For the patient to be in a positive nitrogen balance or anabolic state, the amount of nitrogen taken in by the patient (IV and oral) needs to be more than that excreted. A 24-hour urine collection is needed to measure the amount of urinary urea excreted. A factor of 4 g is added (2 g for fecal losses and 2 g for integumental losses) to measure total nitrogen excretion.

Nitrogen balance is then calculated by subtracting the amount of nitrogen lost from the amount of nitrogen given or taken by the patient:

$$\text{Nitrogen balance} = \frac{\text{Protein intake}}{6.25} - (\text{urine urea nitrogen} + 4)$$

Normally at equilibrium, the following measures reflect the severity of the catabolic state[34]:

- Mild: -5 to -10 g/dL
- Moderate: -10 to -15 g/dL
- Severe: greater than -15 g/dL

The usual goal is to achieve a positive nitrogen balance during nutritional support of $+4$ to 6 g nitrogen/24 h.

Other assessment techniques used include somatomedin activity, prognostic nutritional index, handgrip dynamometry, isotopic methods, imaging techniques, and whole body conductivity and impedence measurements.[16,69]

There is no single indicator of nutritional status. A global assessment of many indices and the patient's clinical status are necessary to determine the incidence and degree of nutritional deficiency. Reassessment is individualized whenever the clinical status changes and throughout the course of nutritional therapy.[48]

Once the nutritional assessment data have been collected and evaluated, the optimal method for nutritional support must be selected. This decision process is depicted in Figure 16-2.

NUTRITIONAL REQUIREMENTS

The practical outcome of the nutritional assessment is to determine the calorie and protein needs of the patient. These requirements are increased during acute, catabolic illness and in some chronic conditions.

Energy Requirements

Nutrient energy requirements are generally expressed in kilocalories (kcal). Numerous methods for determining an individual's nutritional requirements are available, with varying degrees of sophistication. One of the most commonly used is the Harris-

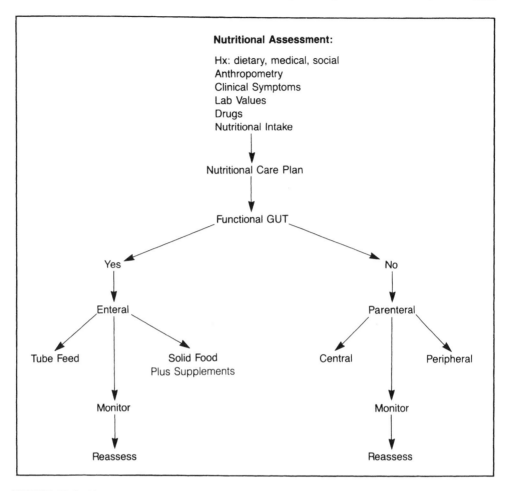

FIGURE 16-2 Nutritional support process. (Courtesy: Grant, DeHoog, Nutritional Assessment and Support, 1991.)

Benedict equation, which was derived from healthy individuals. It estimates basal energy expenditure (BEE) in kilocalories using weight, height, age, and sex with the following equations[39]:

BEE (male) = (66.47 + 13.75W + 5.0H) – 6.76A

BEE (female) = (655.10 + 9.56W + 1.85H) – 4.68A

where W is weight in kg, H is height in cm, and A is age in years. usual body weight is most commonly used.

Because the BEE does not take into account activity or injury, others have proposed activity factors (AF) and injury factors (IF), which take into account the percentage increase in BEE due to injury and stress or decrease due to starvation (Table 16-6). Energy requirements are estimated by multiplying BEE × AF × IF.

TABLE 16-6
Correction Factors for Estimating Nonprotein Energy Requirements of Hospitalized Patients

Clinical Condition	Correction Factor[b]	References
Nutritional status		
Normal	1.3[c]	Feurer and Mullen[12]
Depleted	1.5[c,d]	Kinney,[3] Feurer, and Mullen [12]
Fever	1.0 + 0.13 per °C	
Elective surgery		Kinney[3]
Peritonitis	1.0–1.2	Kinney,[3] Long[14]
Soft tissue trauma	1.2–1.5	Kinney[3]
Multiple fractures	1.14–1.37	Duke et al,[16] Long et al[15]
Major sepsis	1.2–1.35	Kinney,[3] Long et al[15]
Major head injury (with steroids)	1.4–1.8	Kinney,[3] Long et al[15]
Major head injury (without steroids)	1.4–2.0	Clifton et al,[17] Haider et al[18]
Thermal injury[a]	1.4	Young et al[19]
0–20%		Wilmore[6]
20–40%	1.0–1.5	
40–100%	1.5–1.85	
Starvation (adults)	1.85–2.05	Long et al [15]

[a]Total nonprotein energy requirement is estimated from the product of corrections factors × HBE.

[b]Correction factors apply to men and women; figures represent maximum increases and must be adjusted as recovery and convalescence proceed (see Fig 4–1).

[c]Provides allowance for minimal activity above resting.

[d]Estimates additional requirement to achieve anabolism when accompanied by optimal protein intake.

[e]Percent body surface burned.

Silberman, H. (1989). Parenteral nutrition: General principles. In H. Silberman (Ed.), *Parenteral and Enteral Nutrition* (p. 94). Norwalk, CT: Appleton & Lange.

Others have proposed arbitrarily assigning degress of catabolism[5] or levels of stress[11] to the patient's clinical state (Table 16-7). Most patients do not require more than 40 kcal/kg/d.

A third approach that is pragmatic and probably most useful to clinicians is to provide, using actual body weight, 30 kcal/kg/d and 1.5 g/kg/d of protein as a starting point. These are conservative indices, are easy for the clinician to remember and calculate, and will not result in overfeeding. Indirect calorimetry may be used at some institutions, mainly teaching hospitals and research centers. This requires expensive equipment that directly measures oxygen consumption and carbon dioxide production to determine actual energy expenditure. The accuracy of results is determined by the skill of the individual doing the test, accurate calibration of the equipment, and the conditions under which the test is taken.

TABLE 16-7
Metabolic Requirements According to Catabolic Degree/Stress Level[4,10]

Degree of Net Catabolism	Stress Level	Clinical Type	Urinary Nitrogen Loss (g/d)	BEE Multiple	Nonprotein Calories kcal/kg/d	Protein Multiple g/kg/d	Nonprotein Calorie Nitrogen Ratio (kcal:g N)
1	0	Nonstressed starvation	5	1.0	20–25	1.0	125:1–150:1
2	1	Elective surgery (low stress)	5–10	1.3	25	1.5	100:1
3	2	Polytrauma (moderate stress)	10–15	1.5	30	2.0	100:1–90:1
4	3	Sepsis (severe stress)	>15	1.75	35	2.0–2.5	90:1

BEE, basal energy expenditure

Regardless of the method chosen, it is important to avoid overfeeding. The early adage of nutrition support, "the more, the better," is no longer advocated. Overfeeding has deleterious effects on respiritory and hepatic function and should be avoided, especially in the acutely ill patient. Additional calories for desired weight gain should be held until the patient is recovered.

Protein Requirements

Protein requirements for healthy individuals are based on the amount needed to maintain nitrogen equilibrium, assuming energy is being met by nonprotein kilocalories. The recommended daily allowance for healthy adults is 0.8 g/kg/d although elderly adults require at least 1 to 1.2 g/kg/d for nitrogen equilibrium.[63] Protein requirements are increased during illness to meet stress needs for wound healing and immune competence and to replace losses. Because 6.25 g protein yields 1 g nitrogen, in general, 1.5 g/kg/d of protein is required to achieve nitrogen balance with TPN regimens in adults, although up to 2 to 2.5 g/kg/d may be needed.

Calorie/Nitrogen Ratio

Sufficient nonprotein calories to meet energy requirements are needed for protein synthesis. A calorie/nitrogen ratio of between 90:1 and 150:1 has been most often identified, depending on the level of stress—the higher the stress, the lower the calorie/nitrogen ratio.[11,36,68]

Fluid Requirements

Individual fluid requirements vary greatly and can fluctuate on a daily basis. Fluid needs should be carefully assessed when designing the PN formula. The minimum daily requirement for healthy adults is 1 mL/kcal. Factors that may increase fluid needs include fever and increased losses from diuresis, diarrhea, vomiting, and drainage from wounds and fistulas. Environmental factors such as specialized high-airloss beds, ultraviolet light therapy, and radiant warmers increase fluid requirements as well.[84] Humidified air reduces insensible fluid loss and results in lower fluid requirements. Preexisting excess or deficiency states and cardiac and renal function must also be evaluated.

The PN solution can be formulated using concentrated nutrients (70% dextrose, 15% amino acids, 20% lipids) to provide adequate nutrients when fluid restriction is needed. Additional IV fluids may be needed to accommodate increased fluid requirements. Unless the patient is stable, this is best done by giving additional crystalloid IV fluids (D_5W, $D_5 \frac{1}{2}NSS$) by a separate lumen or route. These can be frequently adjusted as necessary without affecting nutrient delivery. They can also be used as additional vehicles for electrolyte corrections.

TOTAL PARENTERAL NUTRITION SOLUTIONS _____

Solutions for TPN contain admixtures of carbohydrates, fats, protein, electrolytes, minerals, vitamins, trace elements, and water. These complex solutions can provide all the necessary nutrients to meet requirements for growth, weight gain, anabolism, and wound healing. The proportion of each component is individualized based on the patient's clinical status, chronic diseases, fluid and electrolyte balance, and specific goals of PN.

Carbohydrates

Glucose is the primary energy source in most PN solutions. Concentrations from 10% to 70% glucose may be used with a final solution concentration of no more than 10% to 12% for peripheral infusion and no greater than 35% for central venous infusion. Parenteral glucose is hydrolized and provides 3.4 cal/g. At least 100 to 150 g glucose is required to meet the obligate needs for glucose by the brain, central nervous system, red blood cells, white blood cells, active fibroblasts, and certain phagocytes, which normally require glucose as the sole or major energy source.[68] No more than 5 to 7 mg/kg/min (equals a maximum of 5–7 g/kg/d, which is easier to calculate) should be given, which is the maximum rate of glucose utilization. Less would be given to the diabetic, hyperglycemic, or critically ill patient—usually no more than 4 g/kg/d.[8,55]

Amounts greater than this in ill and stressed patients will result in conversion of excess glucose to fat, which requires energy (increased oxygen consumption and carbon dioxide production), and leads to fatty liver changes with prolonged use. Fifty to 70% of the daily nonprotein kilocalories are generally given as glucose.

Lipids

Intravenous lipid emulsions are given to prevent essential fatty acid deficiency (EFAD) and as a concentrated source of energy (9 kcal/g fat). EFAD has been detected as early as 3 to 7 days after initiation of fat-free TPN although clinical signs of dietary inadequacy may take 3 to 4 weeks to become evident.[10] Clinical signs include dry or scaly skin, thinning hair, thrombocytopenia, and liver function abnormalities.

Prevention of this deficiency state is desirable because EFAD is associated with decreased ability to heal wounds, adverse effects on red blood cell membranes, and a defect in prostaglandin synthesis.

Lipids generally provide 20% to 50% of the nonprotein calories in TPN solutions but should not exceed 60% or 2.5 g/kg.[36,68] IV fat emulsions are available in 10% (1.1 calorie/mL) and 20% (2 calories/mL) formulations. The 20% solutions are most often used because less volume is needed. Adverse reactions may occur although the incidence is less than 1%. Symptoms include dyspnea, cyanosis, nausea, vomiting, headache, dizziness, increased temperature, sweating, chest or back pain, pressure over eyes, and hyperlipidemia. Administration of IV fat emulsions is contraindicated in patients with disturbances in normal fat metabolism such as pathologic hyperlipidemia, lipoid nephrosis, or acute pancreatitis if accompanied by hyperlipidemia. Lipids are as the main energy source in peripheral parenteral nutrition (PPN) solutions and also further dilute the PPN solution as it enters the vein, decreasing the final concentration and incidence of phlebitis.

The manufacturer's directions should be followed for infusion. Lipids are better tolerated and used if they are infused slowly, not to exceed the manufacturer's recommendations of no greater than 62 mL/h up to a maximum of 12 hours for each bottle (up to 24 hours if a 3-in-1 mixture). Fast infusion rates have been associated with impairment of the reticuloendothelial system function, potentiating the inflammatory response by altering the ability of this defense system to respond to bacterial invasion. When lipids are given at the rate of 1.3 g/kg/d over 24 hours as part of a total nutrient admixture, no impairment of the reticuloendothelial system was seen.[44]

Current lipid solutions contain only long-chain triglycerides, but newer, structured lipids are under investigation and may prove to be beneficial for use in critically ill and septic patients.

Protein

The protein or nitrogen source is provided by synthetic crystalline amino acid solutions. First-generation amino acids were provided as protein hydrolysates and were associated with toxicities, which is not a concern with the current crystalline amino acids.[56] These solutions contain a mixture of essential and nonessential amino acids. Special amino acid formulations for renal failure, hepatic failure, and neonates are available. Some evidence indicates that high branched-chain amino acid formulas may be beneficial during sepsis and severe metabolic stress, but this remains controversial. Use of the special formulas is generally restricted because of the high cost and conflicting reports of efficacy.[2,69]

Electrolytes

Electrolytes are added to TPN solutions to meet individual patient requirements and to correct any deficiencies caused by increased loss, utilization, or requirements, or decreased absorption. They include sodium, potassium, chloride, calcium, magnesium, and phosphorus acetate. Various standard electrolyte solutions are available, as well as individual electrolytes. The requirements of individual patients may vary depending on their nutritional status and underlying disease process. It is important to keep in mind that the activity of electrolytes in the body can occur in interrelated patterns. No one electrolyte can function, be deficient, or be overabundant in the body without affecting others.[48]

Vitamins

Vitamins are organic compounds essential for maintenance and growth that are not synthesized by the body.[45] There are two main groups: fat soluble (A, D, E, K) and water soluble (B complex, C). Vitamins are sensitive to or become inactive with temperature changes and exposure to light. Therefore, they are added before administration and protected from exposure to direct light.

There are commercially available vitamin admixtures. To meet the daily requirements set by the American Medical Association Nutrition Advisory Group, 10 mL of the multivitamin mixture is added to the TPN solution.[59] Vitamin K is not included in adult multivitamins. It may be given weekly or daily in TPN as a trace element (1 mg/d).

Trace Elements

Trace elements are required in very small amounts and are referred to as micronutrients. Those commonly added to TPN solutions include zinc, copper, chromium, manganese, and selenium. They are available individually or as multitrace solutions. Requirements for individual trace elements may be increased in certain situations.

Drugs and Medications

A variety of drugs and medications are compatible with TPN solutions although compatibility studies are lacking for many. The feasibility of mixing drugs with TPN solutions depends on various factors, including the physical compatibility of the admixed components, the chemical stability of the drug, the retention of drug concentration over time, and the bioactivity of the components after admixture. The most commonly added medications are heparin, insulin, and H_2 blockers. It is preferable not to add multiple drugs to the solution. For current information about drug compatibility with PN solutions, refer to Trissel's *Handbook on Injectable Drugs*, which is updated and published yearly, and available in hospital pharmacies. Caution is needed to avoid drug–nutrient interactions. A summation of available information concerning known TPN admixture compatibilities is presented in Tables 16-8, 16-9, 16-10, and 16-11. Note that compatibilities differ depending on whether it is being added to a traditional dextrose and amino acid solution or to a total nutrient admixture (TNA).

Because a designated port is recommended solely for PN, piggybacking medications to TPN solutions is generally not recommended.

Solution Preparation

Safe preparation of PN solutions requires that trained personnel admix the solution under a laminar flow hood using strict aseptic technique. Specific protocols covering all aspects of preparation, storage, and quality assurance should be established. Guidelines may vary from institution to institution but should meet established standards.

Solutions may be prepared as traditional dextrose–amino acid solutions or as TNAs. If dextrose–amino acid solutions are used, the IV lipid emulsions are usually piggybacked to the TPN or administered via a separate route.

TABLE 16-8
Drugs Compatible With Parenteral Dextrose–Amino Acid Solutions

Drug	Reference	Drug	Reference	Drug	Reference
Albumin	103	Dobutamine	104	Methotrexate	104
Amikacin	104	Dopamine	104	Methyldopa	104
Aminophylline	104	Doxycycline	104	Methylprednisolone	104
Azlocillin	104	Erythromycin	104	Metoclopramide	104
Caffeine	130	Famotidine	135	Mezlocillin	104
Carbenicillin*	104	Fluorouracil*	104	Miconazole	104
Cefamandole	131	Folic acid	104	Morphine	104
Cefazolin	104	Furosemide	104	Moxalactam	104
Cefoperazone	104	Ganciclovir	136	Nafcillin	104
Cefotaxime	104	Gentamicin	104	Neostigmine	134
Cefoxitin	104	Heparin	104	Netilmicin	104
Ceftazidime	132	Hydralazine	134	Oxacillin	104
Ceftraxone	133	Hydrochloric acid	137	Oxytocin	134
Cephalothin*	104	Hydromorphone	138	Penicillin G	104
Chloramphenicol	104	Imipenem-cilastatin	139	Phenobarbital	134
Chlorpromazine	134	Insulin, regular (human)	140	Phytonadione	104
Cimetidine	104	Insulin, regular	104	Piperacillin	104
Clindamycin	104	Iron dextran	104	Polymyxin B	104
Cyanocobalamin	104	Isoproterenol	104	Ranitidine*	104
Cyclophospha-mide	104	Kanamycin*	104	Tetracycline†	104
		Lidocaine	104	Ticarcillin*	104
Cytarabine	104	Meperidine	141	Tobramycin	104
Digoxin	104	Metaraminol	104	Vancomycin	142, 143
Dipyridamole	134	Methicillin	104		

*Some data suggest incompatibility under certain conditions.

†Visual compatibility only; tested with parenteral nutrition solution without electrolytes; drug may chelate with divalent cations and cause precipitation.

Dickerson, R. N., Brown, R. O., & White, K. G. (1993). Parenteral nutrition solutions. In J. L. Rombeau & M. D. Caldwell (Eds.), *Clinical nutrition: Parenteral nutrition* (p. 328). Philadelphia: W. B. Saunders.

Total nutrient admixtures, also known as trimix (triple mix) or 3-in-1, consist of all components, including lipids, being mixed together in one large bag. These solutions are used almost exclusively by home care companies and increasingly in many hospitals.

All additives should be added to the PN solution in the pharmacy under sterile conditions. Additives should not be added on the nursing unit or after the bag has been spiked and hung. If additional additives are needed after the bag is hanging, alternate methods or routes should be considered.

TABLE 16-9
Drugs Incompatible With Parenteral Dextrose–Amino Acid Solutions

Drug	Reference
Amphotericin B	104
Ampicillin*	104
Cephradine	129
Metronidazole [with NaHCO$_3$]	104
Phenytoin	104

*Some visual compatibility data suggest compatibility under certain conditions.

Dickerson, R. N., Brown, R. O., & White, K. G. (1993). Parenteral nutrition solutions. In J. L. Rombeau & M. D. Caldwell (Eds.), *Clinical nutrition: Parenteral nutrition* (p. 328). Philadelphia: W. B. Saunders.

Total Nutrient Admixtures

The TNA solutions offer a significant advantage in the ability to provide cost-effective, patient-specific nutritional support. Nursing time is saved by only having one bag to hang each day. Pharmacy admixing is simplified by the use of computerized automixing systems, which also allow for more patient-specific formulations. Potential bacterial contamination of either the solution or line is decreased because of decreased accessing of the line. The increased usage of TNA reflects the trend toward the daily use of lipid emulsions as a daily calorie source.

The stability of TNA is affected by many factors including admixture contents, storage time and conditions, addition of nonnutrient drugs, pH of the solution, and variability in temperature.[20,21] A recent Food and Drug Administration (FDA) alert strongly advises pharmacists to use care in the compounding order of nutrients and advocates the use of a 1.2-µm filter during infusion to avoid problems with calcium-phosphate precipitation.[25] TNA is normally a milky white, opaque solution although a faint yellow hue may be evident with the addition of vitamins. The nurse should examine the solution for any signs of instability before hanging and periodically thereafter. Particulate matter is hard to detect because of the opacity of the solution. Other physical or chemical phenomena may occur and are discussed in Table 16-12. TNA solutions are usually stable for 24 hours after admixing with the addition of vitamins and up to 7 days if vitamins are not added until ready to hang. Further research is in progress.

VASCULAR ACCESS

Administration of hypertonic PN solutions require an easily placed, well tolerated central venous access device (CVAD) that can be used for extended periods of time. Infusion into a large vein with high blood flow to rapidly dilute the solution is desirable to reduce phlebitis, venous thrombosis, pain, and hemolysis.[3,35,64]

TABLE 16-10
Drugs Compatible With Parenteral Total Nutrient Admixture Solutions

Drug	Reference	Drug	Reference
Albumin	94, 126	Heparin	89
Aminophylline*	111	Hydrocortisone	94
Ampicillin	104	Insulin, regular	104
Carbenicillin‡	104	Insulin, regular (human)	140
Cefamandole	104	Isoproterenol	104
Cefazolin	104	Kanamycin	104
Cefoxitin	104	Lidocaine	104
Cephalothin†	104	Meperidine	104
Cephapirin	104	Methicillin†	104
Chloramphenicol†	104	Metoclopramide	94
Cimetidine	104	Nizatidine	146
Clindamycin	104	Norepinephrine	104
Digoxin	104	Oxacillin	104
Diphenhydramine†	104	Penicillin G	104
Dopamine	104	Phytonadione	94
Erythromycin	104	Ranitidine	147
Famotidine	145	Ticarcillin	104
Furosemide	104	Tobramycin	104
Gentamicin	104		

*May cause calcium phosphate precipitation when low concentrations of amino acids and borderline calcium phosphate amounts are used.

†Stable with lipid emulsion alone[144]; no data exist for total nutrient admixture solutions.

‡Some aggregation of lipid globules noted.

Dickerson, R. N., Brown, R. O., & White, K. G. (1993). Parenteral nutrition solutions. In J. L. Rombeau & M. D. Caldwell (Eds.), *Clinical nutrition: Parenteral nutrition* (p. 328). Philadelphia: W. B. Saunders.

The superior vena cava is the vein of choice for PN administration. The subclavian and internal jugular veins are the most common insertion sites for accessing the superior vena cava. Other insertion sites, such as the external jugular and femoral veins, may be necessary in patients with limited venous access. The desirable location for the tip of all CVADs is in the distal superior vena cava, parallel to the vessel wall, just above the right atrium.[3,64,65,80] CVAD insertion should only be performed by an experienced physician to reduce the incidence of insertion complications.

A variety of CVADs are available, for either short-term or long-term access. Short-term access is usually obtained using single- or multiple-lumen percutaneously placed catheters. These are generally used for days to weeks in acute illness, but they may be used for longer periods with meticulous care. Peripherally inserted central venous catheters (PICCs) may be used for either short- or long-term access. Unlike other CVADs mentioned here, PICCs can be inserted by specially trained RNs via the

TABLE 16-11
Drugs Incompatible With Parenteral Total Nutrient Admixture Solutions

Drug	Reference
Amikacin	148
Iron dextran*	94, 149
Methyldopa†	104
Phenytoin	104
Tetracycline‡	104

*Manufacturer data suggest compatibility with smaller doses of iron dextran (eg, 10 mg)[94]

†Visually incompatible with total nutrient admixture (TNA) when reconstituted with 5% dextrose in water; visually compatible when reconstituted with normal saline solution.[150]

‡Compatible with lipid alone; however, may chelate with divalent cations of TNA solution.

Dickerson, R. N., Brown, R. O., & White, K. G. (1993). Parenteral nutrition solutions. In J. L. Rombeau & M. D. Caldwell (Eds.), *Clinical nutrition: Parenteral nutrition* (p. 328). Philadelphia: W. B. Saunders.

TABLE 16-12
Visible Phenomena to Observe for in TNA Solution

Phenomena	Characteristics	Action
Physical phenomena		
Aggregation (stratification)	Rare white "streaks" (early stages of creaming)	Not harmful Readily reverses with *gentle* agitation
Creaming	Dense white color at top of TNA ("cream" layer)	Not harmful Reverses with *gentle* agitation
	Aggregates migrate to top of the solution	If reappears in 1–2 h or < after agitation, it may indicate an unstable emulsion If left undistributed, may begin to coalesce (see below)
Chemical phenomena		
Coalescence/cracking (breaking/oiling out)	Oil globules on the surface of creamed emulsion coalesce or fuse to form larger oil droplets	**Irreversible!** Cannot be dispersed Do not hang
	May appear as an oil layer on top of the solution, as large oil globules, or streaks of oil throughout the solution	If appears while infusing, take down and return to pharmacy immediately!

Adapted from Clintec Nutrition Company. (1992). *Total nutrient admixtures: Clinical and practice guidelines.*

antecubital veins (basilic, cephalic, or median antecubital in order of preference). They are available with single or double lumens.

Long-term central venous access is usually obtained using tunneled catheters or totally implanted venous access ports. Tunneled catheters are available with single or multiple lumens. Implanted ports are currently available as single- or dual-portal septa that can be accessed from either the top or side. These long-term access devices are surgically placed in the operating room and can be used for months to years.

Swan-Ganz catheters are generally not recommended for infusion of PN. However, if no other access is available, the right atrium or proximal port can be used. The side arm of the introducer should not be used because it is short and located in the subclavian vein.

Nurses play a major role during the insertion and use of CVADs. They are responsible for the daily care and are held accountable for preventing or minimizing the many device-related complications, including life-threatening ones. Protocols for the insertion, care, and maintenance of CVADs should be established and followed according to current standards.

Insertion

A thorough explanation of the procedure before insertion will help to alleviate anxiety and ensure patient cooperation during the procedure. Proper teaching beforehand tends to increase patient tolerance and markedly decreases the level of pain experienced during the procedure. It is important to elicit feedback during the teaching so the nurse can assess the patient's level of understanding and eliminate fears. Sedation may be required for children and for highly anxious or combative patients. Adequate hydration is essential to dilate the central veins for successful cannulation. The nurse should make sure that all necessary equipment is gathered before the procedure is started.

Percutaneously placed catheters are inserted at the bedside using strict aseptic technique. The physician should wear mask, gown, and sterile gloves and those assisting should wear a mask. The patient is placed in Trendelenburg (head-down) position to enable the vein to fill more readily. A small towel roll may be placed along the vertebrae to hyperextend the neck and elevate the clavicle for easier access. Sterile drapes are placed around the insertion site to provide a sterile field. Reassure the patient that the face will be only partially covered, allowing easy breathing. A local anesthetic is used and the skin is thoroughly prepped with an antiseptic solution to reduce the risk of infection.

The nurse's responsibility during insertion includes instructing the patient to perform the Valsalva maneuver ("take a deep breath and hold it, bearing down and straining slightly"), observing for breaks in surgical technique, and reassuring the patient. The Valsalva maneuver is used when the needle is open to the air, before and during the threading of the catheter, to prevent possible air embolism. If the patient is unconscious or unable to do the Valsalva maneuver, the nurse can perform it by gently pressing down on the patient's sternum at the appropriate time. If the patient is intubated, the physician can time the threading of the catheter during expiration. Holding the patient's hand on the insertion side, and gently pulling the arm down toward the foot as the needle is inserted under the clavicle will ensure optimal positioning for venous access. During insertion, the patient may experience unusual sensations, including pressure, but should not feel any pain.

A suture is usually placed at the catheter insertion site to secure the catheter and help prevent accidental dislodgment, and a sterile, occlusive dressing is applied. A portable chest x-ray should be taken immediately to determine the location of the catheter tip and rule out any potential complications. Isotonic IV solutions (D_5W, saline) are usually infused at a slow keep-open rate until correct placement is confirmed. Some suggest infusion of 250 to 300 mL of isotonic solution before the x-ray so that a hydrothorax may be detected and corrected before initiating PN.[64] PN should never be initiated until catheter tip placement in the distal superior vena cava has been confirmed. It is unacceptable for the tip to be located in the heart, inferior vena cava, or any extrathoracic vessel. Atrial rupture, valvular damage, myocardial irritability with arrhythmias, and cardiac tamponade are some of the complications reported when the catheter tip is located in the heart. An increased incidence of catheter-induced thrombosis and occlusion is associated with tip placement in the subclavian, jugular, inferior vena cava, or narrower extrathoracic vessels.

Complications are infrequent but the patient should be closely monitored after catheter insertion. Be particularly alert for signs of respiratory distress, pain, slowly increasing hematoma, or any unexplainable symptom. (Specific catheter-related complications are discussed later.) In 1994 the FDA's Central Venous Catheter Working Group released a series of three videotapes titled "Complications of Central Venous Catheters" in an effort to reduce complications through education.

PARENTERAL NUTRITION ADMINISTRATION

All institutions should have specific protocols for the administration, monitoring, and discontinuation of PN, which should be reviewed annually. ASPEN has published standards for nutrition support of hospitalized patients, hospitalized pediatric patients, home patients, and residents of long-term care facilities.[72-76] In addition, the Intravenous Nurses Society (INS) has updated published standards for intravenous therapy, which includes PN.[43] Safe administration of PN depends on strict adherence to these protocols.

Solutions for PN are normally kept refrigerated until they are used. The recommended maximum hang time for PN solutions is 24 hours. PN solutions should be inspected for any signs of precipitate or instability before hanging. The label should also be checked against the PN orders to ensure accuracy. The volume and infusion rate are usually noted on the label by the pharmacy.

Parenteral nutrition should be infused at a constant infusion rate, as ordered. Variable infusion rates can result in wide fluctuations in blood sugar levels. Too-rapid infusion of these highly concentrated dextrose solutions can cause a hyperglycemic reaction or even hyperosmolar, nonketotic coma. Rates should never be adjusted more than ±10%. The use of an infusion pump, preferably volumetric, should be mandatory and will ensure accuracy.

The infusion is started slowly and gradually increased as fluid and glucose tolerance permits. Generally, no more than 250 g glucose should be administered the first day to allow the body to adjust to the increased glucose load (100–150 g if the patient is diabetic or hyperglycemic).[55,57,58] If the blood sugar concentration is less than 200 mg/dL, the glucose load can be gradually increased to the desired goal. There is usually no need to restrict protein or lipids the first day in adults.

Glucose tolerance, may, however, be compromised by sepsis, stress, shock, hepatic and renal failure, starvation, diabetes, pancreatic disease, and administration of some medications, particularly steroids and some diuretics. Age is another variable; the elderly and the very young are particularly susceptible to glucose intolerance. For these patients, administration of exogenous insulin is often necessary. It is preferable to add insulin to the PN solution because it provides a more constant serum insulin level than does periodic subcutaneous administration.[55,57,58] In addition, a sliding scale subcutaneous insulin coverage schedule should be implemented. Adjustments to the insulin added to the PN solutions are generally made based on the amount of additional coverage required the previous day, until glycemic control is obtained. The blood sugar level should continue to be monitored closely because insulin needs may decrease as the stress or sepsis subsides or steroids are decreased and discontinued. Blood sugar concentration should be maintained less than 200 mg/dL during PN administration.

If PN solutions are interrupted or unavailable, standing orders should be available to infuse 5% dextrose solutions at the same rate, either through the central line or peripherally if the central line is removed or lost.[36] This will prevent the sudden hypoglycemia caused by the high endogenous insulin secretion associated with hypertonic PN solutions. Although some institutions and physicians still prefer to use a 10% dextrose solution in these situations, it has been deemed unnecessary.[36]

Many institutions have established standard start times for PN (eg, 4 PM) to simplify nursing management. This also allows the pharmacy to establish standard times for admixing the solutions and delivery to the nursing unit. PN orders are generally required in the pharmacy several hours before the established start time.

Intravenous Tubing and Filters

The IV tubing and filters should be changed every 24 hours according to INS standards and the Centers for Disease Control and Prevention (CDC) guidelines. It is most efficient to standardize the time of tubing and filter changes to coincide with the daily start time for the day's solution. This eliminates additional breaks in the line. Luer lock connections are optimal to avoid accidental disconnection. If not available, the tubing connection should be taped.

The need for in-line filtration of PN solutions is apparent given the recent FDA Safety Alert.[25] A 0.22-μm filter is used for traditional dextrose–amino acid solutions, with the lipids piggybacked below the filter. These filters effectively retain bacteria, fungi, and particulate matter. TNA solutions require use of a 1.2- or 5.0-μm filter, which will effectively eliminate microprecipitates, candida, and some bacteria.[20] Bacterial contamination of PN solutions is rare. The justification for use of in-line filters centers around the removal of microprecipitates rather than microorganisms. Microprecipitates are often not visible on visual inspection, particularly in TNA solutions.

A risk of contamination always exists when IV tubing and filters are changed. Therefore, precautions need to be taken and aseptic technique strictly followed. All connections should be swabbed thoroughly with alcohol or povidone-iodine before the tubing is changed. It is also a good idea to swab the end of the catheter hub to remove any dried blood or sticky residue. Make sure the catheter is clamped before tubing change to avoid the risk of air embolism. If a clamp is not available, the patient should be positioned flat in bed and advised to perform the Valsalva maneuver during the tubing change. PN lines should not be violated by pressure-monitoring devices or transducers, stopcocks, blood drawing, or administration of blood or medications. This practice also reduces the risk of contamination and infection.

Cycling Parenteral Nutrition

Occasionally, PN may be "cycled" to allow the patient periods of time during the day free of the infusion and pump. This also allows for the development of a postabsorptive state that more closely reflects normal nutrition. Cyclic PN is routinely used for HPN patients, allowing them freedom to ambulate and lead a more normal life as their clinical condition permits. It may also be beneficial for certain hospitalized PN patients to allow maximum freedom for ambulation and physical therapy. Duke University Medical Center routinely starts cyclic PN on all patients expected to be on PN for more than 2 weeks early in their clinical course. This practice has been well received by both patients and nurses.[36] Most often, PN solutions are tapered off during the day and all their PN is infused over 12 to 14 hours at night. Cycling from 24 hours to 12 to 14 hours is usually done gradually over several days, with close monitoring. Usually, the infusion rate is decreased by one half during the first and last hours of infusion to allow for tapering up at the beginning and down at the end of infusion. Most patients tolerate this well without developing rebound hypoglycemia. Blood sugar levels during the accelerated infusion rates for cyclic PN may be up to 250 mg/dL. Normoglycemia is usually present during the hours off PN.[82,83]

Discontinuing Parenteral Nutrition

Parenteral nutrition should not be stopped without alternate plans for therapy so that nutritional status can be maintained or continue to improve. The effect of PN on appetite has been controversial and difficult to quantitate. Recent findings suggest that PN does affect appetite.[29] In one animal study, oral intake was diminished for a week or longer after PN was discontinued.[38]

Abrupt cessation of PN should be avoided. It is generally safe to taper the infusion over several hours before stopping.[19] The previous practice of tapering over several days is not usually necessary. If the patient is receiving other sources of adequate carbohydrate either enterally or orally, tapering is not needed. Reductions in PN should not begin until an alternate source of nutrient intake is initiated, such as enteral or oral. As enteral or oral intake increases, PN is gradually decreased. PN should not be discontinued until at least half of the estimated requirements are tolerated enterally or orally. Accurate calorie counts are essential to the successful transition from PN to enteral or oral intake. An algorithm for successful transition to enteral or oral feedings has been proposed (Fig. 16-3).

FIGURE 16-3 Transition to oral feedings. (TF, tube feeding.) (Adapted from DeChicco, R. S., & Matarese. L. E. [1992]. Selection of nutriton support regimens. *Nutrition in Clinical Practice, 7,* 244.)

NURSING MANAGEMENT

Clinical assessment and monitoring are imperative for the safe administration of PN, which should be considered in the same manner as medication administration. The nurse should be familiar with the solution composition, the expected metabolic response, and the potential complications of therapy. A good knowledge base should enable the nurse to identify patients who are at risk for metabolic complications and to better monitor the patient's response to nutrient delivery. Catheter site care and dressing changes are also in the domain of nursing management.

Dressing Change Procedures

Dressing change procedures may vary but all use the same general techniques and rationale. Prepackaged sterile dressing change kits, which include all necessary equipment, are generally used. Some kits may include instructions as well. The bedside table should be cleansed with an antiseptic solution to provide a clean work area. The old dressing should be removed and the site inspected for any signs of erythema, exudate, or edema. The physician should be notified if any of these are observed. The suture should also be examined to ensure it remains intact. Meticulous handwashing should be standard before any dressing change. The nurse generally wears a mask and sterile gloves; gowns and sterile bed drapes are required in some institutions. The entire area to be covered by the dressing should be scrubbed in concentric circles starting at the catheter insertion site and moving out to the periphery (Fig. 16-4). A swabstick touching the periphery should never be returned to the center. The area is first scrubbed with either alcohol or alcohol-acetone swabsticks to clean any debris and defat the skin (acetone). If alcohol-acetone swabsticks are used, care should be taken not to come into direct contact with the catheter itself—acetone is drying and may cause cracks in the catheter. A brisk scrub with three povidone-iodine swabsticks should follow, taking 2 minutes. This can be timed by a watch or may be accomplished by scrubbing each concentric circle two to three times with each swabstick to a 5-inch circumference. Povidone-iodide is both antibacterial and antifungal. It should be allowed to air dry. Sustained antibacterial activity may occur for about 12 hours.[65] It is no longer recommended to remove the povidone-iodine with alcohol. Allergic response to topical povidone-iodine is rare. A recent study showed that the

FIGURE 16-4 Scrub technique using concentric circles starting at the center toward the periphery.

use of 2% aqueous chlorhexidine solution is superior to either alcohol or povidone-iodine in reducing the incidence of catheter-related infection.[53] At this time, there is no practical commercially prepared single-use package of chlorhexidine available in the United States to use for dressing changes.

The use of an antimicrobial ointment at the insertion site remains controversial. There is a lack of conclusive research to show the benefit of ointment use, and existing studies are difficult to compare because of differences in protocol. If an ointment is to be used, povidone-iodine products are recommended as the best for central lines because of their broader spectrum of coverage, including gram-negative bacteria and fungi.[51] The decision to use an antimicrobial ointment should be based on a review of the literature, documentation of the infection rate in the institution, and cost versus benefit. Some practitioners have found that ointment used under transparent dressings affects its adherence and may provide a wetter environment that could support organism growth resistant to the ointment.[3,24]

The choice of dressing material—gauze and tape or transparent—is also controversial. Transparent dressings offer the advantage of being able to observe the insertion site without disturbing the dressing, are more comfortable for the patient, and require less frequent dressing changes. Gauze and tape dressings preclude site inspection, are usually more uncomfortable for the patient, and require more frequent dressing changes. Transparent dressings are routinely changed every 2 to 5 days; gauze and tape dressings should be changed every 48 hours.[64] Both dressings should also be changed immediately if the integrity of the dressing has been compromised. A recent controversial meta-analysis comparing several studies found a significantly increased risk of catheter tip infection with the use of transparent compared with gauze dressings.[41] An increased risk of bacteremia and catheter-associated sepsis was also associated with the use of transparent dressings when compared with gauze. However, the value of this meta-analysis has been questioned because the studies that were compared used different dressing protocols and frequencies of change; use of ointments and catheter uses also varied. A study of high-risk intensive care unit patients showed that when transparent dressings were changed every 48 hours, colonization was minimal and no significant increase in the risk of infection occurred.[54] A careful review of the literature should be done when establishing dressing change protocols. Further research is ongoing and needed to establish more definitive standards and guidelines.

Some protocols use "skin prep" or tincture of benzoin around the perimeter of the dressing area to ensure better dressing adherence and minimize skin shearing on dressing removal.

Monitoring

Accurate daily weights, measured at the same time of day, using the same scale, and with the patient wearing the same amount of clothing, are important. Intake and output should also be scrupulously maintained and recorded. These measures are necessary to assess fluid balance and adequacy of the prescribed nutrients. Vital signs should be obtained and recorded at least every shift and more often if the patient is unstable or the temperature is greater than 100°F (37.7°C) orally or 101°F (38.3°C) rectally. Certain drugs and disease states suppress the normal febrile response and affected patients must be assessed individually.

Monitoring of urine for glucose and ketones every 6 hours assists in detecting any glucose intolerance. It can also be of value in early detection of impending sepsis, which may occur at any time before clinical symptoms appear. Glycosuria should not be allowed to persist without clinical evaluation and treatment.[13,36,84] Although not as accurate as serum glucose determination, urinary glucose monitoring is less invasive and useful for monitoring patients who are glucose tolerant with serum glucose levels less than 200 mg/dL. A urinary glucose level greater than 2+ requires a serum glucose test to obtain a more accurate determination. Diabetic patients, patients with serum glucose levels over 200 mg/dL, and those taking steroids should be on every 4- to 12-hour serum glucose monitoring with coverage. Many institutions now use glucose monitors on some or all nursing units, making fingerstick glucose determinations readily available.

Biochemical monitoring is also important to assess the adequacy of the PN regimen and the presence of any metabolic complications. "Nutritional profiles" or standing laboratory tests are recommended for routine monitoring of PN. Routine laboratory tests and their frequency are outlined in Table 16-13. Ideally a full chemi-

---

TABLE 16-13
Laboratory Monitoring of Parenteral Nutrition

Daily until stable, then	Blood sugar
Monday-Wednesday-Friday	Electrolytes
	BUN
	Creatinine
Baseline, then	Nutritional Profile
weekly (ie, q Monday)	Blood sugar, electrolytes, BUN, creatinine (as above)
	Total protein
	Albumin
	Transferrin
	Calcium
	Phosphorus
	Magnesium
	Total bilirubin
	Alkaline phosphatase
	AST
	ALT
	LDH
	Cholesterol
	Triglycerides
	CBC
	PT

ALT, alanine transaminase; AST, aspartate transaminase; BUN, blood urea nitrogen; CBC, complete blood count; LDH, lactic dehydrogenase; PT, prothrombin time cal profile, including glucose, electrolytes, urea nitrogen, creatinine, albumin, transferrin, calcium, magnesium, phosphorus, liver function, prothrombin time, and complete blood count, should be obtained before PN is initiated. Critically ill and unstable patients may require more frequent monitoring. Other studies may be warranted depending on the clinical status of the patient.

COMPLICATIONS

Complications associated with PN are generally divided into three categories: technical, metabolic, and septic. These complications can be minimized or even avoided with the establishment of and adherence to strict protocols and careful monitoring.

Mechanical Complications

Mechanical complications are related to the insertion or maintenance of CVADs and may be immediate or delayed. Insertion complications are infrequent when the CVAD is inserted by a physician skilled and knowledgeable about anatomy and CVAD insertion. Complications after catheter insertion are depicted in Figure 16-5 and described below.

Malposition

A catheter may be inadvertently advanced into an incorrect vein during placement—most commonly going cephalad into the jugular vein, into the contralateral subcla-

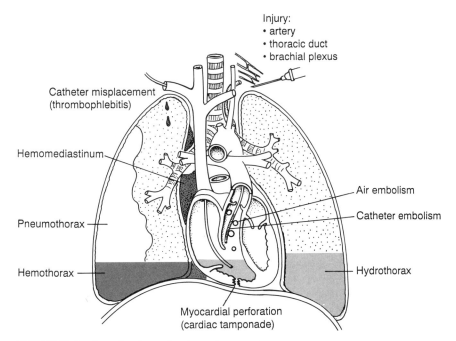

FIGURE 16-5 Complications of catheter insertion (Adapted from Fisher, J. E. [1991]. *Total parenteral nutrition* [2nd ed.]. Permission granted by Fisher and Little, Brown & Co.)

vian vein or smaller vessels, or into the right atrium. The correct placement for the catheter tip is in the distal superior vena cava, parallel to the vessel wall. Malposition of the catheter tip may predispose the patient to complications and can also occur spontaneously at any time after catheter insertion (ie, due to a change in intrathoracic pressure as with coughing or vomiting, a rapid infusion, or random body movement).[64] It is imperative that a chest x-ray be done immediately after insertion and periodically thereafter to ascertain catheter tip location. Malpositioned catheters should be repositioned, most commonly with a guidewire under fluoroscopy.

Arrhythmias
Various cardiac arrhythmias can be precipitated by the guidewire or the catheter, causing irritation to the myocardium. Retracting the guidewire (during insertion) or repositioning the catheter after insertion will correct this problem.

Pneumothorax
Pleural puncture may occur inadvertently because of the anatomic proximity of the lung to the subclavian veins. A tension pneumothorax is an emergent problem. It is most likely to occur in patients on mechanical ventilators, especially those requiring high inspiratory pressure or positive end-expiratory pressure (PEEP).[65] It can be prevented by lowering PEEP or removing from the ventilator and bagging during the procedure. Sharp chest pain, cough, decreased breath sounds, and hypoxia may be present, or the pneumothorax may be evident only radiologically. Treatment is based on the symptoms and the size of the pneumothorax. A chest tube is often indicated although smaller pneumothoraces often resolve spontaneously.

Hemothorax
The subclavian vein or adjacent vessels may be traumatized during venipuncture or later by catheter erosion, causing slow, constant bleeding into the thorax. This is particularly serious if the patient has a bleeding disorder. A hematoma may form, causing respiratory distress from deviation of the trachea. Delayed bleeding, arteriovenous fistula formation, or development of a false aneurysm may occur.[64] Chest tube drainage may be necessary; thoracotomy may be required in some cases.

Hydrothorax/Hydromediastinum
The vein may be perforated, either during insertion or later due to erosion of the catheter through the vein wall, causing IV solutions to be infused directly into the chest. Signs and symptoms depend on the volume and rate of extravasation. Early symptoms include low-grade fever, dyspnea, and chest pain. Hypoxia, respiratory distress, sepsis, and cardiovascular collapse may occur as it progressively worsens.

Inadvertent Arterial Puncture
It is possible to inadvertently enter an artery during the insertion. This can usually be determined by pulsatile or bright red blood return. The presence of hypoxia or hypotension may mask this phenomenon, with diagnosis made by reviewing the chest x-ray. The head of the bed should be elevated and direct pressure applied for 5 to 10 minutes. Hematoma formation may cause deviation of the trachea and respiratory distress. PN solutions should never be infused intra-arterially.[64]

Nerve Injury

Both the brachial plexus and phrenic nerves may be inadvertently damaged during insertion because of their close proximity to the central veins. The phrenic nerve can be damaged in both internal jugular and subclavian insertions by the needle or a malpositioned catheter.[64] A tingling sensation in the fingers, pain shooting down the arm, or permanent weakness may occur. Hemidiaphragm paralysis can result from phrenic nerve injury.

Lymphatic Injury

Lymphatic injury or fistula or chylothorax may occur with puncture or laceration of the lymphatic trunks or thoracic duct. Lymphatic vessels are in proximity to both jugular and subclavian veins. The thoracic duct empties into the left subclavian vein at its junction with the left internal jugular.[64] It is enlarged in cirrhotic patients because of alterations in lymph flow. Clinical manifestations include aspiration of clear fluid on insertion or clear drainage from the insertion site. Removal of the catheter is necessary.

Catheter Embolism

Catheter embolism may occur with improper insertion technique by shearing off a portion of the catheter while withdrawing the catheter through the insertion needle. This practice should be avoided. Removal can usually be accomplished by snaring the fragment under fluoroscopy. Newer over-the-wire techniques of catheter insertion will eliminate this complication.

Air Embolism

Air embolism is fortunately rare because its occurrence is the most lethal complication of catheter insertion. Air embolism is a potential danger whenever the central venous system is open to the air—during insertion, IV tubing or cap changes, accidental disconnection, or through a tract left after catheter removal. This is most likely to occur on deep inspiration when the patient is in an upright position, dehydrated, or hypovolemic. The exact amount of air necessary to cause death remains controversial and also depends on the patient's clinical status. Signs and symptoms vary with the severity and may include dyspnea, apnea, hypoxia, disorientation, tachycardia, hypotension, pulmonary wheeze, or a precordial murmur. Severe neurologic deficits, including hemiplegia, aphasia, seizures, and coma, have been associated with air embolism. This is attributed to direct access of air into the cerebral circulation in most situations.

Immediate treatment is aimed at preventing obstruction of the right ventricular outflow tract by air. The patient should immediately be placed on the left side in deep Trendelenburg position (*right side up*). This keeps the air in the right atrium and out of the pulmonary circulation. Needle aspiration of air through the catheter or by direct intracardiac approach may be necessary.

Precautions should be taken during catheter insertion, tubing and cap changes, and catheter removal to prevent air embolism. Tubing junctions should be properly secured. Catheter removal should be immediately followed by placement of an occlusive gauze dressing with an ointment over the site. This will occlude the tract and as sist with healing. This dressing is usually needed for 24 to 48 hours or until the tract is totally closed.

Cardiac Tamponade/Vein Perforation

This rare but lethal complication may occur within hours of insertion or days or weeks later. Catheters can advance several centimeters during arm, shoulder, or neck movement.[64] Perforation of the vein, right atrium, or right ventricle may occur from the catheter tip eroding through the wall. Clinical manifestations may include retrosternal or epigastric pain, shortness of breath, venous engorgement of the face and neck, restlessness and confusion, hypotension, paradoxical pulse, muffled heart sounds, or cardiac arrest. Chest x-ray may reveal pleural effusions and mediastinal widening. Cardiac tamponade is immediately treatable by discontinuing the infusion, aspirating through the catheter, or performing pericardiocentesis.[64] Treatment must be rapid and aggressive. A high mortality rate is reported because of late diagnosis.

Catheter Occlusion

Partial or complete catheter occlusion may occur as a result of fibrin sheath formation or thrombus at the tip of the catheter, blood clots, lipid deposits, precipitates, kinking or malposition, and device rupture or breakage. Increased difficulty in infusing fluids may be the first indication of fibrin sheath formation. The fibrin sheath may cause a partial occlusion of the catheter by acting as a "flap-valve" to prevent withdrawal of blood but allowing infusions.[3,61] It may eventually encase the entire catheter causing complete occlusion of all lumens. The sheath may also become seeded with microorganisms, serving as a nidus for infection.

Urokinase and streptokinase have been used to restore patency of CVADs occluded by blood or fibrin sheath.[42,46,47] Urokinase is preferred because it is less antigenic. Solutions specifically made for catheter clearance (1:5000 U/mL) are available, and the manufacturer's directions should be meticulously followed.

Occlusion of the CVAD may also occur from drug precipitates or lipid deposition. Precipitate occlusion may occur from inadequate flushing between medications, simultaneous administration of incompatible medications or solutions, and medications admixed in concentrations exceeding that required for stability.[3] Calcium and phosphorus precipitates are a common cause of occlusion with PN solutions.

Occlusions from drug precipitates or lipid deposition typically result in sudden occlusion of the catheter either during or immediately after an infusion.[61] Shulman and colleagues reported the use of 0.1% hydrochloric acid to restore the patency of CVADs occluded by drug precipitates.[67]

Occlusion with lipid depositions has been reported, especially with the use of TNAs. Pennington and Pithie reported successful clearance of four of five catheters with a solution of 70% ethanol in water.[62]

Further studies are needed to validate these reports and to guide the clinician in making appropriate treatment decisions.

Venous Thrombosis

The development of venous thrombosis may occur with any type of CVAD secondary to injury to the vein wall during insertion or by movement of the catheter against the vein wall after insertion. Catheter thrombogenicity may depend on the type of catheter material and the surface characteristics.[3,61] Predisposing risk factors for vein thrombosis include hypovolemia, venous stasis, and hypercoagulable states. Chemically induced thrombosis can result from infusion of hypertonic solutions, including PN, and small-volume antibiotics or chemotherapy admixtures and vesicants administered through CVADs whose tips are in the upper arm or subclavian or innominate veins.[14,61] Intermittent or long-term infusion of these solutions should be delivered through catheters whose tips terminate in the superior vena cava.

Patients with venous thrombosis may be asymptomatic, making careful observation for early signs imperative. Symptoms may include increased anterior chest venous pattern, arm or neck swelling, external jugular distention, or fluid leaking from the insertion site during infusion (caused by backflow). Diagnosis may be made by arm venography, contrast studies through the catheter, Doppler, duplex imaging, magnetic resonance imaging, and radionucleotide studies.[50]

Treatment of catheter-induced venous thrombosis remains controversial and depends on the extent of thrombus formation, the severity of the symptoms, and the risk or likelihood of reestablishment of venous access.[14,61] Conservative treatment without device removal consists of anticoagulant therapy followed by warfarin therapy. Catheter removal followed by anticoagulant therapy may be necessary for more severe symptoms. Bern and colleagues advocate the use of low-dose warfarin to reduce the risk of thrombosis for patients who are at increased risk.[4]

Metabolic Complications

Metabolic complications are the most frequently observed with PN and can be avoided when PN orders are written by knowledgeable physicians and laboratory studies are meticulously monitored. Table 16-14 includes the most frequently observed metabolic complications. Only those most life-threatening ones are discussed more fully below.

Glucose intolerance has already been discussed. The sudden development of hyperglycemia in a patient who was previously glucose tolerant may indicate impending infection or sepsis. Hyperglycemia and glycosuria may precede clinical signs of sepsis by 12 to 24 hours.[13,37,52]

Progressive hyperglycemia, if not detected or if inadequately treated, can lead to the life-threatening complication of hyperglycemic, hyperosmolar, nonketotic coma. Marked hyperglycemia and glycosuria may lead to an osmotic diuresis accompanied by dehydration, electrolyte imbalance, and a decreasing level of consciousness that can result in seizures and coma, leading to death if untreated. Reversal of this state requires immediate discontinuation of the PN solution, aggressive fluid and electrolyte replacement, correction of hyperglycemia by insulin administration, and correction of acidosis with bicarbonates. Frequent monitoring of blood sugar, electrolytes, arterial blood gases, and vital signs during treatment is essential.

Hypoglycemia is chemically defined as a serum glucose level of less than 50 mg/dL. Many patients may be asymptomatic at this level. Symptoms include weakness, headache, chills, tingling in the extremities or mouth, cold and clammy skin, thirst, hunger, apprehension, diaphoresis, decreased levels of consciousness, and changes in vital signs. Hypoglycemia during PN may occur with excess insulin ad-

Text continues on p. 380

TABLE 16-14
Potential Metabolic Complications Associated With Parenteral Nutrition (PN)

Cause(s)	Prevention	Treatment
Hyperglycemia		
Carbohydrate intolerance	Urine S/A q8h	Decrease PN rate or dextrose concentration/amount
Too rapid infusion of PN	Accuchecks q6h	
Too much carbohydrate load	Be aware of meds that may cause glucose intolerance (ie, steroids)	Increase proportion of calories as lipids
Insulin resistance—stress, sepsis, diabetes, steroids	Start PN infusion slowly	Add insulin to the solution and/or use sliding scale insulin coverage
		Maintain blood sugar < 200 mg/dL
Hypoglycemia		
Abrupt decrease or cessation of PN	Wean or slow down PN infusion when stopping	Hang 5% D/W at same rate of PN if unable to hang PN
Excessive insulin administration	Hang 5% D/W at same rate of PN if unable to hang PN	Give IV glucose STAT. 50% dextrose may be needed. Maintain proper flow rate.
	Maintain infusion rate; use an infusion pump	
	Monitor urine/serum glucose levels	
Hyperglycemic hyperosmolar, nonketotic coma		
Untreated glucose intolerance causes hyperosmolar diuresis, electrolyte imbalances, coma, death (40–50% mortality rate)	Appropriate glucose monitoring	Monitor closely
	Frequent chemistry profiles to assess electrolytes, osmolarity	Discontinue PN
Increased risk in elderly, diabetics, malnourished, steroid therapy, and with stress or sepsis		Rehydrate with normal saline or other isotonic solution
		Correct electrolyte imbalances, especially potassium and bicarbonate
		Monitor ABGs
		Insulin as needed
Hyperkalemia		
Excessive potassium replacement	Monitor serum potassium and renal function	Stop or decrease potassium in solution
Renal disease—potassium cannot be excreted	Anticipate that a sodium deficiency may lead to hyperkalemia	Assess for other sources of potassium
Leakage of potassium from cells following severe trauma	Accurate I/O to evaluate fluid balance	Monitor pulse for changes (bradycardia)
		In severe hyperkalemia, dialysis may be necessary

(continued)

TABLE 16-14   (Continued)

Cause(s)	Prevention	Treatment
Hypokalemia		
Excessive potassium losses (increased GI losses with diarrhea, fistulas)	Monitor serum potassium	Add potassium to PN solution
	Anticipate potential potassium depletion with large GI losses	May need additional IVPB potassium run over 4–6 h to correct severe deficiency
Diuretic therapy		
Large doses of insulin	Monitor I/O	Monitor pulse for tachycardia/arrhythmia
Increased requirement with anabolism	Be aware of drugs that cause excessive potassium loss	Monitor for metabolic alkalosis (potassium loss may cause sodium retention)
	Be aware that patients severely malnourished are susceptible (re-feeding syndrome)	
Hypernatremia		
Dehydration	Maintain I/O	Decrease sodium or provide salt-free solution until corrected
Diarrhea	Monitor serum sodium	
Diabetes insipidus	Be aware of drugs that cause sodium retention (ie, steroids)	Provide enough free water to meet needs
Excessive replacement		Treat or correct cause
Hyponatremia		
Diuretics	Accurate I/O	Fluid restriction
GI losses (vomiting, fistula)	Urine specific gravity	Add sodium to PN
CHF, renal failure, cirrhosis	Accurate weights (assess fluid shifts)	Minimize GI loss if possible
Water intoxication		Close metabolic monitoring
Hyperphosphatemia		
Renal failure	Accurate I/O	Low or no phosphate added
Excessive replacement	Monitor serum levels and renal status	May need dialysis
Hypophosphatemia		
Inadequate in PN	Be aware of potential disease states that cause low phosphate levels	Replace phosphate in PN
Insulin therapy		If <1.5 mg/dL—give IVPB replacement over 4–6 h
Disease states:	Frequent lab monitoring, especially if low levels/depleted	
Alcoholism		If <1.0 mg/dL—discontinue PN and correct via IVPB over 4–6 h before restarting PN
Respiratory alkalosis	Be aware of medications that may lower phosphates (carafate, magnesium and aluminum hydroxide, steroids)	
Renal problems		Replace calcium as needed (repletion of phosphate may cause calcium to drop)
Severe diarrhea		Discontinue PN if patient symptomatic
Malabsorption associated with low calcium and magnesium levels		
Increased requirements		

(continued)

TABLE 16-14   (Continued)

Cause(s)	Prevention	Treatment
Hypocalcemia		
Vitamin D deficiency	Monitor serum levels	Replace by adding calcium to PN
Insufficient replacement	Be aware of disease states, medications, malnutrition that can cause hypocalcemia	May require IVPB of calcium to correct severe deficiency
Pancreatitis		Correct hypomagnesemia
Hypomagnesemia		Correct for deficiency caused by hypoalbuminemia
Hyperphosphatemia		
Hypoalbuminemia		
Hypomagnesemia		
Insufficient magnesium in PN	Monitor serum levels closely	Increase magnesium in PN
Excess GI or renal losses (diarrhea, fistula, diuretics)	Be aware of disease states or drugs that can cause hypomagnesemia	If very low, IVPB replacement
Certain drugs (aminoglycosides, diuretics, cisplatin)		Discontinue PN if patient symptomatic
Disease states (chronic alcoholism, pancreatitis, diabetic acidosis, sepsis/infection, burns)		Monitor for cardiac arrhythmia
Hypermagnesemia		
Excess magnesium in PN	Monitor serum levels	Decrease or delete from PN
Renal failure	Monitor renal function	Calcium salts
		Dialysis may be necessary
Metabolic acidosis		
Renal insufficiency; acute/chronic renal failure	Monitor ABGs, electrolytes	Give bicarbonate or replace some or all of chloride with acetate in PN
Diabetic ketoacidosis	Monitor renal function	Monitor vital signs
Diarrhea	Be aware of disease states that may cause metabolic acidosis	
Lactic acidosis (shock)		
Potassium-sparing diuretics		
Massive rhabdomyolysis		

ABGs, arterial blood gases; CHF, congestive heart failure; GI, gastrointestinal; I/O, intake and output; IVPB, intravenous piggyback; S/A, sugar and acetone.

ministration. Insulin needs will decrease when steroids are tapered and discontinued, and as sepsis resolves, and should be adjusted in the PN solution accordingly. Abrupt cessation of PN may also result in hypoglycemia, especially if larger amounts of carbohydrates are used. Tapering of the PN before discontinuation can eliminate this problem.

The infusion of hypertonic dextrose results in the intracellular shift of potassium, magnesium, phosphorus, and calcium. Requirements for these electrolytes, particularly potassium and phosphorus, may be increased. Increased losses or requirements related to the patient's clinical status or treatment may also increase electrolyte requirements. Conversely, the presence of renal failure may require restriction of some or all of these electrolytes. Careful monitoring of electrolytes and adjustments to the PN solution are essential to maintain electrolyte balance.

Hypophosphatemia is another serious, life-threatening complication associated with PN. It is caused by inadequate phosphate replacement, increased requirements due to losses, disease state, and certain medications.[40,66,70] Severe hypophosphatemia and its associated complications can occur in malnourished patients being aggressively refed with PN and has been referred to as the refeeding syndrome. Severe cardiopulmonary decompensation associated with severe hypophosphatemia can lead to seizures, coma, and death. Treatment should be primarily preventive. Early detection and treatment, once it occurs, is imperative. A more thorough review of this serious complication can be found in the literature.[40,66,70]

Frequent metabolic monitoring can ensure that potential metabolic complications will be prevented or documented and treated. The nurse is in a key position to monitor for these changes and report them to the appropriate physician.

Infectious and Septic Complications

Catheter-related sepsis associated with PN is a serious and potentially lethal complication resulting in prolonged hospitalizations and increased morbidity and mortality. The multitude of available studies are difficult to evaluate and compare because there is no uniform definition of catheter-related sepsis and study methods are different.

Reported infection rates vary in institutions, depending on the type of catheter, methods used to evaluate, and the patient's clinical status. Immunosuppressed and critically ill patients are the most susceptible to developing catheter-related sepsis. In addition, a CVAD is a foreign body that alters natural defense mechanisms and induces an inflammatory response.[31]

The most common definition of sepsis differentiates colonization from actual sepsis related to the catheter and can be found in Table 16-15. Appropriate catheter culturing methods should be used to diagnose catheter-related sepsis.[17] The most common organisms causing catheter-related infection include coagulase-negative staphylococci, *Staphylococcus aureus*, and *Candida* species.[3]

Catheter-related infection or sepsis may result from skin contaminants at the insertion site, hub and tubing/device junction contamination, from the hands of health care professionals, and homogeneous seeding from other sources (lungs, urine, abdomen, wounds). The incidence of solution contamination is rare because of meticulous admixing protocols.

Catheter-related sepsis may present in the patient as fever, chills, hypotension, change in mental status, and leukocytosis. Metabolic acidosis and hyperglycemia may be early signs of sepsis in critically ill patients receiving PN.[9] A complete fever work-up is necessary, including culturing of all potential sources of infection.

Options for the management of catheter-related sepsis include exchange of the catheter over guidewire versus removal of the catheter. The decision is determined by the patient's clinical status, culture results, and the nature of the offending organism. Guidewire exchange is associated with fewer risks of insertion-related complications and is safe if the patient is not floridly septic. If the catheter segment culture is positive, this catheter should also be removed and a new catheter placed in a different lo-

TABLE 16-15
Definitions of Catheter-Related Infection and Sepsis[1,51]

1. Contamination	<15 CFU from cultured tip or intracutaneous catheter segment
2. Colonization	>15 CFU from catheter tip or intracutaneous catheter segment or
	no clinical symptoms
3. Insertion site infection	>15 CFU from catheter tip or intracutaneous catheter segment
	External signs of localized infection (drainage, redness)
4. Primary catheter-related bacteremia	>15 CFU from catheter tip or intracutaneous catheter segment
	Positive blood culture with the same organism
	No other identified source of infection
5. Secondary catheter-related bacteremia	>15 CFU from catheter tip or intracutaneous catheter segment
	Positive blood culture with the same organism
	Other source positive for the same organism (urine, lungs, abdomen, wound)

CFU, colony-forming units

cation. If the patient is floridly septic or the blood culture is positive, the catheter should be removed immediately.[9,30] In either of the above situations, empirical antibiotics are often started once all cultures are obtained. Tunneled catheters and implanted ports pose additional problems because they cannot be changed over wire or readily replaced, and they often serve as "lifelines" for patients with limited sites for central venous access. Many of these infections can be successfully treated with antibiotics without removing the catheter.[30] Most consider the presence of *Candida* automatic grounds for catheter removal, regardless of type.

Some institutions have protocols for the routine change of either catheter site or the catheter over guidewire to prevent the incidence of catheter-related sepsis. At least two studies did not demonstrate any advantage to this practice.[7,12]

Catheter site infection should not be confused with catheter-related sepsis. Most catheters under transparent dressings will show some erythema at the insertion site. The presence of erythema or exudate at the site may indicate a localized infection and not necessarily a sign of catheter infection. Conversely, patients may be septic with no signs evident at the catheter site.

Vigilant observation of protocols for insertion, use, and maintenance of CVADs is necessary to minimize the incidence of infection and catheter-related sepsis.[51]

HOME PARENTERAL NUTRITION

Home parenteral nutrition has been a successful alternative for many patients who require prolonged or lifetime PN. The emergence and growth of "high tech" home care infusion companies has facilitated the safe administration of PN in the home environment. This has resulted in shortened hospital stays, reduced costs, and improved patient well-being, both psychologically and physically, by being in the home environment. Standards for home nutrition support have been established and should be used.[73]

Because HPN is expensive, strict policies have been established for reimbursement for HPN. Care must be taken in determining who is eligible for HPN.

Therapy may be provided as either a continuous or cyclic infusion. Cyclic infusion over 12 to 14 hours, as previously discussed, is preferred, especially for ambulatory patients. Most home infusion companies prefer to provide TNAs for HPN. Regardless of the method chosen for a particular patient, the teaching program should be individualized for a patient's learning needs and capabilities and home care environment. The patient should be encouraged to assume as much responsibility for self-care as possible to be able to feel "in control."

Nurses have a primary role in preparing the patient for HPN.[60] The prospect of HPN may seem overwhelming to the patient and the family or caregiver. Thorough preparation and teaching are essential because the procedures are complex. Careful assessment of the patient's and caregiver's willingness and ability to perform the procedures and assume responsibility for the management of this therapy is important. One nurse should be selected as the primary teacher. A lack of consistency can confuse the learner and extends the learning period.[65] Ideally, teaching should be initiated in the hospital and continued in the home if not completed before discharge. Earlier discharge of patients in the managed care environment may shift the focus for education entirely into the home setting.

The education process should include verbal instructions, with demonstration of all procedures. Return demonstration by the patient or primary caregiver is essential to assess competency. A manual of written instructions should be provided to all patients. The verbal and written instructions should include the following[65]:

- All appropriate procedures related to the administration of PN and care and maintenance of the CVAD
- Use, maintenance, and trouble-shooting of the infusion pump
- Storage, management, and disposal of solutions and supplies
- Self-monitoring guidelines (see Figure 16-6 for a sample home health record and guidelines for use) and potential complications
- Problem-solving techniques
- Emergency interventions
- Expectations of home care and medical and nursing follow-up

A social worker, discharge planner, or case manager may be helpful to answer questions and concerns about financial considerations and community resources. Psychosocial support is also essential.

Arrangements for a home infusion provider should be determined as early as possible. Ideally, the home infusion nurse will visit the patient and family in the hospital to establish rapport, discuss learning needs, feelings, status, and the regimen ordered by the physician. In many cases, the home infusion nurse will provide all the in-hospital teaching as well.

Home Health Record

Guidelines For Patient TPN Home Health Record
This form will be available to the Home Health Nurse to help monitor patient's progress.

1. Patient's name.
2. Enter date daily.
3. Enter weight daily (same time).
4. Enter temperature reading twice a day.
5. Enter urine results (if appropriate) per physician's order.
6. Enter blood sugar value (if appropriate) per physician's order.
7. Enter amount of TPN infused.
8. Enter rate/amount of lipids infused.
9. Enter oral intake.
10. Enter urine output.
11. Enter other output.
12. Enter stool frequency/consistency.
13. Note dressing change by a check mark in the box. Indicate appearance of site by use of the key letter:
    C = clean/dry
    R = red
    D = drainage
    P = pain
    S = swelling
    L = loose
14. Enter information as noted in parentheses.
15. Enter any other situations/problems not addressed.
16. Save this record for Home Health Nurse.

Name:							
Date:							
Weight: _____ lbs. _____ kg.							
Temperature: a.m.							
p.m.							
Urine: A							
Sugar and acetone M							
P							
M							
Blood Sugar:							
Intake Rate/amount of TPN infused (cc's/24 hours)							
Lipids							
Albumin							
Antibiotics							
Oral fluid intake/24 hours (Total cc's)							
Output - Urine Other output (cc's) Type							
Stool frequency/ consistency L/F							
Dressing changed/site: C = clean/dry R = red D = drainage P = pain S = swelling L = loose							
General: (include problems, appetite, how you feel, foods eaten, supply problems, etc.)							

FIGURE 16-6 Home health record and guidelines for use for patient receiving TPN at home. (Courtesy: Midwestern Regional Medical Center, Zion, IL)

The benefits of HPN clearly outweigh the risks, and patients today enjoy new freedoms and near-normal life-styles as a result of this added dimension to nutritional support therapy.

SUMMARY

The use of PN in the 1990s requires a high level of sophistication and knowledge on the part of those prescribing, admixing, administering, and monitoring the use of this therapy. The nurse, who sees the patient on a daily basis, is a key member of the interdisciplinary team whose impact on patient management will only be enhanced by an increased knowledge and understanding of PN.

REFERENCES

1. *Arrow multilumen central venous catheters: Nursing care guidelines.* (1994). Arrow International, Inc., pp. 72–80.
2. American Society for Parenteral and Enteral Nutrition Board of Directors. (1993). Guidelines for the use of parenteral and enteral nutrition in adults and pediatric patients. *Journal of Parenteral and Enteral Nutrition (Suppl.), 17*(4).
3. Baranowski, L. (1993). Central venous access devices: Current techniques, uses, and management strategies. *Journal of Intravenous Nursing, 16*(3), 167–194.
4. Bern, M. M., Likich, J. J., & Wallach, S. R., et al. (1990). Very low doses of warfarin can prevent thrombosis in central venous catheters. *Annals of Internal Medicine, 112*(6), 423–428.
5. Blackburn, G. J., & Bistrian, B. R. (1976). Nutritional care of the injured and/or septic patient. *Surgical Clinics of North America, 56*(5), 1195–1225.
6. Blackburn, G. L., Bistrian, B. R., & Maini, B. S., et al. (1977). Nutritional and metabolic assessment of the hospitalized patient. *Journal of Parenteral and Enteral Nutrition, 1*(1), 1–12.
7. Bonawitz, S. C., Hammell, E. J., & Kirkpatrick, J. R. (1991). Prevention of central venous catheter sepsis: A prospective random trial. *Annals of Surgery, 57*, 618–623.
8. Burke, J., Wolfe, R., & Mullany, C., et al. (1979). Parameters of optimal glucose infusion and possible hepatic and respiratory abnormalities following excessive glucose infusion. *Annals of Surgery, 190*, 379–385.
9. Cahill, S. L., & Benotti, P. N. (1991). Catheter infection control in parenteral nutrition. *Nutrition in Clinical Practice, 6*(2), 65–67.
10. Carpentier, Y. A., VanGossum, A., Dubin, E. Y., & Deckelbaum, R. J. (1993). Lipid metabolism in parenteral nutrition. In J. L. Rombeau & M. D. Caldwell (Eds.), *Clinical nutrition: Parenteral nutrition* (pp. 35–74). Philadelphia: W. B. Saunders.
11. Cerra, F. R. (1984). Nutritional requirements. In F. R. Cerra (Ed.), *Pocket manual of surgical nutrition* (pp. 59–85). St. Louis: C. V. Mosby.
12. Cobb, D. K., High, K. P., & Sawyer, R. G., et al. (1992). A controlled trial of scheduled replacement of central venous and pulmonary artery catheters. *New England Journal of Medicine, 327*(15), 1062–1068.
13. Crocker, K. S. (1988). Metabolic monitoring during nutritional support therapy. In J. A. Grant & C. Kennedy-Caldwell (Eds.), *Nutritional support in nursing* (pp. 191–231). Philadelphia: Grune & Stratton.
14. Cunningham, R. S., & Bonam-Crawford, D. (1993). The role of fibrinolytic agents in the management of thrombotic complications associated with vascular access devices. *Nursing Clinics of North America, 28*(4), 899–909.
15. Curtas, S. (1988). Nutritional assessment. In C. Kennedy-Caldwell & P. Guenther (Eds.), *Nutritional support: Nursing core curriculum* (2nd ed., pp. 29–42). Silver Spring, MD: American Society for Parenteral and Enteral Nutrition.
16. Curtas, S., Chapman, G., & Meguid, M. M. (1989). Evaluation of nutritional status. *Nursing Clinics of North America, 24*(20), 301–313.
17. Curtas, S., & Tramposch, K. (1991). Culture methods to evaluate central venous catheter sepsis. *Nutrition in Clinical Practice, 6*(2), 43–48.
18. DeChicco, R. S., & Matarese, L. E. (1992). Selection of nutrition support regimens. *Nutrition in Clinical Practice, 7*, 239–245.
19. Dickerson, R. N. (1985). Question: How fast can I taper TPN in a hospitalized patient? *Hospital Pharmacy, 20*, 620–621.
20. Driscoll, D. F. (1995). Total nutrient admixtures: Theory and practice. *Nutrition in Clinical Practice, 10*, 114–119.
21. Driscoll, D. F., Bhargava, H. N., Li, L., et al. (1995). The stability of total nutrient admixtures. *American Journal of Health-System Pharmacist, 52*, 623–634.
22. Dudrick, S. J., & Wilmore, D. G. (1968). Long-term parenteral feeding. *Hospital Practice, 3*(10), 65–78.
23. *Evaluating total parenteral nutrition.* (1990). Final report and core statement of the Technology Assessment and Practice Guidelines Forum. Program on Technology and Health Care, Georgetown University School of Medicine, Washington, DC.
24. Evans, N. J., Bamba, M., & Rombeau, J. L. (1993). Care of central venous catheters. In J. L. Rombeau & M. D. Caldwell (Eds.), *Clinical nutrition: Parenteral nutrition* (pp. 353–366). Philadelphia: W. B. Saunders.
25. Food and Drug Administration. (1994). Safety alert: Hazards of precipitate associated with parenteral nutrition. *American Journal of Hospital Pharmacy, 51*, 427–428.
26. Forlaw, L. (1988). Nutritional assessment. In J. A. Grant & C. Kennedy-Caldwell (Eds.), *Nutritional support in nursing* (pp. 91–107). Philadelphia: Grune & Stratton.
27. Forlaw, L., & Bayer, L. (1983). *Introduction to nutritional and physical assessment for the nurse* [Monograph] (pp. 1–22). Washington, DC:

American Society for Parenteral and Enteral Nutrition.

28. Frisancho, A., & Flegel, P. (1983). Elbow breadth as a measure of frame size for males and females. *American Journal of Clinical Nutrition, 37,* 311–314.

29. Gil, K. M., Skeie, B., & Koetan, V., et al. (1991). Parenteral nutrition and oral intake: Effect of glucose and fat infusion. *Journal of Parenteral and Enteral Nutrition, 15,* 426–432.

30. Goodman, E. L., Maki, D. G., Farr, B. M., & Mayhall, C. G. (1990). Preventing central venous catheter-related complications: A roundtable discussion. *Infections in Surgery,* 1–13.

31. Grant, A., & DeHoog, S. (1991). Nutritional assessment and support. In A. Grant & S. DeHoog (Eds.), *Nutritional assessment and support.* Seattle: Authors.

32. Grant, J. A. (1988). Historical perspectives in nutritional support. In J. A. Grant & C. Kennedy-Caldwell (Eds.), *Nutritional support in nursing* (pp. 3–28). Philadelphia: Grune & Stratton.

33. Grant, J. P. (1992). Nutritional assessment by body compartment analysis. *Handbook of total parenteral nutrition* (pp. 15–47). Philadelphia: W. B. Saunders.

34. Grant, J. P. (1992). Functional and dynamic techniques for nutritional assessment. *Handbook of total parenteral nutrition* (pp. 49–73). Philadelphia: W. B. Saunders.

35. Grant, J. P. (1992). Vascular access for total parenteral nutrition: Techniques and complications. *Handbook of total parenteral nutrition* (pp. 107–136). Philadelphia: W. B. Saunders.

36. Grant, J. P. (1992). Administration of parenteral nutrition solutions. *Handbook of total parenteral nutrition* (pp. 171–201). Philadelphia: W. B. Saunders.

37. Grant, J. P. (1992). Septic and metabolic complications: Recognition and management. *Handbook of total parenteral nutrition* (pp. 239–265). Philadelphia: W. B. Saunders.

38. Hanson, B. W., DeSomery, C. H., & Hagedorn, P., et al. (1977). Effects of enteral and parenteral nutrition on appetite in monkeys. *Journal of Parenteral and Enteral Nutrition, 1,* 83–88.

39. Harris, J. A., & Benedict, F. G. (1919). *A biometric study of basal metabolism in man.* Washington, DC: Carnegie Institute of Washington, Publication No. 279.

40. Havala, T., & Shronts, E. (1990). Managing the complications associated with refeeding. *Nutrition in Clinical Practice, 5,* 23–29.

41. Hoffman, K. K., Wever, D. J., & Samsa, G. P., et al. (1992). Transparent polyurethane film as an intravenous catheter dressing: A meta-analysis of infection risks. *Journal of the American Medical Association, 267*(15), 2072–2076.

42. Holcombe, B. J., Forloines-Lynn, S., & Garmhausen, L. W. (1992). Restoring patency of long-term central venous access lines. *Journal of Intravenous Nursing, 15*(1), 36–41.

43. Intravenous Nurses Society Revised Intravenous Nursing Standards of Practice. (1990). *Journal of Intravenous Nursing (Suppl.).*

44. Jensen, G., Mascioli, E., & Seidner, D., et al. (1990). Parenteral infusion of long- and medium-chain triglycerides and reticuloendothelial system function in man. *Journal of Parenteral and Enteral Nutrition, 14,* 467–471.

45. Kennedy-Caldwell, C. (1988). Substrate metabolism, vitamins. In C. Kennedy-Caldwell & P. Guenther (Eds.), *Nutrition support: Nursing core curriculum* (2nd ed., pp. 93–103). Silver Spring, MD: American Society for Parenteral and Enteral Nutrition.

46. Lawson, M. (1991). Partial occlusion of indwelling central venous catheters. *Journal of Intravenous Nursing, 14*(3),

47. Lawson, M., Bottino, J. C., & Hurtabise, M. R., et al. (1982). The use of urokinase to restore patency of occluded central venous catheters. *American Journal of Intravenous Therapy and Clinical Nutrition, 9,* 29–32.

48. Leupold-DeCicco, C. (1996). Total parenteral nutrition. In S. Weinstein (Ed.), *Intravenous therapy handbook* (Baxter Laboratories). Publisher pending.

49. Lipkin, E. W., & Bell, S. (1993). Assessment of nutritional status: The clinician's perspective. *Clinics in Laboratory Medicine, 1312,* 329–352.

50. Lowell, J. A., & Bothe, A. (1991). Venous access: Preoperative, operative, and postoperative dilemmas. *Surgical Clinics of North America, 71,* 1232–1246.

51. Maki, D. G. (1991). Infection caused by intravascular devices: Pathogenesis, strategies, for prevention. In D. G. Maki (Ed.), *Improving catheter site care* (pp. 3–28). New York: Royal Society of Medicine Services Limited.

52. Maki, D. G., & Ringer, M. (1987). Evaluation of dressing regimens for the prevention of infection with peripheral intravenous catheters. *Journal of the American Medical Association, 258,* 2396–2403.

53. Maki, D. G., Ringer, M., Alvarado, C. J. (1991). Prospective randomized trial of povidone-iodine, alcohol, and chlorhexidine for prevention of infection associated with central venous and arterial catheters. *Lancet, 338,* 339–343.

54. Maki, D. G., & Will, L. (1984). Colonization and infection associated with transparent dress-

ings for central venous, arterial, and Hickman catheters: A comparative trial [Program and Abstracts]. 24th Interscience Conference on Antimicrobial Agents and Chemotherapy, Washington, DC.

55. Mascioli, E. A., & Bistrian, B. R. (1983). TPN in the patient with diabetes. *Nutrition Support Services, 2*(7), 14–16.

56. Matthews, D. E., & Fong, Y. (1993). Amino acid and protein metabolism. In J. L. Rombeau & M. D. Caldwell (Eds.), *Clinical nutrition: Parenteral nutrition* (pp. 75–112). Philadelphia: W. B. Saunders.

57. McMahon, M., Manji, N., Driscoll, D. F., & Bistrian, B. R. (1989). Parenteral nutrition in patients with diabetes mellitus: Theoretical and practical considerations. *Journal of Parenteral and Enteral Nutrition, 13*(5), 545–553.

58. Michael, S. R., & Sabo, C. E. (1989). Management of the diabetic patient receiving nutrition support. *Nutrition in Clinical Practice, 4*, 179–183.

59. Multivitamin preparations for parenteral use: A statement by the Nutrition Advisory Group. (1979). *Journal of Parenteral and Enteral Nutrition, 3*, 258.

60. Orr, M. E. (1989). Nutritional support in home care. *Nursing Clinics of North America, 24*(2), 437–445.

61. Orr, M. E., & Ryder, M. A. (1993). Vascular access devices: Perspectives on designs, complications, and management. *Nutrition in Clinical Practice, 8*(4), 145–152.

62. Pennington, C. R., & Pithie, A. D. (1987). Ethanol lock in the management of catheter occlusion. *Journal of Parenteral and Enteral Nutrition, 11*, 507–508.

63. Rolandelli, R. H., & Ulrich, J. R. (1994). Nutritional support in the frail elderly surgical patient. *Surgical Clinics of North America, 74*(1), 79–92.

64. Ryder, M. A. (1988). Parenteral nutrition device systems. In J. A. Grant & C. Kennedy-Caldwell (Eds.), *Nutritional support in nursing* (pp. 91–107). Philadelphia: Grune & Stratton.

65. Ryder, M. A. (1988). Parenteral nutrition. In C. Kennedy-Caldwell & P. Guenther (Eds.), *Nutrition support: Nursing core curriculum* (pp. 485–538). Silver Spring, MD: American Society for Parenteral and Enteral Nutrition.

66. Sacks, G. S., Walker, J., Dickerson, R. N., Kudsk, K. A., & Brown, R. O. (1994). Observations of hypophosphatemia and its management in nutrition support. *Nutrition in Clinical Practice, 9*, 105–108.

67. Shulman, R. J., Reed, T., & Pitre, D. (1988). Use of hydrochloric acid to clear obstructed central venous catheters. *Journal of Parenteral and Enteral Nutrition, 12*, 509–510.

68. Silberman H. (1989). Parenteral nutrition: General principles. In H. Silberman (Ed.), *Parenteral and enteral nutrition* (pp. 189–211). Norwalk, CT: Appleton & Lange.

69. Smith, L. C., & Mullin, J. L. (1991). Nutritional assessment and indications for nutritional support. *Surgical Clinics of North America, 71*, 449–457.

70. Solomon, S. M., & Kirby, D. F. (1989). The refeeding syndrome: A review. *Journal of Parenteral and Enteral Nutrition, 14*(1), 90–97.

71. Spiekerman, A. M. (1993). Proteins used in nutritional assessment. In R. F. Labbe (Ed.), *Clinics in Laboratory Medicine, 13*(2), 353–369.

72. Standards of nutrition support, hospitalized patients. (1988). *Nutrition in Clinical Practice, 3*(1), 28–31.

73. Standards for home nutrition support. (1992). *Nutrition in Clinical Practice, 7*(2), 65–69.

74. Standards for nutrition support: Hospitalized pediatric patients. (1989). *Nutrition in Clinical Practice, 4*(1), 33–37.

75. Standards for nutrition support for residents of long-term care facilities. (1989). *Nutrition in Clinical Practice, 4*(4), 148–153.

76. Standards of practice: Nutrition support nurse. (1988). *Nutrition in Clinical Practice, 3*(2), 78–80.

77. Standards of lab practice consensus guidelines: Laboratory support in assessing and monitoring nutritional status. (1994). L. A. Kaplan (Ed.), *National Academy of Clinical Biochemistry.* Pesce Kaplan Publishers, Cincinnati, OH.

78. Tuten, M. B., Wogt, S., Dasse, F., & Leider, Z. (1985). Utilization of prealbumin as a nutritional parameter. *Journal of Parenteral and Enteral Nutrition, 9*(6), 145–147.

79. Twoomy, P., Zeigler, D., & Rombeau, J. (1982). Utilization of skin testing in nutritional assessment: A critical review. *Journal of Parenteral and Enteral Nutrition, 6*, 50–58.

80. Washington Review. (1990). Complications associated with use of central venous catheters. *Nutrition in Clinical Practice, 5*, 39–40.

81. Wilmore, D. W., & Dudrick, S. J. (1968). Growth and development of an infant receiving all nutrients exclusively by vein. *Journal of the American Medical Association, 203*, 860–864.

82. Wolfe, R. R. (1993). Carbohydrate metabolism and requirements. In J. L. Rombeau & M. D. Caldwell (Eds.), *Clinical nutrition: Parenteral nutrition* (pp. 113–132). Philadelphia: W. B. Saunders.

83. Wolfe, R. R., O'Donnell, T. F., & Stone, M. D., et al. (1980). Investigation of factors determining the glucose infusion rate in total parenteral nutrition. *Metabolism, 29*, 892–899.

84. Worthington, P. H., & Wagner, B. A. (1989). Total parenteral nutrition. *Nursing Clinics of North America, 24*(2), 355–371.

REVIEW QUESTIONS

1. Which of the following size filters is appropriate for use with total nutrient admixtures?
   a. 0.2 μm
   b. 1.0 μm
   c. 1.2 μm
   d. 2.0 μm

2. A urinary urea nitrogen is needed for which of the following reasons?
   a. to determine kidney function
   b. to determine efficacy of nutritional support
   c. to determine protein-calorie malnutrition
   d. to determine protein tolerance

3. Each gram of carbohydrate in parenteral nutrition yields how many kilocalories?
   a. 3.4
   b. 4
   c. 7
   d. 9

4. Each gram of fat yields how many kilocalories?
   a. 4.3
   b. 5
   c. 7
   d. 9

5. A 20% lipid emulsion provides how many calories per mL?
   a. 1.0
   b. 1.1
   c. 2.0
   d. 2.2

6. The nonprotein calorie/nitrogen ratio most appropriate for the highly stressed patient is which of the following?
   a. 60:1
   b. 90:1
   c. 100:1
   d. 150:1

7. The type of malnutrition that most commonly occurs acutely in hospitalized patients is referred to as:
   a. kwashiorkor
   b. marasmus
   c. hypoalbuminemia
   d. protein-calorie malnutrition

8. The maximum rate of glucose oxidation is:
   a. 2–3 g/kg/d
   b. 3–4 g/kg/d
   c. 4–5 g/kg/d
   d. 5–7 g/kg/d

9. The appropriate location for the central venous access device tip is in which of the following veins?
   a. superior vena cava
   b. subclavian
   c. innominate
   d. jugular

10. Mechanical complications associated with central venous access devices include all of the following *except*:
    a. malposition
    b. pneumothorax
    c. arrhythmia
    d. sepsis

CHAPTER 17

Transfusion Therapy

Key Terms

Adverse effects	Identification checks	Patient monitoring
Compatibilities	Immunohematology	

Since the last edition of this text, transfusion centers have encountered significant changes in the public's perception of risks and benefits of donating and receiving blood. This is exhibited by an increase in autologous transfusions in various forms and a decrease in allogenic donations. Another is the ability of a transfusion service to successfully adjust to the numerous changes in the managed care model in the health care field. Essentially today's transfusion medicine is more customized for some patients and requires more complex methods of care plans. Prevention of disease transmission through transfusions continues to be a another paramount focus along with more complex informational technology, capitation, and cost containment in a competetive environment.

Rules and regulations governing the procurement, storage, and administration of transfusion therapy have been established through national organizations and the Food and Drug Administration (FDA). The American Association of Blood Banks (AABB) sets standards that represent accepted performance guidelines for the provision of safe transfusion and transplantation. The AABB also provides standards for a safe work environment for personnel. Review of transfusion practice is required by the Joint Commission on Accreditation of Healthcare Organizations. In addition, state and local governing bodies may require practical issues. All staff working in this field should be knowledgeable about their role and accountable for their practice.

Nurses administer transfusions in most hospitals and must acquire a greater knowledge base than what may be taught in the nursing school curriculum because patients are more likely to inquire about various aspects of this integral part of their treatment. Administration of blood should be performed with documented qualifications of personnel who demonstrate continued competence. Serious problems and complications that can lead to death and can result in litigation are associated with the administration of blood and its components. The IV nurse shares with the blood transfusion service the responsibility for providing the safest transfusion therapy. Nurses must incorporate the fundamental principles of immunohematology into their daily nursing care; the indications, advantages, and disadvantages of a large variety of components; proper procedures for their safe administration; and the ability to recognize early symptoms of transfusion reactions and appropriate interventions. Being knowledgeable and maintaining the skills of administering blood and components will help decrease the risks in this important therapy.

With the increase in acuity in medical facilities and the rapid progression of a patient's course of therapy, quality measures surrounding all aspects of transfusion therapy must be monitored through quality improvement programs to be certain standards are met and policies and procedures are followed.

BASIC IMMUNOHEMATOLOGY

Immunohematology is the science that deals with antigens of the blood and their antibodies. An *antigen* is a substance capable of stimulating the production of an antibody and then reacting with that antibody in a specific way.

The ABO system, discovered by Dr. Karl Landsteiner in 1901, is the most important group of antigens for transfusion as well as transplantation. The synthesis of these antigens, which are located on the surface of red blood cells, is under the control of the A, B, and O genes. In the presence of the A gene, an individual makes A antigen and is classified as group A. Group B individuals have B antigens on their red blood cells, group AB individuals have both, and group O persons have neither (Table 17-1). These antigens are genetically inherited and determine the blood group of the individual.

TABLE 17-1
ABO Classification of Human Blood

Group	Cell Antigens A	Cell Antigens B	Plasma Antibodies A	Plasma Antibodies B	% US Population
O	–	–	+	+	45
A	+	–	–	+	40
B	–	+	+	–	10
AB	+	+	–	–	5

Discovered in 1940 by Stetson and Levine, the Rh system is the second most clinically important system for transfusion. About 85% of the Caucasian population has the D antigen on their red blood cells and are classified as D or Rh positive. The D antigen is lacking in the 15% of the population classified as Rh negative. Rh-negative individuals can readily form anti-D after exposure to the antigen. Severe hemolytic reactions and hemolytic disease of the newborn are the result of this antigen–antibody reaction. Other common antigens in the system are C, E, c, and e.

About 50 other known blood group antigen systems containing about 500 antigens are known. Fortunately only a few systems, such as Kell, Duffy, and Kidd, are commonly encountered.

Leukocytes also carry antigens on their surfaces. The most important group of these are human leukocyte antigens (HLA). Individuals who have been exposed to the red blood cells or leukocytes of other people through transfusion or pregnancy (maternal–fetal hemorrhage) may make antibodies to the foreign antigens carried on those cells.

An *antibody* is a protein in the plasma that reacts with a specific antigen. Antibodies are named for the antigen that stimulated their formation and with which they react. For example, an antibody against the D antigen formed after the transfusion of an Rh (D)-positive unit to a Rh (D)-negative recipient is called anti-D. Antibodies formed in response to exposure to foreign antigens are called *immune antibodies*. Some blood group antibodies are formed without exposure to allogenic red blood cells. The most important of these so-called naturally occurring antibodies are anti-A and anti-B. During the first few months of life, infants make IgM antibodies to whichever of the ABO antigens they lack. For example, a group A infant will make anti-B (see Table 17-1). It is these naturally occurring antibodies (the *isoagglutinins*) that can produce rapid hemolysis of red blood cells with the corresponding antigen that form the basis of ABO incompatibility.

MECHANISM OF IMMUNE RESPONSE

When a patient is transfused with allogenic blood bearing "foreign" (ie, non-self) antigens, the immune system may respond by producing antibodies. Phagocytic cells called macrophages play an important role in the defense system of the body. One of their roles in the immune response is to capture and process foreign antigens. It then "presents" the processed antigen to other members of the immune system, namely, the T and B lymphocytes. B cells, with help from T cells, begin to produce antibodies specific for the antigen presented to them by the macrophages. Stimulated by the appropriate foreign antigen, the B cell swells and changes its internal structure and differentiates into plasma cells to produce antibody.[27] Each plasma cell produces large quantities of antibody of the precise specificity and immunoglobulin class genetically programmed into the cell. The antibodies are secreted into a variety of body fluids, including the blood plasma.

The macrophages have also called on the T cells, which act as helpers or suppressors to B-cell function. The intertwined relationship between T and B cells regulates the type and sensitivity of the immune response.

MECHANISM OF RED BLOOD CELL DESTRUCTION

Two mechanisms of red blood cell destruction are known: intravascular hemolysis and extravascular hemolysis. *Intravascular hemolysis* occurs within the vascular compartment. This mode of red blood cell destruction is the result of the sequential binding of antibody to a red blood cell with a foreign antigen on its surface. This antibody then fixes complement. If the entire complement cascade is triggered, a lytic complex is formed on the red blood cell membrane, which leads to rupture of the red blood cell, releasing hemoglobin into the intravascular compartment.

Antibodies that activate complement often agglutinate in vitro and can cause intravascular hemolysis in vivo. The most frequent cause of this type of red blood cell destruction is transfusion of ABO incompatible blood. Anti-A and anti-B are mostly IgM antibodies that are capable of engaging the complement and coagulation and kinin systems when they bind with their corresponding antigen. The consequences of this type of hemolysis are usually immediate and severe and are often fatal.

The other mechanism of red blood cell destruction, *extravascular hemolysis*, is more commonly seen as a result of incompatibities in blood group systems other than the ABO system. Antibodies to these other blood group antigens are usually IgG. They bind to red blood cells with the corresponding antigen. Phagocytic cells of the reticuloendothelial system, particularly in the spleen, bind the IgG-coated red blood cells, ingest them, and destroy them extracellularly; hence the term, extravascular hemolysis. These IgG antibodies may also fix some amount of complement but not enough to lyse the red blood cells. Instead, the complement-coated red blood cells are cleared from the circulation by the phagocytic cells of the liver, the Kupffer cells, and destroyed intracellularly. The consequences after extravascular hemolysis are not as severe as those of intravascular hemolysis but are recognizable by a drop in the hematocrit, an increase in the bilirubin level, and perhaps by the clinical signs of fever or malaise.

BLOOD GROUP SYSTEMS

The best known blood group system is the ABO system. Landsteiner described a classification of human blood based on agglutination reactions between the red blood cells and serum. The ABO system is the only system in which the reciprocal antibodies are consistently and predictably present in the sera of normal individuals whose red blood cells lack the corresponding antigen(s). The ABO system is the foundation of pretransfusion testing and compatibility.

In 1939, Levine and Stetson discovered the Rhesus (Rh) system, so called because of its relationship to the substance in the red blood cells of the Rhesus monkey. The Rh system is the second most important system in transfusion therapy. They found an antibody that agglutinated red blood cells in 85% of the individuals tested. The antigen causing the reaction is known as the Rh or D antigen. A person whose red blood cells have the D antigen is classified as Rh positive; lacking the D antigen, Rh negative. Because of the ease with which antibody D is made, grouping is done on all donors and recipients to ensure that D-negative recipients receive D-negative blood, except for reasonable qualifying circumstances. Rh-positive recipients may receive either Rh-positive or Rh-negative blood.

Antibodies to the Rh antigens are not present unless an individual has been exposed to Rh-positive red blood cells, either through transfusion or pregnancy. Individuals who develop Rh antibodies will have detectable levels for many years. If undetected, subsequent exposure may lead to a secondary immune response.

Occasionally, weak variants of the Rh D antigen are found, which are identified by special serologic tests. These individuals are termed weak D or Du positive, but they are considered Rh positive both as donors and recipients.

Other blood group systems have been defined on the basis of reaction of cells with antibodies. Antibodies to antigens in the Kell, Duffy, Kidd, and Lewis systems are encountered frequently enough to be clinically important. Antibodies to the blood group antigens in most of the other systems are found so infrequently that they do not cause everyday problems. When present, these antibodies may produce hemolytic reactions. Once demonstrated, precautions must be taken to ensure that the patient receives compatible blood lacking the corresponding antigen. When difficulty arises in crossmatching or when a transfusion reaction occurs, these systems acquire special significance.

PRETRANSFUSION TESTING

The Donor

Under ordinary circumstances, a donor may donate blood no more than every 8 weeks. In addition to ABO and Rh group determination and a screen for unexpected antibodies, several other tests are performed on donor blood before it is released for patient use. They are hepatitis B surface antigen (HBsAg), antibody to human T-cell leukemia virus (anti-HTLV-I/II), anti-human immunodeficiency virus (HIV)-1, anti-HIV-2, antibody to hepatitis C virus (HCV), and a serologic test for syphilis (STS). No blood component is issued unless test results are negative. Alanine aminotransferase (ALT) testing is also performed. ALT is an enzyme that is released from damaged cells in an individual with liver injury or inflammation. Donors with elevated ALT levels may be implicated in posttransfusion hepatitis (PTH) to a greater extent than donors with normal ALT concentrations.[13] Individual institutions set established limits for ALT. However, the value of this surrogate test is being discussed. For now, donors will be deferred if results exceed the set limits.

The Recipient

Tests performed on the intended transfusion recipient include ABO and Rh group determination and screen for unexpected antibodies. Before the administration of whole blood or red blood cell components, a major crossmatch (combining donor red blood cells and recipient serum or plasma) is performed to detect serologic incompatibility.

The AABB requires that if a patient has been transfused in the preceding 3 months with blood or a blood component containing red blood cells or has been pregnant within the preceding 3 months or if the history is uncertain or unavailable, the sample must be obtained from the patient within 3 days of the scheduled transfusion.[2] This requirement is made to rule out the possibility that a newly formed antibody is not missed.

In situations in which delay in provision of blood may jeopardize life, blood may be issued before completion of routine tests according to AABB standards.[2]

Recipients whose ABO group is not known must receive group O red blood cells. Physicians must indicate in the record that the clinical condition is sufficiently urgent to release blood before compatibility testing is completed; the tag or label must conspicuously indicate that compatibility testing is not completed; and standard compatibility tests should be completed promptly.

Recipients whose ABO group has been determined by the transfusing facility, without reliance on previous record, may receive ABO group-specific whole blood or ABO group-compatible red blood cell components before other tests for compatibility have been completed.

ANTICOAGULANTS–PRESERVATIVES

Blood is routinely collected in plastic bags that may contain different anticoagulants–preservatives. Whole blood collected in citrate–phosphate–dextrose (CPD) or citrate–phosphate–double dextrose (C-) has an expiration date not exceeding 21 days after phlebotomy. The difference in the solutions is that C- has twice the amount of dextrose. The anticoagulant–preservative system of CPD–adenine (CPDA-1) may be stored for 35 days. The duration for storage is based on the standard that a minimum of 70% of the transfused red blood cells (stored for 35 days) must be present in the bloodstream of the recipient 24 hours after the transfusion. Providing a nutrient biochemical balance to red blood cells during storage is important to maintain viability and function of the components within the blood and to prevent physical changes. To minimize bacterial proliferation, specific temperatures must be maintained.

Each ingredient in the solution has a function. The phosphate acts as a buffer, slowing the drop in pH of the stored cells and improving viability. Sodium citrate, by combining with ionized calcium, inhibits clotting, thus serving as an anticoagulant. Dextrose (glucose) prolongs the life of the red blood cells by providing a nutrient source. Adenine is a substrate from which red blood cells can synthesize adenosine triphosphate (ATP). The red blood cell depends on ATP to maintain cell surface ion pumps.

A second group of anticoagulant–preservative systems is similar to CPDA-1. They differ, however, in that, once the platelet-rich plasma is removed from the unit within 8 hours, an additive solution of 100 mL containing saline, dextrose, and adenine is added to the packed red blood cells. These additive systems permit storage for up to 42 days. FDA-approved solutions are AS-1 (ADSOL®), AS-3 (NUTRICEL®), and AS-5 (OPTISOL®).

Additional solutions such as pyruvate and other compounds have been licensed and may be added to stored red blood cells nearing the end of their shelf-life. Called "rejuvenated" cells, these additives allow units to be stored even longer.

WHOLE BLOOD

Whole blood contains cells (red blood cells, white blood cells, and platelets), plasma (blood proteins, antibodies, water, and waste), and electrolytes.

Transfusions of whole blood are infrequent but may be indicated when an acute massive blood loss has occurred. Massive hemorrhage is usually defined as a patient having more than 25% to 30% blood volume loss. The goal is to restore intravascular blood volume to prevent hypovolemic shock. The patient requires both oxygen-carrying capacity of the red blood cells and plasma for volume replacement. It is imperative to quickly restore the blood volume to improve oxygen delivery. Crystalloid and colloid solutions will only temporarily correct hypovolemia. Patients should be monitored closely for dilutional coagulopathies.

Whole blood, less than 4 to 5 days old, may be indicated for an exchange transfusion in a newborn. The blood may ensure electrolyte concentration limits tolerable for infants.[3]

Autologous transfusion, whereby the patient donates blood for himself, is frequently returned to the patient (donor) as a whole blood infusion. Whole blood has many disadvantages. Patients must receive from their own blood group, which eliminates ABO compatibility between blood groups (Table 17-2).

With the continuous metabolic changes of red blood cells, definite changes occur in stored blood. The potassium leaks out of the cell and into the plasma. Studies have shown that the potassium level rises to approximately 21 mEq/L by day 21 after collection. Infusions of stored whole blood could potentially cause complications to patients with compromised cardiac status or in patients undergoing exchange transfusion. Another problem is the formation of microaggregates. As cells break down, this cellular debris may be detrimental to patients with lung disease although physicians differ in opinion on the significance of microaggregates. Special filters are available and are designed to protect the infusion of this particulate matter.

Modified whole blood is prepared by removing the plasma, collecting the platelets or cryoprecipitate, and then returning the plasma back into the red blood cells. This product may be used for patients with hemorrhage and other clinical conditions when whole blood is warranted. Although this component has the same hemostatic properties as whole blood, a patient may additionally require separate components. Fresh whole blood, defined as being less than 24 hours old, has no valid indications. Although it contains viable platelets and other coagulation factors, a patient's deficit of these components should be specifically replaced with the component to correct the underlying problem. In addition, processing of donor blood is difficult to complete within 24 hours.

TABLE 17-2
ABO Compatibility for Whole Blood

Recipient	Donor
A	A
B	B
AB	AB
O	O

Whole blood is stored at a temperature of 1°C (34°F) to 6°C (43°F). Expiration depends on the anticoagulant–preservative.

The rate of administration for whole blood should be as rapid as necessary to correct and maintain hemodynamic status.

In massive hemorrhage, one or more large-gauge catheters, such as 14 or 16 gauge, will allow a free flow infusion of blood. Electronic infusion devices do not deliver high enough rates to meet the needs of this clinical crisis.

RED BLOOD CELL COMPONENTS

Packed Red Blood Cells

Packed red blood cells are prepared by removing approximately 225 to 250 mL of platelet-rich plasma from a unit of whole blood, either by centrifugation or sedimentation. This process packs the red blood cells and separates most of the platelet-rich plasma. The red blood cell concentrate contains the same red blood cell mass as whole blood, 20% to 30% of the original plasma, and some leukocytes and platelets. Packed red blood cells generally have a hematocrit between 70% and 80%; thus, the viscosity of the unit is increased. One unit of packed red blood cells provides the same amount of oxygen-carrying red blood cells as a unit of whole blood.

The major indication for packed red blood cells is to restore or maintain oxygen-carrying capacity. Because of the reduced volume of the unit, the danger of circulatory overload is less—a definite advantage in patients with renal failure or congestive heart failure. It is also appropriate for elderly or debilitating patients.[3]

Because approximately two-thirds of the plasma is removed, the patient is not subjected to infusions of additional potassium, citrate, or sodium.

Each unit of packed red blood cells is generally expected to raise the hematocrit 3% and the hemoglobin level 1 g/dL in the average 70-kg person. In infants, the hemoglobin level is expected to rise by 1 g/dL when administered at 3 mL/kg.

The expiration time of packed red blood cells is 35 to 42 days depending on the anticoagulant–preservative used.

Because most of the plasma is removed, thereby reducing the amount of anti-A or anti-B agglutinins (or both), group O may be given to other blood groups. In emergency situations, when time does not permit ABO determination, group O red blood cells may be given (Table 17-3).

Leukocyte-Poor Red Blood Cells

Availability of leukocyte-poor red blood cells can be achieved by 1) leukocyte-absorption filters; 2) frozen deglycerolized red blood cells; 3) microaggregate-filtered red blood cells; 4) washed red blood cells; or 5) buffy coat-depleted red blood cells. Thus, the removal of leukocytes from red blood cells requires either centrifugation, washing, or filtration. Filtration is the most effective, achieving a 2- to 3-log reduction in leukocytes, and is the method of choice.

Leukocyte-poor red blood cells are used to restore red blood cells to patients who have previously experienced two or more nonhemolytic febrile reactions and who may have developed antibodies against transfused leukocytes. These reactions

TABLE 17-3
ABO Compatibilities for Red Cell Components*

Recipient	Donor		
	First Choice	Second Choice	Third Choice
O+	O+	O–	
A+	A+	O+, A–	O–
B+	B+	O+, B–	O–
AB+	AB+	AB–, A+, B+	O+, A–, B–, O–
O–	O–	O+	
A–	A–	O–	A+, O+
B–	B–	O–	A+, O+
AB–	AB–	A–, B–, O–	AB+, A+, B+, O+

*Not whole blood, which must be administered ABO *identical*.

may be extremely uncomfortable and may last for several hours. The component may also be considered for patients with diseases such as leukemia and aplastic anemia where it is anticipated that multiple transfusions will be administered. These patients are at risk of becoming refractory to platelet transfusions because of the formation of antibodies to leukocyte antigens, such as HLA antigens, which are also found on platelets. Patients who have a history of allergic transfusion reactions and are IgA deficient are also candidates for this component.

Leukocyte-poor red blood cells must be administered within 24 hours after preparation. Increasingly, special high-efficiency leukocyte removal filters are being used at the bedside.

The rate of infusion and ABO compatibility are the same as for packed red blood cells.

Frozen–Deglycerolized or Frozen–Stored Red Blood Cells

This component undergoes cryopreservation and is prepared by adding a cryoprotectant such as glycerol. Initially, plasma is extracted from the whole blood. The red blood cells are then coated with glycerol and frozen at –85°C until needed. At that time, the unit is thawed and the glycerol is removed by a variety of washing procedures. After thawing, the component should be administered within 24 hours after the washing process occurs. The finished product has virtually all of the plasma and anticoagulant removed. It contains less than 5% of the original donor platelets and leukocytes and has a hematocrit of approximately 80%.

Controversies exist as to the clinical importance and advantages or disadvantages for the use of this component. The major disadvantage is the substantial additional cost related to the process of preparing and storing the component and the cost of personnel involved. The major clinical indication for using frozen deglycerolized red blood cells is to preserve blood from donors with rare blood groups. It is also useful to patients who are sensitized to IgA or other plasma proteins because the cellular components have been removed as well as serving as an alternative method to reduce cytomegalovirus (CMV) transmission for selected patients.[3] Because of the growing concerns over disease transmission, the increase in autologous donations may produce an increase in the number of units frozen if blood is donated more than 35 to 42 days before being needed.

The rate of infusion and ABO compatibility are the same as packed red blood cells.

Platelets

Platelets are available in two preparations: random donor concentrates made from units of whole blood and single donor concentrates obtained by plateletpheresis of a donor. Platelets contain factor III, a phospholipid that enhances the conversion of prothrombin to thrombin, which forms one of the most important steps in the coagulation process.[11]

Clinical conditions that adversely affect platelet function are sepsis, diseases of the liver and kidney, drugs, cardiopulmonary bypass, and certain bone marrow disorders.[3] Platelet transfusions are indicated for thrombocytopenia caused by uremia, massive loss of blood, chemotherapy, leukemia, and unstable patients with thrombotic thrombocytopenia purpura (TTP). The decision to transfuse platelets must be based on the clinical condition of the patient, the etiology of the thrombocytopenia, and the ability of the patient to produce platelets. Platelet transfusions should not be given on the basis of the number of red blood cells infused, but by the platelet count and signs and symptoms of hemorrhage. Platelets are not indicated for patients with thrombocytopenia secondary to TTP and idiopathic thrombocytopenic purpura (ITP).

Platelet concentrate prepared from whole blood contains a minimum of 5.5×10^{10} platelets in at least 75% of the units tested. Each unit contains about 40 to 70 mL and is expected to increase the platelet count by 5000 to 10,000/μL in a stabilized patient. Routinely, random donor platelets (generally 6 U) are pooled and transfused. Patients are subjected to multiple allogenic donors. Due to immune or nonimmune mechanisms, some patients become sensitized and develop platelet-specific and HLA antibodies. These patients are called refractory: they fail to achieve a satisfactory elevation in their platelet count. They are more likely to benefit from single donor platelets. Obtained by the process of plateletpheresis, these platelets may be produced from HLA-matched donors if necessary.[3] Reactions to platelets may include disease transmission, graft-versus-host disease (GVHD); alloimmunization; febrile or allergic effects, and circulatory overload.

Platelet concentrates do not require crossmatching before infusion. Incompatibility between donor plasma and recipient red blood cells is usually clinically insignificant unless large numbers of platelet transfusions are required or if the patient is a small child. Then ABO compatible platelets should be sought. If available, D-negative individuals should receive compatible platelets. An acceptable rate of transfusion is 5 mL/min.

Specific leukocyte removal filters for platelets are available for effective leukocyte removal at the bedside.

Granulocytes

Granulocytes are obtained by the process of leukapheresis and are infrequently administered. Previously prescribed for gram-negative sepsis, new antibiotic regimens, new recombinant growth factors, and improved management of infections have greatly decreased the use of this component. Patients with chronic granulomatous disease or profound neutropenia may be candidates for granulocyte transfusion when it is expected that they will recover. These transfusions will only temporarily improve the patient's condition.

Granulocytes are stored at room temperature (20°–24°C; 68°–75°F) no more than 24 hours and preferably less than 6 hours. Because granulocytes are contaminated with donor red blood cells, they must be ABO compatible with the recipient's plasma.

Patients undergoing granulocyte transfusions are acutely ill and adverse effects are not uncommon. Febrile and pulmonary reactions may occur and CMV transmission and transfusion-associated GVHD (TAGVHD) are of particular concern.

Granulocytes are administered through a set containing the standard blood filter (80–170 μm) over a 4-hour period for adult and pediatric patients. Microaggregate filters should not be used.

PLASMA

Plasma is the liquid content remaining after the red blood cells have been removed from a unit of whole blood. It contains water, electrolytes, proteins (principally albumin), globulin, and coagulation factors.

Liquid Plasma

Single donor liquid plasma is stored 1°C (34°F) for no more than 26 days in CPD or 40 days in CPDA-1.[3]

Plasma plays an important role in the treatment of burns by supplying plasma proteins that are lost from the wound. Some of the clotting factor activity is lost during storage, limiting its use in patients with coagulation problems.

Under ordinary circumstances, single donor plasma should be compatible with the recipient's red blood cells. Because it lacks anti-A and anti-B agglutinins, AB plasma may be used for all ABO groups and in emergencies when the patient's blood group is unknown.

Fresh Frozen Plasma

Fresh frozen plasma (FFP) contains all the normal components of blood plasma including the clotting factors, in addition to 200 to 400 mg fibrinogen. It has a shelf-life of 1 year when stored at a temperature of –18°C or lower. The plasma is separated from the cells and frozen within 8 hours of collection from the donor. The unit is kept frozen until the time of transfusion. It is then thawed in a water bath at 37°C (98.6°F) and optimally should be administered within 6 hours but no more than 24 hours after thawing to minimize the loss of the most labile clotting factors, factor V and factor VIII. To provide factors V and VIII, the component should be used within the first year of storage for treatment of coagulation disorders. After 12 months, FFP may be frozen for 4 more years provided it is relabeled "plasma" because it should not be used for correcting coagulation disorders. If cryoprecipitate has been removed from the plasma, the remaining unit must be labeled as such.

Fresh frozen plasma is beneficial to patients with demonstrated multiple coagulation deficiencies or inherited or acquired bleeding disorders and, on occasion, to treat active bleeding due to vitamin K deficiency. Because FFP is an isotonic volume expander, patients receiving multiple units should be monitored closely to prevent fluid overload. FFP should never be used for volume expansion; this is more safely treated with crystalloid or colloid solutions. They are less expensive than FFP and lack the risk of transmitting disease. Other safer volume expanders are albumin and plasma substitutes, which do not carry the risk of viral disease transmission. Fresh frozen plasma should not be used as a nutrient supplement.

The rate of administration may be 200 mL/h (the approximate volume of each unit) or less if circulatory overload could be a potential complication. The pediatric rate of infusion should be about 1 to 2 mL/min. Although a crossmatch is not required, the component should be compatible with the recipient's red blood cells (Table 17-4).

Cryoprecipitate

Cryoprecipitate is a concentrate containing factor VIII (antihemophilic factor, AHF) extracted from cold-thawed plasma. It is the cold-insoluble portion of plasma after FFP has been thawed. It contains 80 to 120 U factor VIII, 40% to 70% of the plasma von Willebrand factor (vWF) and 150 to 250 mg fibrinogen in a 20- to 30-mL volume. The component is frozen at −18°C for up to 12 months. It should be administered within 6 hours after thawing. Once thawed, the vWF and fibrinogen remain stable but factor VIII is labile.

In the past, this concentrate was predominately used to treat hemophilia A and revolutionized the treatment of this sex-linked bleeding disorder. However, it is associated with the transmission of viral agents and should only be used for specific clinical conditions such as von Willebrand's disease. These patients have a platelet dysfunction and partial deficiency in the ratio of factor VIII to vWF and benefit from infusions of cryoprecipitate. It is the only component available to treat congenital or

---

TABLE 17-4
ABO Compatibility for Fresh Frozen Plasma

Recipient	Donor
A	A or AB
B	B or AB
AB	AB
O	O, A, B, or AB

acquired hypofibrinogenemia; previously available fibrinogen products have been withdrawn because of the increased risk of transmitting hepatitis.

For factor VIII replacement, repeated transfusions are required because the half-life of factor VIII is 8 to 12 hours in the circulation. Single units may be pooled into one container and administered at a rate of 1 to 2 mL/min. Because cryoprecipitate contains few red blood cells, it should be administered under the same guidelines as plasma when large volumes are transfused.

Plasma Derivatives and Plasma Substitutes

Normal Serum Albumin and Plasma Protein Fraction

Albumin comprises about 40% of the plasma protein and can be purified from raw plasma by several procedures. It replaces plasma in many clinical conditions. Albumin is available in two concentrations: 5% in 250 mL saline and 25% in 50 mL saline.

Albumin 5% is isotonic, being osmotically equivalent to an approximately equal volume of citrated plasma. It may be used to provide volume and colloid in the treatment of shock and burns. Initially after a burn, large volumes of crystalloid solution are needed to correct extracellular fluid losses because of fluid leakage into the intracellular compartment. Smaller amounts of colloid are required at this time. After 24 hours, large amounts of albumin are required to maintain intravascular volume and avoid hypoproteinemia, while smaller amounts of crystalloid are infused. Albumin is also used for replacement fluid during plasma exchange.

Albumin 25% is hypertonic and depends on additional fluids, either drawn from the tissues or administered separately for its maximal osmotic effect; 50 mL of 25% albumin is osmotically equivalent to 250 mL citrated plasma. It must be administered with caution because a rapid infusion may cause an increase in intravascular oncotic pressure resulting in circulatory overload or interstitial dehydration particularily to severely dehydrated patients without adequate amounts of supplemental fluid. Controversy exists to its use for protein replacement in severe hypoalbuminemia. Albumin 25% needs to be infused at a slow rate of 2 to 3 mL/min, adjusted to the patient's condition. Albumin may also be beneficial in newborns with hyperbilirubinemia because it will bind with additional bilirubin and reduce the complication of kernicterus.[22]

Administration of 5% and 25% albumin requires strict aseptic and antiseptic handling. Once the container is entered, it must be used immediately or discarded because albumin has no preservatives. Drugs should not be added to albumin nor should albumin be added to IV solutions. Albumin is a good culture medium and although bacterial contamination is rare, the product should be held, the lot number recorded, and the manufacturer and the FDA notified if reactions are suspected. More frequently, adverse reactions are caused by improper administration. Nurses have an important role in assessing the patient's clinical condition, evaluating the patient, and ensuring proper rate of administration.

Both products have been heat treated to eliminate transfusion-transmitted diseases.

Plasma protein fraction is not as highly purified as albumin and consists of 83% albumin and 17% alpha and beta globulins. It is used in a manner similar to albumin

5%. Neither albumin or plasma protein fraction has any clotting factors and should not be considered "plasma substitutes." There is no ABO or Rh matching for albumin or plasma protein fraction.

Factor VIII Concentrate

Concentrates of factor VIII (AHF) are prepared from plasma by a variety of methods. Traditionally, plasma was fractionated by physiochemical techniques to provide factor VIII concentrates. Most recently, factor VIII has been extracted and purified from plasma using monoclonal antibodies to factor VIII. Patients may ultimately be treated with recombinant factor VIII.[23] The newer techniques offer a higher activity of AHF and are less likely to transmit disease, but they are more costly. The levels vary, depending on the technique used to make the component but are usually too low to be useful for treating vWF disease. Various processes used to inactivate viruses have yielded a safer product and greatly decreased the incidences of viral infection after transfusion.

The clinical use of factor VIII concentrate is the treatment of hemophilia A, a congenital deficiency of factor VIII. The stability of the component allows patients to treat themselves at home and maintain a more normal life-style than they have in the past.

Supplied as a lyophilized powder, reconstituted factor VIII concentrate should be administered immediately at a rate of 2 mL/min. Use of the administration set provided with the product is recommended. Direct injection with a syringe is also acceptable.

No ABO or Rh matching is required.

Factor IX Concentrate

Factor IX concentrate is a commercially available lyophilized concentrated complex containing factor IX in addition to factors II, VII, IX, and X, which are vitamin K-dependent clotting factors synthesized in the liver. It is prepared by fractionation from large pools of human plasma. The product is treated by various methods to lower the incidence of transfusion-transmitted disease.

The clinical indication for factor IX concentrate is the prevention and control of bleeding in patients with hemophilia B, also known as Christmas disease. This disorder resembles hemophilia A. Patients have an abnormal gene that causes a defective synthesis of factor IX. Achieving therapeutic levels of factor IX with FFP would require infusion of large volumes. This product is the only concentrated available source for patients with this deficiency. Factor IX is also indicated for treating factor VII or X deficiencies and hemophilia A with factor VIII inhibitors.

The concentrate is provided with a sterile diluent. It should be reconstituted just before administration. The number of units of factor IX is printed on each vial.

The rate of administration is determined by the patient's condition and may be infused by drip or by push but should not exceed 10 mL/min.

Immune Globulin Intravenous

Immune globulin IV is a highly purified solution of human IgG for IV use. Prepared by cold fractionation from large pools of plasma, many preparations are available. Most contain over 90% IgG antibodies and have an approximate half-life of 22 days.

The primary use of immune globulin IV is to supply sufficient amounts of IgG antibodies passively to patients who are unable to produce their own antibodies. Disease states most commonly requiring immune globulin are congenital agammaglobulinemia, severe combined immunodeficiencies, and some clinical situations of acute or chronic ITP. Because IV immune globulin preparations contain no preservatives, administration should begin promptly after the vial is reconstituted. It is recommended to use the infusion kit supplied with the product or transfer contents to a sterile vacuum bottle if one is not supplied. Dosage varies and depends on the patient's response and may be repeated every 3 to 4 weeks. Reactions may occur and appear to be related to the rate. The recommendation for initial infusion is 0.6 to 1.2 mL/kg/h for the first 30 minutes. If tolerated, the rate may be increased to 2.4 mL/kg/h. However, one should refer to manufacturer's guidelines of the specific component being used. Filtration is not required.

Cytomegalovirus immune globulin (CMV-IVIG) is derived from human pooled plasma and contains a high concentration of antibody to CMV. The product is intended to raise the antibody levels of persons exposed to CMV and reduce the incidence of serious CMV disease. The primary clinical indication is for seronegative kidney transplant recipients who receive a kidney from a seropositive donor.

Because CMV-IVIG contains no preservatives, infusion should begin after reconstitution with Sterile Water for Injection and be completed within 12 hours. Dosage will typically begin 72 hours after transplant and taper intermittently for 16 weeks posttransplant.[17] Reactions appear to be rate related. Administration guidelines suggest a maximum rate of 60 mg/kg/h with a volume limit per hour of 75 mL. Transfusionists must refer to manufacturer's guidelines.

Rh Immune Globulin

Rh immune globulin (RhIG) is a concentrate of IgG anti-D derived from plasma. It is administered by intramuscular injection to Rh-negative individuals to prevent Rh alloimmunization after being exposed to Rh-positive cells.

The Rh antibody produced by the Rh-negative mother of an Rh-positive infant is the cause of Rh hemolytic disease of the newborn (HDN). The preparation available, RhoGAM, should be administered within 72 hours after delivery and for other outcomes of pregnancy (abortion, miscarriage) or amniocentesis when a fetal–maternal hemorrhage could occur. Without RhIG protection, the mother has a 7% to 8% risk of developing anti-D. RhIG is also given antepartum at 28 weeks and again postpartum. This prophylaxis reduces the risk of immunization to 0.1%.[3] Mothers are not candidates for RhIG if the fetus is Rh negative or there is evidence of immunization to D not related to antepartum RhIG therapy.[3] Use of RhIG may be appropriate when an Rh-negative recipient receives Rh-positive red blood cells or components, such as platelets or granulocytes, which may contain sufficient cells to cause immunization.

One vial contains 300 µg of anti-D, which will counteract 15 mL of Rh-positive red blood cells transfused.[3] Individual situations will dictate prophylaxis for red blood cell transfusions because the dose required is extremely large and causes discomfort.

Use of RhIG is not associated with viral transmission.[3]

BLOOD ADMINISTRATION

Each year in the United States, approximately 12 million units of whole blood and packed red blood cells are transfused.[24] Because more nurses are responsible for the administration of components, it is particularly important that they be well versed in every phase of the therapy. Nurses should not only be knowledgeable about the administration of components and monitoring patients during and after the transfusion, but they should also be qualified to perform ABO and Rh certification of the components. The patient's safety depends on adherence to specific rules regarding safe administration. Some institutions have delegated the administration of blood and blood components to a restricted group of specially trained nurses, which provides more uniformity in performance of practice. These special groups also act to coordinate activities between transfusion service and patient care units.[5] The transfusionist is responsible for the following:

1. Verifying the presence of a written physician's order for the transfusion
2. Verifying that documented informed consent has been obtained from the patient
3. Explaining the procedure to the patient
4. Verifying ABO and Rh compatibility between donor and recipient
5. Performing procedures relevant to patient–blood identification
6. Inspecting the unit before administration
7. Selecting and using proper technique and equipment
8. Observing the patient for 5 to 15 minutes at the beginning of the transfusion
9. Notifying the attending nurse to monitor the patient throughout the transfusion and for 1 hour after the transfusion
10. Documenting the transfusion according to established policy

Issue and Transfer

Patient–blood identification is of paramount importance in preventing reactions from incompatible blood. The risk of identification errors is reduced by the use of triplicate requisitions or an on-line ordering system. Such requisitions, identifying the patient and indicating the amount and kind of blood and time needed, are sent to the blood bank with the blood sample.

The mode of transfer of blood components to the nursing unit depends on hospital policy. It may involve a pneumatic tube system, a messenger service, hospital personnel, or the individual who will administer the blood. One of the most common causes of hemolytic reaction is the accidental administration of incompatible blood from the wrong container to the patient. To prevent administration of incompatible blood, only 1 U should be transported by a person at a time.

Patient–Blood Identification

Absolute and positive identification of the donor blood and the patient must be made. All personnel handling the blood should be responsible for checking patient–blood identification. The nurse makes the final check and must decide whether to administer the blood or question it. *ABO and Rh compatibility identification* is made by comparing 1) the patient's previous ABO and Rh determination with patient's and donor's ABO and Rh on the compatibility tag and 2) the blood identification number on the blood container with the identification number on the blood tag and the blood unit itself. Some health care facilities have incorporated computer information systems to tie the patient care unit to the blood bank for more reliable checking.

Patient identification is made by checking the name and hospital identification number on the blood tag with the admitting sheet in the patient's clinical record. The patient then must identify himself or herself by complete name. Identity should never be made by addressing the patient by name and awaiting a response. Errors can occur from faulty response of medicated patients. Patients unable to respond should be identified by the primary or attending nurse. Hospital numbers on the identification bracelet must match hospital numbers on the tag to prevent errors in cases of similar names. Any discrepancy must be investigated and corrected before the blood is administered.

Blood must *never* be administered to a patient who has no identification bracelet.

Handling Blood

Barrier protection must be used when exposure to blood may occur. Minimal protection should be gloves when handling any blood component; gowns and protective eyewear may be advisable in emergency and trauma settings. To prevent excessive warming, blood should be administered within 30 minutes of the time it leaves the bank. If blood is not maintained at 1°C (34°F) to 10°C (50°F) while outside the control of the blood bank, it cannot be reissued. Banked blood stored at 1°C (34°F) to 6°C (43°F) will exceed 10°C (50°F) in approximately 30 minutes at room temperature; blood that cannot be administered immediately should be returned to the blood bank within this time.

Blood should never be placed in the patient care unit refrigerators because they are not controlled and contain no alarms to warn of temperature fluctuation.

If warmed blood is ordered, special blood-warming devices that maintain a controlled temperature should be used to warm the blood. Temperatures are not allowed above 37°C. These warming devices should be available in emergency rooms where it is common to administer blood rapidly. Patients receiving cold blood rapidly (ie, 100 mL/min) reportedly have increased incidences of cardiac arrest. Hot water and standard microwave ovens must never be used to warm blood.

Before the blood component is administered, the expiration date should be noted to avoid infusion of an outdated component.

Sodium Chloride Injection, USP 0.9% (normal saline), may be used to initiate the infusion of red blood cells, whole blood, platelets, or leukocytes. Hypotonic or hypertonic solutions should not be used to dilute blood. Extreme hypotonicity causes water to invade the red blood cells until they burst, resulting in hemolysis. Hypertonic solutions dilute blood, resulting in reversal of this process with shrinkage of the red blood cells.

No medication or IV fluid (with the exception of 0.9% sodium chloride) should be added to blood or administered simultaneously through the same set.

Venipuncture

Peripheral veins with an adequate diameter should be used to ensure the flow of viscous components. The lower extremities are avoided in adults because thrombosis and blood pooling may occur. Areas of joint flexion should also be avoided.

Needle-stick reduction devices should be incorporated when accessing any IV system or IV catheter for transfusions to avoid direct needle sticks.

The peripheral IV site should be checked frequently during the infusion for early detection of extravasation. Red blood cells and whole blood can usually be administered through an 18- or 20-gauge catheter although smaller gauges may be used for other components. Often a 23-gauge catheter is used for pediatric patients.

With the sophistication of IV therapy, using centrally placed catheters for the infusion of blood components is acceptable. Increased numbers of peripherally inserted central catheters (PICCs) are being placed in patients receiving long-term IV therapy. In most situations, components will infuse in a timely manner through 20-gauge or larger PICCs. If a dual-lumen catheter has been placed, the larger lumen should be reserved for transfusions. It is necessary to adequately flush the catheter with normal saline at the conclusion of the transfusion. Subclavian and tunnelled catheters or implanted ports are also suitable for the administration of blood and blood components. Use of an electronic infusion device is recommended.

Rate of Infusion

The rate of infusion is governed by the clinical condition of the patient and the viscosity of the component being infused. Infusions should be set at a slow rate for the first 15 minutes to avoid infusion of a large quantity of blood in case of an immediate reaction. Most patients can tolerate infusions of 1 U red blood cells in 1 to 1.5 hours. Patients in congestive heart failure or in danger of fluid overload require infusions given over a longer period of time, but not to exceed 4 hours.

External pressure devices and large-gauge catheters should be used when it is necessary to infuse blood rapidly. Physicians need to be readily available because certain risks are inherent to rapid volume replacement.

Electronic infusion devices designed to administer blood and its components are frequently required for slow rates of infusion to pediatric and neonatal patients.

Blood Filters

A sterile pyrogen-free blood filter of 80 to 170 µm designed to remove debris, including clots, should be used for administration of most blood components. For best results, the entire surface area of the filter should be filled with the component because this provides an improved flow rate. A single filter may be used to infuse 2 to 4 U blood although some institutions have a policy that a new filter is used with each component. Once the blood filter contains debris, it should be discarded. Continued use of such filters may result in bacterial contamination, a slowed rate of infusion, or hemolysis of the blood at room temperature.

Special leukocyte filters for red blood cells and platelets are available and are recommended to prevent febrile nonhemolytic reactions.

Microaggregate filters (20–40 µm) are designed to remove very small aggregates and fibrin. They may be useful in the setting of massive transfusions.

Filters are not required for the infusion of albumin or immune globulin.

Nursing Care

After initiation, the nurse/transfusionist should observe the patient for the initial 5 to 15 minutes of the infusion. Many of the fatal incompatible transfusion reactions produce symptoms early in the course of the infusion. Primary nurses also share a responsibility for safe transfusion administration. They must be familiar with the various transfusion reactions, be able to recognize adverse reactions, and know what procedures to follow.

If venous spasm occurs from the cold blood being infused, a warm pack applied to the vein through which the blood is being infused will relieve the spasm and increase the rate of flow.

Discontinuing the Transfusion

All data relevant to the transfusion should be recorded in the patient's clinical and transfusion records. Note the time the transfusion was complete, the volume of fluid infused, and the condition of the patient. Observation of the patient for 1 hour after the transfusion is recommended. Posttransfusion monitoring of laboratory values ensures that the clinical goal(s) was achieved.

Administration sets used to infuse blood components should be discarded within 24 hours after use. Bacterial growth may occur from the trapped proteins and debris contained in the set.

All transfusion-related equipment should be placed in biohazard waste receptacles. Follow institutional guidelines for observing universal precautions.

TRANSFUSION REACTIONS

Vast improvements in collection and storage methods, together with growing knowledge in the field of immunohematology, have increased the safety of transfusion therapy. However, an inherent risk still exists with every unit of transfused blood. Both the transfusionist and primary nurse should be aware of this fact and be alert to symptoms of untoward events. Reactions to administered blood cannot all be eliminated by ABO and Rh compatibility testing.

Whenever a transfusion reaction is suspected, the transfusion should be terminated and the IV kept open for possible therapeutic treatment. Vital signs should be taken, the physician should be notified, and a blood sample of 10 mL should be sent to the blood bank with the blood container and a completed transfusion reaction report (except for a urticarial reaction). When a hemolytic reaction is suspected, urine should also be sent to the laboratory for urinalysis. Urinary output should be monitored and all urine saved and observed for hemoglobin or bilirubin. Complete documentation of the reaction is important.

Transfusion reactions may be divided into two main classes: immediate and delayed. Both may be further divided into immunologic and nonimmunologic.

Immediate Effects

Immediate adverse effects of transfusion usually occur during or within 1 to 2 hours after the completion of an infusion. Therefore, closely monitor the patient during and after the transfusion to assess and identify signs and symptoms of impending reactions. Most immediate adverse effects are preventable and are caused by improper administration, failure to comply with standards, or lack of knowledge of the procedure or impact of the therapy.

The importance of thoroughly following written procedures and complying with policy are crucial for safe transfusion therapy.

Immunologic

The etiology of these adverse effects in the recipient are antigen–antibody reactions from red blood cells, leukocytes, or plasma proteins. They are usually produced by the body's response to foreign proteins.

Acute Hemolytic Reaction. Acute hemolytic transfusion reactions occur when an antigen–antibody reaction occurs in the recipient caused by an incompatibility between the recipient's antibodies and the donor's red blood cells. Incompatibilities in the ABO blood group system are responsible for most of the deaths from acute hemolytic transfusion reactions.

The interaction of the isoagglutinins and ABO incompatible red blood cells activates the complement, kinin, and coagulation systems. The entire complement system is activated in the ABO mismatch, causing intravascular hemolysis. If the free hemoglobin released from the destruction of red blood cells is greater than the quantity that can combine with haptoglobin in the plasma, the excess hemoglobin filters through the glomerular membrane into the kidney tubules, and hemoglobinuria occurs.

The kinin system is activated by the antigen–antibody complex and produces bradykinin, which increases capillary permeability, dilates arterioles, and causes a fall in systemic blood pressure.

The coagulation system stimulates activation of the intrinsic clotting cascade, causing small clots in the circulation and may trigger disseminated intravascular coagulation (DIC), which in turn can cause formation of thrombi within the microvasculature.

Intravascular hemolytic reactions are often fatal. Investigation of fatal hemolytic transfusion reactions shows that the most common causes are clerical or other identification errors—of the recipient sample sent to the blood blank, of the blood unit, or of the recipient.

Hemolytic transfusion reactions may be accompanied by chills, fever, flushing of face, burning sensation along the vein in which the blood is being infused, lumbar or flank pain, chest pain, frequent oozing of blood at the injection site and surgical areas, or shock. When reactions occur, the transfusion must be stopped at once and the vein kept open with 0.9% sodium chloride. When a Y blood tubing is used, a new setup (container of fluid and a new administration set) should be connected directly to the cannula. DO NOT OPEN THE FLOW TO THE NORMAL SALINE HANGING WITH THE Y BLOOD TUBING. To do so could result in the patient receiving additional incompatible blood cells contained in the Y tubing.

Vigorous treatment of hypotension and promotion of adequate renal blood flow are imperative. Therapy may consist of administration of volume, diuretics, and volume expanders to promote diuresis and to minimize renal damage. Urinary flow rates in adults should be maintained at or over 100 mL/h for at least 18 to 24 hours.[3] Vasopressors, such as dopamine in low doses, dilate the renal vasculature while increasing cardiac output. Their use requires careful monitoring of the patient's urinary flow, cardiac output, and blood pressure. A diuretic agent such as furosemide is recommended to be given concurrently with adequate IV fluid replacement. The drug improves renal blood flow, thus minimizing the possibility of renal tubular ischemia and renal failure. Mannitol is infrequently used because, if ineffective, may cause hypervolemia and pulmonary edema.

The use of heparin therapy for the resulting DIC remains controversial and is dealt with after evaluating all consequences of the acute hemolytic reaction.

One in every 33,000 transfusions accounts for an ABO incompatibility with the recipient. This translates to one per day![26] Prevention is the hallmark of therapy for this severe reaction. This reaction is preventable.

Febrile Nonhemolytic Reaction. Febrile nonhemolytic reactions (FNR) are usually the result of transfusion of cellular components in the absence of hemolysis whereby antileukocyte antibodies in the recipient are directed against the donor's white blood cells.[19] Even though some leukocytes break down rapidly during storage, the membrane fragments are still capable of sensitizing patients in the same manner as intact leukocytes. Patients who have been sensitized by numerous transfusions or multiple pregnancies are more likely to develop FNH.

Febrile nonhemolytic reactions are defined as a rise in temperature of 1°C and usually occur within 1 to 6 hours after the initiation of the transfusion. Febrile reactions may be accompanied by flushing of the face, palpitation, cough, tightness in the chest, increased pulse rate, or chills. As the name implies, no red blood cell hemolysis occurs. Antipyretics are used for treatment. When a patient experiences this reaction, a similar reaction may not occur with the next transfusion.[3] Documentation of the reaction is important for possible prevention of future adverse effects.

Newly developed leukocyte removal filters are increasingly being used for filtration at the bedside. Use of this filter is advised for patients who have had two or more FNH reactions. The filters are an efficient, effective, and convenient method of removing leukocytes and decreasing incidences of FNH; they require minimal inservice to the transfusionist who will administer the component. Other indications for white blood cell reduced components are to prevent or delay alloimmunization to patients who may need transfusion on a long-term basis. This could include hematology and oncology patients.[26] Deglycerolized red blood cells and washed red blood cells are also relatively depleted of leukocytes. All febrile responses should be clinically monitored because other reactions could be occurring.

Anaphylactic Reactions. Fortunately, anaphylactic reactions are rare. They may occur in patients who are IgA deficient and who have developed anti-IgA antibodies.

The two classic signs that an anaphylactic reaction is imminent are symptoms after only a few milliliters of blood or plasma has been infused and absence of fever. The reaction is characterized by bronchospasm, respiratory distress, abdominal cramps, vascular instability, shock, and perhaps loss of consciousness. This medical emergency requires immediate resuscitation of the patient along with administration of epinephrine and steroids.

Prevention includes the use of autologous transfusions or obtaining units from donors who lack IgA. Reducing the plasma content of red blood cell and platelet transfusions may also be effective in reducing the severity of this reaction.

Urticaria. These reactions are relatively uncommon and are based on a hypersensitivity response, probably to protein in donor plasma.

Urticarial reactions are usually mild and characterized by local erythema, hives, and itching. Occasionally, fever may be present. The transfusion is usually interrupted and may be continued after the patient has responded to antihistamine therapy. If the patient develops extensive urticaria or total body rash or fever, the transfusion may have to be discontinued. In these situations, washed or deglycerolized red blood cells may be indicated for future therapy.

Noncardiac Pulmonary Edema. Although this reaction occurs infrequently, it can provoke severe symptoms. The usual etiology is a reaction between donor high-titer antileukocyte antibodies and recipient leukocytes. The reaction can result in leukoagglutination. The leukoagglutinins may become trapped in the pulmonary microvasculature. The reaction causes severe respiratory distress unassociated with circulatory overload and without evidence of cardiac failure. Chest radiography reveals bilateral pulmonary infiltrates consistent with pulmonary edema but without other evidence of left heart failure.

Clinical signs and symptoms other than respiratory distress include chills, fever, cyanosis, and hypotension. Treatment begins by discontinuing the transfusion and providing respiratory support measures. Once the donor has been implicated in such a reaction, that person's plasma should not be used for transfusion.

Nonimmunologic

Immediate nonimmunologic adverse effects are caused by external factors in the administration of blood: bacterial infection of the patient, contamination of the donor blood, improper handling of blood, and administration of a hypertonic fluid with the transfusion. An antigen–antibody reaction is absent.

Circulatory Overload. Circulatory overload may occur when blood or its components are infused too rapidly or given to a patient who has an increased plasma volume. The consequence is hypervolemia. Patients more prone to this adverse effect are the young and elderly and those with cardiac or renal disease.

Symptoms include a pounding headache, dyspnea, constriction of the chest, coughing, and cyanosis. The transfusion must be stopped and the patient placed in a sitting position. Rapid-acting diuretics and oxygen usually relieve the symptoms. If the condition is severe, a therapeutic phlebotomy may be indicated.

Prevention consists of frequent monitoring of those susceptible to congestive heart failure and the administration of concentrated components slowly. This adverse effect is preventable.

Air Embolism. This complication of transfusion therapy has been dramatically reduced with the use of plastic bags. It may result from faulty technique in changing equipment or plastic bags, careless use of Y-type administration sets, or air infused from one of the containers when fluid and blood are being pumped together. If air does enter the patient, acute cardiopulmonary insufficiency occurs.

Symptoms are the same as those for circulatory collapse: cyanosis, dyspnea, shock, and sometimes, cardiac arrest. The infusion should be stopped immediately and the patient turned on the left side, with the head down. This position traps air in the right atrium, preventing it from entering the pulmonary artery; the pulmonic valve is kept clear until the air can escape gradually. It may be necessary for the physician to aspirate the air with a transthoracic needle. This adverse effect is preventable.

Citrate Toxicity. Patients at risk of developing citrate toxicity or a calcium deficit are those who receive large quantities of citrated blood or have severely impaired liver function. The liver, unable to keep up with the rapid administration, cannot metabolize the citrate, which chelates calcium, reducing the ionized calcium concentration. Hypocalcemia may induce cardiac arrhythmia. This adverse effect occurs infrequently but may be encountered in emergency and operating rooms when large amounts of blood (1 U every 5 minutes) and components have been administered. Symptoms of hypocalcemia include tingling of the fingers, muscular cramps, convulsions, hypotension, and cardiac arrest.

Treatment consists of slowing the rate of infusion and the administration of calcium chloride or calcium gluconate solution.

Hypothermia. Hypothermia occurs commonly when large volumes of cold blood are infused rapidly.[20] Rapid infusions may cause chills, hypothermia, peripheral vasoconstriction, ventricular arrhythmias, and cardiac arrest. In many situations, warming blood to 37°C with automatic blood warmers during rapid massive replacement prevents hypothermia. However, time does not always permit the setup of equipment. Many emergency rooms and trauma centers have eliminated blood warmers and instead warm the IV solutions in special regulated warmers. This reaction is preventable.

Bacterial Contamination. Bacterial contamination of blood is the cause of this reaction and may occur at the time of donation or in preparing the component for infusion. In addition to skin contaminants, cold-resistant gram-negative bacteria may contribute to this untoward event. Organisms such as *Pseudomonas* species, *Citrobacter freundii*, and *Escherichia coli* are potential causes. These organisms, capable of proliferating at refrigerator temperatures, release an endotoxin that initiates the reaction. It is potentially fatal when it occurs. Fortunately, it rarely does.

This complication can be prevented by inspecting the unit before administration. Observation of any discoloration of the blood or plasma or obvious clots should be reported.

Clinical manifestations of a septic reaction include high fever, flushing of the skin, "warm" shock, hemoglobinuria, renal failure, and DIC. These signs and symptoms are similar to those of an acute hemolytic reaction, so diagnosis must be made quickly. The transfusion should be discontinued; immediate therapy, including management of shock, steroids, and antibiotics, is required. Cultures obtained of the patient's blood, the suspected component, and all IV solutions will determine whether the bacteremia is caused by the blood or an IV-related infection. This reaction is preventable.

Many of the reactions discussed thus far are preventable. A recent publication notes that "the true incidence of bedside transfusion errors, i.e., those happening when blood products have left the blood bank, is underestimated because published figures rely on reporting of clinically relevant events or on indirect methods."[5] Quality improvement and monitoring measures may assist to avoid error as may more computerized methods of verifying necessary data.

Delayed Effects

These complications occur days, months, or years after the transfusion and usually are the result of alloimmunization or transmitted disease. To a great degree, prevention is unavoidable.

Immunologic

Delayed Hemolytic Reaction. Delayed hemolytic reactions are caused by an immune antibody, produced by the body's response to a foreign antigen. Usually these antibodies are undetectable at the time of transfusion.[4] These reactions are classified as primary and secondary. The primary or initial reaction is generally mild and may occur a week or more after the transfusion. Known as *primary alloimmunization*, it rarely produces symptoms and may be clinically insignificant. The degree of hemolysis depends on the quantity of antibody produced.

The secondary reaction occurs in a patient previously immunized by transfusion or pregnancy. These patients had formed a red blood cell alloantibody in the past, but the level of this alloantibody has become so low that it is serologically undetectable. On a later occasion, when donor red blood cells possessing the corresponding antigen are infused, they provoke the rapid increase in the specific antibody. The incompatible red blood cells survive until ample antibody is present to initiate a rejection response. The reaction is called secondary or *anamnestic (memory) response* and is caused by reexposure to the same antigen. These reactions are rarely caused by ABO incompatibility. A delayed hemolytic reaction is manifested by fever, mild jaundice, and an unexplained drop in the hemoglobin value. These coated cells are removed from the body by the reticuloendothelial system (extravascular hemolysis). A direct antiglobulin test may detect the antibody, but in a rapidly progressing delayed hemolytic reaction, this test may be negative.

Transfusion-Associated Graft-versus-Host Disease. This is a rare complication but presents severe complications and is often fatal. The usual cause is the transfer of immunocompetent T lymphocytes in blood components to a severely immunocompromised patient. It may also occur from transfusion from first-degree family members.[4] The donor lymphocytes engraft and multiply in a severely immunodeficient recipient. These engrafted cells react against the foreign tissue of the host recipient, causing TAGVHD.[3]

Infusions of FFP or cryoprecipitate are largely acellular and do not cause the disease.

The onset of TAGVHD is usually 4 to 30 days after transfusion and begins with a high fever. Generalized erythroderma, anorexia, nausea and vomiting, and profuse diarrhea may follow. TAGVHD is associated with a morbidity and mortality of 75% to 90% of affected patients.[18] Bone marrow suppression and infection are the causes of death.

Prevention is pretransfusion inactivation of lymphocytes by irradiating the blood component and is appropriate to reduce the risk of TAGVHD in the following situations: 1) fetuses receiving intrauterine transfusions; 2) selected immunoincompetent or immunocompromised recipients; 3) recipients of donor units known to be from a blood relative; and 4) recipients who have undergone bone marrow or peripheral blood progenitor cell transplantation.[2]

Nonimmunologic

Hepatitis. Posttransfusion hepatitis (PTH) has been regarded as a complication of receiving blood since the 1940s and remains the most frequent infectious adverse event today.[25] Hepatitis often presents clinically with fever, fatigue, and jaundice but may lead to progressive inflammation of the liver, resulting in cirrhosis or liver cancer. It is predominantly transmitted by the hepatitis B virus (HBV) and the hepatitis C virus (HCV).

Hepatitis B virus accounts for only a small proportion of cases of PTH.[3] The primary reasons for this low incidence are the elimination of paid donors, the screening of donors for behavior that exposes them to viral hepatitis, and the testing of all donations for HBsAg. Increased donor scrutiny and the use of the surrogate tests (ALT) and antibody to hepatitis B core antigen (anti-HBc) may have also contributed to reducing PTH.

The average incubation period for HBV infection is 90 days with a range of 30 to 180 days. The length of the incubation period depends on the amount of HBV the patient has been exposed to and the route of exposure.[3] Hepatitis B can be transmitted directly by percutaneous inoculation of infectious serum or plasma by needle or transfusion of infectious blood. It can be transmitted indirectly by percutaneous introduction of infectious serum, saliva, or semen through minute cuts or abrasions on the skin or mucosal surfaces.[29] It is strongly advised that health care workers be immunized with hepatitis B vaccine to reduce the risk of acquiring HBV infection by these routes. Approximately 1 in 10 health care workers infected with HBV become "chronic carriers."

Manifested by elevated liver enzyme tests, anorexia, fatigue, malaise, dark urine, fever, and jaundice, the disease usually resolves within 4 to 6 weeks.

Greater than 90% of PTH is caused by neither type A nor type B hepatitis viruses and is designated as non-A, non-B (NANB) hepatitis. The major etiologic agent has now been identified as HCV. Approximately 50% of cases are attributable to transfusion, drug abuse, and employment in a health care profession.[1] Since 1990, screening blood donors for antibody to HCV has become routine. The test, an enzyme immunoassay (EIA), is used to identify blood donors who have been exposed to HCV. Donors found to be repeatedly active to EIAs are deferred. Because of the concerns to the lack of sensitivity of the first EIA, a second-generation EIA has been developed and these assays have been used since 1992.[16] Currently no licensed screening confirmatory test to detect HCV is available. A supplemental test, the radioimmunoblot assay, may be used to verify the screening EIA test. Before the test for antibody to HCV was available, surrogate tests were the only means to eliminate donors whose blood might transmit HCV. Donors with elevated ALT concentrations are deferred because these surrogate tests seem to identify donors who have an increased likelihood of transmitting PTH.

Modes of transmission of HCV appear to be similar in part to HBV. However, the route of HCV infection in many infected persons is unknown. The incubation period for HCV is approximately 50 days with a range of 15 to 180 days. The initial and acute illness is usually milder than HBV. Approximately 75% of patients are anicteric. Liver abnormalities persisting after 1 year indicate chronic hepatitis, and progression to cirrhosis in 20% of patients may occur.

Hepatitis from hepatitis A virus (HAV) is an exceedingly rare cause of PTH largely because of the short time that viral particles remain in the circulation.

The incidence of PTH has decreased over the past 10 years because of the screening of donors and the use of laboratory tests to identify at-risk donors.

Cytomegalovirus Infection.   Recognized to be present in blood and transmitted by transfusion, CMV poses little problem to most immunologically intact recipients. Patients predominately at risk of developing serious consequences of the infection are those who have not been previously exposed and are immunoincompetent; these include low birth weight neonates, patients with malignancies who are immunosuppressed as a result of therapy for their disease, patients with acquired immunodeficiency syndrome (AIDS), and recipients of bone marrow and solid candidates. The incidence of clinical disease may double in these patients if CMV-negative components are not issued. Recently, CMV has gained additional attention because it appears to be a possible cofactor in patients with HIV infection.[8] Patients with HIV may have depression of cell-mediated immunity and be predisposed to opportunistic infections. Significant morbidity and mortality result.

Cytomegalovirus is in the herpes family and is transmitted by viable leukocytes in blood. The incubation period after transfusion is 3 to 8 weeks and 3 to 12 weeks after delivery.[29]

As a means to reduce CMV-related infection in specific patient populations, CMV-seronegative blood may be the best avenue of prevention.

Malaria.   Eradicated in the United States and Canada, malaria is still prevalent in South and Central America, Africa, and Asia. The number of cases reported in the United States had increased in the 1980s because of immigrants and travelers. The rate is lower today.[3] Although no practical laboratory test is available, diagnosis of the disease is made by identifying the organism on a blood smear. The patient may develop a high fever, which reflects lysis of the parasite from infected red blood cells and its release into the bloodstream.[22] Malaria parasite can be transmitted by blood transfusion. Prevention is the exclusion of donors from high-risk areas.

After becoming symptomatic, taking antimalarial prophylaxis, or being in an endemic area, donors are deferred for 3 years. Immigrants, refugees, and citizens from endemic countries may be accepted as blood donors 3 years after departure from the area, if they are asymptomatic.[6]

AIDS.   As early as 1983, those involved in transfusion medicine realized that a new disease was capable of being disseminated by transfusion. Aggressive work began to safeguard the blood supply from AIDS. This infectious disease is caused by HIV. HIV is a retrovirus that infects and kills CD4-positive lymphocytes (helper T cells), thereby destroying the immune system. It produces severe immunodeficiency and renders the individual vulnerable to opportunistic infections. The incubation period of the disease may exceed 10 years. As of December 31, 1995, 513,486 cases of AIDS had been reported to the Centers of Disease Control although it is estimated that over one million people are HIV-infected in the United States.[30] All units of blood in the United States and Europe have been tested for antibody to the virus (anti-HIV) since 1985 by enzyme-labeled immunosorbent assays (ELISA). When the ELISA is repeatedly reactive, a Western blot analysis is done as a confirmatory test. As of June 1992, all blood donors in the United States are screened for antibodies to both forms of HIV—HIV-1 and HIV-2. An additional confirmatory test, the recombinant DNA-derived HIV antigen-based immunoblot assay (RIBA-HIV 216) is being used by some agencies as a confirmatory test.[9] The transmission of HIV has been and continues to be a focal point of discussion and research. It is transmitted by three primary routes: 1) sexual contact with an infected person; 2) parenteral exposure to infected blood or blood components (including needles shared among drug users); and 3) perinatally from an infected mother to her child.[14]

Clinical manifestations are weight loss, diarrhea, fever, lymphadenopathy, Kaposi's sarcoma, and opportunistic infections.

Although there has been a significant decrease in patients infected with AIDS by transfusions (1:225,000 per unit of blood transfused)[10,21] or about 2% of those transfused,[7] society is focused on this unfortunate consequence or adverse effect. Data on the disease reflect major geographic incidences. A decline in incidence of AIDS is not predicted at this time. Intense investigation to develop vaccines for active immunization continues. As the sensitivity of screening tests is improved, incidences will become lower.

To reduce the incidence of AIDS in transfusion therapy, the following measures are recommended: 1) the indications for the administration of blood components should be clear; 2) careful screening of donors and testing of donor units should be done; and 3) autologous transfusion should be used whenever possible.

Syphilis. Serologic testing for syphilis (STS) is required by the AABB on all donor blood. Refrigerated blood storage has nearly eradicated the transmission of syphilis because temperatures of 4°C (39°F) have a spirocheticidal effect, thus eliminating treponemas after 72 hours.[3] Most likely, only components stored at room temperature or those administered within 72 hours after donation could transmit the disease.

Other infectious complications of transfusion include babesia, Chagas' disease, toxoplasmosis, and Lyme disease. Specific questions related to these disease are included on donor questionnaires.

AUTOLOGOUS TRANSFUSIONS

Various methods of autologous transfusion are being used to preserve the blood supply, provide a psychological benefit to patients, and minimize exposure to homologous red blood cell transfusions. The techniques of autologous transfusion have increased and are accepted practice for appropriate candidates in a setting based on the patient's clinical condition.[15] Debate continues as the cost benefit of such programs.

Autologous transfusion is the collection, filtration, and reinfusion of one's own blood; thus the donor and recipient are the same individual. The term autologous transfusion takes on several different meanings and methods—each applied to particular clinical conditions. They are predeposit donation (preoperative), hemodilution (perioperative), intraoperative salvage, and postoperative blood salvage.

Autologous transfusion is a conservative approach to transfusion. The primary reasons for this change and increase usage include advances made in technology, blood conservation, public awareness, and the need to decrease the transmission of bloodborne diseases.

Predeposit (Preoperative) Donation

This technique is best used when a patient is planning an elective surgical procedure in which blood use is likely. The patient may plan periodic visits to a donor center for phlebotomies so that the patient's own red blood cells are stored for use later. Autologous transfusions account for an average of 5.7% of collected blood,[12] and, in some donor centers, as much as 20%.[28] As the public is becoming more aware of the hazards of disease transmission by transfusions, many patients will be more at ease knowing that they may receive their own blood through autologous transfusion programs.

Hemodilution (Perioperative)

In this procedure, the patient's blood is collected and stored in the operating room until the end of the procedure. The patient receives infusions of a crystalloid or colloid solution to maintain plasma volume. Commonly done before cardiopulmonary bypass, hemodilution is limited by the patient's blood volume and hemodynamic considerations.[31] The hematocrit is reduced so patients with lung disease or hypo-oxygenation must be monitored closely. After the surgical procedure, the units of blood taken before surgery are infused back to the patient.[31]

Intraoperative Salvage

This method of autologous transfusion has gained acceptance and is being increasingly used. The technique involves aspirating blood from the operative site, washing the blood manually or using cell-washing machines, and reinfusing the blood back to the patient. The process may be performed completely in the operating room. It is most frequently used in cardiovascular, thoracic, orthopedic, neurologic, and hepatic surgery including transplants. The technique makes large volumes of blood immediately available when bleeding occurs in a clean operative procedure. The procedure is contraindicated in patients with malignancy or infection on the basis that reinfusion of "contaminated" cells may disseminate the tumor cells or infectious organism.

Sterile technique is mandated to avoid infectious agents from entering the system. Techniques vary with different equipment. Equipment and personnel costs can be high, but cost savings and improved medical care outweigh the disadvantages. Some programs are developed within hospitals; others may hire outside agencies to do "traveling" intraoperative autologous transfusions.

Postoperative Salvage

This technique involves collecting shed blood from patients after cardiac, trauma, orthopedic, and plastic surgery. Other clinical conditions may also be appropriate. The advantage of this technique is that it can be done for planned surgery or emergency operations and trauma. Blood collected through special equipment is collected, transfused, or discarded within 6 hours of initiating the collection and is not transfused to other patients. This technique is safe, simple, and cost effective. Combined with other methods of autologous transfusions described, the goal of avoiding homologous blood transfusions is closer.

Receiving one's own blood is the safest transfusion, and these modalities will be increasingly encouraged. Careful administration of autologous blood is still required. To avoid any errors, those administering the blood must verify all aspects of the component, including proper identification. Verification procedures should be identical to those for giving homologous transfusions.

In particular, IV nurses can play an important role in autologous transfusion and blood salvage techniques. Specialized training is required to prevent potential complications to collecting, processing and reinfusing the red blood cells. Because of their skill, involvement, and knowledge of transfusions, their abilities translate well to these alternatives to conventional administration of homologous blood component therapy.

The goals of these programs are to conserve blood and prevent reactions, isoimmunization, and disease transmission. The success of these programs requires 1) availability of responsible staff 24 hours a day, especially if more than one machine is available; 2) preferably dedicated operators for each machine; 3) a quality improvement program; and 4) physician support and public awareness programs. The AABB endorses all modalities of blood conservation. All of these methods help in achieving the goals of autologous transfusions.

DIRECTED DONATIONS

Risk of transfusion-transmitted diseases has generated other programs whereby prospective patients may designate their own blood donors. Each donor enters the same process as any other, but the blood is labeled for a specific recipient provided screening tests are appropriate and the unit is compatible. If the blood is not compatible for the intended recipient, the donation is usually entered into the general supply.

The primary benefit of the program may be emotional because the patient feels more comfortable knowing the donors. This aspect is important and appreciated by patients and families. However, no data to date support the idea that the blood is safer than that from anonymous volunteer donors.[3] All of these programs must incorporate finances, staffing, quality assessment measures and legal considerations. Future directions may be written based on what procedures require what type of transfusion therapy or simply, what is the most cost effective.

REFERENCES

1. Alonso, C., Pedroso, M. L., de Sanjose, S., et al. (1994). Hepatitis C virus among blood donors: follow-up study. *Transfusion, 34,* 527–530.
2. American Association of Blood Banks. (1994). *Standards for blood banks and transfusion services* (16th ed., pp. 6, 25, 26, 31, 32). Arlington, VA: Author.
3. American Association of Blood Banks. (1993). *Technical manual* (11th ed., pp. 32, 61, 75, 79, 120, 391, 393, 396, 462, 463, 478, 480, 484–486). Arlington, VA: Author.

4. American Red Cross, Council of Community Blood Centers, American Association of Blood Banks. (1991). *Circular of information for the use of human blood and blood components*, pp. 6–8.

5. Baele, P. L., De Bruyere, M., Deneys, V., et al. (1994). Bedside transfusion errors. *Vox Sang, 66,* 117–121.

6. Balfour, H. H. (1983). Cytomegalovirus disease: Can it be prevented? *Annals of Internal Medicine, 98,* 514–516.

7. Berkman, S. A., & Groopman, J. E. (1988). Transfusion-associated AIDS. *Transfusion Medical Review, 2,* 18–28.

8. Bhumbra, N. A., & Nankeruis, G. A. (1983). Cytomegalovirus infection. *Postgraduate Medicine, 73,* 62–68.

9. Busch, M. P., Amad, Z. E., McHugh, T. M., Chien, D., & Polito, A. J. (1991). Reliable confirmation and quantitation of human immunodeficiency virus type I antibody using a recombinant-antigen immunoblot assay. *Transfusion, 31,* 129–136.

10. Dodd, R. Y. (1994). In: *Blood supply: Risks, perceptions and prospects for the future.* Arlington, VA: American Association of Blood Banks.

11. Guyton, A. C. (1986). *Textbook of medical physiology* (7th ed., pp. 76–77). Philadelphia: W. B. Saunders.

12. Heaton, W. A. L. (1994). Changing patterns of blood use. *Transfusion, 34,* 365.

13. Hollinger, F. B. (1987). Specific and surrogate screening tests for hepatitis. In: S. J. Insalaco & J. E. Menitove (Eds.). *Transfusion-transmitted viruses: Epidemiology and pathology* (pp. 69–86). Arlington, VA: American Association of Blood Banks.

14. Lifson, A. R. (1988). Do alternate modes for transmission of human immunodeficiency virus exist? *Journal of the American Medical Association, 259,* 1353–1355.

15. Maffei, L. M., & Thurer, R. L. (1988). *Autologous blood transfusion: Current issues.* Arlington, VA: American Association of Blood Banks.

16. MacDonald, K. L., Mills, W. A., Wood, R. C., et al. (1994). Evaluation of clinical and laboratory aspects of antibody tests for detection of hepatitis C virus infection in blood donors and recipients from a low-risk population. *Transfusion, 34,* 202–207.

17. Massachusetts Public Health Biological Laboratories. (1990). *Cytomegalovirus immune globulin intravenous (human).* Boston: Author.

18. Mori, S., Matsushita, K., Ozaki, K., et al. (1995). Spontaneous resolution of transfusion-associated graft-versus-host disease. *Transfusion, 35,* 431–435.

19. Oberman, H. A. (1994). Controversies in transfusion medicine: Should a febrile transfusion response occasion the return of the blood component to the blood bank? Con. *Transfusion, 34,* 353–355.

20. Pauley, S. Y. (1987). Massive hemorrhage in trauma. *Journal of the National Intravenous Therapy Association, 10,* 418.

21. Petersen, L. R., Satten, G., Dodd, R. Y., et al. (1992). Current estimates of the infectious window period and risk of HIV infection from seronegative blood donations. In Program and abstracts of the Fifth National Forum on AIDS, Hepatitis and Other Blood-Borne Diseases, Atlanta, GA, March 30, 1992. Princeton, NJ: Symedco, 37.

22. Petz, L. D., & Swisher, S. N. (1989). *Clinical practice of transfusion medicine* (2nd ed., pp. 417, 653, 689, 696, 698). New York: Churchill-Livingstone.

23. Schwartz, R. S., Abildgaard, D. R., Aledort, L. M., (1990). Human recombinant DNA-derived antihemophilic factor (factor VIII) in the treatment of hemophilia A. *New England Journal of Medicine, 323,* 1800–1805.

24. Shulman, I. A., Lohr, K., Derdiarian, A. K., Picukaric, J. M. (1994). Monitoring transfusionist practices: A strategy for improving transfusion safety. *Transfusion, 34,* 11–14.

25. Sirchia, G., Giovanetti, A. M., Parravicini, A., Bellobuono, A., Mozzi, F., Pizzi, M. N., & Almini, D. (1991). Prospective evaluation of posttransfusion hepatitis. *Transfusion, 31,* 301.

26. Sirchia, G., Rebulla, P., Parravicini, A., et al. (1994). Quality control of red cell filtration at the patient's bedside. *Transfusion, 35,* 431–435.

27. Stroup, M., & Tracey, M. (1982). *Blood group antigens and antibodies* (pp. 29–30). Raritan, NJ: Ortho Diagnostics System.

28. Surgenor, D. M., Wallace, E. L., Hao, S. H. S., & Chapman, R. H. (1990). Collection and transfusion of blood in the United States. *New England Journal of Medicine, 322,* 1646–1651.

29. Thompson, J. M., McFarland, G. K., Hirsch, J. E., Tucker, S. M., & Bewers, A. C. (1986). *Clinical nursing* (pp. 1544, 1550). St. Louis: C. V. Mosby.

30. U.S. Dept. Health and Human Services. (1996). *Morbidity and Mortality Weekly Report, 45* (19).

31. Williamson, K. R., & Taswell, H. F. (1991). Intraoperative blood salvage: A review. *Transfusion, 31,* 662.

REVIEW QUESTIONS

1. The antigen in the ABO system that denotes one's blood group is located:
   a. on the red blood cell
   b. in the plasma
   c. in the serum
   d. on body tissue

2. Which of the following may stimulate a reaction?
   I. Antigen A combining with anti-A antibody
   II. Antigen AB combining with anti-AB antibody
   III. Antigen B combining with anti-A antibody
   IV. Antigen D combining with anti-D antibody
   a. I and II
   b. III and IV
   c. I, II, and IV
   d. all of the above

3. Methods to reduce febrile nonhemolytic transfusion reactions include:
   a. washed red cells with standard 80–170 μm filter
   b. packed red cells with leuco-poor filter
   c. packed red cells with standard 80–170 μm filter
   d. all of the above

4. Which of the following are autologous transfusions?
   I. perioperative
   II. preoperative
   III. intraoperative
   IV. postoperative
   a. I and II
   b. I, II, and III
   c. II, III, and IV
   d. all of the above

5. A patient, group O, may receive red blood cells from a donor who is:
   a. group A only
   b. group O only
   c. group A or O
   d. any group

6. A patient, group AB, may receive plasma from a donor who is:
   a. group A, AB, or O
   b. group AB or O
   c. group AB only
   d. any group

7. Intravascular hemolytic reactions are potentially caused by:
   a. ABO incompatibility
   b. Rh incompatibility
   c. ABO and Rh incompatibility
   d. none of the above

8. The primary cause of posttransfusion hepatitis is:
   a. hepatitis A virus
   b. hepatitis B virus
   c. hepatitis C virus

9. A patient experiences the following signs and symptoms 1 hour after a unit of packed red blood cells has been infused: chills, increased pulse rate, fever, flushing of the face. Which of the following adverse reactions is suspected?
   a. citrate toxicity
   b. congestive heart failure
   c. febrile nonhemolytic reaction
   d. anaphylaxis

10. Treatment of choice for this reaction is:
    a. antipyretics
    b. therapeutic phlebotomy
    c. steroids
    d. IV calcium

CHAPTER 18

Drug Administration

Key Terms

Compartment
  model
Half-life
Incompatibility
Idiosyncrasy
Laminar flow

Oxidation
pH
Plasma
  concentration
Pharmacokinetics
Precipitation

Receptor
Reduction
Tachyphylaxis
Therapeutic
  index

ADVANTAGES OF THE IV ROUTE

The vascular route for drug administration offers pronounced advantages:

1. Some drugs cannot be absorbed by any other route; the large molecular size of some drugs prevents absorption by the gastrointestinal route, whereas other drugs, unstable in the presence of gastric juices, are destroyed.

2. Certain drugs, because of their irritating properties, cause pain and trauma when given by the intramuscular or subcutaneous route and must be given IV.

3. The vascular system affords a method for providing rapid drug action.

4. The IV route offers better control over the rate of administration of drugs; prolonged action can be provided by administering a dilute infusion intermittently or over a prolonged period.

5. The vascular route affords a route of administration for the patient who cannot tolerate fluids and drugs by the gastrointestinal route.

6. Slow IV administration of a drug permits termination of the infusion if sensitivity occurs.

HAZARDS

Despite the advantages offered by the vascular route, certain hazards arise that are not found in other forms of drug therapy:

1. The possibility of incompatibilities when one or more drugs are added to the IV solution
2. Speed shock (a systemic reaction to a substance rapidly injected into the bloodstream)
3. Vascular irritations and subsequent hazards
4. Rapid onset of action, with inability to recall a drug once it has entered the bloodstream

Precipitation may occur when one or more drugs are added to parenteral solution.[8] It does not always occur at the time the solution is prepared, which increases the challenge of IV administration. Some drugs, stable for a limited time, degrade and may or may not precipitate as they become less therapeutically active. If administered IV, solutions containing insoluble matter carry the potential danger of embolism, myocardial damage, and effect on other organs such as the liver and the kidneys.

PHARMACOKINETICS

The pharmacokinetic basis of therapeutics requires the drug, route of administration, and frequency to achieve and maintain a proper drug concentration at the *receptor site* wherever it may occur within the body. If an insufficient amount of drug is present at this site, it may appear to be ineffective and therefore be discontinued. Conversely, the right drug may produce toxicity and be discarded simply because excessive amounts are present in the body. Awareness of drug pharmacokinetics is essential in reducing toxicity and potential excess drug dosages.

Therapeutic index is the margin between a drug's therapeutic and toxic concentrations at the receptor site.[6] Pharmacokinetic models describe and predict drug amounts and concentrations in various body fluids and the changes in these quantities over time. Factors influencing the pharmacokinetics of drugs may be found in Table 18-1.

Plasma concentration level (Cp) represents drug that is bound to plasma protein plus drug that is unbound or free. Two factors determine the degree of plasma protein binding. The first is the binding affinity of the drug for the plasma proteins; the second is the number of binding sites presently available or the concentration of plasma protein.[1] An acidic drug such as salicylate or phenytoin may be bound to albumin; a basic drug such as lidocaine or quinidine may be bound to serum globulins. Calculated plasma levels may assist the physician in evaluating effectiveness of therapy. Figure 18-1 notes concentration time curves after IV injection at three different rates.

TABLE 18-1
Factors Influencing the Pharmacokinetics of Drugs

Patient Characteristics	Disease States
Age	Liver disease
Sex	Renal disease
Body weight	Congestive heart failure
Body habits	Infection
Smoking habits	Fever
Alcohol consumption	Shock
Other coingested drugs	Severe burns

The *compartment models* are essential for the IV nurse in understanding pharmacokinetic principles. The "one-compartment model" states that when a drug is introduced into the body, it is rapidly and homogeneously distributed throughout the entire space or compartment. Precise anatomic sites of drug distribution can only be determined by direct analysis of tissue concentrations, which is only possible in animal studies. The "two-compartment model" states that the first compartment is composed of blood volume and those organs or tissues that have a high blood flow. This compartment equilibrates rapidly with administered drug, which is then distributed into the second compartment. Drug behavior in the body depends on both distribution and elimination.[1]

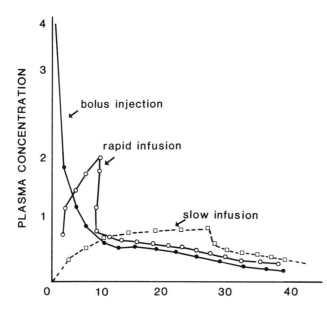

FIGURE 18-1 Concentration time curves following IV injection at three different rates.

TABLE 18-2
Patients Needing Therapeutic Drug Monitoring

Those on combination therapies
Those with renal dysfunction
Those with third-spacing
Those for whom therapeutic failure would prove catastrophic
Those who fail to respond to therapy despite appropriate dosing

THERAPEUTIC DRUG MONITORING

The drug concentration level may be calculated after the initiation of a dosage regimen to ensure that it will produce the target concentration desired. It may also be measured periodically to ensure that it is still producing the desired target concentration or to determine if the therapeutic regimen is failing. Table 18-2 lists the types of patients needing therapeutic drug monitoring; ideal sampling times for various drug classes are listed in Table 18-3.[6]

Loading dose is the initial dose of drug ordered. Designed to produce an immediate target concentration, this is not always practical nor is it safe. An initial dose of lidocaine, calculated to achieve an average target concentration, may produce toxicity after administration as a bolus because it will reach high concentrations in the heart and brain (toxic sites of action) before it is diluted by distribution elsewhere within the body.

Half-life is the time required for the plasma concentration of a drug or the total amount of drug in the body to decline by one-half. Half-life of a drug depends on its volume of distribution (the distribution between the plasma and the various other fluids and tissues and the actual nature of distribution and clearance). During drug administration, it takes one half-life to reach 50% of steady state, two half-lives to reach 75%, three half-lives to reach 87.5%, and four half-lives to reach 93.75%. On discontinuation of a drug or after a drug dosage, it takes one half-life for the plasma concentration to fall to 50% of its initial level.[6]

TABLE 18-3
Ideal Sampling Times

Drug Classification	Sampling Time
Anticonvulsants	Predose
Antidepressants	Predose (lithium, 12 h postdose)
Cardiovascular	Predose (propranolol, 6–10 h postdose [Digoxin])
Antiasthmatics	Predose
Antibiotics	Predose and peak

INCOMPATIBILITIES

The number of possible drug combinations is overwhelming. Manufacturers provide an ever-increasing number of new drug products for the treatment of disease processes. Compounding of drugs for IV administration is generally performed by an IV admixture service as a component of a hospital-based or home infusion pharmacy. Today, admixture programs have expanded their service base, providing compounding service for extended care, ambulatory care, and any clinical setting in which infusion therapies are delivered.

All individuals responsible for mixing and compounding IV drugs must be alert to the hazards involved. Compatibility charts are provided through admixture services to alert the nursing professional to potential problems, particularly when additions to infusions in progress are made on a nursing unit or added in a patient's residence. Factors affecting the compatibility of drugs include order of mixing, quantity of the drug and solution, room temperature, and light. Incompatibilities are not always obvious to the naked eye. They may be classified as physical, chemical, or therapeutic and are described in Table 18-4.

Chemical incompatibilities may be attributed to one or more of several causes. The most common incompatibilities are the result of certain chemical reactions.[2,9,11]

1. *Hydrolysis* is the process in which water absorption causes decomposition of a compound. In preparing solutions of salt, the nurse should understand that certain salts, when placed in water, hydrolyze, forming a strong acid and a weak base or a weak acid and a strong base. Because pH is a significant factor in the solubility of drugs, the increased acidity or alkalinity from hydrolysis of a salt may result in an incompatibility if another drug is added. *Example:* The acid salt sodium bicarbonate when placed in water hydrolyzes to form a strong alkali (sodium hydroxide) and a weak and unstable acid (carbonic acid). Many organic acids are known as weak acids because they ionize only slightly.[7]

2. *Reduction* is the process whereby one or more atoms gain electrons at the expense of some other part of the system.[7]

TABLE 18-4
Types of Incompatibilities

Physical: those in which an undesirable change is physically observed (eg, sodium bicarbonate and calcium chloride forming an insoluble precipitate)[2,9]

Chemical: those occurring in the molecular structure or pharmacologic properties of a substance. *Note:* They may or may not be physically observed (eg, penicillin and ascorbic acid lowering the pH).

Therapeutic: those in which an undesirable reaction results from the overlapping effects of two drugs given together or closely together (eg, penicillin and tetracycline inhibiting the bactericidal effect of penicillin)

TABLE 18-5
Factors Affecting Stability of IV Drugs and Solutions

1. Precipitation of parenteral solution
   - Some commonly prescribed drugs precipitate when added to IV solutions.
   - Differences in the physical and chemical properties of each of these solutions may affect the stability of any drug introduced.
   - A compound soluble in one solution may precipitate in another. Sodium ampicillin deteriorates in acid solutions. This drug, when added to isotonic sodium chloride at a concentration of 30 mg/mL, loses less than 10% activity in 8 h. However, when it is added to 5% dextrose in water, usually a more acid solution, its stability is reduced to a 4-h period.

2. pH
   - A broad pH range (3.5–6.5) of dextrose solutions is allowed by the United States Pharmacopeia (USP). A drug may be stable in one bottle of dextrose 5% in water and not in another.[2]

3. Additional drugs
   - One drug may be compatible in a solution, but a second additive may alter the established pH to such an extent as to make the drugs unstable.[6]

4. Buffering agents in drugs
   - Presence of buffers or antioxidants, which may cause two drugs, however compatible, to precipitate. For example, ascorbic acid, the buffering component of tetracycline, lowers the pH of the product and therefore may accelerate the decomposition of a drug susceptible to an acid environment.

5. Preservatives in the diluent
   - Sterile diluents for reconstitution of drugs are available with or without a bacteriostatic agent.
   - The bacteriostatic agents usually consist of parabens or phenol preservatives.
   - Certain drugs, including nitrofurantoin, amphotericin B, and erythromycin, are incompatible with these preservatives and should be reconstituted with sterile water for injection.

6. Degree of dilution
   - Solubility often varies with the volume of solution in which a drug is introduced. For example, tetracycline hydrochloride, mixed in a small volume of fluid, maintains its pH range over 24 h. However, when added to a large volume (1 L), it degrades after 12 h, becoming less therapeutically active.

7. Period of time solution stands
   - Decomposition of substances in solution is proportional to the length of time they stand. For example, sodium ampicillin with the high pH of 8–10 becomes unstable when maintained in an acid environment over a period of time.

8. Order of mixing
   - The order in which drugs are added to infusions often determines their compatibility.

9. Light
   - Light may provide energy for chemical reactions to occur.
   - Certain drugs, such as amphotericin B and nitrofurantoin, once diluted must be protected from light.[6]

10. Room temperature
    - Heat provides energy for reactions.
    - After reconstitution or initial dilution, refrigeration prolongs the stability of many drugs.

3. *Oxidation* is the corresponding loss of electrons occurring when reduction takes place. Antioxidants are often used as preservatives to prevent oxidation of a compound.[7]

4. *Double decomposition* is the chemical reaction in which ions of two compounds change places and two new compounds are thus formed.[7] A great many salts act by double decomposition to form other salts and probably represent the largest number of incompatibilities. *Example*: Calcium chloride is incompatible with sodium bicarbonate; the double decomposition results in the formation of the insoluble salt calcium carbonate.

PH AND ITS ROLE IN DRUG STABILITY

Because pH plays an important role in the solubility of drugs, it may be well to define it. pH is the symbol for the degree of concentration of hydrogen ions or the acidity of the solution. The weight of hydrogen ions in 1 L pure water is 0.0000001 g, which is numerically equal to 10^{-7}. For convenience, the negative logarithm 7 is used. Because it is at this concentration that the hydrogen ions balance the hydroxyl ions, a pH of 7 is neutral. Each unit decrease in pH represents a tenfold increase in hydrogen ions.

It appears likely that the largest number of incompatibilities may be produced by changes in pH.[7] Precipitation occurs when a compound is insoluble in solution. The degree of solubility often varies with the pH. A drastic change in the pH of a drug when added to an IV solution suggests an incompatibility or a decrease in stability. Solutions of a high pH appear to be incompatible with solutions of a low pH and may form insoluble free acids or free bases. A chart denoting the pH of certain drugs and certain solutions to be used as a vehicle is helpful in warning of potential incompatibilities.

Factors Affecting Stability or pH

Many factors may affect the stability or pH of drugs (Table 18-5 p. 425).

VASCULAR IRRITATION

The hazards of IV therapy can be reduced by taking adequate precautions.

Vascular irritation is a significant hazard of drugs administered IV. Any irritation that inflames and roughens the endothelial cells of the venous wall allows platelets to adhere; a thrombus is formed. Thrombophlebitis is the result of the sterile inflammation. When a thrombus occurs, the inherent danger of embolism is always present.

If aseptic technique is not strictly followed, septic thrombophlebitis may result from bacteria introduced through the infusion cannula and trapped in the thrombus. This is much more serious because of the potential dangers of septicemia and acute bacterial endocarditis.

Preventive Measures

The following precautions must be observed to diminish the potential hazards of vascular irritation:

1. Veins with ample blood volume should be selected when infusing hypertonic solutions or solutions containing irritating compounds.

2. The cannula should be appreciably smaller than the lumen of the vein. A large cannula may occlude the lumen, obstructing the flow of blood; the solution then flows undiluted, irritating the wall of the vein.

3. The venipuncture should be performed at the distal end of the extremity to allow each successive puncture to be executed proximal to the previous. Hypertonic solutions, when allowed to flow through a traumatized vein, cause increased irritation and pain.

4. Veins in the lower extremities are susceptible to trauma and should be avoided.

5. Isotonic solutions should, when possible, follow hypertonic solutions to flush irritating substances from the veins.

6. The rate of infusion may contribute to the irritation. In a large vein, slow administration permits greater dilution of the drug with the circulating blood. In a small vein lacking ample circulating blood, a slow drip prolongs the irritation, increasing the inflammation.

7. Prolonged duration of an infusion increases the risk of phlebitis. After a 24-hour period the danger increases. Periodic inspection of the injection site to detect developing phlebitis is important. After 48 to 72 hours, the injection site should be changed consistent with institutional policy.

8. Precautions should be observed to avoid administering solutions containing particulate matter by:
   a. Proper reconstitution and dilution of additives
   b. Inspection of parenteral fluids before administration
   c. Use of freshly prepared solutions
   d. Use of a set with a filter when danger of precipitation exists
   e. Periodic inspection of solutions containing additives
   f. Avoidance of administration of cloudy solutions unless affirmed by the manufacturer

APPROVED DRUG LISTS

Lists of drugs approved for administration by nursing professionals in all clinical environments in which care is provided must be readily available. In the inpatient setting, the institution's pharmacy and therapeutics committee is the group that generally approves such lists. IV nursing professionals are often members of this committee, and protocols are brought to this group for approval before a drug is added to the list. The committee ideally provides a list of approved drugs for administration by professional nurses, a list of drugs approved for addition to infusions in progress, and a list of investigational agents approved for administration.[4] In the alternative care environment, home health agencies and clinics should also develop lists that are subsequently approved by their medical directors before acceptance by the nursing community.

Controlled Substances Act

This act established five categories of controlled substances, known as schedules, based on their possible potential for abuse, the medical indications, and the potential for dependence on the drug. Many of the drugs administered for pain control are Schedule II drugs with specific prescription and record-keeping requirements.[2]

THE PHYSICIAN'S RESPONSIBILITY

A licensed physician writes and signs all orders for IV drugs and solutions. A complete order includes the drug or solution, route of administration, rate of administration in milliliters per hour, or the approximate length of time of administration of the infusion.

The physician also administers the drugs not on the approved drug list. The determination of who may administer IV drugs is based on nurse practice acts (see Chapters 2 and 4).

ADMIXTURE

Intravenous additives and solutions are best prepared in an IV additive station of the institution's pharmacy. Aseptic technique is best observed when a "clean room" approach is used. A laminar flow hood, proper illumination, and handwashing facilities are readily available in such a setting.

Use of Laminar Flow

Laminar flow is airflow in which the entire body of air within a confined area moves with uniform velocity along parallel flow lines.[3,4] Laminar flow hoods have a vital role in eliminating the hazard of airborne contamination of IV solutions and admixtures. Nurses should be familiar with the general operating guidelines of the hood. Vertical and horizontal hoods are available. Laminar flow hoods should be used within state and federal guidelines as well as the recommendations of the American Society of Health System Pharmacists.

Extreme care in the preparation of solutions diminishes the risk associated with IV therapy.

The IV policy and procedure addressing admixing should define potential hazards, compatibility, stability requirements, and the types of admixtures within the scope of practice. Safeguards should be implemented to protect personnel from potential health hazards associated with the admixing of medications.

1. *Aseptic technique is imperative.* Bacterial and fungal contamination of drug products and parenteral solutions must be avoided.
2. *Proper dilution of lyophilized drugs is essential.* Two special cautions to ensure complete solubility in the reconstitution of drugs must be observed.
   a. The specific diluent recommended by the manufacturer should be used.
   b. The drug should be initially diluted in the volume recommended.
3. *Introduction of extraneous particles into parenteral solutions must be avoided.* Fragments of rubber stoppers are frequently cut out by the needles

used and accidentally injected into solutions. Large-bore (15-gauge) needles are practical for use in the nurses' station and appear to have fewer disadvantages than the smaller needles.

    a. Smaller needles may encourage particles that may be difficult to see on inspection.

    b. The small particles may be of a size capable of passing through the indwelling cannula.

    c. Filter aspiration needles, used when preparing admixtures, can remove particles.

4. A solution that on inspection contains fragments of rubber must be discarded.

Procedure in Compounding and Administering Parenteral Solutions

The following steps should be carried out in the preparation of solutions for infusion:

1. Inscribe order for drug additive directly from original order to medication label.

2. Substantiate drug orders with the drug product and the parenteral solution.

3. Inspect solution for extraneous particles.

4. Check drug product for:

    a. Expiration date—Outdated drugs should not be used because loss of potency or stability may have occurred.

    b. Method of administration

        (1) Intramuscular preparations are not usually used for IV administration; they may contain certain components such as anesthetics or preservatives not meant for administration by the vascular route.

        (2) Some are packaged in multidose vials, which may contribute to contamination.

        (3) The dosage by the intramuscular route may not coincide with that for IV use.

5. With an accepted antiseptic, clean rubber injection site of both the drug product and the diluent.

6. Use sterile syringe and needle.

7. Reconstitute according to manufacturer's recommendation. See Box 18-1 for a list of drugs that have increased adsorption when infused in polyvinylchloride (PVC) containers.[8]

8. Check diluted drug for complete solubility before adding to parenteral solution.

9. After adding to solution, invert solution container to mix the additive completely.

10. Clearly and properly label solution container with:

    a. Name of patient

    b. Drug and dosage

Box 18-1
Drugs With Increased Adsorption When Infused
via PVC Containers

Hydralazine (Apresoline)

Insulin

Nitroglycerin

Phenothiazine tranquilizers (Thorazine, Compazine)

Vitamin A acetate (nonpalmitate form)

Warfarin (Coumadin)

---

    c. Date and time of compounding

    d. Expiration date

    e. Signature

11. As an added precaution to prevent errors, recheck label with used drug ampules before discarding ampules.

12. Inspect solution for precipitates; if any precipitates are present, discard the solution.

13. Substantiate identity of patient with solution prepared.

14. Perform venipuncture consistent with institutional policy and standards of the Intravenous Nurses Society.[4]

15. Observe patient for a few minutes after the initial IV administration of any drug that may cause anaphylaxis.

16. Use added caution in administering any drug whose fast action could produce untoward reactions.

17. Ensure first-dose delivery of drug in a clinically monitored environment.

18. Consideration should be given to the use of latex gloves in preparing medications and in administering IV therapy. The incidence of latex allergies has caused manufacturers of gloves to create alternative glove materials to lessen this concern.

General Safety Rules

The following safety rules for preparation and IV administration of drugs by nurses should be adhered to at all times:

1. Nurses will, on written order, prepare and administer only those solutions, medications, and combinations of drugs approved in writing by the pharmacy and therapeutics committees.

2. No IV infusion that is cloudy, discolored, or contains a precipitate should be given.

3. All IV infusions must be used or discarded within 24 hours of the time the container is opened.

4. Any question regarding chemical compatibility or the relative safety of any drug added to an IV infusion should be directed to the director of the pharmacy.

DRUG DELIVERY SYSTEMS

Manufacturers have kept pace with demands for improved drug delivery systems for use in all clinical settings in which infusion therapy is administered. Standard methods of drug delivery and terminology still apply.[10]

Intermittent infusion allows drugs to be administered on an intermittent basis through a slow keep-open infusion using a secondary container, single-dose additive, or multidose admixture connected to a controlled-volume set. The intermittent infusion may also be given through a self-contained administration system such as an elastomeric pump. Intermittent infusions are often given through an *intermittent infusion device* (*heparin lock*) to conserve veins, allow freedom of motion between infusions, and provide a minimal amount of infusate for the patient whose intake may be restricted. Peripheral and central IV catheters are adaptable as intermittent infusion devices by the addition of a catheter plug or resealable adapter. Patency of these lines is maintained by administering an amount of flush solution sufficient to fill the internal diameter of the line in use. Dilute heparin solution (hence, heparin lock) is most often used. Saline solution may also be used, and the use of antibiotic flush in the immunocompromised patient is gaining support in the medical and nursing communities.

Intravenous push is the direct injection of a medication into the vein. It may be administered through the distal Y site of an administration set, through the intermittent infusion device, or via cannula. The terms "IV push" and "bolus" may be confusing. Drugs such as radiopaque dye used to visualize the cardiac chamber must be injected as a bolus (defined as a discrete mass). Most medications ordered as an IV push or bolus must be administered slowly, up to 30 minutes, depending on the drug itself. Rapid injection increases the drug concentration in the plasma, which may reach toxic proportions, flooding the organs rich in blood—the heart and the brain—and resulting in shock and cardiac arrest. The rate of administration, included with the order for the medication, can reduce any misconceptions and prevent the potential risk of a life-threatening reaction from too-rapid administration of the drug.

Because the IV push allows instant increased drug levels in the blood, it offers immediate relief to the patient. Nurses in many special care units are trained and authorized to administer specific IV pushes. In the past, the IV push was restricted to the intensive care unit, where the patient was monitored and where a potential crisis might arise requiring its immediate use in the absence of a physician. Today, nurses frequently administer IV push injections.

Many drugs, given as IV injections, can be potentially dangerous to the patient. The nurse must understand the action of the drug and assess the patient's condition before administering the medication (see Response to Treatment).

Continuous administration is the term applied to medications mixed in a large volume of infusate and infused over a time period in excess of 2 hours.[11]

Decreased tolerance to the drug can result from factors in the patient's condition:[4]

1. Decreased cardiac output
2. Reduced renal flow or poor glomerular filtration
3. Diminished urinary output
4. Pulmonary congestion
5. Systemic edema

Greater dilution of the drug and a longer injection time can prevent drug accumulation, reduce venous irritation caused by a low pH, and allow time to assess the patient's response and detect early reactions. Use of the manufacturer's recommended diluent is most important because different drugs require different diluents.

Response to Treatment

Knowledge of the expected therapeutic effects of the medication, the recommended dosage range, the side effects, and the toxic symptoms is essential.

Side effects may be manifest as gastrointestinal distress including nausea, vomiting, and diarrhea; as allergic skin reactions; and as central nervous system dysfunction.[5]

Major reactions may consist of respiratory distress, anaphylaxis, cardiac arrhythmias, and convulsions.

Reactions must be detected and reported at once so that proper treatment can be administered (Table 18-6).

TABLE 18-6
Untoward Drug Responses

Response	Clinical Effect	Example
Accumulation	Rate of administration greater than rate of metabolism	Usual adult dose of gentamicin is administered to a renal failure patient
Dependence	Continued administration of drug required to avoid withdrawal symptoms	Visible tremors, restlessness occur in patient receiving hydromorphone
Drug allergy	Hypersensitivity; adverse response to drug resulting from previous exposure	Penicillin administered to a patient with penicillin allergy
Idiosyncrasy	Unpredictable response not attributed to hypersensitivity	Development of aplastic anemia in patient receiving chloramphenicol
Tachyphylaxis	Rapidly developing drug tolerance	May occur after administration of nitroprusside
Tolerance	Patient requires increasing amounts of drug to gain some therapeutic effect	Pain unrelieved by morphine sulfate infusion

TABLE 18-7
List of Available Antidotes

Drug	Clinical Indications
Lidocaine hydrochloride (Xylocaine)	Ventricular arrhythmias; certain hyperactivity
Epinephrine (Adrenalin)	Relief of hypersensitivity reactions; respiratory distress caused by bronchospasm; cardiac arrest after anesthesia reaction
Diphenhydramine hydrochloride, USP (Benadryl)	Allergic skin manifestations
Diazepam (Valium)	Convulsions
Trimethobenzamide hydrochloride (Tigan)	Antiemetic agent

Antidotes

Nurses who administer IV medications should have a knowledge of various antidotes and their use.

Emergency supplies of antidotes should be readily available. Many are available in prefilled syringes for emergency use. Sterile cartridge needle units, with accurately machine-measured doses, provide a closed-injection system ready for instant use (Table 18-7).

IMPORTANT CHECKPOINTS IN IV DRUG ADMINISTRATION

The Drug

1. Understand the expected therapeutic effect of the medication.
2. Know the recommended dosage range and the length of time required for administration.
3. Understand the side effects and toxic symptoms that can occur.
4. Be knowledgeable in the use of the proper antidote and its location.

The Patient

1. Make positive identification of the patient. Do not rely on the patient's verbal identification of himself or herself.
2. Ascertain allergy history (food and drug).
3. Assess the patient's condition and be aware of any factors that can affect the drug action.
4. Know what medications the patient is receiving; be aware of therapeutic incompatibilities that may occur between any other medication the patient is receiving and the IV push medication.
5. Watch for the patient's response during and after the injection.

Preparation of the Medication

1. Check and recheck the order with the drug label.
2. Check the expiration dates of the drug and of the diluent.
3. Use the drug manufacturer's recommended diluent.
4. Clarify any questions or doubts with the patient's physician.

The Injection

1. Make sure that the cannula is within the lumen of the vessel.
2. Make sure that the drug is compatible with the IV solution if it is administered through a primary line. If incompatible, clamp the set and flush the injection port with compatible fluid. Do not use sterile water.
3. Ascertain the compatibility of the medication with heparin when a heparin lock is used. If incompatible, flush the lock with a compatible fluid before and after the IV injection.
4. Administer the medication at an evenly divided rate over the length of time recommended by the manufacturer, using a watch with a second hand.
5. Document the medication, time administered, dosage, time span for administration, any required flushing, the patient's response, and your initials.

Responsibilities of the Health Care Facility

Any institution that authorizes nurses to administer IV medications should provide:

1. Written policies for the IV injection of medications by nurses
2. A list of drugs with the recommended dosage range and rate of administration for each drug
3. A list of drugs that may be incompatible with IV injection medications
4. An educational agenda that includes information on the major reactions of the medications, their antidotes, their proper usage, nursing implications for use of drugs, and assessment and monitoring of patients

Drug delivery systems today provide a wealth of administration sets, delivery vehicles, and approaches to safe delivery of infusion therapies to patients. Each nursing professional *must* assume responsibility for becoming familiar with specific equipment used by the institution to provide safe drug therapy for all patients.

DRUG CALCULATIONS

An integral component of IV nursing practice is the ability to perform the mathematical calculations required to administer correct doses of medication and solution to patients. Accuracy in the administration of medications is a special concern when medications are administered IV.

Flow Rate Calculations

Flow rate calculations require the following base of information: amount of solution to be infused, duration of the administration, and drop factor of the set to be used. First, determine the amount of solution to be administered; then divide that number by the delivery time:

$$\frac{1000 \text{ mL}}{8 \text{ h}} = 125 \text{ mL/h}$$

Next, note the drop factor of the set being used. A macrodrip set takes 10, 15, or 20 drops to deliver 1 mL solution.

$$\frac{\text{No. drops/mL of set}}{60 \text{ (min in an h)}} \times \text{total hourly volume} = \text{no. drops/min}$$

$$\frac{\text{mL/h} \times \text{drop factor of set}}{60} = \text{drops/min}$$

For microdrip or pediatric systems, the equation is:

$$\frac{\text{mL/hr} \times \text{drop factor}}{60} = \text{drops/min}$$

Drug Dosage Calculations

Ratio and proportion or "desired over have" (D/H) may be easily applied to calculation of drug dosages for infusion therapy.[12] Rate of administration of IV drugs may be calculated in units per hour. For example, there are 12,500 U heparin sodium in 250 mL IV solution. The dose ordered is 800 U/h.

$\times$ = 250 divided by 12,500

$\times$ = 0.02

Then, calculate the rate of the prescribed dosage:

0.02 mL $\times$ 800 U = 16 mL/h

In this example, you have 200 mg drug in 500 mL of 5% dextrose in water. You want to know the number of milligrams of drug your patient is receiving per hour. Determine the amount of drug per milliliter of solution by placing D/H or:

$$\frac{500}{20} = 25$$

$$\frac{200}{25} = 8 \text{ mg/h}$$

Percent Solutions

The relationship between the amount of solute and the total quantity of solution is expressed as a percentage or ratio. Percentage strength of solution may be calculated in one of three ways:

1. Percent weight in weight (W/W)—the weight of the solute (drug) compared to the weight of the solution (g drug/100 g solution)

TABLE 18-8
Phases of Clinical Trials

---

1. Phase I: Clinical Pharmacology and Therapeutics
   a. Evaluate drug safety.
   b. Determine an acceptable single drug dosage or levels of patient tolerance for acute multiple dosing.
2. Phase II: Initial Clinical Investigation for Therapeutic Effect
   a. Evaluate drug efficacy.
   b. Conduct a pilot study.
3. Phase III: Full-Scale Evaluation of Treatment
   a. Evaluate the patient population for which drug is intended.
4. Phase IV: Postmarketing Surveillance
   a. Provide additional information about the efficacy or safety profile.

---

2. Percent weight in volume (W/V)—the weight of the solute compared to the volume of the total solution (g drug/100 mL solution)
3. Percent volume in volume (V/V)—the volume of the solute compared to the volume of the total solution (mL drug/100 mL solution)[12]

EXPIRATION DATES

Drug container expiration dates identify the date when a medication or product is no longer acceptable for use. Institutional policy and procedure should state that medications should not be administered beyond their expiration dates. Expiration dates should be verified by the nursing professional before drugs and infusates are given to patients.

ADMINISTRATION OF INVESTIGATIONAL DRUGS

State and federal regulations govern the administration of investigational agents. Signed informed consent is required before patients can participate in the investigation. An informed consent must be written by the investigator, approved by the insti-

---

TABLE 18-9
Elements of Informed Consent

- Written by the investigator
- Approved by the institution's review board or ethics committee
- Signed by the subject (patient or volunteer) or authorized representative
- Witnessed

---

tutional review board, signed by the subject, and witnessed. Before approval by the United States Food and Drug Administration (FDA), drug studies are conducted in four stages (Table 18-8).[2]

Policies and procedures should be developed pertaining to the administration of investigational agents, regardless of the clinical setting in which care is provided. Table 18-9 provides elements of informed consent.[2]

REFERENCES

1. American Hospital Formulary Service. (1995). Bethesda, MD: American Society of Health System Pharmacists.
2. Baldwin, D. (1995). Pharmacology. In J. Terry (Ed.), *Intravenous therapy clinical principles and practice* (p. 191). Philadelphia: W. B. Saunders.
3. Edward, M. (1967). pH—An important factor in the compatibility of additives in intravenous therapy. *American Journal of Hospital Pharmacy, 24,* 442.
4. Revised intravenous nursing standards of practice. (1990). *Journal of Intravenous Nursing* (Suppl.), S52–S53.
5. McGill, D. (1973). Giving IV push. *Nursing,* 73(3) 15–18.
6. Needham Clinical Laboratories. (1983). *Therapeutic drug monitoring* (p. 11). Needham Heights, MA: Author.
7. Pelissier, N. A., & Burgee, S. L. (1968). Guide to incompatibilities. *Lippincott's Hospital Pharmacy, 3,* 15.
8. Phillips, L. D. (1993). *Manual of IV therapeutics* (pp. 369–370). Philadelphia: F. A. Davis.
9. Sackheim, G. L., Lehman, D. D., & Schultz, R. M. (1978). *Laboratory chemistry for the health sciences* (3rd ed., pp. 70, 71, 79). New York: Macmillan.
10. Weinstein, S. M. (1992). Electronic drug delivery in the 1990s and beyond: A nursing perspective. *Pharmacy and Therapeutics, 17*(2), 228–231.
11. Weinstein, S. M. (1990). Math calculations for intravenous nurses. *Journal of Intravenous Nursing, 13*(4), 231–236.
12. Weinstein, S. M. (1991). *Nurses' handbook of intravenous medications* (pp. 605–606). Philadelphia: J. B. Lippincott.

REVIEW QUESTIONS

1. Chemical interactions that cause the most common incompatibilities include all of the following EXCEPT:
   a. hydrolysis
   b. decomposition
   c. reduction
   d. oxidation

2. The process that causes certain salts, when placed in water, to decompose, thereby altering the pH is:
   a. decomposition
   b. hydrolysis
   c. oxidation
   d. reduction

3. Factors that may affect the pH of drugs include all of the following EXCEPT:
   a. additional drugs
   b. buffering agents
   c. body temperature
   d. order/method of mixing

4. To diminish the potential hazards of vascular irritation, the nursing professional should do which of the following?
   a. avoid veins in lower extremities
   b. use a cannula smaller than the lumen of a vessel
   c. use the largest vein possible
   d. use the largest cannula possible

5. Which of the following are nursing responsibilities in the administration of drugs that potentially cause anaphylaxis?
   a. question patient regarding sensitivity
   b. observe patients following initial dose
   c. ensure administration of initial dose in a monitored environment
   d. have physician administer the drug

6. What special cautions should be observed to reduce the risk of particulate matter?
   a. dilute lyophilized drugs
   b. use filter as needed
   c. avoid use of powdered drugs
   d. observe before administration

7. Which of the following are advantages of IV administration?
   a. quicker drug action
   b. avoids reabsorption problems associated with gastrointestinal tract
   c. useful for patients without functioning gastrointestinal tract
   d. reduces trauma associated with intramuscular and subcutaneous delivery

8. Which of the following best describes laminar flow?
   a. entire body of air within confined area moves with uniform velocity along parallel flow lines
   b. guarantee elimination of airborne bacteria
   c. guidelines for use are provided by the CDC
   d. 50% of the air in a confined area moves along vertical flow lines

9. Patients in need of therapeutic drug monitoring include those with:
   a. combination therapies
   b. renal dysfunction
   c. skin disorder
   d. third-spacing

10. Factors influencing the pharmacokinetics of drugs include all of the following EXCEPT:
    a. smoking
    b. alcohol
    c. habitus
    d. height

CHAPTER 19

Pain Management

Key Terms

Analgesia	Peristaltic	Systemic
Epidural	Implanted	Sympathetic
Intrathecal	Opioids	Septum

ACUTE PAIN

Acute pain is caused by an illness, injury, or surgery. This type of pain gradually improves as the body heals. Acute pain affects millions of patients worldwide. If it is not managed properly, acute pain increases the cost of health care by increasing the length of hospitalization, increasing the length of time in intensive care settings, and increasing patient morbidity and mortality. Effective control of acute pain is one of the most important issues in postoperative care today.[2] The following factors influence the incidence, intensity, and duration of postoperative pain:

- Site, nature, and duration of surgical procedure
- Type of incision
- Degree of intraoperative trauma
- Physiologic and psychological features of the patient
- Preoperative preparation
- Amount of preoperative pain
- Presence of complications
- Anesthetic management before, during, and after surgery
- Quality of postoperative care

Box 19-1
Options for Pain Control
- Systemic analgesics and adjuvant drugs (administered orally, intramuscularly, IV, subcutaneously, by continuous infusion, or as patient-controlled analgesia)
- Intraspinal opioids
- Regional analgesia
- Electrical analgesia through transcutaneous electrical stimulation or electroacupuncture
- Psychological analgesia in the form of hypnosis, relaxation techniques

---

The amount of postoperative pain varies among individuals. We must pay attention to the needs of each patient to control the pain effectively. We must be cognizant of individual variability and listen to what the patient is telling us. We cannot assume that, because a particular surgery is performed, the patient will experience an expected amount of pain. Postoperative pain is more severe after intensive surgery such as upper abdominal, intrathoracic, renal, and lower abdominal surgery; extensive surgery of the spine; and surgery of the major joints and of the large bones in the hand and foot.

We are fortunate today to have an abundance of innovative options for postoperative pain management. Acute pain services have been developed in health care institutions nationwide to provide daily assessment and intervention. Box 19-1 lists the pain control treatment options available.

The importance of quality postoperative pain control cannot be emphasized enough. When an individual's pain is not well controlled, the sympathetic system becomes dominant. It commands the body to produce more glucocorticoids and catecholamines. This, in turn, imposes an increased workload on the heart. Other physical stresses include a more rapid respiratory rate with shallower respirations, hyperglycemia, and decreased peristaltic action. These changes lead to postoperative complications such as hypoventilation, hypoxemia and atelectasis, cardiac arrhythmias, congestive heart failure, deep-vein thrombosis, and paralytic ileus. Postoperative pain control also influences the ability to cough, deep breathe, and ambulate after major surgery. Fortunately, much progress has been made in the field of postoperative pain management over the last few years.

Box 19-2
Opioid Receptors
1. Mu
2. Kappa
3. Sigma
4. Delta
5. Epsilon

CHRONIC PAIN

Chronic pain is defined as pain that either remains at the same level of intensity or becomes more intense over time, instead of healing or fading. It is associated with progressive cancer and long-term disability or illnesses. Chronic pain is complex and cannot be managed simply with one treatment. The technologic expertise and knowledge the IV nurse has in infection control assists the team to care for patients using highly technologic means of pain control.

Patients who benefit from the use of pain control technology for the treatment of chronic pain include patients with central nervous system or spinal cord injuries and patients with cancer pain that is refractory to conventional methods of pain control. The use of ambulatory devices facilitates the administration of pain medications. An oncology patient who in the past would have been hospitalized for pain control is able to be maintained safely on an outpatient basis for an extensive time period.

OPIOIDS

Narcotics or opioids are effective when they bind with particular opioid receptors in the body (Box 19-2). This chapter addresses only the mu and kappa receptors. Mu is the most powerful opioid receptor and requires stimulation when serious pain control is required. Particular opioids combine with the mu receptor, for example, morphine sulfate, meperidine HCl, hydromorphone, and fentanyl citrate. Other opioids combine with the kappa receptor; nalbuphine and buprenorphine HCl (Buprenex) are examples. An opioid that combines with the mu receptor used with an opioid that combines the kappa receptor will compete with each other for the mu receptor. Clinically, when an patient is receiving a morphine sulfate infusion of 3 mg/h, and the nurse administers a high dose of nalbuphine, the morphine sulfate is ineffective and pain intensifies. If the patient is physically dependent, he or she may go through physical withdrawal. Opioids that combine with the kappa receptor are weaker analgesics.

Side Effects

Side effects and complications associated with narcotics include:

- Respiratory depression
- Mental status changes
- Urinary retention
- Nausea
- Pruritus
- Constipation

Respiratory depression (8–10 respirations/min breath sounds) is caused by an accumulation of carbon dioxide in the blood, which communicates with the brain (medulla oblongata) to slow respirations until the carbon dioxide level returns to normal. An individual may experience respiratory depression and simultaneous apnea during regular sleep patterns. Institutional protocol should address assessment of respiratory depression during sleep because apnea monitors may disrupt normal sleep.

Oxygen saturation monitors are reliable indicators of the patient's oxygen level in the blood; however, the monitors do not measure the level of carbon dioxide. The oxygen saturation may remain normal for 2 to 4 minutes of apnea. More sophisticated continuous carbon dioxide monitors are needed. Nothing replaces bedside nursing assessment.

Mental status changes are indicative of significant levels of narcotic in the blood and impending respiratory depression. Mental status change may be reflective of hyponatremia or infection, especially in the elderly. Good nursing assessment will differentiate symptoms. Knowledge of the patient's baseline mental status, respiratory rate, blood chemistries, amount and type of narcotic, and other clinical diagnoses or potential diagnoses may assist the nurse in making an accurate assessment.

Urinary retention may be related to narcotic administration, caused by the relaxation of the detrusor muscle located in the floor of the bladder. The patient will feel the urge to void. Administration of bethanecol contracts the bladder, allowing it to empty. Catheterization is another option for immediate relief of urinary retention; however, rate of nosocomial infection increases.

Nausea may be reversed by either narcotic antagonists, such as nalbuphine HCl (Nubain) or naloxone HCl (Narcan), or by antiemetics. If narcotic antagonists are used, the doses should be kept low to prevent reversal of analgesia. If reversal of nausea is not accomplished with antiemetics or low-dose narcotic antagonism, the physician should be notified and further evaluation performed.

When narcotics are administered systemically, histamine is released and pruritus occurs; this may be relieved with antihistamines and possibly a change in medication. When narcotics are administered intraspinally (epidural or intrathecal), resultant pruritus is related to the action of the narcotic at the spinal cord and may be reversed with low-dose narcotic antagonists.

Narcotics slow the peristaltic action of the bowel; so does pain. Adequate pain control, with close bowel monitoring and possible administration of both a stool softener and a peristaltic agent, will alleviate constipation.

Methods of Opioid Administration

Routes of administration include IV patient-controlled analgesia (IV PCA), subcutaneous analgesia, and intraspinal analgesia. Each of these routes requires specific nursing assessment, planning, implementation, and evaluation.

INTRAVENOUS PATIENT-CONTROLLED ANALGESIA

Patient-controlled analgesia allows the patient to control IV delivery of an analgesic and to maintain therapeutic serum drug levels. The physician's order for PCA should include:

1. Loading dose, given IV push at initiation of therapy
2. Lock-out interval, during which the PCA device cannot be activated
3. Maintenance dose

4. Bolus dose

5. Maximum amount the patient may receive within a given time

The loading dose of opioid is achieved through a technique called "titration to effect." This technique calls for administering small doses of narcotic frequently to obtain a level of analgesia. Titration to effect usually occurs within 40 minutes and the patient is monitored during this time by observing mental status, level of pain relief, respiratory rate, and amount of narcotic. The nurse should be qualified to manage this technique; training is often provided by an anesthesiologist. For IV PCA to be effective, the loading dose must be given. Once the loading dose is given and analgesia is increasing, the IV PCA can be piggybacked into the proximal port on the IV tubing.

The lock-out interval is a safety system that prohibits the patient from frequently administering narcotic without giving the narcotic adequate time to achieve analgesia. The usual amount of time between patient-controlled boluses is 5 to 10 minutes.

The maintenance dose is the amount of narcotic that is infusing on a continuous basis. For example, an average, middle-aged, 70-kg adult would receive morphine sulfate at a rate of 1 mg/h. This maintenance dose is usually administered for the first 12 to 24 hours, after which the rate is reduced or the infusion is stopped and analgesia is maintained through self-boluses. This dosage is determined by the patient's age, weight, renal function, history of chemical abuse, and level of pain rating.

The maximum amount of narcotic the patient may self-administer within a given time is determined by the anesthesiologist, surgeon, or primary care physician. This amount is programmed into the infusion pump and offers another safety system that protects the patient from an overdose of narcotic.

The PCA device has an integral system to activate the bolus. A variety of devices are available. Factors to be considered in device selection include:

- Compatibility with currently used IV systems, poles or ambulatory quality
- Battery life
- Memory retention
- Display features
- Security and safety features
- Cost effectiveness
- Delivery mode (bolus versus continuous infusion)
- Durability
- Ease of use

Ambulatory Electronic Infusion Devices

A discussion of ambulatory infusion systems is contained in Chapter 10. These devices have greatly enhanced our ability to manage acute, postoperative, and chronic pain in the hospital or alternative care setting. Devices such as the CADD-PCA (Figure 19-1) are flexible; are programmable in milligrams or milliliters for use with a diversity of drugs and concentrations; are appropriate for subcutaneous, IV, and epidural delivery; are safe to use; are comfortable; and provide a total system of pain management and comprehensive support.

FIGURE 19-1 CADD-PCA® Ambulatory Infusion Pump. (Property of: Sims-Deltec, St. Paul, MN)

SUBCUTANEOUS NARCOTIC INFUSIONS

The subcutaneous infusion of narcotics provides analgesia to patients when IV access is unacceptable or not available. The level of analgesia obtained through subcutaneous infusions of narcotics is similar to that obtained through IV infusions of narcotics. The selection of narcotic is important to the success of subcutaneous infusions. Morphine sulfate and hydromorphone HCl are drugs of choice. The goal of a subcutaneous infusion is to offer a reduced volume of more concentrated solution with minimal chemical irritation. The quality of analgesia is limited to the amount of absorption of narcotic at the subcutaneous site. The conversion from oral narcotic to subcutaneous is equal to the conversion from oral narcotic to intramuscular. Table 19-1 shows the appropriate conversions.

TABLE 19-1
Conversion to Subcutaneous Narcotic

	Equianalgesic Dose (mg)	
Analgesic	Oral	IM or SC
Morphine sulfate	30.0	10.0
Hydromorphone HCl	7.5	1.5

IM, intramuscular; SC, subcutaneous

The technique for subcutaneous access is simple; however, the use of proper equipment and stabilizing methods enhances patient comfort and compliance. Supplies needed for subcutaneous access include a small-gauge scalp-vein needle or cannula, transparent dressing, povidone-iodine swab stick, and an adhesive bandage. The site of choice is commonly the subclavicular area, abdomen, or anterior chest wall. The site is prepped with povidone-iodine and the needle is inserted either at an angle or perpendicular to the skin, depending on the needle used. The needle is then stabilized using the manufacturer's recommended methods.

Trouble-Shooting Techniques

The most common problem with subcutaneous infusion of narcotics is local irritation at the needle insertion site and subcutaneous scarring. These can be minimized through frequent site changes (every other day) and by reducing the infusion volume.

The development of transdermal fentanyl enables a subcutaneous deposit of narcotic through diffusion of a rate-controlling membrane in the Duragesic (Janssen) patch. Doses of fentanyl are 25, 50, 75, and 100 μ/h. When applied to the torso of the patient's body, the patch takes 12 to 15 hours to reach its peak. The patch provides analgesia for 72 hours, with subsequent changes providing steady-state analgesia without the initial 15-hour peak delay. The patient may require fast-acting narcotic through another route until the dose is adjusted to provide steady-state analgesia. The character of the skin is important with transdermal fentanyl; the skin surface must be dry and body hair clipped, not shaved. The patch will not adhere to oily skin. To prevent boluses of fentanyl, the skin surface should be free of abrasions.

INTRASPINAL ANALGESIA

Epidural administration of pain medication offers analgesia, lower narcotic dosages, and less sedation; facilitates earlier ambulation; and enhances patient comfort. A working knowledge of relevant anatomy and physiology will ensure a high level of care. *Epi* refers to the outside and *dura* refers to the covering of the spinal cord, enclosing the cerebrospinal fluid (CSF). This is the part of the spinal canal outside the dura mater enclosed by connective tissue covering the vertebrae and ligamentum flavum. Extending from the base of the skull to the coccyx, it ends at about S-1 in many patients (the spinal cord ends at about L-1) (Figure 19-2).

The epidural space contains a network of large-bore and thin-walled veins. It also contains fat (directly proportional in amount to a person's body fat). The epidural space also contains extensions for nerves that travel from the spinal cord on out. Other terms used to identify the epidural space are peridural and extradural space.

The intrathecal space, containing CSF and bathing the spinal cord, runs parallel to the epidural space. They are separated by the dura mater. Other terms used to identify the intrathecal space are subarachnoid space and spinal space. The term intraspinal is used to describe both the epidural and intrathecal space.

When the epidural space is accessed, the anesthesiologist must penetrate the needle between the spinous processes, through the ligaments, and enter the epidural space with a technique called "loss of resistance." Loss of resistance occurs when the needle enters the epidural space and the pressure placed on the plunger of the syringe allows the contents of the syringe to empty into the epidural space, thus expanding

FIGURE 19-2 Close-up of L-1 epidural catheter placement.

the space. When an anesthesiologist accesses the intrathecal space, the needle penetrates through the same route into the epidural space and continues through the epidural space until it punctures through the dura mater and enters the intrathecal space. The intrathecal space contains CSF, which can be aspirated by the syringe attached to the accessing needle.

Elimination of narcotics from the intraspinal space occurs through two mechanisms: diffusion up the neuraxis in the CSF and vascular uptake in the epidural space. Drug action occurs within the spinal cord at the location of the substantia gelatinosa of the dorsal horn. Opiate receptors are located at the substantia gelatinosa and bind with the intraspinal narcotic, blocking the pain pathway through the dorsal horn to the brain.

The lipid-soluble nature of the narcotic determines the amount of narcotic used, the volume needed, the time to produce analgesia, and the elimination time.

Extremely lipid-soluble narcotics have a more rapid action than water-soluble narcotics. Lipid-soluble narcotics create analgesia in a narrow segment, following the dermatomes that are surrounding the level of narcotic injection. Water-soluble narcotics create a wider spread of analgesia, take longer to create analgesia, and have an increased elimination time. An example of a water-soluble narcotic is morphine sulfate; fentanyl citrate is an example of a lipid-soluble narcotic.

Local anesthetics are sometimes used to create analgesia in the epidural space. Pain transmission is blocked at the sympathetic chain ganglion, which lies on either side of the spinal cord and runs parallel to the spinal cord. When local anesthetics are used, a sympathetic blockade results and the patient benefits by a reduction of the amount of narcotic required to create analgesia, increased peristaltic action of the bowel, reduced workload on the heart, increased tidal volume of the lung, and an increased vascular graft flow, which reduces the incidence of deep-vein thrombosis. Potential side effects are a significant reduction of blood pressure and numbness to the lower extremities.

Delivery Methods

Epidural access may be achieved through the placement of a percutaneous epidural catheter, a fully implantable epidural access portal system, or a fully implantable drug infusion pump. The epidural space is accessed by using a special needle (eg, the Touhy needle). The needle is placed between the spinous processes and penetrates through the ligaments entering the epidural space through "loss of resistance." When the needle is properly placed, the catheter is threaded through the needle. When the epidural catheter is used for temporary analgesia, the catheter is taped to the back and the catheter is connected to the external infusion pump. When the epidural catheter is used for long-term analgesia, the catheter is connected to the implantable pump, port, or external catheter for connection to an external infusion pump.[3,4,7]

Before the epidural catheter is placed, the patient should be informed of the potential risks involved and *informed consent* should be obtained. Bleeding could occur within the epidural space and could exit out the insertion site of the catheter. Patients receiving anticoagulant therapy or with liver damage should have a bleeding time determined. If the bleeding time is less than 10 minutes, the catheter is safe for placement.

Sterile technique is used during catheter placement, consistent with established standards of practice. The physician should be notified if a patient is febrile before placement.

Patients express concerns related to placement, care, and potential problems. They should be told the catheter is placed into the tissue around the spinal cord, not into the spinal cord.

They need to know that their blood pressure may decrease because of muscle relaxation and sympathetic blockade when local anesthetic is injected. This is usually remedied by the administration of fluids.

A spinal headache may occur if the needle enters the CSF or intrathecal space. Spinal headache is caused by discharging CSF into the epidural space. This leak decreases the fluid padding around the brain and a headache results. Classic spinal headaches are "positional" in nature, that is, the patient experiences a headache in the upright position and but not when lying down. The location of the headache varies. Spinal headache may be relieved with a blood patch, a procedure in which the anesthesiologist realigns the needle in the epidural space close to the dural puncture site. The anesthesiologist then withdraws 10 to 15 mL blood from the patient's arm and injects the blood into the epidural needle. The epidural needle is removed and the patient is instructed to avoid the Valsalva maneuver either through lifting or bearing down for 24 hours. The blood patch plugs the leaking dural membrane and increases pressure in the epidural space, forcing the CSF in the intrathecal space toward the brain to relieve the headache soon after the patch is performed.

Epidural Catheters

A small-lumen, temporary catheter made of nylon or Teflon is initially placed. Long-term delivery is possible through the use of a long-term epidural catheter. The average duration of use is 104 days. The longest duration with the DuPen catheter[9] (Figure 19-3) is 972 days and ongoing). The epidural port may also be used.[6]

Potential candidates for epidural pain management should be evaluated for the following:

- Confirmed patient response to epidural medications
- Normal bleeding parameters
- Absence of active, untreated bacterial infection
- Acceptance of the therapy and understanding of potential side effects
- Adequate support systems to meet the patient's needs[5,8,10,11]

FIGURE 19-3   DuPen Eupucath. (Courtesy: Davol, Inc., Subsidiary CR Bard Inc., Salt Lake City, UT)

Care and Management of the Epidural Catheter

Consistent with Intravenous Nurses Society (INS) Standards of Practice, the delivery of medications and maintenance of epidural catheters should be established in IV policies and procedures specific to the Nurse Practice Act. Policies and procedures for obtaining, delivering, administering, documenting, and discarding medication should be in accordance with state and federal regulations.

All medications administered by an epidural catheter should be preservative free. Alcohol is contraindicated for site preparation or when accessing the catheter because of the potential for migration of alcohol into the epidural space and possible resultant nerve destruction. Betadine may be used; however, it can be irritating to the nerves if it migrates into the epidural space. A 0.2-μ filter without surfactant should be used for medication administration. Before use, the catheter should be aspirated to determine the absence of CSF. Epidural catheters may be placed for short- or long-term use.

Mechanical problems may occur with the epidural catheter system, including leaking catheter hub, disconnected catheter, occluded catheter, or leaking at the skin site. Leakage at the catheter hub is a common problem with temporary epidural catheter systems. The patient experiences breakthrough pain due to leakage of medications. Bedding or clothing will be wet. The nurse must tighten the hub or replace

FIGURE 19-4   Epidural catheter and points at which damage may occur. 1 = Tighten catheter; 2 = Leak may occur.

the hub if it is cracked. Clean technique is acceptable for manipulating the catheter hub (Fig. 19-4).

When the catheter is disconnected from the medication infusion, it may be in the patient's bed or on the floor. If the catheter is not grossly contaminated, a sterile scissors can be used to clip the catheter ½ inch from the end distal to the patient. The new end may then be reconnected to the hub of the catheter and tightened. If the catheter is found on the floor, the epidural catheter must be removed and another form of analgesia used. No alcohol or betadine is necessary for this procedure.

When the epidural catheter is occluded, the infusion pump should stop and the alarm should sound. Nursing interventions include ensuring that all clamps are open and checking the tubing to see if kinking has occurred. Loosen the hub and retighten to secure the hub to the catheter and restart the infusion.

The dressing over the catheter exit site may be damp due to leaking at the skin site. The nurse needs to assess whether the patient is experiencing pain or not. If the patient is comfortable, no treatment is necessary other than to replace the wet dressing. If the patient is uncomfortable, remove the dressing to see if the catheter has pulled out of the epidural space. The physician should be notified.

Aspiration of the Epidural Catheter

Aspiration of the epidural catheter is required when the catheter is displaced, either in an epidural vein or in the CSF. Aspiration of the catheter is, however, not a guarantee of either condition and should not be considered conclusive data. The physician should be notified. If the patient is oversedated, the epidural catheter may have migrated into the intrathecal space. If the patient is receiving epidural local anesthetic and feels numbness in the toes only, the catheter may be intrathecal. Aspiration of a small amount of blood (1–2 mL) is also inconclusive because the pool of medication in the epidural space may have mixed with a pool of blood in the epidural space that resulted from the trauma of the insertion. However, if the syringe fills with greater than 3 mL blood and the patient is receiving inadequate analgesia, it can be concluded that the epidural catheter is in an epidural vein. If so, the epidural catheter needs to be pulled back out of the vein and into the epidural space. There is always the risk of pulling the catheter out of the epidural space. The patient needs to be advised of this risk and that an alternative form of analgesia will then be necessary. If there is more than 5 mL clear fluid, the nurse can assume this is CSF unless there is a high-volume infusion of medication and poor diffusion through the dura resulting in higher pools of medications in the epidural space. The clear fluid can be tested to determine glucose level. Higher level of glucose indicates CSF and the physician should be consulted.

Flushing With Preservative-Free Saline

Flushing is performed to determine patency of the catheter; 3 mL preservative-free saline is instilled. If resistance is met, the connector to the epidural catheter should be loosened and a second attempt to flush should be made. If leaking occurs, the epidural catheter connector should be tightened.

Breakthrough Pain

Breakthrough pain may indicate that the pump is programmed incorrectly, the epidural catheter is disconnected and leaking, the epidural catheter is no longer epidural, the catheter has migrated into an epidural vein, or the patient is being underdosed. Despite the reason for breakthrough pain, intervention must be initiated to give the patient pain control. Breakthrough pain with the epidural catheter is treated by administration of 2 to 4 mg morphine sulfate, IV, every 20 minutes as needed. If the patient is sensitive to morphine sulfate, 12.5 to 25 mg meperidine may be substituted, IV, every 20 minutes as needed.

The Epidural Port

The epidural port consists of the portal and catheter and contains a 60-μm filter to remove large particulate matter. The catheter of the portal is positioned in the epidural space by percutaneous introduction, and a subcutaneous pocket is prepared for the portal over a bony prominence. The system is intended for repeated injection or infusion of preservative-free morphine sulfate into the epidural space (Figure 19-5).

Implanted Pumps

Advancements in medical technology have facilitated convenient alternatives to conventional methods of drug delivery. Systems such as the implanted pump (including pump, catheter, and optional access port) are implanted surgically and require peri-

FIGURE 19-5   Epidural port (Courtesy: Sims-Deltec, St. Paul, MN)

FIGURE 19-6 SynchroMed® Pump. (Courtesy: Medtronic, Minneapolis, MN)

odic refilling. The pump weighs approximately 6 oz and stores and releases prescribed amounts of medication into the body (Figure 19-6). A computer programmer may be used by the physician or nurse during refill and checkup sessions to communicate with the pump and to set the prescription as ordered. The pump delivers a controlled amount of medication through a catheter to the area in the body where it will be most effective. These pumps are battery operated and generally last 3 to 4 years. Potential risks include infection at the implant site, catheter plug or kinking, dislodgment, and leaking.

Patients should be cautioned to report redness, swelling, and pain near the incision and to avoid such activities as scuba diving, which would result in pump under-infusion and diminished drug effect. Diathermy and ultrasound treatments should be applied away from the pump site. Flow rates may be affected by atmospheric pressure, body temperature, blood pressure, and concentration and viscosity of the medication.

Possible complications include cessation of therapy caused by battery depletion, migration of the catheter access port, pocket seroma, rupture of the port connector at high injection pressures, complete or partial catheter occlusion, CSF leak, and drug toxicity. The use of needles larger than 22 gauge may compromise the self-sealing properties of the septum. Huber-type needles are recommended to minimize septal damage. The IV nurse is cautioned to follow procedures for the use of implanted pumps, consistent with manufacturer's guidelines and institutional policy.

Patient Identification Card

When the pump is implanted, the surgeon should complete the patient registration and implantation record. The manufacturer will issue the patient a wallet-sized identification card containing information pertinent to the implanted pump. The physician should fill in the space provided for any medical emergency instructions. This card should be carried by the patient at all times.

Postimplantation Care

Patients should be monitored carefully after implantation to confirm proper pump performance, wound healing, and favorable response to therapy. The pump should not be used for the administration of drugs for several days after implantation to allow for adequate wound healing. Instructions for patients with implanted pumps are listed in Box 19-3.

Pump Refill Procedure

The pump will require refills at specific intervals, depending on the volume of the reservoir and the rate of administration. The technique used to refill the pump should be sterile.

The necessary equipment includes:

Sterile fenestrated drape (1)	Sterile extension tubing with clamp (1)
Sterile towel (1)	Sterile gloves (1 pair)(1)
50-mL syringe with drug solution	Sterile 2 × 2 inch sponge (1)
Sterile empty 50-mL syringe (1)	Povidone-iodine swabs (3)
Sterile noncoring needle (1)	Heating pad (1)

The procedure is as follows:

1. Warm 50-mL syringe with drug solution to 15° to 35°C (59°–95°F) with the heating pad.

Box 19-3
Instructions for Patients With Implanted Pumps

Action

1. Avoid traumatic physical activity.
2. Avoid long hot baths, saunas, and other activities that increase body temperature.
3. Consult physician during febrile illness.
4. Consult the physician before air travel or change of residence.
5. Avoid deep sea or scuba diving.
6. Report any unusual symptoms or complications relating to the specific drug therapy or the device.
7. Return at the prescribed time for pump refill.

Result

1. Prevent tissue damage around the implant site.
2. Increased drug flow.
3. Assess the effects of increased drug flow.
4. Adjustments in drug dosage may be required to compensate for anticipated change in drug flow.
5. Dosage may require modification.
6. Ensure safety.
7. Ensure compliance.

2. Identify the outer perimeter of the pump by palpating the pump pocket. Locate pump septum.

3. Wash hands thoroughly and dry.

4. Using sterile technique, place all sterile items on opened sterile towel.

5. Put on sterile gloves.

6. Disinfect pump site with povidone-iodine. Use *three* separate preps. Start at the center of the pump and work outward beyond the periphery of the pump.

7. Place fenestrated drape over prepped pump site. Sterile template may be aligned over septum.

8. *Securely* connect *barrel* of empty 5-mL syringe and extension tubing to the noncoring needle. Close clamp.

9. Using a perpendicular angle, insert needle into center of septum.

10. Open clamp. Lower syringe barrel to below patient level and allow pump to empty.

11. Close clamp. Record returned volume, adding 1 mL for amount of drug remaining in extension tubing. Disconnect and discard syringe barrel.

12. *Securely* attach air-purged syringe with drug solution to extension tubing. Open clamp.

13. Using both hands, inject 5 mL solution into pump. Release pressure and allow drug to return to syringe. This test confirms proper needle placement. Continue to inject and check needle placement at 5-mL increments until syringe is emptied.

14. Pull needle out quickly and apply digital pressure with sterile sponge. If necessary, apply a sterile adhesive bandage.

Stationary Infusion Devices

Abbott Laboratories' LifeCare PCA Classic and PCA Plus II meet the needs of the sedentary patient receiving pain management. The Classic is a single-mode PCA device for low-cost PCA procedures. The Plus II has the ability to dose in micrograms or milligrams (Figure 19-7).

STAFF EDUCATION

Although information on the safe administration of epidural medication and monitoring of potential side effects is available, little has been written about preparing the registered professional nurse for administering and monitoring epidural analgesia. The initial step is to establish criteria and rationale on which the policy and procedure for administration of epidural analgesia would be based, as outlined in Table 19-2.

Development of a care plan illustrating potential side effects and appropriate nursing interventions is an essential component of the process. A sample care plan is detailed in Figure 19-8.

The clinical program should be intensive, and ideally, skills checklists may be used to identify criteria for assessing appropriate techniques.

Text continue on page 460

FIGURE 19-7 LifeCare PCA Plus II Infuser for pain management. (Courtesy: Abbott Laboratories, North Chicago, IL)

TABLE 19-2
Criteria and Rationale for RN Administration of Epidural Analgesia

Criteria	*Rationale*
Only postoperative patients would have epidural narcotics administered by RNs.	Chronic pain patients often require high doses that increase the risk of side effects.
Epidural medication would be limited to preservative-free morphine sulfate (MS).	The onset and duration of action of MS is well-known. Other medications would be administered by anesthesiologists.
RNs will only administer narcotics through epidural, not intrathecal, catheters.	There are greater risks of respiratory depression during intrathecal administration.
An apnea monitor would be used for the first 24 h or longer until dosage has been stabilized.	Respiratory depression is most likely to occur within this time.
The anesthesiologist would be notified when: There is minimal or no pain relief following epidural administration. Clear or bloody fluid is aspirated from the catheter before injecting. Patient experiences pain on injection. Clear drainage is noted on the dressing.	These events indicate problems with the catheter.
Anesthesiologist will change the epidural dressing every 48 h.	Epidural catheters are not sutured into place. The risk of dislodgment at time of dressing change is high.

(Reprinted from the *Oncology Nursing Forum* with permission from the Oncology Nursing Press, Inc. Camp-Sorrell, D., Fernandez, K., and Reardon, M. B. [1990]. Teaching oncology nurses about epidural catheters. *Oncology Nursing Forum, 17*[5], 683-689.)

Init. date	NURSING DIAGNOSIS/PATIENT PROBLEM / DESIRED OUTCOME	ACTIONS/INTERVENTIONS SET & REVIEWED W/PATIENT/FAMILY [ ] YES [ ] NO	TARGET DATE	DATE OF DAILY REVIEW/INITIALS	RESOLUTION DATE / EVALUATION
Initials	1. Knowledge deficit related to the use of epidural analgesia for post-operative pain control	1. Describe the placement of the catheter, its use, who will administer pain medication and the use of an apnea monitor for immediate post-op period			
	Patient demonstrates knowledge related to epidural catheter use for post-operative pain control and verbalizes understanding of need to report pain as soon as perceived				
	2. Potential for injury due to catheter displacement (i e intrathecal space)	1. RN will monitor: a The patency of the catheter b The condition of the dressing c Observe catheter site of intactness and hash marks indicating length d Negative aspiration before each medication administration			
	Catheter will remain in epidural space or will be removed immediately if dislodged				
	3. Potential for ineffective breathing pattern related to respiratory depression secondary to epidural analgesia	1. Maintain apnea monitor for first 24 hours or until a baseline dose is established to maintain patient comfort			
	Patient will exhibit effective breathing pattern: • respirations of six or greater, regular and non-labored				

Initials	RN Signatures	Initials	RN Signatures

Primary Nurse

Social Worker:

Other

FIGURE 19-8 Patient care plan for postoperative pain control using epidural analgesia. *(continued)*

455

Init. date	NURSING DIAGNOSIS/PATIENT PROBLEM DESIRED OUTCOME	ACTIONS/INTERVENTIONS SET & REVIEWED W/PATIENT/FAMILY [ ] YES [ ] NO	TARGET DATE	DATE OF DAILY REVIEW/INITIALS	RESOLUTION DATE EVALUATION
Initials	3 Potential for ineffective breathing (Continued)	2 Have Naloxone (Narcan) 4mg available at all times while epidural narcotics are being used			
		3 Maintain IV access at all times while epidural catheter is in place			
		4 Monitor for signs of restlessness, miosis			
	4 Potential urinary retention related to atonic bladder from sacral analgesia	1 If urinary catheter not in place, measure intake and output every four hours for first 24 hours and every eight hours thereafter			
	.. Patient will demonstrate adequate urinary elimination				
	5 Potential for alteration in comfort related to displacement or dysfunction of the catheter	1 Use visual analog scale and Pain Flow Sheet to monitor patient comfort level every four hours			
	.. Patient will report adequate pain control	2 Administer medication as ordered or notify anesthesiologist of inadequate pain control * Note: No other narcotics, tranquilizers or sedatives may be given unless ordered by anesthesiologist			

Initials	RN Signatures	Initials	RN Signatures

Primary Nurse

Social Worker:

Other

FIGURE 19-8 (Continued)

In date / Initials	NURSING DIAGNOSIS/PATIENT PROBLEM DESIRED OUTCOME	ACTIONS/INTERVENTIONS SET & REVIEWED W/PATIENT/FAMILY [ ] YES [ ] NO	TARGET DATE	DATE OF DAILY REVIEW/INITIALS	RESOLUTION DATE	EVALUATION
	6 Potential for discomfort related to pruitis secondary to release of histamine from the morphine effect	1 Administer antipruritic as ordered by anesthesiologist PRN				
	:Patient will inform caregiver when itching begins. Patient will report relief of itching					
	7 Potential for hypotension related to vasomotor disturbance	1 Monitor vital signs every four hours while epidural is in use				
	:Blood pressure will be maintained at adequate level	2 Maintain adequate intravenous or oral fluid intake				
		3 Elevate lower extremities				
		4 When getting OOB, allow patient to dangle at bedside first				
	8 Potential for injury related to infection secondary to epidural catheter.	1 Monitor catheter insertion site every shift for redness, edema, drainage				
	:Patient will remain infection-free as evidenced by absence of purulent drainage, redness or tenderness at catheter insertion site	2 Maintain strict sterile technique during preparation and administration of medications				
		3 Monitor temperature and WBC to detect possible infection.				

Initials	RN Signatures	Initials	RN Signatures

Primary Nurse

Social Worker:

Other

FIGURE 19-8 (*Continued*) Reprinted from the *Oncology Nursing Forum* with permission from Oncology Nursing Press, Inc. (Camp-Sorrel, D. Fernandez, K., & Reardon, M. B. [1990]. Teaching oncology nurses about epidural catheters. *Oncology Nursing Forum, 17*[5], 683-689.)

PAIN ASSESSMENT FLOW SHEET

DATE: _____
MEDICATION ORDERED: _____
CONTINUOUS RATE: _____
PCA DOSE: _____
LOCKOUT: _____

CHECK ONE:

EPIDURAL: _____
INTRATHECAL: _____
IV-PCA: _____

(Addressograph Plate)

Checks Made Here - See Nurse's Notes:

Date	Time	Sed. Scale	Respir. Rate	Med. Inf. As Ordrd. Tubing Secure	Pain Scale	B.P. / Pulse Lying	B.P. / Pulse Sitting	No Loss Of Sens. Lower Extrem.	Drsg. Dry Intact. No Edema S/S of Inf.	Urinary Ret.	Pruritis	Break Through Pain	Catheter Checked For Placement	Drsg. Chg. (Kit Utlzd.)	Catheter Flushed 3cc NS.	Nausea Vomiting	Pulse Ox.	R.N.'s Initials

1 Hour Assessment / 4-HOUR ASSESSMENT / Local Anesthetic

RN SIGNATURE / INITIALS: _____ _____ _____ _____ _____

N/V ECOG SCALE:
0 - No Nausea or Vomiting
1 - Nausea/Vomiting X 1/day
2 - Nausea/Vomiting Less Than X 6/day
3 - Vomiting X 6/day
4 - Dehydration - IV Therapy

PAIN SCALE:
0 - No Pain
1 - 2 - Discomfort
3 - 4 - Mild Pain
5 - 6 - Distress
7 - 8 - Severe Pain
9 - 10 - Excruciating Pain

SEDATION SCALE:
0 - No Sedation-Pt. Found Awake.
S - Normal Sleep-Easy To Awake.
1 - Mild Drowsy, Easy To Arouse.
2 - Moderate, Frequently Drowsy, Still Able To Arouse.
3 - Severely Somnolent, Unable To Arouse.

FIGURE 19-9 Pain assessment form. (Courtesy: Midwestern Regional Medical Center, Zion, IL)

PAIN ASSESSMENT ORDERS:

_____

_____

_____

_____

_____

_____

_____

_____

NURSE'S NOTES:

_____

_____

_____

_____

_____

_____

_____

_____

_____

_____

_____

_____

_____

_____

_____

_____

_____

_____

_____

_____

_____

_____

_____

FIGURE 19-9   _(Continued)_

PATIENT–CONTROLLED ANALGESIA
Sample Flow Sheet

HOSPITAL I.D.	PATIENT I.D.

DATE_____
MEDICATION—————

LOADING DOSE_____
(IF APPLICABLE)

TIME	12MN	2A	4A	6A	8A	10A	12N	2P	4P	6P	8P	10P
DOSE VOLUME (ML)												
LOCK–OUT												
4 HR LIMIT (ML)												
# DOSE DEL.												
TOTAL VOL. DEL.												
SEDATION (1–5)												
PAIN (1–5)												
RESP. RATE												
NURSE'S SIG.												

ADMIN. SET CHANGE _____

NEW PCA UNIT _____

CONDITION I.V. SITE _____

SCALES

SEDATION	PAIN
1 = WIDE AWAKE	1 = COMFORTABLE
2 = DROWSY	2 = IN MILD DISCOMFORT
3 = DOZING INTERMITTENTLY	3 = IN PAIN
4 = MOSTLY SLEEPING	4 = IN BAD PAIN
5 = ONLY AWAKENS WHEN AROUSED	5 = IN VERY BAD PAIN

FIGURE 19-10   Sample flow sheet for patient-controlled analgesia.

DOCUMENTATION

Documentation should include the type of pain management provided, route of administration, methods used, IV or other access route, site care and maintenance, assessment of pain and degree of pain relief, and problems encountered in dealing with the particular type of access used. Flow sheets facilitate accuracy of documentation and provide a guideline for all areas of concern, including pain rating (intensity) and level of consciousness (Figure 19-9).

TABLE 19-3
American Pain Society Quality Assurance Pain Relief Standards

- Recognize and treat pain promptly.
  - Chart and display pain and relief. (Process)
  - Define pain and relief levels to initiate review. (Process)
  - Survey patient satisfaction. (Outcome)
- Make information about analgesics readily available. (Process)
- Promise patients attentive analgesic care. (Process)
- Define explicit policies for use of advanced analgesic technologies. (Process)
- Monitor adherence to standards. (Process)

When PCA systems are implemented, the nurse records the date, time, medication, patient's name, room number, physician's name, and his or her name on an appropriate flow sheet. The continuous nature of the injection does not permit the nurse to record the exact dosage administered on standard control sheets found in many health care institutions. Many such facilities have developed individualized flow sheets specifically for PCA control (Figure 19-10).

The American Pain Society[6] has developed quality assurance standards for pain relief (Table 19-3).

REFERENCES

1. Ackerman, W. E., Juneja, M. M., Kaczorowski, D. M., & Colclough, G. W. (1989). A comparison of the incidence of pruritus following epidural opioid administration in the parturient. *Canadian Journal of Anaesthesia, 36*(4), 388–391.
2. Bonica, J. J. (1990). Management of post-operative pain. In J. J. Bonica (Ed.), *The management of pain* (2nd ed., pp. 461–480). Philadelphia: Lea & Febiger.
3. Caballero, G. A., Ausman, R. K., & Himes, J. (1986). Epidural morphine by continuous infusion with an external pump for pain management in oncology patients. *American Surgeon, 8*(52), 402–405.
4. DuPen, S. L. (1987). A new permanent exteriorized epidural catheter for narcotic self-administration to control cancer pain. *Cancer, 59,* 986–993.
5. Hassenbusch, S. J., Pillay, P. K., Magdinec, M., Currie, K., Bay, J. W., Covington, E. C., Tomaszewski, M. Z. (1990). Constant infusion of morphine for intractable cancer pain using an implanted pump. *Journal of Neurosurgery, 73*(3), 405–409.
6. Max, M. (1990). American Pain Society quality assurance standards for relief of acute pain and cancer pain. In M. R. Bond, J. E. Charlton, & C. J. Woolf (Eds.), *Proceedings of the VI World Congress on Pain* (pp. 196–189). Amsterdam: Elsevier.
7. Paice, J. A. (1987). New delivery systems in pain management. *Nursing Clinics of North America, 22*(3), 715–726.
8. Patt, R. B. (1989). Interventional analgesia: Epidural and subarachnoid therapy. *American Journal of Hospice Care,* March/April, 11–14.
9. Product literature. Davol, Inc. Subsidiary of C. R. Bard, Inc., P.O. Box 8500, Cranston, RI ONC 60290–88810M.
10. Waldman, S. D. (1990). The role of spinal opioids in the management of cancer pain. *Journal of Pain and Symptom Management, 5*(3), 163–168.
11. Yablonski-Peretz, T., et al. (1985). Continuous epidural narcotic analgesia for intractable pain due to malignancy. *Journal of Surgical Oncology, 29,* 8–10.

REVIEW QUESTIONS

1. Pain management may be provided by which of the following?
   a. systemic analgesics
   b. continuous infusion
   c. intraspinal opioids
   d. regional analgesia

2. Breakthrough pain during IV PCA should be treated by:
   a. increasing medication dose consistent with physician's orders
   b. increasing medication dose consistent with nursing judgment
   c. oral narcotic dosing
   d. intramuscular dosing

3. Nausea may be reversed by narcotic antagonists, such as which of the following?
   a. Nubain
   b. Narcan
   c. Neupogen
   d. Naloxone

4. Epidural morphine has been associated with a high incidence of:
   a. pruritus
   b. nausea
   c. diarrhea
   d. urinary incontinence

5. Alcohol is contraindicated for site preparation or when accessing the catheter because of the potential for:
   a. migration into the epidural space
   b. possible nerve damage
   c. obliterating the catheter
   d. damage to the Silastic

6. Mechanical problems associated with the catheter include:
   a. occlusion
   b. disconnection
   c. leaking at hub
   d. leaking at site

7. Indications for aspiration of the epidural catheter include:
   a. adequate pain control
   b. inadequate sedation
   c. inadequate pain control
   d. oversedation

8. Clear fluid in the syringe after aspiration is an indication of:
   a. catheter patency
   b. catheter kinking
   c. catheter migration
   d. catheter damage

9. Quality assurance pain relief standards have been developed by which of the following?
   a. American Pain Society
   b. American Epidural Society
   c. American Association for Pain
   d. American Pain Control

10. Factors to be considered in device selection include:
    a. battery life
    b. memory retention
    c. display features
    d. safety features

CHAPTER 20

Antineoplastic Therapy

Key Terms

Alkaloid	Bolus	Histology
Alkylating	Cell cycle	Immunocompromised
Alopecia	Cellular kinetics	Investigational
Anticancer	Cytotoxic	Toxicity
Antihemolytic	Extravasation	Vesicant
Antimetabolite		

Cancer chemotherapeutic agents present a real challenge to nurses responsible for their administration. Many nurses point to the reputation of antineoplastics as intimidating and express anxiety about administering them. Success with these substances usually is ensured, however, for clinicians with refined IV skills, sensitive patient preparation practices, and keen awareness of how and why chemotherapy works.

Successful administration of a chemotherapeutic regimen depends on the depth of patient preparation and education, the competence and skill of the nurse, mutual understanding of both patient and clinician on the current goal of therapy (control or palliation), and, finally, a healthy respect for the powerful chemicals themselves.

In fact, there seems to be a direct relationship between the IV therapy skills of the nursing clinician and the "tolerability" of a patient's cancer experience. A new opportunity awaits the professional who chooses to participate in this aspect of cancer care.

EDUCATION

Clinicians

The privilege of administering antineoplastic agents is preceded by extensive exposure to standardized educational preparation and practical experience. To provide consistently safe, high-quality, and appropriate patient care, many centers mandate comprehensive training programs leading to credentialing in chemotherapy administration.

The Oncology Nursing Society (ONS) provides a standardized framework for this credentialing, via *Cancer Chemotherapy Guidelines*, a series of five modular professional education tools.[20,22,23] These guidelines provide structured recommendations for a combined theoretical and clinical curriculum, specific to acute, outpatient, or home care settings. Each module calls for a didactic core curriculum followed by a clinical practicum.

The didactic component includes basic information on the biology of cancer, pharmacology and principles of cancer chemotherapy, specific antineoplastic agents, the major principles governing chemotherapy administration, and patient assessment and management. Then the information is applied during the practicum phase, where clinical skills are exercised and evaluated. Successful candidates are credentialed as qualified to safely and confidently administer chemotherapy.

The following sample course outline provides the major subjects necessary to prepare for chemotherapy credentialing, whether to practice in a specific institution or to prepare for professional certification through the ONS.[20,23,32,33]

    I. Audiovisual Component
        A. Historical overview of cancer chemotherapy
        B. Cell cycle
        C. Cellular kinetics
        D. Indications for antineoplastics use
        E. Drug actions and classifications
        F. Drug development and investigative trials
        G. Therapeutic intent with combined modality therapy
        H. Side effects associated with cytotoxic agents
        I. Drug calculations, handling, preparation, storage, and disposal
        J. Normal dose ranges
        K. Drug administration techniques

    II. Didactic Component
        A. Individual facility policy statement and legal aspects
        B. Pharmacology of antineoplastics
        C. Drug calculation and reconstitution
        D. Drug administration principles and techniques
        E. Management of side effects and common problems
        F. Education materials and teaching strategies for patients and families
        G. Documentation
        H. Patient and family resources

    III. Individual Handout Materials
        A. Nursing qualifications
        B. Policy and procedures

    C. List of drugs approved for administration by nurses
    D. Samples of written education tools for patients
    E. Nomogram to calculate body surface area
    F. Math test
    G. Pretest
    H. Class evaluation
    I. Bibliography

IV. Clinical Practicum
    A. Drug calculation
    B. Drug preparation and handling
    C. Drug storage and transport
    D. Drug administration techniques
    E. Complications management
    F. Appropriate documentation
    G. Patient and family teaching and follow-up

Safe delivery of IV antineoplastic agents is only a part of caring for chemotherapy patients. A nurse who specializes in medical oncology needs a solid foundation of special knowledge. Following is a list of suggested areas for special emphasis in a basic education program for oncology nurses.

I. Patient Evaluation
    A. Performance status
    B. Nutritional status
    C. Hematologic assessment
    D. Psychosocial assessment
    E. Systems review
        1. Cardiac
        2. Renal
        3. Hepatic
        4. Pulmonary
        5. Gastrointestinal
    F. Diagnostic evaluation

II. Treatment Selection
    A. Histology
    B. Location, size
    C. Prior therapy
    D. Therapeutic intent
        1. Cure
        2. Control
        3. Palliation
    E. Treatment type
        1. Primary
        2. Adjuvant
        3. Combined modality
    F. Drug calculation, scheduling, and dose modifications
    G. Treatment response

III. Principles of Cancer Chemotherapy
   A. Pharmacology
   B. Drug classifications
   C. Cellular kinetics
   D. Drug interactions
   E. Drug delivery (route, rate)

IV. Complications and Toxicities
   A. Short-term
      1. Alopecia
      2. Gastrointestinal reactions
      3. Bone marrow
      4. Allergic reactions
      5. Phlebitis and extravasation
      6. Psychosocial
   B. Long-term
      1. Genetic
      2. Oncogenetic
      3. Immunosuppressive
      4. Reproductive
      5. Psychosocial
   C. Specific organ toxicities
      1. Cardiac
      2. Renal
      3. Pulmonary
      4. Hepatic
      5. Gastrointestinal
      6. Neurologic
      7. Dermatologic
      8. Reproductive

V. Nursing Care
   A. Early detection and prevention of complications
   B. Delivery of expert care
   C. Patient and family education
   D. Psychosocial support (newly diagnosed, remission, recurrence, terminal)
   E. Follow-up support needs

The remarkable progress of antineoplastic agents as a major treatment modality poses a growing series of particular challenges to administering clinicians. Ongoing and vigorous clinical investigations from cooperative groups are dedicated to discovering new therapeutic methods of cytotoxic drug delivery. Nurses who specialize in medical oncology have a responsibility to maintain their up-to-date expertise through study of current professional literature along with continuing education programs. The ONS recommends development of an institutional mechanism for annual evaluation of clinicians' knowledge and skills relative to chemotherapy administration. It requires renewal of its professional certification through formal examinations every 4 years.[20]

Legal Considerations

A thorough understanding of legal implications (outlined in Chapter 2) is an essential element of professional education for nurses administering antineoplastic agents. Some legal considerations pertinent to cancer chemotherapy:

1. *Clinical education.* Before treating any patient, documentation of the clinician's successful training in IV fluid and drug administration should be available in personnel files.

2. *Lines of supervision.* The clinician should have a clear, written statement of the lines of supervision.

3. *Standards of care.* The clinician should have a clear, written statement of the employing facility's "standards of care," including a definition of "reasonable care" in each pertinent area of practice.

4. *Patient and family education.* The clinician should have completed the process of initial patient and family education regarding all medications in the treatment regimen, including their side effects, with subsequent assertions and documentation of the patient understanding.

5. *Informed consent.* Although gaining informed consent is a physician responsibility in most states,[3] a nurse should ensure that consent has been granted before administering chemotherapy. "If consent has not been obtained, the hospital or institution may be held liable if treatment is administered. Failure to obtain a patient's consent may constitute 'battery.' Battery may be defined as any physical contact of a patient without his permission."[6]

It is in a clinician's best interest to request a written definition of the institution's scope of practice and to explore details of medical liability insurance covering the practice. Many employers provide adequate coverage for care administered when the nurse is on duty. Independent practitioners, instructors, or those working in physicians' offices may opt for personal malpractice coverage. As nurses assume greater responsibility in administering cancer chemotherapy, there may be increased incidence of litigation involving nurses. Meticulous adherence to the details of defined statutes and standards of care may minimize that risk.

The following organizations provide more details on legal statutes that govern nursing practice pertaining to chemotherapy administration:

- American Nurses Association
- Individual state departments of professional regulation (for data on state's Nurse Practice Act)
- Intravenous Nurses Society[14]
- Oncology Nursing Society

Because a patient's clinical record contains legally binding information that can be used as evidence in litigation, it is a crucial nursing responsibility to ensure that documentation is accurate and comprehensive. Miller aptly describes the essentials of adequate documentation, which include time of a significant incident, a thorough and objective description of the care provided, patient status, and the exact nature of physician involvement.[17]

The expert oncology nurse frequently practices more autonomously than colleagues in other specialties, which may imply increased legal vulnerability. For example, extensive telephone contact is common with oncology patients; the nurse should therefore be mindful of the accepted "scope of practice" when responding to patient needs.

The nurse commonly is a key clinician involved in clinical trails that call for take-home investigational drugs. By law, only a pharmacist or physician may dispense medication. Therefore, packaging and delivery of investigational drugs is not a legal function for nurses.

Finally, knowledge of common dosing and scheduling of each common chemotherapeutic agent is the best protection (for patient and nurse) from delivering an incorrect (possibly lethal) drug dosage.

Clients

Experience indicates that treatment acceptance and response usually are more favorable when the patient is actively involved in the therapy program. When administering cytotoxic agents, the nurse should invite open communication with the patient in all phases of care, even to the extent of actively soliciting patient assistance in clinical functions such as assessing vein status. The wise clinician will listen to, and be guided by, patient statements like: "The nurse tried that vein two times last week, and it didn't work." In addition to providing a sense of patient involvement and control, the nurse can capitalize on a patient's intimate knowledge of his or her own body.

It is wise to inform a patient that, as IV solutions are infused, it is normal to detect a sense of coolness along the venous pathway. Likewise, it is prudent to alert a patient to early extravasation signs (pain, burning, stinging, a feeling of tightness, tingling, numbness, any other unusual sensations) when vesicant agents are infused because patients often are able to detect them before they are apparent to the clinician.

Some antineoplastics can be associated with localized and generalized anaphylactic reactions; when reported early and treated properly, their course can be reversed or minimized. Particularly with these agents, patients should be encouraged to report unusual symptoms of generalized tingling, chest pains or sensations, shortness of breath, or light-headedness. The sensitive clinician will assess the patient's overall anxiety level in deciding the best way to impart this information.

These levels of participation run the risk that some patients will aggressively seek to direct their own care. Patient statements like these are not uncommon: "This is the vein we'll use today" or "I'll give you one try, but then you'll have to find someone else." Professional clinicians know that such patient behavior can be traced to understandable anxiety and do not allow it to undermine self-confidence. Several minutes spent explaining the rationale and process of vein selection may eliminate the problem.

Once a working rapport is established, the nurse usually finds that patient behavior shifts to implicit trust in the skill and judgment of the clinician with whom he or she is most familiar. In fact, personal attachment to a particular clinician often begins during the patient education phase of treatment, even before drugs are administered. It is in the patient's best interest for the clinician to encourage a wholesome and balanced professional relationship from the outset, before any unwholesome dependence develops.

Patients are best served when encouraged to tap their own resources and empowered to endure therapy without inordinate focus on the personality of the treatment provider. Ideally, a healthy partnership develops in which the patient is a valued contributor to the nurse's plan of care.

Nurses administering chemotherapy have a tremendous opportunity to minimize treatment-related morbidity (and thus to enhance their patients' quality of life) through competent patient education. Patient, family, and caregiver education is as integral to the cancer treatment regimen as is optimum selection of veins for agent infusion.

The primary focus of this chapter is, of course, the technique of chemotherapy administration. At the same time, it is important to recognize that safe, skilled, efficient craftsmanship in delivery of antineoplastics is only about half the job of contemporary IV therapy nursing professionalism. The more sensitive (and sometimes more influential) part of the art revolves around intuitive patient and family education, fashioned to address a particular patient's situation. Some guidelines are presented. Brown and Hogan[3] proposed the following key assessment considerations when tailoring a teaching plan for an individual patient.

1. The nurse assesses and identifies what the patient and family need and want to know about the disease and treatment and takes steps to ameliorate their impact.

2. The nurse and patient and family agree on education goals focused on individual patient and family needs (not clinician convenience or habit).

3. The nurse selects educational methods and materials consistent with patient and family learning needs and abilities.

4. The nurse considers how, when, and by whom teaching will be done.

5. The nurse continuously evaluates the patient's and family's learning level, with reference to original education goals.

6. The nurse conscientiously documents all components of the education process. (An organized and systematic form in the medical record is an efficient and effective way to ensure that this phase is up to date.)

Multiple psychosocial, emotional, and physiologic barriers come into play because of the nature of the disease and of public perception of cancer and cancer therapy (Table 20-1).[24,30] A nurse's primary concern is that the patient has absorbed (not only "been provided") sufficient information to provide legitimate "informed consent."[3]

Some barriers to patient education can be overcome by such simple means as teaching in a physical environment that reduces anxiety, including the family in the educational process, and providing patient-appropriate materials. Often it is wise to allow a span of time between a scheduled teaching session and treatment itself to allow the patient opportunity to assimilate important information.

Certainly patient education is an ongoing process, from the outset and for the duration of therapy. The process often sorts itself into a natural division of three phases. Table 20-2 summarizes the essential components of the education process.

Somerville[26] provides the following guidelines for nurses involved in patient education. They are designed to evaluate teaching content and technique by assessing the degree to which expected patient outcomes are achieved.

1. Patient demonstrates knowledge related to diagnosis and disease process.
   a. States diagnosis and explains disease process
   b. Describes previous experience with cancer and treatments

---

TABLE 20-1
Examples of Potential Barriers to Successful Education of Patients Receiving Chemotherapy

Barrier Type	Examples
Emotional	Anxiety related to cancer diagnosis, anticipation of cancer therapy, cost issues
	Depression related to disease process and treatment
	Denial, used as coping mechanism
	External locus of control—learned helplessness and powerlessness
Physiologic	Biochemical imbalances causing nausea and vomiting, fatigue, restlessness, irritability
Psychosocial	Altered consciousness caused by disease process and/or medications
	Cultural attitudes/beliefs/values that may yield unwillingness to learn ("My wife takes care of this kind of thing.")
	Refusal to claim ownership of self-care—attention to "self" perceived as "selfish" and culturally unacceptable
	Lack of inquisitiveness in effort to be seen as "good patient"
Functional	Compromised literacy level or language differences
	Being overwhelmed by new information (names of drugs, disease jargon, personnel names, schedules, etc.)
	Age, decreased retention or memory
Environmental	Busy, rushed, and distracting clinics
	Foreign, high technology, and threatening surroundings
	Close proximity to other patients can be restricting and depersonalizing

(Prepared by M. M. McCluskey from Somerville, E. T., Padilla, G. V., & Bulcavage, L. M. [1991]. Theories used in patient/health education. *Seminars in Oncology Nursing, 7*(2), 87–96; Villejo, L., & Meyers, C. [1991]. Brain function, learning styles, and cancer patient education. *Seminars in Oncology Nursing, 7*[2], 97–104.)

---

   c. Acknowledges need for treatment

   d. States alternatives to prescribed treatment

2. Patient demonstrates knowledge related to rationale for chemotherapy treatment.

   a. Verbalizes need for chemotherapy

   b. Verbalizes attitude toward and expectations about cancer treatment

   c. States understanding of use of chemotherapy alone or in conjunction with other treatment modalities, if applicable

   d. Identifies treatment protocol

3. Patient demonstrates knowledge related to potential therapeutic side effects of chemotherapy.

   a. States diagnosis and expected response to treatment

   b. Identifies specific effect of treatment with chemotherapeutic agents

4. Patient demonstrates knowledge of treatment plan and schedule.

   a. Identifies drugs to be given

   b. States frequency and duration of treatment

TABLE 20-2
Educational Essentials for Patients Receiving Chemotherapy
COMMON GOAL TO ALL PHASES: TO LESSEN PATIENT'S KNOWLEDGE DEFICIT RELATED TO CHEMOTHERAPY

Phase	Goal	Nursing Actions
Pretreatment	To provide sufficient information to:	Provide written, patient-appropriate educational materials containing specific chemotherapy agents before treatment is initiated; make allowances for extended learning period, if necessary
	Facilitate patient's ability to provide valid informed consent	Thoroughly discuss expectations of therapy
	Provide nonthreatening environment conducive to learning and to accepting chemotherapy treatments confidently	Discuss anticipated procedures and administration technique, potential side effects, and planned interventions for symptom management
		Encourage patient involvement in decision-making regarding care and treatment plan
		Conduct patient teaching in a quiet, comfortable, and private environment
		Provide opportunity for patient and family to tour treatment area
		Provide opportunity to meet IV nurse assigned to case
		Provide nutritional counseling
		Provide opportunity for patient to express fears, concerns, and comprehension
		Emphasize variability and reversibility of side effects such as alopecia; offer patient assistance and alternatives
		Be absolutely honest with patient
Treatment	To provide sufficient information to:	Explain how chemotherapy works—cytotoxicity
	Enable patient to cope effectively with immediate effects of chemotherapy	Instruct patient to report immediately any discomfort, pain, or burning during the administration of chemotherapy
	Achieve patient sense of participation in and control over care	Review antiemetic schedule, foods to avoid, and hydration requirements
		Identify known side effects of each drug in use; instruct in precautions for thromboyctopenia—use of electric razors, nonabrasive toothbrush, ways to avoid constipation/Valsalva maneuver
		Review drug and food allergy history and record before first treatment—assess for multiple drug therapy complications—incompatibilities, and communicate to physician (eg, ASA-containing medications)
		Provide calendar with schedule of treatments, appointments with physicians and labs, and expected time line for neutropenia/thrombocytopenia to occur
		Assist patient in energy conservation program and in setting realistic goals for work and social activities
		Discuss need for contraception and potential for infertility
		Discuss potential need for central venous access
		Instruct patient in oral hygiene and use of nonalcohol-based mouth rinses
		Encourage patient to bring written lists of questions to office/clinic visit, to avoid anxiety-related omission

(continued)

Phase	Goal	Nursing Actions
Posttreatment (ongoing)	To provide sufficient information to: Allow patient to demonstrate self-management, interventions to control side effects Allow patient to function to maximum realistic potential	Provide information regarding medical self-care in managing side effects of each drug treatment Explain reasons for follow-up studies to evaluate disease response Remind patient not to travel alone immediately after treatment (in most cases) Instruct patient to report temperature >101.0°F (38°C), to report signs and symptoms of infection, increased bruising, blood in urine or stool, bleeding gums, rashes, fatigue, shortness of breath, sore throat, oral lesions, change in bowel habits, numbness or tingling in fingers or toes Stress importance of good personal hygiene; handwashing; and avoidance of rectal thermometers, enemas, and people with communicable diseases Encourage patient to call for assistance with any new or unusual medical developments and provide information on how to reach appropriate health care personnel 24 h/d Confirm return appointments and assist with patient transport services, if needed or possible Phone patient after first and subsequent treatments, when problems are possible Solicit questions regarding response to treatment, patient concerns, comprehension, and self-care regimen Review and reinforce previous information related to diagnosis, disease, and treatment

TABLE 20-2 *(Continued)*

(Prepared by M. M. McCluskey from McNally, J. C., Somerville, E. T., Miaskowski, C., & Rostad, M. [Eds.]. [1991]. *Guidelines for oncology nursing practice* [2nd ed.]. Philadelphia: W. B. Saunders; Groenwald, S. L., Frogge, M. H., Goodman, M. S., & Yarbro, C. H. [1990]. *Cancer nursing: Principles and practice* [2nd ed.]. Boston: Jones & Bartlett.)

    c. Identifies studies, tests, and procedures required before treatment

    d. Identifies follow-up tests, studies, and procedures needed to evaluate treatment results

5. Patient demonstrates knowledge of drugs' potential side effects.
    a. States mechanism of drugs' actions
    b. States reason for side effects
    c. Identifies specific side effects that may occur with each drug
    d. States self-management interventions to control side effects
    e. States signs and symptoms reportable to health care professionals
    f. Identifies procedures for reporting signs and symptoms

6. Patient demonstrates knowledge of techniques to manage chemotherapy treatment.
    a. Maintains nutritional status to best of ability
    b. Follows oral, body and environmental hygiene measures

      c. Maintains optimal rest and activity pattern

      d. Uses safety precautions to prevent injury

      e. Seeks and uses resources as necessary

      f. Verbalizes reduced anxiety related to chemotherapy treatment

      g. States intention to comply with treatment plan

7. Patient demonstrates knowledge relative to various access devices, if applicable.[26]

Wise oncology clinicians are encouraged to refer to the comprehensive works of colleagues who have provided outlines of nursing responsibilities to ensure patient and family education in the disease process, treatment, toxicities, and symptom management.[3,11,19,25,26]

CHEMOTHERAPEUTIC AGENTS

Drug Preparation, Safe Handling, and Disposal

Administering cancer chemotherapy carries some occupational risks. Adherence to recommendations for safe handling of these agents minimizes risks such as skin, mucous membrane, and eye irritation; light-headedness; facial flushing; headache; nausea; and alopecia. These manifestations appear in direct relationship to the time, amount, and method of exposure to specific classes of antineoplastics. Until more definitive studies are produced, prudent health care professionals will minimize their own potential health risks by strict adherence to guidelines in antineoplastic policy and procedure development, along with cautions during drug preparation and handling.[3,10,20,21,29] Because of the teratogenic, mutagenic, and carcinogenic properties of antineoplastic agents, these guidelines should be followed strictly, especially by nurses who are pregnant, planning pregnancy, or breast-feeding (Table 20-3 and Figure 20-1).[2]

Successful administration of chemotherapy calls for seasoned and keen judgment based on scientific evidence. It is not safe to administer these agents without clear understanding of why they are used and how they work. Expert technical skills aside, a basic understanding of *indications for use* and *mechanisms of action* are pivotal to the quality of patient care an IV nurse provides.

Indications for Use

Nitrogen mustard was the first modern chemical used therapeutically to treat the uncontrolled cellular proliferation that characterizes cancer. This lucky discovery resulted from scientific observation that bone marrow depletion (hypoplasia) occurred in soldiers exposed to mustard gases during World War II. In years that immediately followed, patients with leukemia and lymphoma were treated with nitrogen mustard; short-term but significant antitumor activity resulted. A subsequent synthesis of various analogues to nitrogen mustard led to what now is the mainstay in treatment of malignancies.[15]

Before these anticancer chemicals were discovered, surgery and radiotherapy were primary cancer treatment techniques. These modalities remain useful in treating

TABLE 20-3
Guidelines for Safe Handling and Disposal of Antineoplastic Agents

A. Drug Preparation
1. All antineoplastic drugs should be prepared by specially trained individuals in a centralized area to minimize interruptions and risks of contamination.
2. Drugs are prepared in a class II biologic safety cabinet (vertical laminar airflow hood) with vents to the outside, if possible. The blower is left on 24 h/d, 7 d/wk. The hood is serviced regularly according to the manufacturer's recommendations.
3. Eating, drinking, smoking, and applying cosmetics in the drug preparation area are prohibited.
4. The work surface is covered with a plastic absorbent pad to minimize contamination. This pad is changed immediately in the event of contamination and at the completion of drug preparation each day or shift.
5. The prescribed drug is prepared using aseptic technique according to the physician's order, other pharmaceutic resources, or both.
6. Disposable surgical latex unpowdered gloves are used when handling the drugs. Gloves should be changed hourly or immediately if torn or punctured.
7. A disposable long-sleeved gown made of lint-free fabric with knitted cuffs and a closed front is worn during drug preparation.
8. A thermoplastic (Plexiglas) face shield or goggles and a powered air-purifying respirator should be used if a biologic safety cabinet is not available.
9. Because exposure can result when connecting and disconnecting IV tubing, when injecting the drug into the IV line, when removing air from the syringe or infusion line, and when leakage occurs at the tubing, syringe, or stopcock connection, priming of all IV tubing is carried out under the protection of the hood.
10. Other measures to guard against drug leakage during drug preparation include venting the vial and using large-bore needles, luer lock fittings, and sterile gauze or sponge around the neck of the vial during needle withdrawal. Aerosolization may also be minimized by attaching an aerosol protection device (CytoGuard, Bristol-Myers) to the vial of drug before adding the diluent.
11. Once reconstituted, the drug is labeled according to institutional policies and procedures; the label should include the drug's vesicant properties and antineoplastic drug warning.
12. Antineoplastic drugs are transported in an impervious packing material and are marked with a distinctive warning label.
13. Personnel responsible for drug transport are knowledgeable of procedures to be followed in the event of drug spillage.

B. Drug Administration
1. Chemotherapeutic agents are administered by registered professional nurses who have been specially trained and designated as qualified according to specific institutional policies and procedures.
2. Before administering the drugs, the nurse ensures that informed consent has been given and clarifies any misconceptions the patient might have regarding the drugs and their side effects.
3. Appropriate laboratory results are evaluated and found to be within acceptable levels (eg, complete blood count, renal and liver function).
4. Measures to minimize side effects of the drugs are carried out before drug administration (eg, hydration, antiemetics and antianxiety agents, and patient comfort).
5. An appropriate route for drug administration is ensured according to the physician's order.
6. Personal protective equipment is worn, including disposable latex surgical gloves and a disposable gown made of a lint-free, low-permeability fabric with a closed front, long sleeves, and elastic or knit closed cuffs (optional).
7. The work surface is protected with a disposable absorbent pad.
8. The drug or drugs are administered according to established institutional policies and procedures.
9. Documentation of drug administration, including any adverse reaction, is made in the patient's medical record.
10. A mechanism for identification of patient's receiving antineoplastic agents is established for the 48-h period following drug dispensing.
11. Disposable surgical unpowdered latex gloves and a disposable gown are worn when handling body secretions such as blood, vomitus, or excreta from patients who received chemotherapy drugs within the previous 48 h.
12. In the event of accidental exposure, remove contaminated gloves or gown immediately and discard according to official procedures.
13. Wash the contaminated skin with soap and water.
14. Flood an eye that is accidentally exposed to chemotherapy with water or isotonic eye wash for at least 5 min.
15. Obtain a medical evaluation as soon as possible after exposure and document the incident according to institutional policies and procedures.

(continued)

TABLE 20-3 *(Continued)*

C. Drug Disposal

1. Regardless of the setting (hospital, ambulatory care, or home), all equipment and unused drugs are treated as hazardous and disposed of according to the institution's policies and procedures.
2. All contaminated equipment including needles are disposed of intact to prevent aerosolization, leaks, and spills.
3. All contaminated materials used in drug preparation are disposed of in a leak-proof, puncture-proof container with a distinctive warning label and are placed in a sealable 4-mil polyethylene or 2-mil polypropylene bag with appropriate labelling.
4. Linen contaminated with bodily secretions of patients who have received chemotherapy within the previous 48 h is placed in a specially marked laundry bag, which is then placed in an impervious bag that is marked with a distinctive warning label.
5. In the event of a spill, personnel should don double surgical latex unpowdered gloves; eye protection; and a disposable gown made of a lint-free, low-permeability fabric with a closed front, long sleeves, and elastic or knit closed cuffs.
6. Small amounts of liquids are cleaned up with gauze pads, whereas larger spills (>5 mL) are cleaned up with absorbent pads.
7. Small amounts of solids or spills involving powder are cleaned up with damp cloths or absorbent gauze pads.
8. The spill area is cleaned three times with a detergent followed by clean water.
9. Broken glassware and disposable contaminated materials are placed in a leak-proof, puncture-proof container and then placed in a sealable 4-mil polyethylene or 2-mil polypropylene bag and marked with a distinctive warning label.
10. Contaminated reusable items are washed by specially trained personnel wearing double surgical unpowdered latex gloves.
11. The spill should be documented according to established institutional policies and procedures.

(From Goodman, M. S. [1991]. Delivery of cancer chemotherapy. In S. B. Baird [Ed.]. *Cancer nursing: A comprehensive textbook* [p. 294]. Philadelphia: W. B. Saunders.)

FIGURE 20-1   An oncologic pharmacist prepares the drug, using aseptic technique, in a class II biologic safety cabinet (vertical laminar air-flow hood).

localized tumors, which can either be surgically removed or destroyed by radiating the genetic material within the cancer cells.

Cancer often is a systemic disease, however, that requires systemic therapy. By nature, cancer cells deviate from normal cells in structure, function, and production; therefore, cancer has the characterizing ability to invade blood and lymph vessels and to spread beyond the localized region of the primary disease site.[5] The ability of these aberrant cells to metastasize is the foundation on which systemic anticancer therapy is based. Although immunotherapy is a promising systemic approach to cancer, chemotherapy is the primary systemic modality in clinical use today.

Mechanisms of Action

Chemotherapy controls cancer with cytotoxic chemical agents designed to kill rapidly dividing cancer cells with minimal impact on cells with normal, healthy mitotic characteristics. Table 20-4 shows that chemotherapy is responsible for cure in about 12% of human cancers and has a significant effect on improved survival in another 40% to 50%. Remaining cancers are less responsive to chemotherapeutic intervention as a "curative modality."[5]

Palliation is a legitimate chemotherapeutic goal for patients with advanced or incurable disease. Even when there is no real hope of complete cure, cancer cells often remain somewhat sensitive to antineoplastic agents, so disease progression can be slowed. Agents often can control pain caused by tumor pressure, can ease fluid obstruction, and can "quiet" hypercalcemia and other organic processes.

Agents are grouped according to their specific effect on cancer cell chemistry and the cell cycle phase in which they interfere. (The cell cycle refers to the time required for a single cell to reproduce itself.[11])

Antineoplastic agents fall into two categories: *Cell cycle phase-specific agents* are active only during a particular point in the cell replication cycle; *cell cycle phase-nonspecific agents* are active at any point in that cycle. Regardless of the drug's timing and impact location, the basic mechanism of antineoplastic action is the same—chemotherapeutic drugs inhibit DNA synthesis. This disables cell reproduction, so cancer cells die.

Chemotherapies are further categorized into six major groups: alkylating agents, antimetabolites, plant alkaloids, antitumor antibiotics, hormones, and now taxanes. Within each of these categories is a spectrum of agents of various toxicities, all relating to their antineoplastic properties.

Drug toxicities can be appreciated with understanding that agents are designed to destroy rapidly dividing cells. It is logical, therefore, that other cells that divide rapidly—bone marrow, hair follicles, gastrointestinal mucosa, reproductive tissues—also are most vulnerable to drug action. Therefore, the most frequent side effects of these drugs include cytopenia, alopecia, mucositis, nausea, vomiting, and infertility.

Figure 20-2 demonstrates these relationships in systemic therapies. Of course, these toxicities are linked to malignancy type, patient age, performance status, and level of health before and during therapy.[5]

Table 20-5 provides a quick reference guide for basic drug preparation, handling and administration, plus frequently experienced toxicities, according to organ systems (eg, hematologic, dermatologic, gastrointestinal, genitourinary, hepatic, and

TABLE 20-4
Classification of Tumors According to General Sensitivity to Chemotherapy
TUMORS RESPONSIVE TO CHEMOTHERAPY

Tumors Curable in Advanced Stages by Chemotherapy

Choriocarcinoma

Acute lymphocytic leukemia
(in children and adults)

Hodgkin's disease

Diffuse large cell lymphoma

Lymphoblastic lymphoma
(in children and adults)

Follicular mixed lymphoma

Testicular cancer

Acute myelogenous leukemia

Wilms' tumor

Burkitt's lymphoma

Embryonal rhabdomyosarcoma

Ewing's sarcoma

Peripheral neuroepithelioma

Neuroblastoma

Small cell cancer of the lung

Ovarian cancer

Tumors Curable in the Adjuvant Setting by Chemotherapy

Breast cancer

Osteogenic sarcoma

Soft tissue sarcoma

Colorectal cancer

Tumors Responsive in Advanced Stages but not yet Curable by Chemotherapy

Bladder cancer

Chronic myelogenous leukemia

Chronic lymphocytic leukemia

Hairy cell leukemia

Multiple myeloma

Follicular small-cleaved cell lymphoma

Gastric carcinoma

Cervical carcinoma

Soft tissue sarcoma

Head and neck cancer

Endometrial cancer

Adrenocortical carcinoma

Medulloblastoma

Polycythemia rubra vera

Prostate cancer

Glioblastoma multiforme

Insulinoma

Breast cancer

Carcinoid tumors

Tumors Poorly Responsive in Advanced Stages to Chemotherapy

Osteogenic sarcoma

Pancreatic cancer

Renal cancer

Thyroid cancer

Carcinoma of the vulva or penis

Colorectal cancer

Non–small-cell lung cancer

Melanoma

Hepatocellular carcinoma

(From DeVita, V. T. [1989]. Principles and practice of cancer chemotherapy. In V. T. DeVita, S. Hellman, & S. A. Rosenberg [Eds.], *Cancer: Principles and practice of oncology* [p. 297]. Philadelphia: J. B. Lippincott. Used with permission.)

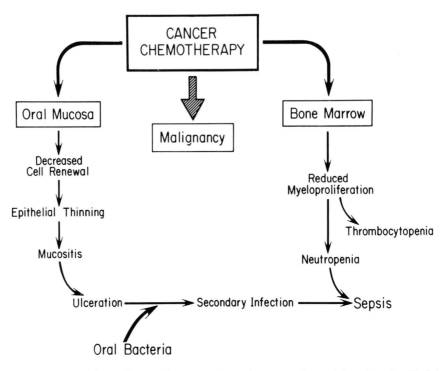

FIGURE 20-2   Effects of systemic cancer chemotherapy on the oral, basal, and epithelial cells and on the bone marrow stem cells. (From Sonis, S. T. [1989]. Oral complications of cancer therapy. In V. T. DeVita, S. Hellman, & S. A. Rosenberg [Eds.], *Cancer: Principles and practice of oncology* [3rd ed., p. 2146]. Philadelphia: J. B. Lippincott. Used with permission.)

neurologic). Comprehensive tables are available and should be used for more detailed information on indications for use, routes of delivery, pharmacokinetics, and dosing, which vary extensively as new protocols indicate the use of new combinations of existing drugs.[5-7,11]

Combined Modality Therapy

Although any treatment modality can be used alone, often they are used in combination with one another. Frequently chemotherapy is used as adjuvant treatment to assist in curing or controlling disseminated disease. Combining the available modalities is done in an effort to optimize cancer cell kill while minimizing associated toxicities.[11]

With the exception of oral alkylating agents, used for chronic leukemias, single-agent chemotherapy regimens are rare in contemporary medicine.[16] Simultaneous multiagent use capitalizes on synergistic drug actions on the cell cycle, to maximize their antitumor effects. Combining agents also modifies dose-limiting toxicities.

Table 20-6 provides a list of common combinations of cytotoxic agents.[18] A classic example of combination chemotherapy is the MOPP regimen (mechlorethamine

Text continues on p. 496

TABLE 20-5
Quick Reference to Commonly Administered Parenteral Chemotherapeutic Agents

Drug	Amt/Vial	Diluent	Final Concentration	Usual Dose	Usual Administration Technique	Comments and Major Toxicities
Asparaginase Enzyme Nonchemo- therapeutic agent	10,000 IU	5 mL SWI 2 mL SWI	2000 IU/mL 5000 IU/mL	15–25,000 U/m^2 as a single dose	IVP slowly over 30 min IVPB (D5W, NS) in up to 1000 mL. IM	Acute liver dysfunction. Nausea and vomiting common and may be severe Hypersensitivity rxns Depression, lethargy, and drowsiness
Bleomycin Antitumor Antibiotic	15 U	7.75 mL NS	2 U/mL	10–20 U/m^2 qwk or twice weekly IM, IV or SQ. Constant infusions over 3–7 days at 20 U/m^2/day	IVP, IM or SQ IVPB (rare)	Pulmonary fibrosis Hypersensitivity rxns, fever and chills (premedicate with Tylenol) Skin rxns common (especially pruritic erythema) Reversible alopecia Mucositis, stomatitis, and mild nausea and vomiting
Carboplatin Platinum complex	450 mg 150 mg 50 mg	45 mL SWI 15 mL SWI 5 mL SWI	10 mg/mL	360–400 mg/m^2 q4wk	IV infusion ONLY (D5W, NS) May dilute to as low as 0.5 mg/mL	Leukopenia and throm-bocytopenia nadir at day 21; recovery by day 28–30 Nausea and vomiting (less severe than with Cisplatin) Increase in serum creatinine and BUN DO NOT USE ALUMINUM NEEDLES
BCNU (carmustine) Alkylating agent	100 mg	3 mL of provided diluent. Then 27 mL SWI.	3.3 mg/mL	150–200 mg/m^2 q6wk	IVPB ONLY (D5W, NS) Infuse in 100–250 mL of fluid over 1–2 hr	Delayed leukopenia 4–5 wks after admin-istration, with nadir lasting 1–2 wks Thrombocytopenia with nadir 4–5 wks after administration lasting 1–2 wks Nausea and vomiting common occurring 2–6 hr after adminis-tration and lasting 4–24 hr

(continued)

TABLE 20-5 *(Continued)*

Drug	Amt/Vial	Diluent	Final Concentration	Usual Dose	Usual Administration Technique	Comments and Major Toxicities
						Painful venous irritation during administration.
						Dose-related pulmonary fibrosis
						Dose-related renal failure
Cisplatin Platinum complex	50 mg AQ 100 mg AQ	Already in solution	1 mg/mL	20–40 mg/m² day × 3–5 days q 3–4 wks 20–120 mg/m² given as a single dose q 3–4 wk	IV infusion ONLY (D5W, NS) 250–1000 mL Infuse over 1–8 hr Ensure adequate hydration	Nausea and vomiting—often severe starting about 1 hr after treatment and lasting 24 hr
						Nephrotoxicity is dose related
						Ototoxicity with tinnitus and/or hearing loss is dose dependent
						Moderate leukopenia and thrombocytopenia with a nadir on day 18–23 and recovery by day 39
						Alopecia and electrolyte imbalances
						PROTECT FROM LIGHT.
						USE 5-μM FILTER FOR SOLNS CONTAINING MANNITOL
						DO NOT USE ALUMINUM NEEDLES
Cyclophosphamide (Cytoxan) Alkylating agent	1000 mg 500 mg	50 mL SWI 25 mL SWI	20 mg/mL	500–1500 mg/m² q 3–4 wks	IVP over 5–10 min. (usually doses <750 mg). IVPB (D5W, D5NS) infuse in 100–150 mL over 15–30 min	Acute hemorrhagic cystitis in poorly hydrated individuals at doses of 1–2 g/m² FORCE FLUIDS Leukopenia with a nadir of 8–14 days and recovery in 18–25 days; nausea and vomiting with an onset within 4–6 hr after treatment and lasting 8–10 hr

(continued)

TABLE 20-5 *(Continued)*

Drug	Amt/Vial	Diluent	Final Concentration	Usual Dose	Usual Administration Technique	Comments and Major Toxicities
						Alopecia in 50% occurring approx. 3 wk after treatment
						Medium to low risk of pulmonary toxicity
						Cardiac necrosis with high dose
						Nail and skin hyperpigmentation
						Nasal stuffiness during administration
						Testicular atrophy and amenorrhea
Cytarabine (ARA-C) Antimetabolite	1000 mg 500 mg	10 mL SWI 10 mL SWI	100 mg/mL 50 mg/mL	100–150 mg/m^2 IV or SQ for 5–10 days	IVP (low dose) over 1–2 min	Leukopenia and thrombocytopenia with a nadir in 5–7 days
				20–30 mg/m^2 intrathecally	IVP (D5W, NS) in up to 1000 mL fluid for high-dose therapy	Nausea and vomiting dose related
				High dose: 3 g/m^2 q12hr for 6 days		Medium to low risk of pulmonary toxicity
						Stomatitis and diarrhea
						Lethargy and keratoconjunctivitis with high doses (use dexamethasone eye drops)
						Alopecia (occasional)
						Cerebellar toxicity
DTIC (dacarbazine) Alkylating agent	200 mg 100 mg	19.7 mL SWI 9.9 mL SWI	10 mg/mL	75–125 mg/m^2/day for 10 days repeated q 4 wk	IVP over 1 min IVP (D5W, NS) in up to 250 mL	Leukopenia and thrombocytopenia with a nadir at 21–25 days
				50–250 mg/m^2/day for 5 days repeated q 3 wk	Infuse over 30 min	Severe nausea and vomiting common. Occurs 1–3 hr after treatment usually lasting up to 12 hr
				650–1450 mg/m^2 as a single dose q 3–4 wk		Anorexia
						Flulike symptoms with high doses
						Alopecia and facial flushing

(continued)

TABLE 20-5   *(Continued)*

Drug	Amt/Vial	Diluent	Final Concentration	Usual Dose	Usual Administration Technique	Comments and Major Toxicities
						IRRITANT: avoid extravasation. Local pain at injection site. Slow rate of infusion to decrease pain from venous spasm.
						PROTECT FROM LIGHT
Dactinomycin Antitumor Antibiotic Vesicant	0.5 mg	1.1 mL SWI	0.5 mg/mL	*Adults* 1–2 mg/m^2 q 3 wk or 0.25 mg/m^2 day × 5 days q 3–4 wk *Children* 0.25–0.5 mg/m^2 day × 5 days. Not to exceed 0.5 mg/day	IVP slowly over 2–3 min IVPB (D5W, NS) in 50–100 mL over 20–30 min	Leukopenia and thrombocytopenia occurring in 7–10 days with nadir at approx. 3 weeks Nausea and vomiting common and severe occurring immediately or a few hours after treatment lasting 4–20 hr—may be prolonged Erythema, hyperpigmentation and alopecia Stomatitis, dysphagia, proctitis and diarrhea Skin irritation or even necrosis in previously irradiated areas ("radiation recall")
Daunorubicin (Cerubidine) Antitumor Antibiotic Vesicant	20 mg	4 mL SWI	5 mg/mL	30–60 mg/m^2/day for 2–3 days q 3–4 wks	IVP slowly over 2–3 min Continuous infusion IVPB (D5W, NS) in 50–100 mL to infuse over 20–30 min	Leukopenia with nadir between 1–2 wk, recovery in 2–3 wk Thrombocytopenia less significant with nadir at 4–15 days and recovery in 2–3 wk Nausea and vomiting commonly occurring 1 hr after dose and lasting for several hours Diarrhea and stomatitis Rash, alopecia totalis

(continued)

TABLE 20-5   *(Continued)*

Drug	Amt/Vial	Diluent	Final Concentration	Usual Dose	Usual Administration Technique	Comments and Major Toxicities
						Cumulative cardio-toxicity at max. lifetime dose of 500–600 mg/m^2 (aggravated by concurrent radiation)
						Fever
						Red urine—advise patient
						PROTECT FROM LIGHT
Dexrazoxane (Zinecard) Cardioprotectant Antidote	250 mg, 500 mg	0.167M (M/6) Sodium lactate	10 mg/mL	Dosage ratio of 10:1 of Dexrazoxane: doxorubicin	Slow IVP, rapid IV infusion (NS, D5W) In final conc. of 1.3–5 mg/mL	Give doxorubicin after completing dexrazoxane, but no later than 30 min from start of dexrazoxane dose
						Dexrazoxane may add to myelosuppression caused by chemotherapeutic agents
Doxorubicin (Adriamycin) Antitumor Antibiotic Vesicant	200 mg MDV	Already in solution	2 mg/mL	60–75 mg/m^2 as a bolus injection of a continuous infusion over 2–4 days q 3–4 wk 30 mg/m^2 daily for 3 days q 3–4 wk	IVP slowly over 20–30 min IVPB (D5W, NS) in 50–100 mL over 20–30 min Continuous infusion over 24–96 hr via IV fluid or EID	Leukopenia and thrombocytopenia with a nadir at 10–14 days and recovery in 21 days
						Alopecia (usually complete), hyperpigmentation of nailbeds and dermal creases
						Nausea and vomiting, sometimes severe, anorexia, stomatitis—especially with daily × 3 schedule
						Radiation recall: irritation of previously irradiated areas
						Arrhythmias and ECG changes

(continued)

TABLE 20-5 *(Continued)*

Drug	Amt/Vial	Diluent	Final Concentration	Usual Dose	Usual Administration Technique	Comments and Major Toxicities
						CHF due to cardiomyopathy related to total cumulative dose (risk greater at doses above 550 mg/m^2
						May enhance cyclophosphamide cystitis
						Advise patient of red discoloration of urine occurring up to 24 hrs after administration
						"Adria" flare may occur: erythematous streak up the vein
						Incompatible with heparin and 5-FU
						PROTECT FROM LIGHT
Doxorubicin Liposomal (Doxil) Anthracycline	20 mg	Liposomal dispersion	2 mg/mL	20 mg/m^2/every 3 weeks	IVPB (D5W). Infuse in 250 mL over 30 min	Same toxicities as doxorubicin HCL, but less frequent fever and nausea
						Acute Infusion Reaction: rate-related: flushing, SOB, facial swelling, chest tightness, hypotension—decrease rate or stop
Etoposide (VP-16) Plant alkaloid	100 mg	Already in solution	20 mg/mL	50–100 mg/m^2/day × 5 days	IVPB (D5W, NS) ONLY in 250 mL over at least 30 min to 1 hr	Leukopenia (dose-related), primarily granulocytopenia; nadirs within 7–14 days and recovery within 20 days. Thrombocytopenia uncommon
						Alopecia: mild and reversible
						Nausea and vomiting: mild; anorexia in 10%–13%

(continued)

TABLE 20-5 *(Continued)*

Drug	Amt/Vial	Diluent	Final Concentration	Usual Dose	Usual Administration Technique	Comments and Major Toxicities
						Hyperbilirubinemia and increased transaminase levels more common with high dose protocols
						Peripheral neuropathy
						TRANSIENT HYPOTENSION ASSOCIATED WITH RAPID ADMINISTRATION: INFUSE OVER 30 MIN TO 1 HR
						Discontinue infusion if hypersensitivity/bronchospasm occurs.
Fluorouracil (5-FU) Antimetabolite	500 mg	Already in solution	50 mg/mL	300–450 mg/m²/day IVP × 5 days q 28 days 300–750 mg/m² IVP weekly or every other week 1000 mg/m² infused over 24 hr × 4–5 days	IVP at any convenient rate Continuous infusion (D5W, NS) CADD pumps over 5 days Intraocular 1 mg/0.1 mL in preservative-free NS	Leukopenia nadir at 9–14 days, with recovery in 21–25 days. Thrombocytopenia nadir at 7–14 days with recovery by approx. day 30. Both are dose limiting and less common with continuous infusion. Dermatitis, nail changes, hyperpigmentation, alopecia and chemical phlebitis with long term infusion (see Figure 24-12). Nausea, vomiting, and anorexia. Diarrhea (may be severe) can be dose limiting. Stomatitis is more common with 5-day infusion. Pharyngitis Cerebellar ataxia and headache PROTECT FROM LIGHT

(continued)

TABLE 20-5 *(Continued)*

Drug	Amt/Vial	Diluent	Final Concentration	Usual Dose	Usual Administration Technique	Comments and Major Toxicities
Fludarabine (Fludara) Antimetabolite	50 mg	2mL SWFI	25 mg/mL	25 mg/m^2/day for 5 consecutive days May repeat course q28 days	IVPB, IV infusion (NS, D5W) Infuse in 50 to 125 mL, in a glass container	Dose-dependent CNS toxicity—delayed blindness, coma, death—can occur up to 21 to 60 days after the last dose Hematologic: neutropenia, anemia, thrombocytopenia GI: nausea, vomiting, diarrhea, anorexia Tumor lysis syndrome associated with large tumor burdens Pulmonary: cough, pneumonia, dyspnea General: chills, fever, infection, malaise
Idarubicin (Idamycin) Antitumor Antibiotic Vesicant	10 mg 5 mg	10 mL NS 5 mL NS	1 mg/mL	12 mg/m^2/day for 3 days 8–15 mg/m^2 as a single dose q 3 wk sometimes used	IVP over 10 to 15 min IVPB (D5W, NS) in any convenient volume	Myelosuppression, dose limiting Nausea, vomiting, diarrhea, and stomatitis Alopecia, extravasation reactions, and rash Transient arrhythmias, decreased LVEF, and CHF PROTECT FROM LIGHT
	1 gm 3 gm 200 mg	20 mL SWI 60 mL SWI Already in solution	50 mg/mL 100 mg/mL	1–1.2 g/m^2 over 5 consecutive days q 3–4 wk Higher doses have been given over 2–3 days 20% of Ifosphamide dose given just before 4 and 8 hr after Ifosphamide	IVPB ONLY (D5W, NS, D5NS) in 250–1000 mL over 30 min or more IVP over 5 min. IVPB (D5W, NS) 50–100 mL over any convenient time	Leukopenia, thrombocytopenia (dose limiting); anemia Nausea, vomiting, anorexia, constipation, and diarrhea Alopecia, rash, and urticaria Increased ALT, AST, and hyperbilirubinemia

(continued)

TABLE 20-5 *(Continued)*

Drug	Amt/Vial	Diluent	Final Concentration	Usual Dose	Usual Administration Technique	Comments and Major Toxicities
						Hemorrhagic cystitis and hematuria. Encourage ample fluids: HYDRATION OF >2 L/DAY TO MAINTAIN URINARY OUTPUT AND FREQUENT VOIDING. USE OF MESNA RECOMMENDED.
Ifosphamide (Ifex) Alkylating agent Mesna						Somnolence, lethargy, disorientation, confusion, dizziness, and malaise
						Chemical thrombophlebitis
Uroprotective agent (non chemotherapeutic agent)						MESNA: Nausea, vomiting, diarrhea, abdominal pain, and altered taste
						Rash and urticaria
						Lethargy, headache, joint or limb pain, fatigue
Leucovorin, Calcium Tetrahydrofolic acid derivative Nonchemotherapeutic agent	350 mg 50 mg	17.5 mL SWI 5 mL SWI	20 mg/mL 10 mg/mL	Methotrexate rescue: 10–25 mg/m^2 q 6 hr × 6–8 doses To potentiate the effect of 5 FU: 20–500 mg/m^2/dose	IVP at any convenient rate IM PO IVPB (D5W, NS) 50–250 mL over 15 min	Rare hypersensitivity reactions
Mechlorethamine (Nitro Mustard) Alkylating agent Vesicant	10 mg	10 mL SWI	1 mg/mL	Hodgkin's disease: 6 mg/m^2 on days 1 and 8 of a monthly cycle (MOPP regimen) Up to 0.4 mg/kg as a single agent monthly	IVP over 1–3 min into the tubing of a rapidly running IV	Leukopenia and thrombocytopenia within 24 hr, with a nadir at 6–8 days to 3 wk Severe nausea and vomiting beginning 1–3 hr after treatment and lasting approx. 8 hr. Diarrhea Discoloration of infused vein and phlebitis

(continued)

TABLE 20-5 *(Continued)*

Drug	Amt/Vial	Diluent	Final Concentration	Usual Dose	Usual Administration Technique	Comments and Major Toxicities
						Alopecia and stomatitis
						Vesicant: use of the antidote sodium thio-sulfate is indicated if extravasation occurs
						Advise patient of metallic taste
						Amenorrhea and impaired spermato-genesis
						Mechlorethiamine is incompatible with other antineoplastic agents and IV fluids due to its instability.
Methotrexate Antimetabolite	200 mg 50 mg 1 g	Already in solution preserv. free 19.4 mL SWI	25 mg/mL 50 mg/mL	Solid tumors: 20–40 mg/m² every 1–2 wk Leukemias and lymphomas: 200–500 mg/m² every 2–4 wk Intrathecal: Usually 12 mg in preserva-tive-free NS	IVP (<100 mg) at any convenient rate IVPB (D5W, NS) in up to 500 mL over 30 min to 1 hr Intrathecally IM	Leukopenia and throm-bocytopenia with high dose Stomatitis, sore throat, and pruritis with high dose Diarrhea can be severe with melana. Hematemesis Nausea and vomiting uncommon with low-dose therapy Renal dysfunction with high dose. Hepatic dysfunction more likely in patients receiving long-term continuous or daily treatment. Encephalopathy with multiple intrathecal doses. Confusion, ataxia, tremors, irritability, seizures, and coma Hypersensitivity rxns associated with fever, chills, and rash

(continued)

TABLE 20-5   *(Continued)*

Drug	Amt/Vial	Diluent	Final Concentration	Usual Dose	Usual Administration Technique	Comments and Major Toxicities
						Skin erythema, depigmentation or hyperpigmentation, alopecia, and photo-sensitivity
						Doses >80 mg/wk should be accompanied by leucovorin rescue (see under leucovorin)
Mitomycin C Antitumor Antibiotic Vesicant	20 mg 5 mg	50 mL SWI 10 mL SWI	0.5 mg/mL	10–20 mg/m² q 6–8 wk	IVP over 1–5 min IVPB (D5W, NS) in up to 250 mL over 30 min	Leukopenia and thrombocytopenia: delayed, cumulative, and dose limiting; anemia. Leukopenia nadir at day 25, recovery by day 32–39. Thrombocytopenia nadir at day 28, recovery by day 42–49
						Stomatitis, alopecia, dermatitis, and pruritis
						Nausea, vomiting, anorexia, and diarrhea
						Hepatomegaly and liver failure
						Parasthesias, fatigue, lethargy, weakness, and blurred vision
						Interstitial pneumonitis. Discontinue drug if acute bronchospasm occurs.
						Nephrotoxicity with high doses (>50 mg/m²)
						Pain on injection and phlebitis
Mitoxantrone Antitumor Antibiotic	20 mg 25 mg 30 mg	Already in solution	2 mg/mL	10–12 mg/m²/day × 5 days for induction therapy for ANLL	IVP has been used (over 3 min. or more), but IVPB preferred route	Leukopenia and thrombocytopenia nadirs at 10–12 days, with recovery on day 21

(continued)

TABLE 20-5 *(Continued)*

Drug	Amt/Vial	Diluent	Final Concentration	Usual Dose	Usual Administration Technique	Comments and Major Toxicities
				Other: 12 mg/m^2 q 3–4 wk	IVPB (D5W, NS) in at least 50 mL over not <3 min	Alopecia (mild), pruritis, and dry skin Nausea, vomting, diarrhea, and stomatitis (mild) Cumulative cardiomyopathy (CHF), arrhythmias, and chest pain (occasional) Hypersensitivity rxns may include hypotension, uticaria, and rash Advise patient of blue/green discoloration of urine, stool, and sclerae for 24–48 hr after treatment May also discolor veins Fever, conjuctivitis, phlebitis, and amenorrhea
Paclitaxel (Taxol) Antitumor agent	30 mg	in solution	6 mg/mL	Ovarian: 135 mg/m^2 every 3 wk Breast: 175 mg/m^2 every 3 wk	IV infusion (NS, D5W, D5 NS, D5 Ringers) Ovarian: over 24 hr Breast: over 3 hr Prepare to conc of 0.3–1.2 mg/mL in glass Do not allow contact of the undiluted Taxol concentrate with plasticized PVC equipment Use in-line filter @ 0.22 micron or less, and a polyethelene-lined administration set	Hematologic: Do not repeat course until patient's neutrophil is at least 1500 cells/mm^3 and platelet count at least 100,000 cells/mm^3; thrombocytopenia, leukopenia, neutropenia, anemia, bleeding Premedicate to avoid hypersensitivity reaction, with dexamethasone, diphenhydramine, and ranitidine (or cimetidine) Cardiac: Hypotension and bradycardia—monitor vital signs during 1st hour of administration; ECG abnormalities

(continued)

TABLE 20-5 (Continued)

Drug	Amt/Vial	Diluent	Final Concentration	Usual Dose	Usual Administration Technique	Comments and Major Toxicities
						General: Infection
						Neurologic: dose-dependent peripheral neuropathy, arthralgia/myalgia
						GI: nausea, vomiting, diarrhea, mucositis
						Dermatologic: alopecia, rash, flushing
						Pulmonary: dyspnea
Plicamycin (Mithracin) Antitumor agent Antibiotic	2500 mcg	4.9 mL SWFI	500 mcg/mL	Testicular tumor: 25–30 mcg/kg/day for 8 to 10 days Hypercalcemia: 25 mcg/ky/day for 3–4 days	IV infusion (NS, D5W). Infuse in 250 to 1000 mL over 4–7 hr Premedicate with antiemetics if using shorter infusion time IVP, through a running infusion over 5 min	GI symptoms: anorexia, nausea, vomiting, diarrhea, stomatitis—use antiemetics if using shorter infusion time Dose-related hemorrhagic syndrome: Epitaxis first sign, monitor platelet count, prothombin, and bleeding times Renal: Nephrotoxicity Hypocalcemia Parenteral irritant—avoid extravasation
Streptozocin Antitumor Antibiotic Nitrosourea	1000 mg	9.5 mL NS	100 mg/mL	500–1000 mg/m²/day × 5 days q 3–4 wk 1–1.5 g/m² weekly	IVP over 15 min or more IVPB (D5W, NS) in up to 250 mL over 1–2 hr Continuous infusion × 5 days	Anemia (common). Leukopenia and thrombocytopenia (rarely dose limiting). Eosinophilia Nausea and vomiting common and occasionally severe; anorexia, diarrhea, and abdominal cramps Nephrotoxicity common (dose related) with proteinuria

(continued)

TABLE 20-5 *(Continued)*

Drug	Amt/Vial	Diluent	Final Concentration	Usual Dose	Usual Administration Technique	Comments and Major Toxicities
						Vein irritation during administration; slow infusion to minimize pain
						Transient increases in ALT, AST, alk phos, and LDH.
						Glucose intolerance and glycosuria
Teniposide (VM-26)	50 mg	in solution	10 mg/mL	Refractory to cytarabine regimen: 165 mg/m^2 BIW for 8–9 doses Refractory to vincristine/prednisone regimen: 250 mg/m^2 weekly for 4–8 wk	IV infusion (NS, D5W) Infuse in concentration of 0.1, 0.2, 0.4 or 1 mg/mL, over 30 to 60 min or longer	Contains 30 mg benzyl alcohol/amp—use with caution in premature infants Anaphylaxis may occur GI: mucositis, nausea, vomiting, diarrhea
Thiotepa Alkylating agent	15 mg	1.5 mL SWI	10 mg/mL	Nontransplant: 12–16 µg/m^2 q 1–4 wk Transplant: 900 mg/m^2 Intrathecal: 1–10 mg/m^2 q 1–2 wk Bladder instillation: 30–60 mg q 1–4 wk Intracavitary: 0.6–0.8 mg/kg through the same tubing used to remove fluid from the cavity	IVPB (D5W, NS) in 50–100 mL over 10 min Bladder instillation: in 50 mL NS	Thrombocytopenia (more prominent) and leukopenia with nadirs at 14 days and recovery after 2–4 wk. Anemia Alopecia (rare with low dose) Hypersensitivity rxns include hives, rash, and pruritis Nausea, vomiting, anorexia, and stomatitis dose dependent Headache, dizziness, and weakness of lower extremities Paresthesias associated with intrathecal administration

(continued)

TABLE 20-5 *(Continued)*

Drug	Amt/Vial	Diluent	Final Concentration	Usual Dose	Usual Administration Technique	Comments and Major Toxicities
						Azoospermia and amenorrhea
						Pain at site of injection
Vinblastine (Velban) Plant Alkaloid Vesicant	10 mg	10 mL NS	1 mg/mL	6–10 mg/m^2 q 2–4 wk	IVP over 1 min IVPB not recommended, but stable in NS at a concentration of 20 mg/mL Continuous infusions have been given over 96 hr or longer through a central venous catheter	Marked leukopenia with early nadirs. Thrombocytopenia and anemia
						Alopecia. Skin and soft tissue damage if extravasated (treat with SQ injections of hyaluronidase and application of heat to disperse drug). Rash and photosensitivity
						Nausea, vomiting, and constipation; abdominal pain, anorexia, diarrhea, and stomatitis
						Peripheral neuropathy, myalgias, headache, seizures, depression, dizziness, and malaise
						Acute bronchospasm more common when administered with Mitomycin C
						Severe jaw pain
						Phlebitis and vein discoloration
						Azoospermia and amenorrhea
Vincristine (Oncovin) Plant alkaloid Vesicant	1 mg	Already in solution	1 mg/mL	0.5–1.4 mg/m^2 q 1–4 wk Usually the maximum dose is 2 mg	IVP over 1 min Occasionally given as a continuous infusion (D5W, NS) over 96 hr via a central line	Leukopenia (mild and rare), thrombocytopenia (rare)

(continued)

TABLE 20-5 *(Continued)*

Drug	Amt/Vial	Diluent	Final Concentration	Usual Dose	Usual Administration Technique	Comments and Major Toxicities
						Alopecia; skin and soft tissue damage if extravasated (use SQ hyaluronidase and applicaton of heat to disperse drug); rash
						Nausea, vomiting (rare); constipation (place patient on bowel regimen). Abdominal pain, anorexia, and diarrhea
						New labeling requirements must specify "for IV use only" (intrathecal administration is fatal)
						Peripheral neuropathy, parasthesias, constipation, paralytic ileus, and myalgias
						Acute bronchospasm more common when administered with Mitomycin C
Vinorelbine (Navelbine) Mitotic inhibitor	10 mg, 50 mg	In solution	10 mg/mL	30 mg/m^2/wk	IV syringe (NS, D5W), IV bag (0.45 NS, NS, D5W, D5 0.45 NS, Ringer's, Lactated Ringer's) Syringe: conc @ 1.5–3 mg/mL, IV bag: conc @ 0.5–2 mg/mL, infuse over 6–10 min into side port of a free-flowing IV closest to the IV bag, then flush with 75 125 mL of solution	Hematologic toxicity: granulocyte counts should be >1000 cells/mm^3 prior to administration of vinorelbine Pulmonary: acute shortness of breath (most common in patients receiving concurrent mitomycin therapy), severe bronchospasm Myelosuppression: dose-limiting Dermatologic: mild alopecia, injection site erythema, pain, phlebitis

(continued)

TABLE 20-5   *(Continued)*

Drug	Amt/Vial	Diluent	Final Concentration	Usual Dose	Usual Administration Technique	Comments and Major Toxicities
						GI: mild nausea, constipation, diarrhea, stomatitis
						Hepatic: transient elevated LFTs
						Neurologic: peripheral neuropathy

The information here is provided as guidance only. Nurses should always consult the manufacturer's current prescribing information before administering drugs. ALT, alanine aminotransferase; ANLL, acute nonlymphocytic leukemia; AST, aspartate aminotransferase; alk phos, alklaline phosphatase; BUN, blood urea nitrogen; CHF, congestive heart failure; ECG, electrocardiographic; IVP, intravenous push; IVPB, intravenous piggyback; LDH, lactate dehydrogenase; LVEF, left ventricular ejection fraction; MDV, multiple-dose vial; NS, normal saline; rxn(s), reaction(s); SQ, subcutaneous; SWI, sterile water for injection.

(As revised by Jane Leung-Vega, RPH, MS, Merck-Medco Managed Care. Prepared by Christopher Charlton, RPH, and M. M. McCluskey, RN, OCN, CRNI, St. Joseph Hospital, Chicago IL [1992]. From: Dorr, R., & Fritz, W. [1980]. *Cancer chemotherapy handbook*. New York: Elsevier; Hubbard, S. M., Seipp, C. A., & Duffy, P. L. [1992]. Administration of cancer treatments: Practical guide for physicians and oncology nurses. In V. T. DeVita, S. Hellman, & S. A. Rosenberg [Eds.]. *Cancer: Principles and practice of oncology* [3rd ed., pp. 2371–2375]. Philadelphia: J. B. Lippincott; ECOG drug information sheets [1992]. [4th ed.]. Madison, WI: Eastern Cooperative Oncology Group.)

TABLE 20-6
Anticancer Drug Combinations

ABVD	Doxorubicin + bleomycin + vinblastine + dacarbazine
CHOP	Cyclophosphamide + doxorubicin + vincristine + prednisone
CMF	Cyclophosphamide + methotrexate + fluorouracil
COPP	Cyclophosphamide + vincristine + procarbazine + prednisone
CVP	Cyclophosphamide + vincristine + prednisone
CY–VA–DIC	Cyclophosphamide + vincristine + doxorubicin + dacarbazine
FAC	Fluorouracil + doxorubicin + cyclophosphamide
FAM	Fluorouracil + doxorubicin + mitomycin
MOPP	Mechlorethamine + vincristine + procarbazine + prednisone
MPL + PRED	Melphalan + prednisone
MTX + MP + CTX	Methotrexate + mercaptopurine + cyclophosphamide
VAC	Vincristine + dactinomycin + cyclophosphamide
VBP	Vinblastine + bleomycin + cisplatin
VP–L–Asparaginase	Vincristine + prednisone + asparaginase

(From National Cancer Institute. [1990]. *Chemotherapy and you—A guide to self-help during treatment*. Bethesda, MD: U.S. Department of Health and Human Services. Used with permission.)

[Mustargen], vincristine [Oncovin], procarbazine, and prednisone) used to treat Hodgkin's disease.[11]

The specific and fixed sequence in which drugs are administered yields specific and predictable toxicities. Figure 20-3 illustrates this regimen's depletion of bone marrow, which results in neutropenia (the "nadir").[3,11]

Combining cytotoxic agents, then combining them with one or more additional therapy modalities, potentially provides the greatest collective benefit of each therapy, thus, the greatest likelihood of cure. A combination of therapies, either for cure or control, may expose a patient to significant toxicity. Most patients (especially

MOPP/ABV ± D Administration Schedule and Corresponding White Blood Cell Count Nadirs

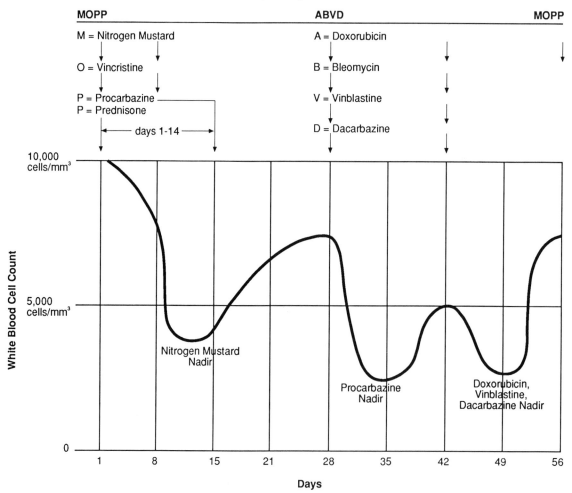

FIGURE 20-3 MOPP/ABV ± D administration schedule and corresponding white blood cell count nadirs. (From Goodman, M. S. [1986]. *Cancer: Chemotherapy and care* [p. 16]. Evansville, IN: Bristol-Myers. Used with permission.)

those who have been cured) reported that the discomfort caused by these toxicities was well worthwhile.[5]

Goodman underscores the importance of the nurse's own positive attitude when educating patients about chemotherapy's toxicities and side effects, by offering hope to patients and their families in stressing the dramatic potential benefits of treatment.[9]

Routes and Modes of Administration

Proper pretreatment evaluation can have an enormous impact on the efficacy of the nurse's care plan and on the patient's chemotherapy experience. The nurse should ascertain answers to the following questions before proceeding with treatment:

1. Does the patient understand enough to provide fully informed consent?

2. Is the patient being treated with chemotherapy for the first time? If not, is the record complete regarding previous chemotherapy experience (physical and emotional response, experience with and management of side effects, and so forth?)

3. Is assessment of the patient's and family's ability to manage at home complete? Is the patient familiar with resources to assist with sequelae of chemotherapy?

4. Has the nurse assessed and reviewed the patient's physical history before administering treatment? Have all compromised organ systems been considered in dose calculation (especially liver and kidneys, which metabolize and clear the agents)?

5. Has the patient mobilized available coping mechanisms? Is the patient "ready for therapy?"

6. Is the patient prepared for potential hair loss?

7. Has an antiemetic regimen, both medical and dietary (in clinic, in home), been explained and initiated?

8. Does the patient have special hydration and electrolyte replacement needs? Have replacements been ordered? Does the patient understand the need to continue supplementing fluids after treatment? Is the patient capable of fulfilling this requirement?

9. In the past 48 hours, have laboratory values been obtained (eg, blood counts, platelets, blood urea nitrogen, creatinine, liver function studies)? Are they within normal limits?

10. Does the nurse have therapy protocol or written/signed physician order that specifies patient name, drug name(s), dosage per square meter of body surface area, total dose, and rate, frequency, and route of administration?

11. Is the patient as physically comfortable as possible, with easy access to a nurse call light?

12. Are all necessary treatment supplies at hand (eg, safe handling equipment, IV therapy materials, and hazardous waste containment)? Is light adequate to facilitate venipuncture and patient observation? Is environment conducive to privacy, especially in the event of emesis? (See Figure 20-4.)

FIGURE 20-4 An environment conducive to successful chemotherapy administration is well lit and contains the necessary equipment, including adjustable infusion chair with arm rests, easily reached IV therapy equipment and materials, biohazardous waste container, safe handling materials, emesis basin, sphygmomanometer, emergency and extravasation equipment, and available nurse-call system.

13. Is the nurse prepared for anaphylaxis or extravasation? Is proper emergency equipment readily available? (See Tables 20-7 and 20-8.) Are necessary professionals available in the event of patient emergency?

14. Does the patient have adequate venous access?

Successful chemotherapy treatment relies on proper preparation in these areas. Individual patients often require extended pretreatment evaluations for special needs, for example, those who are exceptionally anxious, who lack family or social support, who are cognitively challenged, or who are scheduled to receive investigational antineoplastic agents. When chemotherapeutic protocols change, any or all of these steps must be repeated or modified to update patient education.

When the nurse and patient have combined their resources to satisfy these questions, administration of chemotherapy may begin.

Systemic Drug Delivery

Although chemotherapy can be administered through a variety of routes, oral and IV continue to be most common. Antineoplastic agents are delivered orally if they can be tolerated and absorbed by the gastrointestinal tract. Only a few agents fall into this category. IV administration is far more common. Successful IV administration demands careful vein selection and venipuncture.

Vein selection depends on the purpose and length of infusion and the vesicant and irritant properties of the drugs. Peripheral veins may be used for bolus or short-term infusion. Central venous access is preferred for patients scheduled for long-term infusions or those at risk of extravasation caused by vein fragility or inaccessibility.

For peripheral venous access, patients should be positioned comfortably in a chair with extended armrests, with hand and arm stabilizers. Successful IV nurses allow ample and unhurried time to assess both arms and hands to avoid areas of scle-

TABLE 20-7
Emergency Drugs and Equipment

Drugs	Strength	Volume
Epinephrine 1:1000 (1 mg/mL)	1:10,000	10 mL
Anhydrous theophylline	400 mg	100 mL
Diphenhydramine	50 mg	1 mL
Hydrocortisone	2 mL	100 mL
Dopamine (200 mg)	800 µg	250 mL
Levarterenol bitartrate	2 mg	500 mL
Sodium bicarbonate	8.4%	50 mEq/50 mL
Furosemide	40 mg	4 mL
Diazepam	10 mg	2 mL
Lidocaine	100 mg	5 mL
Naloxone hydrochloride	0.1–0.4 mg	5 mL
Nitroglycerine (sublingual)	0.15 mg	

Equipment

Suction machine with catheters

Oxygen tank with nasal and face mask

Ambu bag with adult–child face mask

Syringes and needles

Standard resuscitation equipment

Check daily and restock as necessary.

(From Goodman, M. S. [1991]. Delivery of cancer chemotherapy. In S. B. Baird [Ed.], *Cancer nursing: A comprehensive textbook* [p. 295]. Philadelphia: W. B. Saunders. Used with permission.)

rosis, thrombosis, hematoma, or phlebitis. The examination of both arms also gives the nurse a baseline reference should changes occur during treatment.

If veins are obscure, comfortably warm, moist compresses may be applied to the patient's hands and forearms. Clothing can be loosened to allow full view of the IV site. Watches and tight jewelry should be removed if they constrict the venous pathway or impede the smooth flow of drugs along the venous network.

Alternating arms, from treatment to treatment, often minimizes vascular irritation and phlebitis associated with IV administration of chemotherapy agents; it also allows time for healing. Documentation should specify which arm was used for each treatment. If not informed of this procedure, and if treated by various nurses, a patient may unwittingly prefer to have all treatments in one arm, increasing the risk of phlebitis.

Aseptic techniques—including sterile venipuncture procedures, universal precautions, and safe handling of antineoplastics—require a nurse's constant vigilance, especially because of the susceptibility of these patients to systemic contamination caused by leukopenia.

TABLE 20-8
Extravasation Kit: Items and Quantities

Needles	18 gauge (2)
	25 gauge (2)
	filter needle (1)
Tape	1 inch paper
Telfa pads	4 × 4 in (4)
Sterile gauze dressing	4 × 4 in (2)
Alcohol wipes	(4)
Syringes	Tuberculin
	3 mL
	5 mL
	10 mL
	20 mL
Local anesthetic	Ethyl chloride
Diluent	Sterile saline: 10 mL (1) preservative free
	Sterile water: 10 mL (1)
Steroid cream	1% topical lotion (optional)
Antidotes	10% sodium thiosulfate (10 mL)
	Hydrocortisone solution (100-mg vial)
	Dexamethasone: 4 mg/mL
	Hyaluronidase (150 U) (in refrigerator)
	Dimethyl sulfoxide (50–100%) topical
Latex gloves	
Hot pack	
Cold pack	
Policy and procedure for extravasation management	
Extravasation record	

Restock kit after each use. Kit should be available wherever vesicant drugs are being administered.

(From Goodman, M. S. [1991]. *Delivery of cancer chemotherapy.* In S. B. Baird [Ed.], *Cancer nursing: A comprehensive textbook* [p. 295]. Philadelphia: W. B. Saunders. Used with permission.)

A clinician should follow a pattern for venipunctures, using the most distal veins first, moving proximally with successive venipunctures from hand to forearm.[28] For example, if a forearm venipuncture was unsuccessful, or if blood was drawn earlier, cytotoxic agents administered to the hand of the same arm might leak into tissue surrounding the recent proximal puncture. With vesicants, necrosis could result.

Large veins along the distal forearm (cephalic, median, and basilic) are easy to access and may provide safe, convenient venipuncture sites. Using these larger veins diminishes the risk of chemical phlebitis from antineoplastics' caustic properties, especially with bolus (IV push) administration.[13] In the event of extravasation, this area also offers greater mass of soft tissue (than over the hand, for example) that may be more easily grafted, thereby avoiding functional impairment.[9]

Because IV solutions often contain admixtures incompatible with cytotoxic drugs (eg, heparin sodium combined with doxorubicin), there is potential for precipitates to develop, which can result in vein irritation and phlebitis. Compatibility considerations are imperative to consider, not only with antineoplastics but with any adjunctive therapies such as antiemetics or corticosteroids.

Vesicant chemotherapy should not be administered using previous IV sites. The following precautions must be considered if an existing IV line is the only available site for nonvesicants:

1. Remove nontransparent dressing completely and ensure venous patency before treatment.

2. Change tubing before and after any chemotherapeutic treatment using admixtures.

3. Flush with approximately 50 to 100 mL fluid before and after treatment. (For patients with fluid restrictions, the nurse must ascertain that the additional volume is allowable.)

When establishing a new IV line, joint flexion areas (eg, wrist, antecubital fossa) should be avoided whenever possible. The chosen vein should feel smooth and resilient, not hard or cordlike.[13] Several factors contraindicate use of the antecubital fossa:

1. The area includes important anatomic structures (eg, median nerve, brachial artery), which could suffer serious complications if necrosis occurs, sometimes even amputation. At minimum, extensive tissue necrosis could require complicated, costly, and psychologically difficult reconstructive efforts.

2. Prolonged infusions restrict arm mobility because elbow function is limited during infusion.

3. Phlebotomists favor antecubital fossa veins for drawing blood specimens. If repeated needle insertions and agent infusions fibrose the tissue, future blood sampling may become difficult.

4. The area's fat and tissue volume make it difficult to visualize and detect early subcutaneous infiltration.[17]

Despite the nurse's technical competence, usable veins sometimes are difficult to locate and access. An arbitrary limit of three unsuccessful venipunctures is suggested before a nurse seeks assistance from a coworker. Repeated venipunctures increase anxiety levels for both patient and nurse and may decrease the likelihood of successful vein cannulation.

Lower extremities or an arm with impaired circulation should not be used for cytotoxic agents. Stagnant or sluggish blood flow delays the agent's reaching general circulation; it also can potentiate any local reaction. Impaired circulation in the extremities can result from an invading neoplasm, existing phlebitis, varicosities, axillary node dissection on the side of a mastectomy, an immobilized fracture, or even extensive hematomas or inflamed areas.

Most chemotherapy regimens can be administered on an outpatient basis. When treating an outpatient peripherally, a stainless steel winged infusion needle is preferred. Often nurses must cannulate veins in elusive areas, such as between the knuckles, or the cephalic vein at the arch over the radial wrist bones. The nurse may choose to tape the tube (rather than the wings) securely to the skin in difficult areas like these to ensure needle stability in the vein.

Bolus (IV push) administration of some medications may threaten insertion because of the needle's short bevel. The small scalp-vein needle's wings should be secured to the skin, whenever possible, with a short strip of tape. Tape should be applied so that the needle insertion site and immediate surrounding area are clearly visible. A common extravasation site is just above the insertion site. If obscured, subtle infiltration evidence may go unnoticed. Tubing should be taped independently, then looped so that blood return can be checked during administration. When the needle is securely in place, the remainder of the IV set should be arranged to remain intact and functional, even in the event of sudden movements like vomiting.

Before cytotoxic drug administration, an IV fluid-flush is tested to ensure venous patency. If a fragile vein bursts, or if a needle has perforated its wall, conventional IV fluids are absorbed without damaging surrounding tissue. A patient with a heparin lock or permanent central venous catheter requires a flush-solution infusion before chemotherapy administration to avoid drug incompatibilities. At least 10 mL IV of fluid between drugs will avoid inopportune chemical interactions. Likewise, approximately 50 mL IV fluid as a final flush will clear the line and vein after antineoplastic administration is complete.

Bolus (IV push) administration calls for slow, even pressure. Small-gauge needles offer greater resistance than larger needles. Any unusual resistance calls for cessation of infusion while the cause is sought. If the bevel of the needle is resting against the vein wall, careful repositioning may resolve the problem. If the clinician applies too much force, the patient may experience pain or venous spasm. A fast, forceful infusion may even cause nausea or exaggerated hypersensitivity sensations (eg, nasal congestion with Cytoxan). Most adverse reactions can be avoided, however, with even "push" pressure and constant supervision of all administration process.

Figure 20-5 illustrates standard procedure for drug delivery via the scalp vein, which uses either a two-syringe technique or a side port of a freely flowing IV line. Short-term chemotherapy may also be delivered with a conventional mini-infusion (piggyback) approach. When injecting vesicants, needle stability and adequate blood return must be checked every 1 to 2 mL, regardless of administration method. Immediate cessation of drug administration is required if there is any doubt about venous patency. With vesicants, the complicated site should be treated as an extravasation; with nonvesicants, treatment can be resumed with a new cannulation site.

After chemotherapy treatment, the cannula is removed with a dry sterile sponge. The extremity is elevated and pressure applied until bleeding stops. Then a dressing is applied to the site. Because thrombocytopenia is a common result of chemotherapy, blood leakage into subcutaneous tissues can result in hematomas that are painful, unsightly and, until reabsorbed, preclude use of the site. Patients also should be cautioned not to handle heavy items with the treated arm or hand.

Venous access devices may be required for patients with a vesicant in their treatment programs or with impaired peripheral venous vasculature.[10,25] Such devices (tunneled, nontunneled, or implanted subcutaneously) can be used for either long- or

Apply tourniquet to mid-forearm, palpate radial pulse and loosen tourniquet if pulse cannot be felt. Have patient open and close fist for venous distention.

Cleanse injection area and hold patient's hand, using thumb to keep skin taut and anchor vein. Place needle in line with vein, bevel up, about one-half inch below proposed entry site.

Insert needle through skin and tissue at 45° angle, relocate vein, decrease needle angle slightly and slowly enter vein with a downward then upward motion.

Remove tourniquet and tape scalp vein tubing.

Attach syringe of saline, aspirate to remove air and irrigate.

Remove saline syringe, attach chemotherapy syringe and inject slowly, checking for blood return and swelling.

Flush catheter with saline solution.

Remove needle, apply pressure to prevent bleeding and apply Band-Aid.

If administering agent via sidearm of continuously running IV, establish intravenous access and freely dripping fluid. Cleanse sidearm, insert needle of chemotherapy syringe and administer drug, maintaining even pressure.

FIGURE 20-5 Venipuncture and peripheral administration of chemotherapeutic drugs. (From Goodman, M. S. [1986]. *Cancer: Chemotherapy and care* [p. 21]. Evansville, IN: Bistol-Myers. Used with permission.)

short-term treatment plans. They can be percutaneously inserted, either centrally or peripherally, eventually to dwell in the superior vena cava or above the junction of the right atrium.[8] They have become state of the art in chemotherapy administration because of their ease of placement, convenience, and safety benefits. As important, they eliminate peripheral venipuncture, dramatically enhancing patient serenity and comfort. Other advantages include:

1. Peripheral venous system is preserved.

2. The device also can be used for blood and nutritional products, antibiotics, analgesics, antiemetics, and cytotoxic agents, singly or in tandem.

3. It allows home infusions of vesicants and multiple drug therapies that otherwise are safely administered only in clinical settings within acute care facilities.

Potential disadvantages include costs of insertion and maintenance, thrombus consequent to improper or inadequate irrigation, infection or sepsis, air embolism,

---

TABLE 20-9
Types of Venous Access Devices and Indications for Their Use

Silastic Atrial Catheters

Frequent venous access required for blood sampling, blood products, therapy, etc.

Bone marrow transplant recipient

Patient with leukemia

Single bolus injections of chemotherapy

TPN and antibiotic therapy

Short- or long-term chemotherapy infusions (vesicant or nonvesicant)

Inpatient/outpatient chemotherapy infusion

Significant other or patient capable of caring for device

Small-Gauge Central Venous Catheters

Short-term infusion chemotherapy (2–3 mo)

Short-term infusion of vesicant chemotherapy

Inpatient/outpatient infusion therapy

Single bolus injections of chemotherapy

Frequent venous access needed for chemotherapy

Infrequent blood sampling via peripheral vein

Brief life expectancy

Significant other or patient capable of caring for device

Implanted Ports

Infrequent venous access required

Single bolus injections of chemotherapy

Inpatient/outpatient infusion of nonvesicant chemotherapeutic agents

Short- or long-term chemotherapy

Used for TPN, blood transfusions, fluid replacement, or antibiotics

Infrequent blood sampling required

Patient physically unable to care for VAD

A young child: frequent venous access not required

Cosmesis/patient preference

TPN, total parenteral nutrition; VAD, venous access device.

(Adapted from Goodman, M. S., & Wickham, R. [1984]. Venous access devices: An overview. *Oncology Nursing Forum, 11*[5], 16–23.)

and catheter severing or migration. Before discharge, patients and families need meticulous training in device maintenance, including take-home written instructions. These devices afford dramatic quality-of-life advantages, but they demand extraordinary patient responsibility and maintenance activities. If improperly instructed, patients may experience catheter occlusions caused by inadequate irrigation, infections, or air embolism caused by line mismanagement (eg, poorly taped connections, mishandled clamps), which usually require device removal.

Table 20-9 lists various devices for long-term venous access. Device selection depends on frequency of access need, treatment duration, administration mode, venous integrity, and patient preference.[25] Criteria for patient assessment are featured in Table 20-10. Common placement sites appear in Figure 20-6. Although IV therapy is

---

TABLE 20-10
Patient Assessment Criteria for a Vascular Access Device

Criteria

Frequency of venous access
Longevity of treatment
Mode of administration
Venous integrity
Patient preference

Low Priority	High Priority
Infrequent venous access	Frequent venous access
Short-term therapy	Long-term indefinite treatment period
Intermittent single injections	Continuous infusion chemotherapy
Administration of nonvesicant/ nonirritating drugs	Home infusion of chemotherapy
No previous IV therapy	Administration of vesicant/ irritating drugs
Both extremities available	Venous thrombosis/sclerosis due to previous IV therapy
Venous access with two or fewer venipunctures	Venous access limited to one extremity
Patient does not prefer VAD	Prior tissue damage due to extravasation
	Multiple (>2) venipunctures to secure venous access
	Patient prefers VAD

VAD, vascular access device.

(From Goodman, M. S., & Wickham, R. [1984]. Venous access devices: An overview. *Oncology Nursing Forum, 11*[5], 16–23.)

the primary use of these devices, they also can be placed intra-arterially for organ profusion or intraperitoneally for "belly baths."[9,16]

Implanted venous access devices offer an alternative to central venous lines. Advantages include reduced infection risk, no care requirements for external catheters, and diminished risk of drug infiltration or vein sclerosis from irritating drugs administered peripherally.[7] Implantable devices are available from a variety of manufacturers; an example appears in Figure 20-7.

Long-term infusions of vesicant drugs (eg, Adriamycin, Mitomycin, or Oncovin)

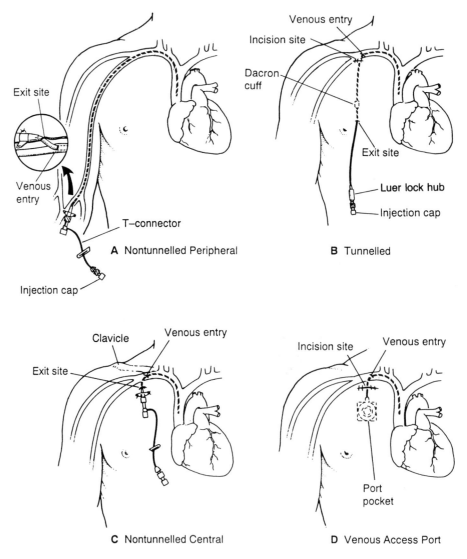

FIGURE 20-6 Common sites for long-term venous access devices. (From Wickham, R. [1987]. Techniques for long-term venous access. In Fifth National Conference on Cancer Nursing Proceedings, [p. 10]. Atlanta: American Cancer Society. Used with permission.)

Huber point needle — syringe
— self sealing septum
skin line — sleeve
suture — cuffs

FIGURE 20-7 (**A**) PORT-A-CATH® Implantable Access System (Property of Sims-Deltec, Inc., St. Paul, MN) (**B**) A subcutaneously implanted port with Huber point needle penetrating the skin and the injection septum. (From Hubbard, S. M. Seipp, C. A., & Duffy, P. L. [1989]. Administration of cancer treatments: Practical guides for physicians and oncology nurses. In V. T. DeVita, S. Hellman, & S. A. Rosenberg [Eds.], *Cancer: Principles and practice of oncology* [3rd ed., p. 2382]. Philadelphia: J. B. Lippincott. Used with permission.)

— muscle

usually are not administered through implanted devices because of the risks of needle dislodgment and consequent extravasation. Because proper needle placement is assessed and documented at least every 8 hours with these vesicants, a patient with a implanted device requires inpatient care. This is not the case with vesicant administration via indwelling Silastic central venous catheters, like the Hickman, Broviac or Groshong devices.

In fact, venous access devices are so simple and reliable that there is a real risk of complacency for nurses treating these patients. Individual manufacturer recommendations for care and maintenance should be followed strictly, particularly because specific diameters, volumes, lumen sizes, and clamping procedures vary among models.

Complications are rare and usually avoidable if normal professional standards and chemotherapy administration practices are observed. When they do occur, they are severe and often life-threatening.

Infusion Systems

Venous access devices provide another key benefit to patients requiring continuous or intermittent chemotherapy; they allow treatment at home. External ambulatory infusion systems for antineoplastics reduce inpatient admissions and costs and allow patient autonomy in familiar home surroundings.

All external ambulatory infusion systems are self-powered (independent of household electrical current); they may (or may not) be mechanical. Generally they are battery powered, lightweight, and reusable. They infuse either through a piston-valve (Autosyringe) or a peristaltic mechanism (CADD; Figure 20-8). Administration rate is controllable. Mechanically powered pumps feature alarm systems that detect any back pressure that might occur with occlusion or infiltration. These pumps also detect air in the line; an alarm sounds when the fluid reservoir is empty. The Travenol Infuser system, on the other hand, exerts positive pressure when its balloon, containing the drug, deflates into the venous access device. Infusion rate is determined by balloon pressure.

Any list of ambulatory infusion systems products and technologies might be obsolete within weeks of publication. IV clinicians are better served to keep abreast of manufacturer-provided instructional materials, patient education information, and trouble-shooting support services of the devices currently favored in one's own clinical setting.

Clinicians must be intimately familiar with system operations, also, to educate patients and families in early detection of complications, including line occlusion, thrombosis, infiltration or extravasation, and system failure. The ONS provides course contents and clinical practicum recommendations for nursing education and practice, which clinicians may find helpful in preparing patients to succeed with these systems.[22]

Following is a list of assessment factors to consider when recommending use of an ambulatory infusion system:

1. Level of patient and family understanding of pump and alarm features and functions; level of patient and family compliance, reliability, dexterity, and comfort with the device; patient and family eyesight keen enough to see pump function clearly

FIGURE 20-8 CADD-I Ambulatory Infusion pump, model 5100 HFX. (Property of: Sims-Deltec, Inc., St. Paul, MN)

2. 24-hour proximity to health care provider in the event of pump failure or occlusion

3. Drug regimen that matches device capacities and features

4. Insurance coverage of unit rental or purchase costs

Infusion systems can be attached by belt or shoulder strap to ease patient movement. Mechanical systems generally call for hands-on programming and reprogramming, requiring an on-site visit from a nurse when changes are needed.

The same is true for replenishing fluid and drug reservoirs. Upcoming developments to ease ambulatory infusions (eg, pump reprogramming by computer and over-phone lines, without hands-on human intervention) are promised for the near future.

Regional Drug Delivery

Although systemic IV administration of chemotherapy is most common, some tumors respond better to local exposure to antineoplastics. Alternative methods of drug administration have been established to deliver high concentrations of chemotherapeutic agents locally, into a body cavity or into the organ site of the tumor. A drug can be directed into the area of known malignancy, such as intraperitoneal, to treat malignant ascites or metastatic seeding of peritoneum from ovarian carcinoma, intravesical to treat bladder cancer; intrathecal or intraventricular for cancers known to have invaded the central nervous system; intrapleural for malignant effusions and sclerosing purposes; topical for early malignancies of the integumentary; or intra-arterial for the regional delivery of chemotherapy into the liver through the hepatic artery.[12]

Another advantage of the regional delivery of these infusions is that they can "bathe" the affected body cavity or organ without imposing toxic effects on the whole system.

The most likely alternative route of antineoplastic administration involving the IV nurse is the intra-arterial infusion that uses a totally implanted infusion pump (Figure 20-9). This route generally is used to treat primary hepatic tumors or hepatic metastasis or colorectal, stomach, esophageal, pancreatic, breast, lung, or malignant melanoma.[28] Intra-arterial infusion also is used to treat large localized disease in primary head and neck tumors, brain tumors, and widespread metastatic disease in the pelvis; large drug concentrations are administered through arteries that supply these areas.[3]

The Infusaid Pump is the most common totally implantable drug-delivery system. The Food and Drug Administration (FDA) approved its commercial use for 5-fluorouracil (5-FU), methotrexate, floxuridine (FUDR), heparin, morphine sulfate, insulin, and some aminoglycosides. Volatile fluorocarbon vapor pressure powers the pump using bellows to force the fluid from the drug chamber at a specified rate. Vapor pressure is influenced by changes in body temperature, atmospheric pressure, and drug viscosity. Because the pump's flow rate increases by roughly 10% for each degree Centigrade increase in body temperature, patients must agree to report any fever, so that pump refill schedules can be assessed and adjusted.

Because infection and thrombosis are the most common complications, patients also are instructed to report pain, changes in temperature of the skin over the pump, color, sensation, or fluid leakage.[13]

FIGURE 20-9 (**A**) Infusaid Pump for chemotherapy administration. (**B**) Internal components of Infusaid Pump. (Courtesy: Intermedics Infusaid, Inc., Norwood, MA)

About every 1 or 2 weeks, the pump is refilled (with either active antineoplastics or saline) for constant area perfusion by percutaneous injection. The device's side port device may be used for direct intra-arterial access. The nurse must be intimately familiar with techniques and risks of this route of drug delivery, with strict adherence to details available from manufacturer data and institutional policy and procedure before attempting pump accessing or filling.

These devices also support effective pain management when used to infuse low-dose narcotics or intrathecal or subcutaneous delivery modes.

Intrathecal therapy is another alternative route of cancer chemotherapy that might call for IV nurse involvement. A cerebrospinal access device, like the Ommaya reservoir, is subcutaneously implanted to avoid repeated lumbar punctures in treating

FIGURE 20-10 Cerebrospinal fluid reservoir (Ommaya type) facilitates repeated intraventricular administration.

meningial carcinomatosis, the infiltration by cancer of the leptomeninges of the brain. The reservoir provides access to the cerebrospinal fluid through a burr hole in the skull (Figure 20-10).

Hubbard and coworkers[13] described the nursing procedure to use and maintain these devices.

First, the reservoir is pumped several times to fill the device with spinal fluid. Then, the skin is prepared and the reservoir is obliquely punctured, using sterile technique, with a 25- to 27-gauge scalp-vein needle. Sufficient spinal fluid is removed for laboratory studies and to keep exchanges isovolumetric. Then, a chemotherapeutic agent is injected slowly through a scalp-vein needle into the reservoir, which next is flushed with Elliott's B solution.

After the needle is removed, the reservoir is pumped to distribute the drugs into the intraventricular space. Preservative-free morphine sulfate also can be administered into an Ommaya reservoir for prolonged pain relief.

CONTROVERSIAL ISSUES

Some elements of antineoplastic administration therapy and procedure have earned unanimous consensus. Others are handled in various ways, depending on personal experience, preference, opinion, and talent. Until further investigation leads to definitive direction, some controversy will remain in a few areas of chemotherapy theory and practice.

The ONS acknowledges the controversies among practicing clinicians. Several issues that require further investigative studies are listed, without judgment, below:

    A. Use of the antecubital fossa for administration of antineoplastic agents
        1. Favoring the use of the antecubital fossa
            a. Larger veins permit more rapid drug infusion and administration.

      b. Larger veins permit potentially irritating agents to reach general circulation sooner, with less threat to smaller veins.

    2. Discouraging the use of the antecubital fossa

      a. Arm mobility is restricted when needle is in place.

      b. Extravasation risk is increased with patient movement (eg, coughing, vomiting).

      c. Infiltration could require extensive reconstruction, limiting arm use during healing, possibly resulting in decreased function and increased morbidity risk.

      d. Early assessment of infiltration is difficult because of subcutaneous tissue.

      e. There is potential for vein fibrosis from chemotherapeutic agents at site commonly used for laboratory blood draws.

B. Needle size

    1. Favoring the use of larger gauge (eg, 19- and 21-gauge) scalp-vein needles

      a. Potentially irritating chemotherapeutic agents reach general circulation quickly, without irritating peripheral veins.

      b. Administration time is decreased, reducing patient exposure to potentially stressful environment.

    2. Favoring the use of smaller gauge (eg, 23- and 25-gauge) scalp-vein needles

      a. Less likelihood of small-vein wall puncture

      b. Less likelihood of scar formation

      c. Less pain on needle insertion

      d. Increased blood flow around a smaller-bore needle increases agent dilution.

      e. Smaller-bore needle minimizes risk of mechanical phlebitis.

      f. Nausea and vomiting threats are decreased by slow infusion.

C. Drug sequencing

    1. Favoring vesicant administration first

      a. Vascular integrity decreases over time.

      b. Vein is most stable and least irritated at start of treatment.

      c. Initial assessment of vein patency is most accurate.

      d. Patient awareness of symptomatic changes is most acute.

    2. Favoring vesicant administration last

      a. Vesicants are irritating and may increase vein fragility.

      b. Venous spasm can occur at the beginning of bolus (IV push) therapy.

D. Side arm versus direct push administration

    1. Favoring side arm administration

      a. Freely running IV lines allow maximum dilution of potentially irritating drugs.

      b. Administration can be readily interrupted while maintaining venous access.

    2. Favoring direct push administration

      a. Vein integrity can be assessed more easily and signs of extravasation noted earlier.[20]

COMPLICATIONS

Regardless of clinician skill and standards, sometimes patients experience problems unique to administration of cytotoxic agents.

Venous Fragility

Elderly, poorly nourished, and debilitated patients often have fragile veins. Unskilled nurses may unwittingly cause painful and unsightly hematomas that eliminate use of treatment area until reabsorption is complete. Nurses should attempt to cannulate fragile veins without a tourniquet because distention and rapid engorgement may cause the vein wall to rupture when the tourniquet is released.

A second clinician may apply gentle hand pressure directly above the venipuncture site to distend it. Other distention alternatives include application of moderate heat or even inviting the patient to clench or pump the fist. Gravity flow may be may be maximized if the patient dangles the hand and arm. Or the clinician may lightly finger tap the site to distend the vein.

Regardless of chosen technique, fragile veins require a cautious approach, allowing ample time to prepare for successful venipuncture on the first attempt.

Localized Acute Allergic Reactions

The clinician should be prepared for allergic reactions in any IV cytotoxin administration. Localized allergic reactions, "flares," often are associated with administration of doxorubicin hydrochloride.[31] The first manifestation may be erythema along the venous pathways. Blotchiness, hivelike urticaria, or the rapid appearance of welts also may appear. The patient may report itchiness, stinging, or an increasing sensation of heat in the area. Some suggest the reaction is caused by intercellular release of histamines, which increases permeability of cell membranes. This permeability may allow drugs to leak into subcutaneous tissues.[31] Other possibilities include drug interactions, contaminants, or molecular extravasation through vascular endothelium.

Preventive measures include additional drug dilution, either by adding the drug to 100 to 200 mL solution or by administering the drug piggyback. Table 20–5 lists some common administration techniques. The nurse should always consult and follow manufacturer's recommendations, however.

Many practitioners discontinue treatment when a localized allergic reaction occurs to prevent chemical cellulitis. Before removing the IV needle, additional drug-free fluid is infused to limit and resolve erythematous reaction. The medications listed below can be used to treat localized sensitivity reaction. All drugs require physician order before they are infused:

Hydrocortisone sodium succinate (Solu-Cortef). Slow IV push, 25 to 50 mL, anti-inflammatory agent.

Benadryl. IV push, 25 to 50 mg, antihistamine.

Venous Spasm

Some cytotoxic agents are known to produce pain or spasm along the venous pathway. Carmustine (BiCNU) is diluted with absolute alcohol, which may be the offending agent. The breakdown products from photodegradation or dacarbazine (DTIC) may be responsible for acute local burning associated with the drug's use. Mechlorethamine hydrochloride (Mustargen) also can cause pain, especially in patients who have been treated chemotherapeutically over extended time spans.

Although there are many special cautions for special drugs, it is important to re-member that *any* agent can cause venous pain, in any patient, at any time. Venous pain and spasm also can result from bolus (IV push) pressure too forceful for a small-gauge needle. Venous pain and spasm can be alleviated with these measures:

1. Slowing drug infusion rate

2. Diluting the antineoplastic agent

3. Applying warm or cool arm compresses during infusion. (Some patients respond better to cool compresses, some to warm. Care must be taken to avoid second-degree burns.)

4. Administering Xylocaine 1%–0.25 mL (3 mL total), as needed. (Patient allergy history and physician order are required before administration.)

The chemical phlebitis risk exists with most IV cancer chemotherapy agents, but the risk increases when two or more antineoplastics are combined. Early phlebitis can be associated with pain, erythema, occasional limb edema, and a sensation of warmth in the affected extremity. As acute symptoms subside, venous pathways may retain dark bluish to brown discoloration for some time, while arm use is restricted. Acute phlebitis reactions can interrupt sleep patterns and interfere with a patient's routine living activities.

Noninvestigational drugs associated with phlebitis include:

Actinomycin	Mechlorethamine hydrochloride
Carmustine	Mitomycin C
Cisplatin	Streptozotocin
Dacarbazine	Vinblastine
Daunorubicin	Vincristine
Doxorubicin hydrochloride	

Nurses must exercise utmost caution to prevent phlebitis because some treatment regimens must be terminated if phlebitic reactions occur. When a time-sensitive and aggressive treatment program must be suspended until treatment sites are healed, the patient's long-term disease control may be jeopardized. Sometimes it is possible to substitute nonsclerosing agents from the same drug category as the offending agent. Occasionally a patient with history of phlebitic treatment sites will manifest reactions to any IV drug administrations.

In addition to preventive measures suggested in the section on vascular irritation (see Chapter 7), the nurse may adopt these measures to diminish the threat of phlebitis:

1. Administer hydrocortisone sodium succinate (Solu-Cortef), 25 to 50 mg, slow IV push. After ensuring vein patency, half the dose is administered before an-tineoplastic administration; the other half is delivered after the final flush, im-mediately before the needle is removed. (A physician's order is required before this drug can be administered.)

2. Reduce the concentration of the cytotoxic agent with saline solution.

Repetitive needle insertions for blood sampling and antineoplastic administrations increase the likelihood of both phlebitis and thrombosis. In fact, some patients develop phlebitis despite the most meticulous clinical efforts to avoid them. Once phlebitis has occurred, these therapeutic measures may be indicated:

1. Elevation of the affected extremity
2. Application of topical heat
3. Administration of systemic analgesics (with physician's order)

A patient's venous status should be assessed carefully before chemotherapy is administered. If veins are deep, difficult to visualize and palpate with tourniquet distention, if peripheral veins are extraordinarily small, or if the proposed treatment plan is long, a central venous access device should be considered.

Generalized Anaphylactic Reaction

A clinician should be prepared for anaphylactic reaction at any time, with any drug, in any patient. Before initiating any treatment, the clinician should be well aware of the institution's policies regarding emergencies arising from administration of cytotoxic agents and the location of emergency supplies and equipment. For example, some hospital policies preclude a nurse from administering chemotherapy unless a physician is present. Others may not permit the administration of investigational drugs until they have been approved by the institution's pharmacy and therapeutics committees because nurses should not be accountable for managing unpredictable side effects that might arise during treatment.

To prepare for the possibility of anaphylaxis, the nurse should be vigilant for any signs of flushing, shaking, sudden agitation or anxiety, nausea, vomiting, urticaria, hypotension, generalized pruritus, respiratory distress (wheezing, coughing, shortness of breath, or asthma-type reaction). If undetected, a generalized anaphylactic reaction might cause seizure or cardiopulmonary arrest.

Before therapy begins, the nurse should position the patient in a reclining position that eases management of an anaphylactic event (see Figure 20-4). If the patient is seated at a table not adjacent to a bed, for example, anaphylaxis is unnecessarily difficult to handle. An emergency cart with all appropriate medications, plus stethoscope and sphygmomanometer (see Table 20-7), also should be at hand.

The procedures of some facilities call for a "standing order" sheet to be signed by the responsible physician before treatment. This timesaving and prudent procedure allows the clinician to begin emergency treatment even before the physician arrives.

The nurse also should record a baseline blood pressure reading before treatment. If a patient normally is hypotensive, a normal blood pressure reading is useful, should shock symptoms occur. The same is true for a baseline reference point of the patient's mental status. Particularly with metastatic brain disease or other mental alterations, early symptoms of anaphylaxis—agitation, anxiety, speech disorders, mental confusion—can be misleading without a clear picture of the patient's pretreatment mental state.

Regardless of whether a patient displays mild reaction (eg, generalized pruritus) or sustains complete cardiovascular collapse, the nurse should be prepared to:

1. Recline the patient, smoothly, safely and quickly.
2. Administer basic cardiopulmonary resuscitative measures.

3. Maintain a patient IV line for emergency drug administration.

4. Provide calm reassurance.

5. Administer appropriate drugs, as ordered.

6. Monitor patient until the reaction subsides.

Anaphylaxis prevention is an important goal in administration of any cancer chemotherapy. Nevertheless, the nurse must be aware of which agents are associated with anaphylaxis and prepared to administer those agents as recommended in product brochures:

1. *Bleomycin sulfate (Blenoxane)*. Package insert recommends treatment with 2 U or less with the first two doses as test doses.

2. *Cisplatin (Platinol)*. No specific recommendations for dose attenuation or treatment duration. Product brochure lists suggestions for symptom management.

3. *Asparaginase (Elspar)*. Before the first dose of Elspar, before retreatment of any patient manifesting positive reactors, and after careful assessment of hypersensitivity risk, the clinician should consider performing desensitization.

Even though a physician may have ascertained an allergy history, the nurse should solicit and chart the same information. When the potential exists for anaphylactic reaction, these precautionary measures might be useful:

1. Test dosing

2. Antihistaminic, steroidal, or anti-inflammatory or antipyretic pretreatment

3. Uninterrupted dosing to preclude significant reactive-antibody build-up

Extravasation

Controversies surround appropriate treatment of local infiltrations of chemotherapy agents. No treatments show well documented efficacy.[6] Controlled clinical trials are lacking because of the low number of accruable patients treated by skilled clinicians and because of ethical issues associated with a control or "no-treatment" arm. In fact, it often is difficult to ascertain that an infiltration actually has occurred. Table 20-11 outlines the venous reactions compared with actual extravasations. Obviously, skilled clinicians do not allow infiltration of sclerosing agents to continue to any obvious point. Therefore there is a real ethical and moral question surrounding involving a patient in "intentional" extravasation research. Because of its particularly morbid tissue effect, most extravasation studies on animals have been conducted using doxorubicin hydrochloride (Adriamycin). Among patient consequences of extensive tissue necrosis (Figure 20-11):

1. *Pain*. Extensive necrotic areas often require narcotics for pain management.

2. *Physical defects*. Necrosis may preclude a patient from work for indefinite periods. If a patient's job requires full range of motion, for example, permanent functional compromise may severely impinge upon quality of life. Cosmetic defect may result in severe emotional impact (see Figure 20-12).

TABLE 20-11
Nursing Assessment of Extravasation Versus Other Reactions

Assessment Parameter	Extravasation		Irritation of the Vein	Flare Reaction
	Intermediate Manifestations of Extravasation	Delayed Manifestations of Extravasation		
Pain	Severe pain or burning lasting min or hr, eventually subsiding; usually occurs while the drug is being given and around needle site	48 h	Aching and tightness along the vein	No pain
Redness	Blotchy redness around needle site, not always present at time of extravasation	Later occurrence	The full length of the vein may be reddened or darkened	Immediate blotches or streaks along vein, usually subsides within 30 min with or without treatment.
Ulceration	Develops insidiously, usually 48–96 h later	Later occurrence	Not usually	Not usually
Swelling	Severe swelling usually occurs immediately	48 h	Not likely	Not likely; wheals may appear along vein line
Blood return	Inability to obtain blood return; presence-rate	Good blood return during drug administration	Usually	Usually
Other	Change in the quality of infusion	Local tingling, sensory deficits	—	Urticaria

(From Oncology Nursing Society. [1992]. *Cancer chemotherapy guidelines: Module V, Recommendations for the management of vesicant extravasation, hypersensitivity and anaphylaxis.* Pittsburgh.)

3. *Medical expenses.* Patients themselves may be responsible for the financial costs of their care, so multiple or lengthy hospitalizations or costly plastic surgeries may pose economic challenges. Debilitation may require additional healing time or secondary medical problems may occur.

4. *Disease control.* Valuable time may be lost if a patient is unable to sustain scheduled chemotherapy treatment plans to control the disease process. Myelosuppression from previous cancer treatments may promote secondary infection of the necrosed area, postponing the treatment plan even further.

5. *Time.* Patients with work or school responsibilities may be kept from "normal life" until healed. Income suspension poses additional financial hardship to the patient and family.

6. *Psychological impact on clinician and patient.* The "incident" and its aftermath may strain trust and communications between patient and nurse.

FIGURE 20-11 Extensive tissue necrosis following vesicant therapy. (Courtesy: Sharon Weinstein, CRNI, MS)

Prevention

Of course, years of experience in treating patients with antineoplastics perfect the clinician's technique and are good patient safeguards. It is important to keep in mind, however, that extravasation of tissue-sclerosing agents can occur, even to the most skillful IV nurse. This concept is underscored to allay the anxiety of all nurses responsible for administering antineoplastics. The emphasis should be on perfecting IV technique and safety while using prudent preparation measures in case an extravasation should occur. Although there are no guarantees for any clinician, there can be reasonable confidence that an astute nurse can minimize its impact with early detection and treatment. Details are outlined in Table 20-12.

Patient Education

The patient must be informed of possible consequences when chemotherapy agents are administered, so "informed consent" is comprehensive and legitimate. A sensitive clinician will convey the risks in such a way that the patient can react to the information appropriately and without unnecessary fear.

Constant clinician attendance is required by patients who are irrational, unconscious, or in some way unable to perceive or report early signs of extravasation. Alert and cooperative patients may report stinging, burning, pain at the cannula insertion site, or any unusual sensation. On the other hand, it is important to keep in mind that extravasation can occur even without perceptible symptoms.

General Precautions

When administering any antineoplastics, clinicians should heed these guidelines:

1. *Anticipate the possibility of extravasation.* Before any treatment, the clinician should be familiar with the agents known to produce tissue necrosis (see Table

Text continues on page 523

TABLE 20-12

Extravasation of Vesicant Antineoplastic Agents: Preventive Strategies

Risk Factor	Preventive Strategy	Rationale
Skill of the Practioner	Chemotherapy administration only done by registered nurses who are specifically trained and supervised.	Procedures for management of extravasation vary according to the drug infiltrated. Certain drugs (streptozocin or BCNU) may cause a burning sensation during infusion, which is normal. However, it is abnormal and indicative of a problem if burning occurs during infusion of drugs such as doxorubicin and mitomycin.
	No attempts by practitioner to do procedures beyond his or her expertise.	
	Practitioners are skillful in venipuncture.	Procedures change rapidly. Techniques need to be learned and mastered before assuming responsibility for administration of chemotherapy.
	Practitioners are knowledgeable of the signs and symptoms of extravasation and drug therapy.	
	Practice is based on institutional policies and procedures that are routinely updated to meet the changing standards and methods of practice.	The definition of customary care in the community helps dictate standard of practice.
Condition of the Veins Small fragile veins Access limited owing to axillary surgery, vein thrombosis, prior extravasation Long-term drug therapy Multiple vein punctures	Use conventional methods for venous distention such as heat and percussion.	Risk of vesicant drug seepage exists with repeated venipuncture.
	Assess all available arm veins. Assess veins in a methodical fashion, taking time to select the most appropriate vein.	Multiple vein injections lead to thrombosis and limited availability.
	If practitioners do not feel confident in their ability to cannulate a person's veins successfully, they should seek the assistance of a colleague.	
	After attempting one or two injections without success, the practitioner should seek the assistance of a colleague before trying again.	
	A patient who consistently needs two or more attempts to secure venous access should be considered a candidate for a VAD.	Before the advent of vascular access devices (VADs), multiple venous injections to administer a drug might have been accepted as the only method of drug administration. This is no longer the case. Instead, treatment should be delayed until a VAD can be placed.
	The time to place a VAD is before an extravasation, not after.	Most VADs can be used immediately or within 24–48 h, so delay in drug therapy is not usually an issue.
Drug Administration Technique	Vesicant agents are never given as continuous infusions into a peripheral vein.	The risk of infiltration of a vesicant from a peripheral vein infusion is great owing to the following: Blood return is not assessed frequently.

(continued)

TABLE 20-12   *(Continued)*

Risk Factor	Preventive Strategy	Rationale
		The longer the infusion, the greater the possibility of needle dislodgment.
		The patient can move the extremity, which could dislodge the IV cannula.
		Even a small amount of vesicant can cause tissue damage.
		Infiltration can be subtle and difficult to detect until a large volume has infiltrated.
		The patient may be sedated from an antiemetic and be unable to report sensations associated with extravasation.
	If peripheral line is on a controlled infusion pump, disconnect pump before injection of chemotherapy.	The pump forces drug into the tissues.
	When a vesicant is to be given as a continuous injection, the drug should be infused via an external based central venous catheter whenever possible.	When an implanted port already exists, the patient is taught to check the needle three times a day to ensure placement during continuous infusion of a vesicant.
		The incidence of vesicant drug extravasation from ports used for continuous infusion is well documented and presents a risk to be avoided, if possible.
	Vesicant agents are most commonly administered using the two-syringe technique or through the side port of a free-flowing peripheral intravenous line.	The two-syringe technique allows for proper assessment of blood flow and resistance in the vein.
		A scalp-vein needle causes minimal vein irritation.
	Two-Syringe Technique	
	Select an appropriate vein.	
	Begin a new IV line using scalp-vein needle (25 or 23 gauge).	
	Access vein using a single approach.	A subtle leak can be caused by accidentally piercing the vein before accessing it; avoid searching for a vein with repeated approaches.
	Flush line with 8–10 mL saline. Assess for brisk, full blood return and any evidence of infiltration. Check for swelling at the site, redness or pain, and lack of blood return.	
	Once access is ensured, switch to syringe of chemotherapy.	
	Dilute drugs according to the package insert.	Increasing the diluent increases the time it takes to administer the drug, thus increasing risk of infiltration.
	Inject drugs slowly and with minimal resistance.	The speed of the injection is determined by the resistance in the vein. Resistance will vary depending on the size of the needle used.

(continued)

TABLE 20-12   *(Continued)*

Risk Factor	Preventive Strategy	Rationale
	Assess for blood return every 1–2 mL infusion. Flush with 3–5 mL of saline between each drug and 8–10 mL at the completion of the infusion of the drug or drugs.	
	Side-arm Technique Ensure proper venous access site. The IV fluid should be additive free. Cannula used to access the vein should be at least a 20 gauge to ensure an adequate blood return and fluid flow. Secure cannula but do not obstruct entrance site. Pinch off tubing and assess for blood return. Test the vein with 50–100 mL to ensure an adequate and swift drip of infusion. With IV fluid continuing to drip, slowly inject vesicant into IV line. Do not allow vesicant to flow backward. Do not pinch off tubing except to assess for blood return. Assess for blood return every 1–2 mL injection. Flush scalp-vein needle with saline at the completion of injection.	The rationale for the side-arm technique is the added dilution of the drug by the continuous drip of the IV fluid. Common pitfalls: Not using a large enough cannula for a brisk infusion of infusate. Vesicant backs up into IV line. IV line has to be pinched off to inject vesicant, which defeats the purpose. Clinician tends to take eyes off of the site of drug infusion to watch fluid drip more than with two-syringe technique.
Order of Vesicant Drug Administration (*Note:* Sequencing is probably unimportant. The most critical issue is adequately testing the vein with saline [8–10 mL] before administering any drug [vesicant or nonvesicant]).	Give vesicant first. Give vesicant between two nonvesicants. Give vesicant last.	Vascular integrity decreases over time. Practitioner's assessment skills are most acute initially. Patient may be more sedated from antiemetic and less able to report changes in sensation at infusion site as time goes on. Chemotherapy is irritating to the veins. Nonvesicants are presumed to be less irritating than vesicants. Because venous spasm occurs early during the injection, it is less likely to be confused with pain of extravasation if vesicant is given last. It is assumed that because the vein tolerated the nonvesticants, it will also tolerate the vesicant.

(continued)

TABLE 20-12   *(Continued)*

Risk Factor	Preventive Strategy	Rationale
Site of Venous Access: Choosing the Best Vein	VADs, including tunneled catheters, implanted ports, and nontunneled central venous catheters, are indicated when patients have small, frail veins and are in need of long-term indefinite chemotherapy, continuous infusion of vesicant drugs, or both. Although a VAD is a good way to prevent extravasation, it is not indicated just because someone is receiving a vesicant drug. Peripheral access is optimal in the large veins of the forearm, especially the posterior basilic vein. After these, the metacarpal veins of the dorsum of the hand are easy to access and stabilize. The veins over the wrist are risky because of potential damage to tendons and nerves should extravasation occur. *Note:* A large straight vein over the dorsum of the hand is preferable to a smaller vein of the forearm. The antecubital fossa is to be avoided for vesicant drug administration. If the antecubital fossa appears to be the only vein available for access, the patient needs an access device. Hold chemotherapy—insert VAD.	VADs are important options for patients with poor venous access. Externally based catheters are ideal for continuous infusion of vesicant chemotherapeutic agents because the risk of extravasation is very minimal. Expert technique and a knowledgeable clinician are the most cost effective and safe means of administering vesicant drugs. Veins in the forearm are large and adequately supporting by surrounding tissue. Adequate tissue exists around veins to provide coverage and promote healing should a problem occur. The area is dense with tendons and nerves. Seepage of a vesicant can be subtle and go unnoticed. Damage here can result in loss of structure and function. Risking extravasation and subsequent tissue damage is not worth the temptation to give "just one more treatment" before considering other options. There is no evidence that delayed chemotherapy for 24 h in selected cases is detrimental to the overall outcome.
	Avoid administering chemotherapy in lower extremities.	Risk for thrombosis is increased when chemotherapy is given in lower extremities.
Using a Preexisting IV Line	Do not use a preexisting peripheral intravenous line if any of the following are true: The IV cannula was placed more than 12 h earlier. The site is reddened, swollen, or sore, or there is evidence of infiltration. The site is over or around the wrist. Evidence of blood return is sluggish or absent. IV fluid runs erratically and the IV seems positional.	It is unreasonable to disregard the potential for a perfectly adequate venous access line because it was not started by the person administering the vesicant drug. Our ability to assess the vein and evidence of blood return should be adequate to ensure the practitioner of an adequate and safe venous access.

(continued)

TABLE 20-12   *(Continued)*

Risk Factor	Preventive Strategy	Rationale
Using a Preexisting IV Line (Continued)	If the IV fluid runs freely, the blood return is brisk and consistent; and the site is without redness, pain, or swelling, then there is no reason to inflict unnecessary pain by injecting the patient again.	
	Prior dressings must be carefully removed over the cannula insertion site to fully visualize the vein during injection of the vesicant agent.	Dressings and tape can severely impede both visually and tactilely an assessment for an extravasation.

(From Goodman, M. S. [1991]. Delivery of cancer chemotherapy. In S. B. Baird [Ed.], *Cancer nursing: A comprehensive textbook* [pp. 300–302]. Philadelphia: W. B. Saunders. Used with permission.)

20-5). A chart listing vesicants and their recommended antidotes should be conveniently posted (Table 20-13), with antidotes readily available for administration. (Studies reveal that delay in antidote administration increases the severity of the local tissue reaction.) The institution's policy regarding hot or cold emergency compresses should be established in the clinician's mind. If standing emergency orders are available, they should be signed by the responsible physician and placed in the patient's chart.

2. *Infuse saline to test venous patency before administering cytotoxic agents.* Administering IV antineoplastics should be postponed until the clinician is absolutely confident that fluids are flowing unimpeded into the vein. A flush of at least 5 to 10 mL normal saline will ensure venous patency and needle placement before antineoplastic agents are administered. If an immediate second venipuncture is difficult or ill-advised, the therapist may choose to infuse additional normal solution into the original site, to prove the vein competent beyond doubt. Only then should the cytotoxic agent be administered. If for any reason the clinician suspects the agent is not infusing properly, administration should be interrupted and further assessment undertaken. It is logical that the greater the extravasation volume, the more severe is local tissue destruction. *When in doubt, stop the infusion.*

3. *Be alert to signs of slow leak or insidious infiltration.* If the needle punctures the vein's posterior wall, chemotherapy agents can leak into deep subcutaneous tissues. If small-gauge needles are used, particularly when there is large volume of subcutaneous fat, infiltration is more difficult to detect. This risk underscores the need for early comparison and assessment of the venipuncture site and immediate surrounding skin.

4. *Monitor drug and blood flow rates frequently.* When administering agents with the bolus (IV push) technique, the nurse should pull back on the syringe's plunger approximately 3 to 4 mL to check blood backflow. Although a good blood return does not *always* guarantee that extravasation has not occurred,

TABLE 20-13
Recommended Antidotes for Vesicant/Irritant Drugs

| Chemotherapeutic Agent | Antidote | | Antidote Preparation |
	Pharmacologic	Nonpharmacologic	
Mechlorethamine Nitrogen Mustard, (Mustargen)	Isotonic sodium thiosulfate	Cold compresses	Mix 4 mL 10% Na thiosulfate with 6 mL sterile H_2O for injection. (⅙ molar solution results.) If using Na thiosulfate 25% mix 1.6 mL with 8.4 mL sterile H_2O for ⅙ molar solution.
Vincristine (Oncovin) Vinblastine (Velban) Vindesine (Eldisine) Teniposide (VH-26) Etoposide (VP-16)	Hyalouronidase (Wydase)	Warm compresses	Mix with 1 mL NaCl (150 U/mL)
Cisplatin (Platinol) Note: Large extravasations of concentrated solutions produce tissue necrosis.	Isotonic sodium thiosulfate		Mix 4 mL of 10% Na thiosulfate with 6 mL sterile H_2O for injection. (⅙ molar solution results.) If using Na thiosulfate 25% mix 1.6 mL with 8.4 mL sterile H_2O for ⅙ molar solution.

SQ, subcutaneous.

(From Oncology Nursing Society [1992]. *Cancer chemotherapy guidelines: Module V, Recommendations for the management of vesicant extravasation, hypersensitivity and anaphylaxis.* Pittsburgh.)

any changes in blood backflow should be investigated promptly. It may be necessary to adjust and reposition the needle if the bevel is resting against the vein wall. Because infiltration is the most frequent complication of IV therapy, it is prudent to make observations every 2 to 3 minutes, particularly when vesicants are infused. Vesicants' requirements for clinician vigilance pose special problems for nurses in inpatient units because the needs of patients in other rooms often preclude guarantees of adhering to vesicants' 2- to 3-minute infusion monitoring requirements. In fact, most facilities promulgate policies that disallow vesicant administration with mechanical infusion devices or without constant attendance by a clinician.[21]

5. *Replacement nurses should have thorough, patient-centered orientation.* If it is even remotely possible, a replacement nurse should be on the job, working alongside the predecessor nurse, ideally until he or she is entirely familiar with the medical regimen in place. To gain baseline pretreatment reference points for each patient, a successor nurse should have an opportunity to review and examine IV sites; check for venous patency; and review charts, histories, drugs, and infusion rates. This opportunity offers enormous psychological

Method of Administration	Comments	References	
		Humans	*Animals*
1. Inject 1–4 (⅙ molar) through existing IV line cannula. 2. Administer 1 mL for each mg extravasated 3. Inject SQ if needle removed.	1. Na thiosulfate neutralizes mechlorethamine. 2. Initiate treatment immediately. 3. Avoid multiple injections of antidote. Irrigate area with single injection as effectively as possible.	26 33	34
1. Inject 1–4 mL through existing IV line cannula. 2. Administer 1 mL for each mL extravasated. 3. Inject SQ if needle removed.	1. Enhances absorption and dispersion of the extravasated drug. 2. Warm compresses increase systemic absorption of the drug.	35 36	11 37 38 39
1. Inject 1–4 mL (⅙ molar) through existing IV line cannula. 2. Administer 1 mL for each mL extravasated. 3. Inject SQ if needle removed.	1. Inactivates cisplatin on contact. 2. Treatment not recommended unless a large amount of a highly concentrated solution is extravasated.	40 41	42 39

benefits for nurses and patients alike and promises that a consistent quality of care can be maintained.

6. *During vesicant infusion, a patient should remain in the treatment area.* Nurses in inpatient units should ensure that no diagnostic studies or therapies are scheduled to take a cancer patient off the unit during infusion of vesicants. If it is essential that the patient leave the treatment area, saline solution should be substituted while the infusion of the cytotoxic agent is temporarily discontinued. Alternatively, the nurse may accompany the patient to supervise drug infusion while diagnostic or therapeutic services are conducted off the treatment unit.

Treatment

By their very nature, some infiltrations are difficult to detect in early stages. It bears repeating: If vesicant extravasation is *suspected*, it should be treated as a *presumed* extravasation. Tables 20-14 and 20-15 offer general guidelines for treating vesicant extravasations. Some common antidotes are listed in Table 20-13.[23] Although clinicians' opinions and experiences differ regarding infiltration management, most agree that ice should be applied 15 to 30 minutes four times daily for most antineoplastic extravasations; the exceptions are the vinca alkaloids, which call for local heat application.

Clinicians should keep in mind that detailed charting of an extravasation should be completed as soon as possible after emergency needs have been met. Not only is this important for medicolegal purposes, comprehensive documentation is important for any incident review activities. Litigation rarely reaches a court until several years after an event. Because a clinician-witness is permitted to review medical documents before testimony, records should be as complete and precise as possible. Documentation should include:

1. Facility's nurse
   a. Date
   b. Time
   c. Type of venous access (needle type and size)
   d. Insertion site
   e. Number of venipuncture attempts and location
   f. Drug(s)
   g. Drug sequence
   h. Drug administration technique
   i. Approximate drug volume extravasated or suspected of extravasation
   j. Patient statements, complaints, reports
   k. Nursing management of extravasation
   l. Photo documentation (per institution policy)
   m. Appearance of site
   n. Physician notification
   o. Plastic surgery consultation/notification, if indicated

---

TABLE 20-14
Rationale for Use of Heat and Cooling for Extravasations

I. Heat
  A. The desired effect is to:
    1. Increase blood supply and increase the dispersion of the enzyme hyaluronidase (Wydase) into the subcutaneous tissues.
    2. Promote healing after the first 24 h by increasing blood supply.
    3. Enhance the absorption of the vesicant agent (theoretic effect of vasodilation).
  B. Opponents of the use of heat feel that vesicant agents injure the cells' metabolic mechanisms. Heat increases metabolic demands and therefore may decrease cellular destruction.*

II. Cooling
  A. The desired effect is to:
    1. Decrease the blood supply and decrease the absorption of drugs into the subcutaneous tissues.
    2. Constrict peripheral veins which decrease blood supply to the area and thereby minimize localized pain.
    3. Decrease the absorption and diffusion of the vesicant agent, thereby resulting in local tissue "pooling" (theoretic effect of vaso-constriction).
  B. Proponents of the use of a cooling maneuver feel that it decreases many enzymatic reactions and decreases the destructive effect of released white cell components (eg, lysozymes). Cooling also slows cellular metabolic rates and may improve survival of marginally injured tissues.*

(*Personal communication. V. Hentz, M.D., Plastic Surgery, Stanford University Medical Center, Stanford, California. In S. A. Miller [1980]. Oncology Nursing Forum, 7[4], pp. 8–16. Reprinted with permission.)

TABLE 20-15
Suggested Guidelines for the Treatment of Extravasation Associated With Vesicant Agents

Procedure	Rationale
1. Stop the infusion.	1. To prevent further drug leakage into the subcutaneous tissues.
2. Aspirate back remaining drug in the needle and tubing by drawing back on the syringe.	2. To remove any residual drug.
3. Superimpose normal saline.	3. To dilute the extravasated agent.
4. Administer by IV push suggested antidotes (physician's order needed). (See Table 20-13.)	4. To intentionally extravasate the antidote via the same route as the extravasated drug.
5. Remove the needle.	5. To facilitate step 6. The site can no longer be used as an IV route.
6. Administer suggested antidotes (see Table 20-13) SQ with multiple punctures into the suspected extravasation site.	6. Direct infiltration of the antidote into area of greatest concentration.
7. Elevate extremity.	7. To minimize swelling.
8. Apply cooling or heat pack.	8. See Table 20-14.
9. Apply topical antidotes.	9. To minimize surface (skin) inflammatory and erythematous reactions.
10. Obtain a plastic surgery consult.	10. Early plastic surgery intervention with wound débridement is mentioned by several authors when doxorubicin HCl has extravasated. When doxorubicin was initially introduced clinically, the necrotic ulcers from extravasation were followed without débridement. The ulcers showed no tendency to heal spontaneously. It is believed that doxorubicin attaches to the DNA molecule and causes cell death. It is thought that the drug is then released to attach to adjacent living cells with further cellular destruction. Early excision is advised to stop this progression.
11. Document in writing in official patient record.	11. To enhance later recall and for medicolegal purposes.
12. Maintain contact with patient.	12. To follow symptomatology and ensure that appropriate interventions are initiated.

SQ, subcutaneous.

---

     p. Follow-up instructions to patient
     q. Date of return visit
     r. Nurse's signature[12]
  2. Extravasation record (Figure 20-12)
  3. Incident report

As nurses, much of our success, like that of most medical disciplines, results from a combination of science, art, and perseverance. Administering antineoplastic

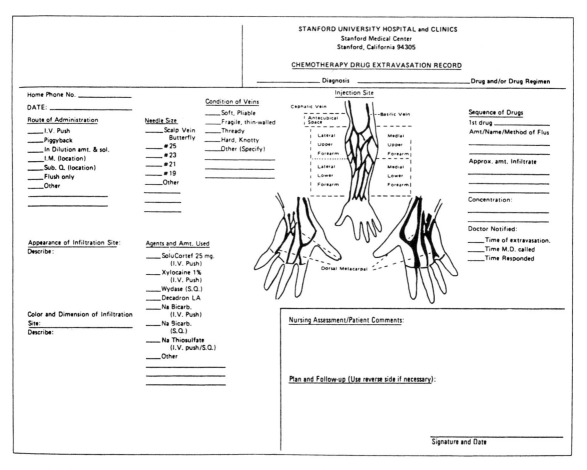

FIGURE 20-12 Extravasation record used at Stanford University Hospital and Clinic. (From Miller, S. A. [1980]. *Oncology Nursing Forum, 7*[4], 8–16. Used with permission.)

therapy is among the many privileges one may have in sharing our patients' cancer experience, which is unique to each person who must endure it. It calls for sophisticated skills of head, hands, and heart. What is a formidable task to some becomes a refined skill to the professional who commits to knowing all that is necessary to efficiently and safely infuse the substances that attempt to control and kill cancers.

REFERENCES

1. Bender, C. M. (1987). Chemotherapy. In C. R. Ziegfeld (Ed.), *Core curriculum for oncology nursing* (pp. 225–235). Philadelphia: W. B. Saunders.
2. Bingham, E. (1985). Hazards to health workers from antineoplastic drugs. *New England Journal of Medicine, 313,* 1220–1221.
3. Brown, J. K., & Hogan, C. M. (1990). Chemotherapy. In S. L. Groenwald, M. H. Frogge, M. S. Goodman, & C. H. Yarbro (Eds.), *Cancer nursing: Principles and practice* (2nd ed., pp. 230–273). Boston: Jones & Bartlett.
4. Crudi, C., & Larkin, M. (1984). *Core curriculum for intravenous nursing.* Philadelphia: J. B. Lippincott.
5. DeVita, V. T., Hellman, S., & Rosenberg, S. A. (Eds.). (1989). *Cancer: Principles and practice of oncology* (3rd ed.). Philadelphia: J. B. Lippincott.

6. Dorr, R. T. (1980). *Cancer chemotherapy handbook*. New York: Elsevier.

7. Fischer, D. S., & Knobf, M. T. (1989). *The cancer chemotherapy handbook* (3rd ed.). Chicago: Year Book Medical Publishers.

8. Goodman, M. S., & Wickham, R. (1984). Venous access devices: An overview. *Oncology Nursing Forum, 11*(5), 16–23.

9. Goodman, M. S. (1986). *Cancer: Chemotherapy and care*. Evansville, IN: Bristol Laboratories.

10. Goodman, M. S. (1991). Delivery of cancer chemotherapy. In S. B. Baird (Ed.). *Cancer nursing: A comprehensive textbook* (pp. 291–320). Philadelphia: W. B. Saunders.

11. Guy, J. L. (1991). Medical oncology—the agents. In S. B. Baird (Ed.), *Cancer nursing: A comprehensive textbook* (pp. 266–290). Philadelphia: W. B. Saunders.

12. Holleb, A. I. (1991). *American Cancer Society textbook of clinical oncology*. Atlanta: American Cancer Society.

13. Hubbard, S. M., Seipp, C. A., & Duffy, P. L. (1989). Administration of cancer treatments: Practical guide for physicians and oncology nurses. In V. T. DeVita, S. Hellman, & S. A. Rosenberg (Eds.), *Cancer: Principles and practice of oncology* (3rd ed., pp. 2369–2402). Philadelphia: J. B. Lippincott.

14. Revised intravenous nursing standards of practice. (1990). *Journal of Intravenous Nursing* (Suppl.).

15. Johnson, B. L., & Gross, J. (Eds.). (1985). *Handbook of oncology nursing*. New York: John Wiley & Sons.

16. Lokich, J. J. (1987). *Cancer chemotherapy by infusion*. Chicago: Precept Press.

17. Miller, S. A. (1980). Legal implications for the nurse involved in cancer chemotherapy administration. In R. T. Dorr & W. L. Fritz (Eds.), *Cancer chemotherapy handbook* (pp. 743–754). New York: Elsevier.

18. National Cancer Institute. (1990). *Chemotherapy and you—A guide to self-help during treatment*. Bethesda, MD: U.S. Department of Health and Human Services.

19. Oncology Nursing Society and American Nurses Association. (1987). *Standards of oncology nursing practice*. Kansas City: American Nurses Association.

20. Oncology Nursing Society. (1988). *Cancer chemotherapy guidelines: Modules I–IV*. Pittsburgh: Author.

21. Oncology Nursing Society. (1989). *Safe handling of cytotoxic drugs: Independent study module*. Pittsburgh: Author.

22. Oncology Nursing Society. (1989, I & II). (1990, III). *Access device guidelines, recommendations for nursing education and practice. Module I, catheters; Module II, implanted ports and reservoirs; Module III, pumps (infusion systems)*. Pittsburgh: Author.

23. Oncology Nursing Society. (1992). *Cancer chemotherapy guidelines: Module V, recommendations for the management of vesicant extravasation, hypersensitivity and anaphylaxis*. Pittsburgh: Author.

24. Padilla, G. V., & Bulcavage, L. M. (1991). Theories used in patient/health education. *Seminars in Oncology Nursing, 7*(2), 87–96.

25. Petersen, J. (1991). Chemotherapy. In S. B. Baird (Ed.). *A cancer sourcebook for nurses* (6th ed., pp. 73–83). Atlanta: American Cancer Society.

26. Somerville, E. T. (1991). Knowledge deficit related to chemotherapy. In J. C. McNally, E. T. Somerville, C. Miaskowski, & M. Rostad (Eds.), *Guidelines for oncology nursing practice* (2nd ed., pp. 57–61). Philadelphia: W. B. Saunders.

27. Suddarth, D. S. (Ed.). (1991). *Lippincott manual of nursing practice*. Philadelphia: J. B. Lippincott.

28. Tennenbaum, L. (1989). *Cancer chemotherapy: A reference guide*. Philadelphia: W. B. Saunders.

29. U.S. Department of Labor, Office of Occupational Medicine, Occupational Safety and Health Administration. (1986). *Work practice guidelines for personnel dealing with cytotoxic (antineoplastic) drugs* (Publication No. 8.1.1). Washington, DC: Author.

30. Villejo, L., & Meyers, C. (1991). Brain function, learning styles, and cancer patient education. *Seminars in Oncology Nursing, 7*(2), 97–104.

31. Vogelzang, N. (1979). Adriamycin flare: A skin reaction resembling extravasation. *Cancer Treatment Reports, 63*, 2067–2069.

32. Welch-McCaffery, D. (1985). Rationale, development and evaluation of a chemotherapy certification course for nurses. *Cancer Nursing, 8*, 255–262.

33. Ziegfeld, C. R. (Ed.). (1987). *Core curriculum for oncology nursing*. Philadelphia: W. B. Saunders.

REVIEW QUESTIONS _____

1. Which of the following is NOT a goal of cancer chemotherapy?
   a. cure
   b. control
   c. palliation
   d. surgery

2. Which of the following actions may prevent anaphylactic reactions during administration of antineoplastic agents?
   a. obtain an allergy history
   b. have an emergency cart available
   c. obtain and record baseline vital signs
   d. establish baseline mentation assessment

3. Which of the following statements concerning extravasation is true?
   a. may occur in presence of a blood return
   b. never occurs in presence of blood return
   c. may be prevented by using central veins
   d. never occurs with peripherally inserted central catheters

4. If a second venipuncture site is needed and the patient's other arm may not be used, the second site should be located:
   a. distal to the original
   b. proximal to the original
   c. in the lower extremity
   d. in a central line

5. All of the following drugs are established vesicants EXCEPT:
   a. dactinomycin
   b. daunorubicin hydrochloride
   c. doxorubicin
   d. dacarbazine

6. All of the following elements of documentation of extravasation are essential EXCEPT:
   a. number of attempts at venipuncture
   b. date and time of treatment
   c. antineoplastic agents and their sequence
   d. approximate quantity of drug extravasated (or suspected of extravasation)

7. Knowledge of which of the following areas is essential to effectively administer antineoplastic therapy?
   a. clinical pharmacology
   b. safe drug calculations
   c. proper disposal
   d. preparation and handling

8. Which of the following is NOT a barrier to a patient's thorough understanding of cancer treatment with antineoplastic therapy?
   a. anxiety
   b. compromised literacy
   c. denial
   d. familiar environment

9. Which of the following precautions should NOT be taken when preparing and handling IV antineoplastic agents?
   a. wear protective equipment, consistent with OSHA guidelines
   b. prepare drug in class II biologic safety cabinet
   c. label all syringes and containers
   d. clip all needles carefully

10. All of the following factors should be considered before establishing a venipuncture site on a patient receiving antineoplastic agents EXCEPT:
    a. avoid areas of impaired lymphatic drainage
    b. drug sequencing
    c. baseline reference points of vital signs and mental status is required
    d. patient education

PART V

Special Applications of Intravenous Therapy

CHAPTER 21

Pediatric Intravenous Therapy

Key Terms

Developmental	Intraosseous	Play therapy
Gestational	Metabolic rates	Umbilical
Intractable diarrhea	Neonate	

This chapter focuses on features of IV therapy unique to pediatric patients. This group can be further divided into developmental stages by age: infant (0–12 months), toddler (1–3 years), preschool (4–5 years), school-age (6–12 years), and adolescent (12–18 years).[25] A subdivision of the infant group includes neonates, or newborns from 0 to 28 days, which must also include the unique IV therapy needs of the premature infant.[39]

PRELIMINARY CONSIDERATIONS

How do the needs of a pediatric patient differ from those of an adult? Body circumference of the adult alters relatively little from the onset of adulthood through the remainder of life, whereas body circumference of a child must accommodate more than a threefold increase in length and approximately a 20-fold increase in weight between birth and adolescence.[2] Thus, the stress levels and basal metabolic rates of a child are exceedingly higher than those for an adult. A more subtle area of concern is the child's developmental needs, which require patience, education, and understanding from the IV nurse. A full comprehension of the child's developmental stage according to age enables the health care team to provide appropriate, nonthreatening care. Furthermore, understanding the child's developmental stage enhances the ability of the staff to recognize that needs of children vary markedly, not only by stress levels but also by growth and developmental levels.

Some common reasons for IV therapy in the pediatric patient include:

1. *Maintenance of fluid and electrolyte balance.* The younger the child the greater the risk not only of fluid and electrolyte imbalance but also of fluid overload and congestive heart failure. Rehydration of a child with diarrhea may seem routine, but complexities can arise even in a child who requires fluid for rehydration when experiencing respiratory distress, altered electrolyte balance, or other complications. In this situation, manipulations according to actual fluid restriction are made.

   Because fluid therapy is often short lived and can be advanced quickly to oral rehydration therapy, a peripheral catheter is often the IV device of choice. If hypertonic solutions or chronic fluid therapy is indicated, a central access device may be recommended.

2. *Antibiotic therapy.* The most common pediatric disease requiring antibiotic therapy is sepsis. Even before a child who displays the symptoms of sepsis (ie, increased heart rate, irritability, temperature spikes) is actually diagnosed, prophylactic IV antibiotics are routinely administered while a complete sepsis work-up is in progress (eg, urine cultures, throat cultures, blood cultures, wound cultures, and so forth). If the sepsis work-up reveals a positive blood culture, the IV antibiotics are continued for a complete 10-day course of therapy. If the sepsis work-up is negative, the prophylactic IV antibiotics are discontinued. Antibiotic therapy is also used for treatment of cystic fibrosis, meningitis, osteomyelitis, and many other indications.

   Length of antibiotic therapy differs according to diagnosis, so choice of IV device is based on those factors, as well as vein availability of the child. For short-term therapy (1–2 weeks), a peripheral IV may suffice, whereas for more than 2 weeks, a midline or peripherally inserted central catheter (PICC) may be indicated.[60]

3. *Medication therapy.* In addition to antibiotics, many medications used in adults are also used in children. These include drugs such as aminophylline; insulin; cimetidine (Tagamet); ranitidine (Zantac); electrolytes; anticonvulsants and sedatives; vasoactive drugs such as dopamine (Intropin), and isoproterenol (Isuprel); immunosuppressant agents such as cyclosporine (Sandimmune); and a host of other IV medications. In many cases, drugs have not yet been approved for pediatric IV administration, but they are used based on ongoing and published research studies, experience in adults, and the emergency status of the child. For this reason, children are often referred to as "therapeutic orphans," indicating a lack of information regarding interaction between a medication and the body processes of the child.[3] Emergency medications and fluids for respiratory and cardiac arrest may be administered

by the intraosseous (IO) route (discussed later in this chapter) versus the IV route if IV access cannot be obtained.

4. *Anticancer drugs.* Most chemotherapy or anticancer drugs required for treating childhood cancers use the IV route because of efficacious absorption. There are many more IV protocols designed for the child with cancer compared to the adult, primarily because most childhood cancers are unique to children (eg, Wilms' tumor, neuroblastoma, and retinoblastoma). Precision in regulating the specific IV chemotherapy along with monitoring IV clearance is crucial in this group because of the incremental risk of fluid overload, electrolyte imbalances, and chemotherapy side effects.

   Many children with cancer benefit from the flexibility of single- or double-lumen nontunneled, tunneled, or implanted central access devices.

5. *Nutritional support.* Supplemental parenteral nutrition is often used for short-term benefit as an adjunct therapy to enteral or oral intake and is usually given through a peripheral IV. Total parenteral nutrition (TPN) is used for the child whose gut is not functional for congenital or acquired reasons such as prematurity, short-bowel syndrome, acquired immunodeficiency syndrome (AIDS), or cancer. TPN is administered via some type of central access device, described later in this chapter. Parenteral nutrition has been a lifesaver in the pediatric milieu, but it is not without risks, so close monitoring is necessary.

6. *Transfusion therapy.* Blood components most often used in children include packed red blood cells, platelets, and fresh frozen plasma. In addition, components derived from a unit of plasma may be administered to children with special needs, as in the use of cryoprecipitate for treatment of hemophilia A and coagulation factor concentrates for treatment of factor deficiencies. Gamma globulin therapy has expanded because of the availability of IV IgG versus intramuscular gamma globulin.

   Transfusions of blood and blood components may be administered to a child through a peripheral IV for one-time or infrequent transfusion or through a central device for chronic transfusion needs. Because transfusion carries the risk of iron build-up, IV chelating agents are often prescribed in addition to transfusion therapy.

   A procedure unique to the neonatal population is exchange transfusion, where blood volume is gradually removed and replaced to correct such conditions as hemolytic disease of the newborn (HDN).

   Exchange transfusions are optimally undertaken using two IV sites or an IV and intra-arterial site. These can be a combination of peripheral, central, or umbilical access devices. The procedure for exchange transfusion is described later in this chapter.

   Although transfusion therapy is covered fully in Chapter 17, an overview of the therapeutics unique to pediatric patients is presented in this chapter.

Two of the main considerations in administration of IV therapy to children are emotional preparation of the child and initiation of IV access. The next several sections look at these topics in detail, including special nursing considerations for treating pediatric patients. Specific IV therapeutic modalities are described, after emotional considerations and peripheral and central IV access are discussed.

EMOTIONAL CONSIDERATIONS

What other considerations are essential to maintain the highest caliber of care in children? Even though children of varied ages and intellectual capacities all receive similar IV therapies, pre- and post-IV therapy education must be given, taking these variables into account. A child's capacity for understanding the significance of IV therapy, including the importance of not manipulating the IV site, usually occurs between the ages of 3½ to 5 years, depending on the individual child. Explanations of all procedures must be given to the child and the parent.

Establishing Trust

To gain insight into the problems of establishing trust, the practitioner should recognize the child's viewpoint. A thought-provoking question for practitioners is, "How can I expect the child to totally trust me when I am about to hurt him or her by performing a venipuncture?" Usually it is best to tell the child that the venipuncture will hurt but only for a short time. Define the term *time* not by minutes—young children will not understand this—but by comparison to other procedures, for example, "The actual IV puncture takes about the same time as it takes me to take your temperature, get you a glass of orange juice, or for you to finish your dinner." Inform the child that even though this therapy may be painful initially, it should make him or her feel better like before the illness. *Always be honest* with a child.

Specifically, do not promise a certain number of IV attempts or "only one stick" because a child will lose trust if several attempts are necessary. Give the child the opportunity to cry, providing as much privacy as possible. If old enough, let the child participate in the therapy; a child's ability to rip tape, open alcohol swabs, and hold tubing may provide tasks and distraction, particularly in the school-age group. Fear of needles may be assuaged by telling a child that once the IV is in place, the needle is no longer there, and only a small "straw" is in the vein. This theory can be reinforced during play therapy.

Play Therapy

Play therapy, consisting of practicing IV therapy on a doll, is an ideal teaching strategy that allows emotional preparation through acting out. It may not, however, always be practical because of the urgency of IV therapy or the availability of dolls. When it is pragmatic, nurses certainly can participate in this form of play therapy for teaching purposes, or they may seek such assistance from the child-life workers.

A "coping basket," filled with items for various age groups is easy and inexpensive to put together. The basket can include a Slinky, a clear sealed acrylic "magic wand" with floating sparkles, a kaleidoscope, a "Kush" ball, and a bottle of bubbles for blowing.[32] The items are cleanable and small enough for a spot in the treatment room of a hospital, a pediatric care office, or the equipment bag of a home infusion nurse. An adolescent my find a portable stereo with headphones useful as a distraction during IV insertion.

Establishing Rapport

Another important aspect of IV therapy is establishing rapport with the family and child through good communication. Communication differs with all age groups according to the child's intellectual level.

An IV therapy teaching tool with pictures and large print words in simple language can help the preschool-age child understand the procedure. The learning tool can be used as a hospital coloring book.[64]

Adolescents, in particular, require a great deal of individual attention and allowance for their independent nature versus their dependent situation. Adolescents feel grown up and desire the opportunity to assess their disease status; they deserve the opportunity to participate in the decision-making aspect of their care. Adolescents are easily hurt when criticized. They feel that they are grown up but lack the experience and knowledge of the adult. Therefore, educational techniques practiced with adolescents should encompass a commonsense approach, permitting each adolescent an opportunity to deal with IV therapy to the best of his or her ability. Over-expectation and performance pressure from the IV practitioner can result in emotional conflicts and depression in this age group.

Nursing assessments should include developmental level of the child, influence of the disease process and IV therapy on the child's psyche and body image, previous experience with venipuncture, and desire of parents or parental figures to be present during IV initiation. The presence of parents during a painful or invasive procedure is controversial and needs to be evaluated on a case-by-case basis. Parents may provide emotional support and represent security during an actual procedure, but they should not be used to restrain a child unless no other assistance is available (ie, home care). If a parent chooses to not accompany a child into the treatment room for the IV insertion, this decision should be honored by the IV nurse and parents should not be made to feel guilty. Provision of comfort and praise after an IV insert provides an ideal means of parental involvement after the procedure is completed.

Pain Reduction

By using pain reduction techniques, such as imagery and the coping basket, the anxiety associated with IV insertion can be reduced. In addition, local anesthetics, such as topically applied Emla cream or intradermal saline at the IV site may decrease pain sensation in children.[52]

PREPARATION FOR VENIPUNCTURE

From infancy to adolescence, children go through different developmental stages, and pre- and post-IV care should be geared to these stages, including preparation for the procedure, IV site protection, and mobility and safety needs. Infants are provided with comfort, such as a pacifier during IV insert, and observed for aspiration if feeding occurred just before the procedure. Toddlers and preschool-age children are prepared immediately before the IV start in simple, positive terms, such as "We are going to start the IV now." School-age children can be prepared slightly in advance, afforded with privacy and small tasks, and allowed to cry, but hold still. Adolescents can be prepared well in advance and encouraged to make decisions regarding their care, such as having an IV restarted later in the day so they can go out on pass from the hospital for several hours, and participating in self-care, such as monitoring for IV site complications, maintaining intake and output with supervision, and even setting up home TPN or accessing an implanted port. The teenage population may test caregivers and express the need for independence by not always being compliant with therapy, so monitoring and encouragement are still needed, and planning a schedule with the teenager may be beneficial.

Care must be taken to assess each child individually, not just according to age or physiologic development. In some cases, children have disease processes that cause reduction in growth, such as in children with renal disease. Psychological age and ability must be considered when looking at the emotional needs of a child.

When hospitalized, children tend to regress and exhibit behaviors more common to a younger age group (ie, a child who is toilet trained may regress back to the diaper stage when hospitalized). Developmental landmarks are resumed again after treatment is discontinued or stabilizes.

Preparation for IV insert in children should be geared toward developmental stage as follows[25]:

Infant (0–12 months)
Trusts others to fulfill needs.

- Preparation for venipuncture includes discussion with parent or caregiver regarding site, usage, and appearance of IV.
- Provide comfort with pacifier.
- Avoid IV insert immediately after feeding or aspiration may occur.

Toddler (1–3 years)
Increased mobility, self-discovery, separation anxiety; the "no" stage.

- Prepare for IV insert immediately before procedure with simple explanations.
- Do not offer choices. Say "We're going to do your IV now," not "Can we do your IV now?"
- Provide comfort by allowing child to hold favorite toy, security blanket, or object.
- Usually need an assistant to help restrain a toddler

Preschool (4–5 years)
Thinking is magical; child may fantasize about procedures based on their understanding. This age group fears invasive procedures and loss of blood, such as for a lab test.

- Prepare child just prior to IV insert.
- Allow child to touch equipment.
- Use medical play, for example, putting IV in a doll.
- Allow child to cry.
- May need help to hold still; use a fellow caregiver if possible.

School Age (6–11 years)

More independent and mastering new skills; body image starts to become important, and fear of bodily mutilation develops.

- Prepare child same day as procedure.
- Child may help to set up equipment or do small tasks (ie, rip tape).
- Allow for privacy.
- Do not force child to be brave; "don't be a cry baby" is not appropriate.
- Allow child to cry.
- Maintain privacy during IV start.

Adolescent (12–18 years)

Wavers between need for independence and dependence on others for care. Has adult learning abilities and reasoning, but not the maturity of experience; body image and peer acceptance are important.

- Prepare several hours to days in advance to allow for assimilation of IV insert information and formulation of questions.
- Allow choices, for example, "Can the IV be started after I go out on pass to the mall?"
- Maintain privacy and consider body image in choice of site whenever possible.

PERIPHERAL AND CENTRAL INTRAVENOUS ACCESS

Let us now analyze sites and devices appropriate for IV therapy, from peripheral to central locations. Depending on the child's age, a site for administering IV drugs is typically more difficult to find than in an adult. Both hydration status and previous IV therapy may be used as predictors of difficulties in obtaining an intact venous access. In the child, the site selected for IV therapy should involve minimal risk and allow maximum efficiency and safety.[10]

Peripheral IV Sites

When selecting the optimal site for IV therapy, certain basic strategies should be followed. An excellent site in the neonate and infant is the head because the scalp has an abundant supply of superficial veins (Figure 21-1). The bilateral superficial temporal veins just in front of the pinna of the ear or the metopic vein, which runs down the middle of the forehead, are generally easy to find and involve minimal patient risk.

Scalp veins are readily available until about 12 to 18 months of age, when hair follicles mature and superficial layers of skin thicken, making venous access difficult. When inserting an IV in the scalp, one must be aware of artery location, because it is difficult to distinguish veins from arteries in this area. Inadvertent arterial puncture reveals bright red blood, pulsation, and blanching of skin caused by arteriospasm when the IV device is flushed.[17] The IV device should be removed and pressure held

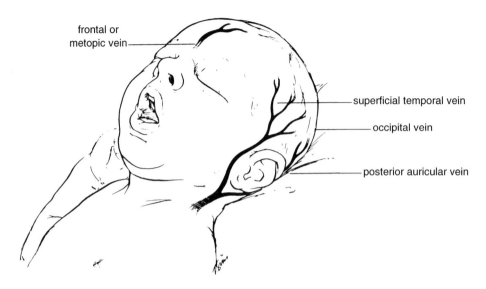

frontal or metopic vein

superficial temporal vein

occipital vein

posterior auricular vein

FIGURE 21-1 Sites for scalp vein infusions.

on the site until bleeding stops. Use of an "arterial" IV could result in damage to the artery and the area to which oxygenated blood is delivered. The scalp as an IV site can also be distressing to parents, who may believe that the IV is in the brain. If the head must be shaved, shave or clip the smallest area possible, saving this hair for the parents as the child's first haircut, thus alleviating some distress at the use of this site.[17] A scalp IV can restrict mobility and be easily dislodged; with the advent of small IV catheters for peripheral access, scalp veins are no longer the first choice for IV access in babies.

Other favorable peripheral IV sites include the hand, forearm, upper arm, foot, and antecubital fossa, moving from distal to proximal locations (Figure 21-2). Some unusual sites such as axilla, abdomen, and popliteal area have also been used when chronically ill infants and children exhibit greatly diminished peripheral venous access from long use (Table 21-1). Foot veins are used up to walking age and occasionally in older children where other usual sites are not available, such as in burn or multiple trauma patients. Depending on the regulations of the state's Board of Nursing and institutional policy, external jugular and femoral veins are used for IV access and obtaining blood samples, although these last two sites are usually reserved for IV access by a physician, nurse practitioner, or emergency personnel.

Peripheral Intravenous Devices

Before and during the 1970s, the device of choice for pediatric IV access was the winged infusion needle. This device was used for short-term IV therapy and withdrawal of blood samples for laboratory analysis. In the late 1970s, 22-gauge catheter-over-needle devices made of plastic, then Teflon, became available and could be used for longer lasting IV access in pediatric patients.[2] Winged infusion needles are still used for blood sampling in many pediatric institutions because the vacuum withdrawal method of blood sampling used in adults is often too aggressive for tiny pediatric veins.

FIGURE 21-2 Pediatric venipuncture sites. (Used with permission from Fay, M. J. (1983). Special challenges of Pediatric IVs. *Dimensions of Critical Care Nursing.* Hall-Johnson Communications. Photo by Randi Boyette)

Catheter-over-needle device design has advanced to include thin-wall cannulas (Figure 21-3) for greater flow rates, smaller gauge size (24 and 26), shorter length, nonkinking material, and devices made of Aquavene™, an elastomeric hydrogel that expands in gauge and length after 30 minutes in the vein, allowing a smaller catheter to be inserted and a longer dwell time than traditional catheters.[56] Small-gauge catheters such as the 26 and 24 for neonates and the 24 and 22 for children and adolescents are the choice when up to 2 weeks of IV therapy is prescribed.[70] After this time, peripheral access sites diminish and use of a longer lasting or central device may be warranted.

INTRAVENOUS INSERTION TECHNIQUES _____

Peripheral Intravenous Insertion

General IV insertion techniques have been described previously and will not be discussed in this chapter; however, some special techniques for achieving venous access in children are highlighted.

TABLE 21-1
Peripheral Intravenous Access Sites for Pediatric Patients*

Preferred Sites	Veins
Hand	Digital, metacarpal
Forearm	Supplementary cephalic, basilic, median antebrachial
Antecubital fossa	Median basilic, median cephalic, median cubital
Upper arm (below axilla)	Basilic, cephalic
Foot (before walking age)	Greater saphenous, lesser saphenous
Scalp (before 18 mo)	Occipital, frontal, temporal
Lower leg (before walking age)	Greater saphenous, lesser saphenous

Secondary Sites†	Veins
Wrist	Superficial veins: infiltration in this area may result in pressure on the radial nerve
Abdomen	Superficial veins: rarely used, usually limited to neonates and chronically hospitalized patients; infiltration may result in damage to abdominal wall
Axilla	Axillary vein: usually limited to neonates; infiltration may cause pressure on structures in chest cavity
Knee	Popliteal vein: usually limited to neonates due to decreased mobility

*Sites listed in order of preference; consider individual characteristics
†Secondary sites should be considered only when preferred sites are not available.

To dilate veins in children, a smaller tourniquet may be necessary, and in neonates, a rubber band with a tape tab provides an easily removable tourniquet for scalp IVs (Figure 21-4). In some cases, no tourniquet is used.[17] Additional aids to vein location and dilatation may include warm soaks or transillumination.[46] Insertion of IVs in children requires stabilization of the extremity before venipuncture, so that movement of the child does not dislodge the newly inserted device and require subsequent sticks. An

FIGURE 21-3   Small gauge thin-walled Teflon peripheral IV catheter, suitable for use with children. (Courtesy: Critikon, Inc., Tampa, FL)

FIGURE 21-4 Rubberband used as a tourniquet on baby's scalp. (Courtesy: A. M. Frey)

armboard usually is an adequate restraint (Figure 21-5) and can be taped to the treatment room table to provide passive restraint during IV insertion.

A firm but gentle insertion technique is necessary for a successful venipuncture in a child because blood return in the flashback chamber may not appear as readily and the characteristic "pop" of entering a vein may not be felt. Choose the nondominant extremity first for IV access when possible; in unusual sites such as scalp and abdomen, the rule is to place the IV in the direction of venous flow or toward the heart.

Equipment and supplies are set up before venipuncture, usually in a treatment room if possible, thus preserving the child's room and bed as a "safe" place, where invasive procedures are not performed.[55] In an intensive care environment, supplies may be prepared away from the bedside so as not to cause undue anxiety before the

FIGURE 21-5 An armboard is used to support the area of the IV site and provide light restraint during IV insertion. (Courtesy: A.M. Frey)

actual venipuncture. In the home, supplies are usually set up in an area where lighting is maximized and a flat surface, such as a kitchen table, can be used as a work area.

Equipment for IV insertion includes the following[55]:

IV tubing with volume control device as warranted by age of child and type of infusion:

Volumetric pump

Microdrop calibrated chamber

Smallest container that will last for 24 hours

Stabilization equipment:

Armboard

Site protector

Short extension tubing with Luer lock connections

Tourniquet or rubber band

Antimicrobial solution for site cleansing

Adhesive tape

Sterile gauze or transparent dressing

Injection cap

1 to 3 mL of flush solution in a syringe

Gauze

Gloves

IV pole (if necessary)

IV device ranging from 25 to 20 gauge depending on size of child and viscosity of infusate

The number of attempts at IV access should be no more than two or three, except in extreme emergency. Limiting venipuncture attempts decreases physical and emotional trauma to a child and can preserve venous integrity. Occasionally in children, threading of the IV catheter can be difficult. Threading of the catheter into the vein can be facilitated by making sure the catheter tip has entered the vein lumen after flashback of blood, by advancing the IV device slightly. Other measures include attaching a small connector tubing with flush solution, and flushing gently as the catheter is advanced. Sometimes, just waiting a few seconds until the child has calmed down can decrease the incidence of venous spasm and facilitate catheter threading. IV insertion in children requires patience and practice until the learning curve is diminished and skill level increases. Figures 21-6 through 21-9 demonstrate IV insertion in a 5-month-old baby with meningitis who is receiving IV antibiotics intermittently through a heparin lock.

Once venous access has been obtained, the next strategy involves stabilization of the IV.

Stabilizing the Intravenous Line

Stabilization is essential, primarily in the younger child whose level of comprehension concerning the importance of not manipulating the IV site is minimal. All IVs placed in the head are taped in a U-shaped chevron pattern, and the extension tube is

FIGURE 21-6 Blood enters the flashback chamber of the IV catheter, then the 24-gauge catheter is advanced slightly. (Courtesy: A. M. Frey)

looped into a coil so that if the child pulls on the IV, the tension of the pull will affect the coil, not the IV site. A small, open-ended paper cup is placed on top of the site to act as a protective covering. Sites requiring stabilization include the hand and the arm, both of which generally require armboard support. The advantage of this type of stabilization is that it restricts the child's range of movement, thereby decreasing the risk of dislodgment of the IV needle. The foot also demands stabilization, primarily to use saphenous vein. Venous accessibility in the foot is not only more difficult, but it results in mobility restriction from the stabilizing legboards that are used to keep young children, especially under age 2, from manipulating the needle (Figure 21-10). An important aspect of IV access in the foot involves maintenance of normal joint configuration by placing padding under the foot, thus maintaining the natural

FIGURE 21-7 The catheter is advanced fully, stylet is pulled back, and tourniquet is removed. (Courtesy: A. M. Frey)

FIGURE 21-8 The stylet is removed and T connector is attached to hub of IV catheter. Catheter is flushed gently to assess patency. (Courtesy: A. M. Frey)

bend at the ankle and avoiding foot drop or contracture injuries. Coverings such as stretch netting may keep little fingers away from the IV site, while providing easy visualization. The top "ribbed" portion of a sweatsock, slipped over the IV, can serve the same function for home IV access. A roller bandage should not be used to cover an IV site because it is time consuming to unravel and makes site assessments difficult. Surgical cutdown is less popular now that smaller, long-term IV devices are available.

FIGURE 21-9 Clear sterile dressing is applied, the site is labeled, and the injection cap is attached to T connector. Fingertips and IV site remain visible. (Courtesy: A. M. Frey)

FIGURE 21-10 Foot IV site. Note that joint configuration is maintained and toes and IV site are visible. (Courtesy: A. M. Frey)

Use of Restraints

In younger children, especially those in the toddler group, great care must be taken to protect the IV site. In general, restraints are seldom used at children's medical centers because it is not only confining but also creates a sense of frustration and mistrust in the child. Only on a rare occasion, with an extremely uncooperative child or a child who may injure himself or remove the IV, may restraints be used.

Postinsertion Care of the Peripheral IV

Dressing changes are usually only done when the IV site is changed, every 48 hours as recommended by the Intravenous Nurses Society (INS) Standards of Practice.[35]

Although 48 hours is the currently recommended site change interval, a recently published survey indicated that the majority (71.9%) of children's hospitals surveyed indicated that peripheral IV sites were changed only when necessary.[4]

One study done in a pediatric critical care unit demonstrated that peripheral IV sites could be left in place up to 6 days.[21]

Flushing techniques for peripheral and central devices are also a controversial topic. Few studies involved pediatric patients until recently. These studies indicate that saline alone may be efficacious in maintaining patency of 22-gauge catheters in children; however, the numbers of 24-gauge catheters reported was small, and one study demonstrated increased patency in 24-gauge catheters when a dilute heparin flush was used.[12,30,48] The most common practice is to irrigate peripheral IVs with 1 mL of a solution of 10 U heparin per mL normal saline every 8 hours.[4]

Removal of the IV should be done carefully, without the use of scissors near the site. IV complications in children are similar to those of the adult and are described earlier in this textbook. The most common peripheral IV complication is infiltration, which can lead to an extravasation injury. Current pediatric treatment modalities include the application of cold, elevation of the extremity, and local pharmaceutical intervention with such agents as hyaluronidase, phentolamine, and glyceryl trinitrate.[6,19]

Emergency Intravenous Access

Surgical Cutdown

If routine vein accessibility is extremely difficult, a surgical cutdown performed by the surgical team may be indicated. The most common cutdown sites are the saphenous vein of the foot and the cephalic vein in the forearm. Because this procedure requires venous laceration or minor surgery, the site must be cleaned subsequently with antiseptic solution of povidone-iodine and povidone-iodine ointment at least biweekly to prevent local infection. Surgical cutdown is less popular now that smaller, long-term IV devices are available.

Intraosseous Access

Obtaining successful IV access is essential to provide efficacious pediatric advanced life support. In many cases, during a "code" situation, peripheral veins have collapsed because of cardiac arrest and poor perfusion. Time for performance of a surgical cutdown can range from 2 to 40 minutes, with a median time of 8 minutes.[36] IV access should be obtained within 5 minutes from the start of a resuscitation effort. After traditional routes have been attempted, often simultaneously, IO access is a realistic goal. *Intraosseous infusion* is defined as infusion of blood, fluids, or drugs through a rigid needle directly into the bone marrow cavity.[43] From 1922, when first described by Drinker and colleagues,[13] through the 1940s to 1960s, this technique was widely used. As IV device technology improved, facilitating peripheral venous access, IO technique lost popularity. Since 1983, interest in IO therapy has increased because of a letter to the editor of *American Journal of Diseases in Children* that questioned the abandonment of this route.[66]

Intraosseous technique is based on the fact that fluid injected into the medullary cavity of the bone is quickly taken up by the extensive network of venous sinusoids, and drugs given by the IO route and the central venous route are equally effective, working faster than those administered by peripheral IV.[43] The best site for IO infusion in children up to 5 or 6 years old is the anterior medial aspect of the tibia, 1 to 3 cm below the tibial tuberosity, thus avoiding the growth plate at the end of the bone[36,43,51] (Figure 21-11).

Other sites include distal medial tibia, midanterior distal femur, iliac crest, humerus, and sternum in children less than 3 years of age, before which time, the sternum is too thin to support the IO needle.[51] Contraindications to IO access include site infections, fractures, burns, and bone disorders, such as osteogenesis imperfecta (brittle bone disease) and osteopetrosis (marble bone disease), where bones may fracture easily.[43,51]

Intraosseous access is indicated during emergency situations, such as respiratory or cardiac resuscitation efforts or when two attempts at peripheral IV access are unsuccessful.[43] A short rigid needle with a stylet is used to obtain IO access (Figure 21-12); alternately, a lumbar puncture needle may be used for infants although this needle can bend easily and is awkward to insert. Disposable bone marrow aspiration needles are now manufactured for IO access; 16, 18, or 20 is the recommended gauge size because a small-lumen needle can become blocked with bone fragments or bend on insertion. After antimicrobial cleansing of the desired site, the IO needle is inserted perpendicular to the bone surface at a slight angle away from the epiphyseal plate. A screwing motion is used to insert the needle into the bone until decreased re-

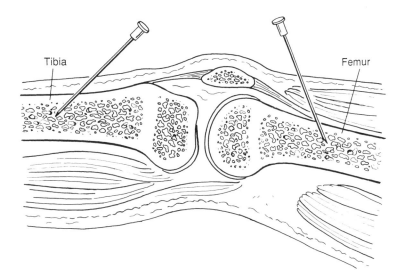

FIGURE 21-11 The anterior medial aspect of the tibia (lateral view) is the best site for intraosseous access in the child under 6 years of age.

sistance is noted and the needle stands without support, usually at a depth of 1 cm in an infant or child. Further advancement may cause penetration of the opposite wall of the bone and result in extravasation of infusates. Some IO needles are now manufactured with a premarked shaft to indicate depth. After insertion, the stylet is removed and bone marrow content, similar to blood, is aspirated; this sample may be used for readings of $PaCO_2$ and pH, important parameters indicating success of resuscitative efforts.[43] A short connector tubing and flush solution, similar to that used with IV catheters, is connected to the hub of the IO needle and a split sterile gauze dressing and tape are placed to secure the site. If the child is awake, intradermal anes-

FIGURE 21-12 Intraosseous needle with Diekmann modification (two laterally opposed side ports, positioned near distal tip to ensure flow if tip is obstructed by bone fragment). (Courtesy: Cook Critical Care, Bloomington, IN)

thesia before IO needle placement is advised. The site should be observed for infiltration of infusates into surrounding tissues; the same bone should not be used for repeated access if infiltration occurs.

Types of infusions given by the IO route are listed in Table 21-2. Infusates may be administered by gravity, manual pressure, or infusion pump.

Complications are relatively rare. Increased chance of osteomyelitis has been related to long-term use of the IO route, as well as infusion of hypertonic solutions. Other complications can include cellulitis, abscess, or local necrosis; fat embolism, although a possibility, has not been reported in children, probably because of the low fat content of bone marrow in children, especially those under the age of 4.[43] Success rates with IO therapy have been reported to be as high as 97%.[58] However, further studies are needed, and replacement of the IO needle with IV access is recommended as soon as conventional IV access is feasible.

TABLE 21-2
Intraosseous Infusions

Fluids	Medications	Blood Products
5%, 10%, and 50% dextrose	Analgesics	Whole blood
Saline	Anesthetics	Packed red blood cells
Lactated Ringer's solution	Anticonvulsants	Plasma
Parenteral nutrition	Antisera	Albumin
	Antibiotics	Dextran
	Catecholamines	
	Miscellaneous	
	Atropine	
	Calcium	
	Dopamine	
	Dobutamine	
	Epinephrine	
	Heparin	
	Insulin	
	Lidocaine	
	Levarterenol	
	Phenytoin	
	Sodium bicarbonate	
	Contrast media	

(From Glaesser, P. N., & Losek, J. D. [1986]. Emergency intraosseous infusions in children. *American Journal of Emergency Medicine, 4,* 35; Miccolo, M. A. [1990]. Intraosseous infusion. *Critical Care Nurse, 10,* 35–47; Mofenseon, H. C. [1988]. Guidelines for intraosseous infusions [Letter to the editor]. *Journal of Emergency Medicine, 6,* 145–146; Arbeiter, H. I., & Greengard, J. [1944]. Tibial bone marrow infusions in infancy. *Journal of Pediatrics, 25,* 1.)

Intermediate-Term Midline Intravenous Access

In recent years, use of IV devices that are placed peripherally, but are of longer length, and are left in place for a longer period of time, has become popular. As with most medical equipment, adult-sized versions of these devices are tested initially, and then research in children is commenced. The INS Standards of Practice define central IV devices as those whose proximal tip is located in the subclavian, superior vena cava, or inferior vena cava.[35] Peripheral IV site changes should be done frequently to avoid infectious complications. However, in cases where intermediate-term IV therapy is desired and surgically placed central lines are not indicated, midline-located IV catheters have fulfilled a need. In children, these catheters have been efficacious for treatment of such disorders as cystic fibrosis, osteomyelitis, Lyme disease, Crohn's disease, and a variety of other conditions that require several weeks of IV antibiotic, antifungal, or nutritional therapy, where peripheral IV access with short traditional catheters would be impractical.

A sample of such catheters currently available includes the Landmark™ catheter in 24 and 22 gauge, with a length of 3 to 6 inches. This catheter is made of Aquavene™, the same material as the longer dwelling, short peripheral catheter that expands in size and length. The Landmark™ catheter is placed in the veins of the antecubital fossa, above or below the bend of the elbow, and threaded into the upper arm, where larger vein lumen and increased blood flow provide dilution of the infusate.[28] In addition, PICCs have been inserted so that the tip is purposely placed in a vein in the upper arm.[69] Varying degrees of success have been reported with use of these devices; more research, particularly in the pediatric population, is certainly a mission for the IV nurse. Follow manufacturers recommendations for use of such catheters.

Central Intravenous Access

When long-term IV access is desired because of unavailability of peripheral sites or a need for long duration or lifelong therapy is identified, central venous access is indicated. Many types of devices exist for this purpose, including umbilical catheters, PICCs, surgically placed cuffed tunneled catheters, and totally implanted devices. Choice of device depends on the duration and type of therapy prescribed, patient and family input, and disease process. Although these devices are described in detail in earlier chapters, features unique to the pediatric population are outlined.

Umbilical Catheterization

Most sites for neonatal IV therapy are similar to those for children discussed earlier in this chapter. However, a catheter unique to the neonatal population is the umbilical vessel catheter. Umbilical catheterization is common practice in many neonatal and intensive care units for treatment of acutely ill infants. This mode of therapy provides an easy route for IV administration. The risks include thrombosis, embolism, vasospasm, vascular perforation, infection, and hemorrhage.[7] To prevent these complications, a specially designed umbilical catheter with the following features should be selected:

1. Flexibility
2. Relatively rigid walls for accurate pressure monitoring
3. A single end-hole to avoid clotting in the tip

4. Smoothness of the tip to prevent perforation of the vessel wall during catheter insertion

5. Radiopaqueness to radiographically visualize the location of the tip of the catheter

6. Small capacity so that only a small amount of blood need be withdrawn to clear the catheter for blood sampling

7. Size from 3.5 to 5 Fr catheter

Arterial Versus Venous Umbilical Catheterization. Let us now examine the difference between arterial and venous umbilical catheterization. Within minutes of birth, the umbilical arteries normally constrict; delays in the process, however, occur in states of hypoxia and acidosis. The vast majority of infants are catheterized in the first day of life because umbilical catheterization is generally not possible past the fourth day of life.

The procedure for umbilical catheterization begins with the physician or nurse practitioner's preparation for asepsis, including handwashing, gloving, masking, and gowning. This step precedes the preparation of the umbilical stump with an iodine solution, followed by cleansing with alcohol, and subsequently draping of the sterile field and exposing the umbilical area. Dissection begins at the umbilical cord around 1.5 cm from the skin until the umbilical vessels are identified. Two thick-walled, pin-point-sized arteries are easily distinguishable from a large, thin-walled vein. The heparinized catheter is passed through either the umbilical artery or vein, depending on the type of therapy desired.

Arterial catheterization accomplishes five goals: 1) blood sampling; 2) measurements of arterial pressures; 3) parenteral or antibiotic therapy in the vascularly compromised child; 4) exchange transfusions; and 5) arterial pH and blood gases. Venous umbilical catheterization accomplishes four goals, including (1) and (3) above as well as providing a means for a direct measurement of central venous pressure and a route for the infusion of TPN.[39]

Placements differ between the umbilical venous route and the arterial route. Ideally, the tip of the umbilical venous catheter should be positioned in the inferior vena cava near the right atrium in good position for central venous pressure and TPN administration. Comparatively, the umbilical arterial catheter is best positioned above the level of aortic bifurcation in good position for arterial measurements and exchange transfusions.

Once the catheter is placed correctly and position is confirmed radiographically, a suture may be placed superficially through the stump, tying it firmly to the catheter for anchorage.[38] The catheter is generally connected to a three-way stopcock for pressure monitoring, blood drawing, and fluid administration. When fluid administration is not necessary, the line may be heparinized. It is of the utmost importance to maintain patency of the indwelling catheter because blood clots can otherwise form. Flushing with heparin (1 U/mL IV fluid) should be done frequently.

Increased thrombosis when administering fluids through an umbilical artery has been reported; therefore this mode of therapy should be used with caution. The nursing assessment for pending complications should include the following:

1. Examine buttocks to detect blanching caused by arterial spasms.

2. Closely monitor the umbilical line with Luer lock attachments to prevent disconnection of the tubing with resultant hemorrhage.

3. Closely monitor peripheral edema, unequal femoral pulses, and respiratory distress, which could indicate emboli formation.

4. Perform daily dressing changes with the application of povidone-iodine ointment to decrease the risk of sepsis.

5. Observe and document the quality of the arterial waveform on the monitor; change in quality or dampening of the waveform may indicate a problem with the umbilical arterial line.

If complications arise, report them immediately to the appropriate physician so immediate medical attention can be provided. Early intervention can reduce the risk of morbidity and mortality when using the umbilical access for IV therapy.

Because of the risk of complications and the short duration when using the umbilical vessel for IV therapy, many physicians now prefer to use an alternate peripheral site, such as the scalp or hand, or other central venous access.

Nontunneled Central Catheters

Nontunneled catheters include subclavian, jugular, and femoral catheters, as well as PICCs. These catheters are referred to as "nontunneled" to distinguish them from longer-dwelling cuffed Silastic catheters that are surgically tunneled under the skin. Nontunneled subclavian catheters usually have small lumens and a short length and may have from one to four lumens (Figure 21-13). These catheters are made of a stiffer material such as polyvinylchloride for easier insertion the short distance through the skin into the vein. In children, these catheters may be inserted nonsurgically, using a local anesthetic, in such sites as the internal or external jugular vein, the subclavian vein, or the femoral vein. If a child is very apprehensive, anxious, or uncooperative, a sedative such as chloral hydrate may be indicated before the procedure.

Catheter stiffness, high incidence of thrombus, and easy dislodgment limit use of these catheters to a relatively short period of time, ranging from a few days to up to 4 weeks.[67] Catheters may be changed over a wire if lumens become blocked or sepsis is suspected although benefit of this practice is yet to be definitely proven and it remains controversial. In children, subclavian catheters are often used for IV access in

FIGURE 21-13 Subclavian double-lumen catheter. (Courtesy: A. M. Frey)

critical situations, such as a multiple trauma patient brought to the emergency room or children in the pediatric intensive care unit, where several weeks of IV access and possible need for parenteral nutrition exists. Catheters placed in jugular and femoral locations can be occluded by anatomy because infants tend to have a shortened neck and frequently adduct their legs, causing kinking in the catheter placed in the neck or groin. Femoral location is also the diaper area and the dressing may become soiled frequently and exposed to infective organisms prevalent in this region. Subclavian catheter insertion in neonates is technically difficult and can result in life-threatening complications such as pneumothorax, hydrothorax, hemothorax, and massive hemorrhage.[14] Fortunately, alternate choices for central venous access are available, and the PICC is one of these choices for neonates to adults.

The PICCs were fairly common in the adult intensive care unit in the 1960s and have made a comeback in recent years.[67] Newer versions come in tiny sizes (27, 25, and 23 gauge) for neonates and infants to larger sizes (20, 18, and 16 gauge) for older children and adults. Double-lumen PICCs are also available, but large introducer and catheter size negates use of these in young children and those with tiny veins. PICCs are associated with fewer complications than surgically placed catheters[10] and insertion can be done without the risks of general anesthesia. Pediatric-sized PICCs are manufactured of polyurethane, elastomeric hydrogel, or softer Silastic-type material shown to have low incidence of irritation and thrombus formation, allowing PICCs to remain in place for months to years.[45] These catheters may be inserted in children in the hospital, outpatient, or home setting (Figure 21-14). In neonates, PICCs are inserted into the veins of the antecubital fossa, as well as axillary, saphenous, popliteal, and external jugular veins[9] (Figure 21-15). In older children who have reached walking age, the basilic and cephalic veins in the antecubital fossa, or slightly above or below this site, are ideal. Insertion of PICCs is covered in Chapter 11; the technique is similar in adults and children, although a child may be more anxious and less likely to be cooperative, and may need restraint and use of local anesthetic for easier insertion.

FIGURE 21-14 PICC in place prior to dressing application, in left median cubital vein of a 3-year-old with repeat surgery for Hirschsprung's disease; after surgery, child was NPO on TPN. (Courtesy: A. M. Frey)

FIGURE 21-15   PICC in place, with dressing on site, in left basilic vein of neonate with hypoplastic ventricle. Patient is receiving prostaglandin infusion via the PICC. (Courtesy: A. M. Frey)

The complication rate with PICCs in children is minimal and includes clotting or occlusion as the most documented complication, particularly in neonates, where small gauge size and low flow rates may lead to catheter blockage. This complication has led several researchers to recommend use of flow rates greater than 2 mL/h, as well as addition of heparin (1 U/mL) to IV fluids.[9] Other complications include phlebitis, leaking, edema, erythema, and suspected or confirmed sepsis. Sepsis rates range from 0% to 11% in studies of infants.[22] In one study comparing peripherally and surgically placed central catheters in neonates, complication rate and dwell time were the same.[59] In addition to neonates, PICCs are also used for intermediate (2 weeks to several months) IV access in infants through adolescents for treatment of such conditions as cystic fibrosis, Crohn's disease, osteomyelitis, joint infections, brain abscesses, inflammatory bowel disease, pancreatitis, and any other condition requiring intermediate-term antibiotic, antifungal, or parenteral nutrition therapy, as well as therapies required by pediatric oncology patients.

Tunneled Central Venous Catheters

Tunneled catheters are most often chosen for long-term venous access, as are implanted ports, which will be discussed in the next section. In the early 1970s, Broviac developed the first tunneled catheter for patients who required long-term TPN.[5] Broviac catheters (Bard/Davol) have since become frequently used when long-term central IV access is needed, such as with children who have cancer. The Groshong catheter (Bard/Cath Tech), developed in the 1980s, is also tunneled, but is made of more thin-walled silicone than the Broviac.[71] Single- and double-lumen Broviacs and single- and double-lumen Groshongs are used in children; the triple-lumen Broviac tends to be somewhat large for pediatric use. Both catheters contain a Dacron polyester cuff that anchors the catheter in place subcutaneously several weeks after insertion[8] (Figure 21-16). Both catheters have a Luer-locking proximal hub(s) outside the patient; the Broviac has an open distal tip on the internal portion, whereas the distal

FIGURE 21-16   Neonatal- and pediatric-sized Broviac catheters with and without Dacron cuff and Vitacuff. (Courtesy: Bard Access Systems, Cranston, RI)

tip of the Groshong is closed with a two-way slit valve. More detailed descriptions of tunneled catheters are provided in Chapter 12.

If no contraindications to general anesthesia exist, tunneled catheters are often inserted in the operating room or radiology suite by a surgeon or interventional radiologist. Local anesthesia and possibly a sedative medication may be used in older children for catheter placement in the treatment room or at the bedside. Often, several procedures are coordinated with catheter insertion to avoid unnecessary trauma while the child is awake; for example, a newly diagnosed leukemia patient may have one visit to the operating room for Broviac insertion, bone marrow biopsy, and lumbar puncture.

In the larger child, the catheter is usually inserted percutaneously into the subclavian vein. In infants and neonates, because of the small size of the subclavian vein, this approach can be extremely dangerous. Therefore, in infants and children under age 5, the catheter is usually inserted through the facial vein or the external or internal jugular vein to the superior vena cava (Figure 21-17).

After proper placement is verified by chest radiography, subcutaneous tunneling of the catheter is done—either up the parietal occipital area or down the chest wall to the fourth or fifth intercostal space, depending on the catheter type. This distal exit site from the original phlebotomy site provides a barrier from infection,[49] facilitates catheter maintenance, and provides the child with full-range neck mobility.

In some children, chest access sites are not available because of many previous central lines and vein thrombosis, or other surgery or complications. An alternate site for catheter placement is the femoral vein to the inferior vena cava, particularly in children under walking age. The proximal portion of the catheter is then tunneled under the skin of the abdomen or out onto the thigh.

Care of tunneled catheters is described in detail in previous chapters, and includes dressing changes, flushing to maintain patency, and prevention of infection and dislodgment. Care of tunneled catheters is continually researched, and procedures for

FIGURE 21-17 Example of inserted pediatric infant-sized Broviac catheter. Note that the catheter is threaded into the external jugular to the right atrium and tunneled subcutaneously down the chest wall.

children are based on manufacturers' guidelines, catheter volume, experience with adults, and ongoing and previously published research studies. Dressing materials range from use of no dressing in the well healed nonimmunocompromised patient, to an adhesive bandage, gauze pad, or transparent dressing. Dressing changes are usually done using clean or sterile technique two to three times a week. Catheter patency is maintained with saline or heparinized saline in the strength of 10 to 100 U/mL, given from once or twice daily to once weekly.[44] These protocols vary among institutions and are continuously reviewed based on research studies and the needs of the child.

The complications most frequently reported for tunneled catheters in children include infection, occlusion, and dislodgment, with the toddler age group exhibiting the highest complication level.[34] Broviac infection rates can range from 5% to 31.6% and are usually reported in terms of rate per 1000 catheter days to maintain consistency of data.[13] The most common organisms reported include *Staphylococcus aureus* and *Staphylococcus epidermidis*, as well as some gram-negative organisms, many of which are normal body flora.[11] Because of the high infection rate attributed to tunneled catheters, activities such as swimming and showering, where exposure to organisms can occur, may be prohibited, and alternate activities should be carefully planned for the child with a tunneled catheter in place. Occlusion may be corrected with urokinase (Abbokinase) or hydrochloric acid, depending on the cause of the occlusion.[33] Dislodgment may be avoided by carefully looping the external "tail" of the catheter under the dressing or to the chest; wearing of a T-shirt for all age groups with tunneled catheters is recommended. If breakage occurs, temporary repair may be done with a blunt-tip needle or IV catheter, so sterility and patency can be maintained until a more permanent splicing procedure can be accomplished.[67]

Implanted Ports

Venous access ports are implanted in the chest, upper abdomen, or in the forearm, with the catheter threaded into a central vein. Low-profile pediatric ports have been available for several years and are made of stainless steel, titanium, or plastic, or a

FIGURE 21-18   Low profile pediatric implanted port accessed with 22-gauge, ¾ inch, 90° angle, noncoring needle. (Courtesy: A. M. Frey)

combination of those materials (Figure 21-18). Ports are a good choice for long-term venous access for the pediatric patient older than 3 years because before that age, lack of subcutaneous tissue may cause the port to erode through the skin. Because the port requires access at least monthly with a needle, this is an important consideration when advising patients and family about venous access devices. A port is ideal for the child who requires intermittent therapy, can tolerate the needle access, and does not like the inconvenience of an external catheter, such as patients with cancer, short-bowel syndrome, or cystic fibrosis.[44]

Ports are accessed from the top or side, depending on the design, with a noncoring needle; a 22-gauge, ½-inch needle for a forearm port and a 22-gauge, ¾- to 1-inch needle for a chest port are usually adequate for the viscosity and flow of pediatric infusions. Needles are changed every 7 to 10 days while the port is being used; dressings over the accessed port can be changed with the needle change or more frequently. When the port is not being used for infusion of medications, parenteral nutrition, transfusion therapy, or blood sample withdrawal, patency is maintained by flushing the port with heparinized saline, usually in the volume of 3 to 5 mL and the strength of 100 U/mL on a monthly basis.[31,44]

Complications reported with ports are similar to those identified for tunneled catheters, but the reported infection rate is lower (0–9%) than with externalized catheters.[34] Although risk of port dislodgment is minimal, the noncoring needle may be dislodged and cause infiltration and possible tissue injury if vesicant drugs are being administered. Slight discomfort has been reported with needle access of the port, but this diminishes in time, and a high level of satisfaction has been reported with this device.[57] The port may be accessed by a hospital or home IV nurse, by the parents, or in some cases, by patients themselves, after return demonstration of correct technique. Of consideration in the cystic fibrosis population is use of the arm port versus the chest port because chest physiotherapy, involving percussion of the chest, is a large part of the treatment plan for cystic fibrosis, and a chest port may obstruct therapy. Complete port description and care may be found in Chapter 12.

Of consideration to children and parents is catheter care, safety, cost, and body image. For instance, in toddlers, catheter dislodgment may easily occur; an infant may bite through the catheter during the teething period. A child who is extremely afraid of needles may not do well with an implanted port, which has to be accessed with a needle periodically. Conversely, an older child or adolescent may choose an implanted port over a tunneled catheter to avoid disturbance of body image. If the central device is to be used for continuous infusions or cycled daily therapies, such as TPN, a Broviac may be a better choice; if intermittent treatments are prescribed, a port might be the better device. Pediatric hospitals often employ clinical nurse specialists who can demonstrate pros and cons of each device, assist families in their choice of venous access, introduce children with similar devices, and help decrease anxiety about insertion and care of the device.

PEDIATRIC INTRAVENOUS THERAPIES

Primary indications for pediatric IV therapy include fluid balance, medication administration, cancer therapy, nutrition support, and transfusion therapy. Although these topics are covered fully in other chapters, features unique to the neonatal and pediatric patient are highlighted here.

Fluid Therapy

Fluid requirements during IV therapy are a concern. At what rate should IVs be administered to a child? Obviously, the answer to this question is determined by the child's stature and metabolic rate. The amount of fluid required for maintenance levels depends on insensible water loss from lungs, skin, urine, and stools and from metabolic expenditures from both internal or external stress levels.

Assessing Fluid Needs

Before deciphering fluid requirements, familiarization with the three different methods for assessing 24-hour maintenance fluids is crucial: namely, the meter squared, caloric, and weight methods. The methods listed below are according to the guidelines from Graef and Cone.[24]

1. The *meter squared* method has an arbitrary estimate of requirement of 1500 to 1800 mL fluid per square meter. The advantage of this method is its simplicity; its disadvantage is in the accessibility of a visual nomogram.

2. The *weight* method uses the child's weight in kilograms to estimate fluid needs. The advantage of this method also is its simplicity; the disadvantage is that it is less accurate in the patient who weighs more than 10 kg.[24]

3. The *caloric* method calculates that the usual expenditure of fluid is approximately 150 mL for every 100 calories metabolized. This method too is simple, but not totally accurate unless actual calorie requirements and energy intake are continuously assessed.

Maintenance fluid requirements for neonates and children differ in volume allowed in 24 hours, but fluid needs of both groups are calculated in milliliters per kilogram weight (Table 21-3).

The methods just discussed only address maintenance replacement according to insensible losses and do not address the additional metabolic expenditures that require further replacement therapy. For example, the most common cause of incre-

> **TABLE 21-3**
> **Guide to Protein, Caloric, and Fluid Requirements per Day for the Pediatric Patient**

Age	Protein/kg	Calories/kg
Premature	2.5 g	120–150
Term newborn	2.5 g	100–120
1–3 y	1.5–2 g	70–100
4–6 y	1.5 g	70–100
7–10 y	1–1.5 g	70–100
11–14 y	1 g	50–100
15–18 y	1 g	50–70

Fluid Requirements by Weight

0–10 kg	100 mL/kg
11–20 kg	100 mL/kg—first 10 kg
	50 mL/kg—second 10 kg
21 kg and up	100 mL/kg—first 10 kg
	50 mL/kg—second 10 kg
	20 mL/kg—after 20 kg

(From Goldberg, M., & Tyrala, E. [1981]. *Parenteral nutrition guide* [3rd ed., p. 19]. Philadelphia: St. Christopher's Hospital for Children. Used with permission of the authors.)

mental fluid and caloric needs is temperature elevation. An increase in temperature elevation by 1°C increases the child's caloric needs by 12%. Conversely, a child who is hypothermic has a caloric decrease of 12% per degree Celsius, which decreases the fluid requirements.

Other conditions that affect incremental fluid requirements include gastrointestinal losses, small intestinal drainage, and ongoing diarrhea. The physician and the nurse should assess the entire metabolic situation before prescribing the amount and type of IV therapy a child needs. A precise intake and output record is the most valuable assessment tool for determining fluid requirements. When abnormal losses occur via the kidneys, it is wise to determine the extent of the loss and replace it rather than estimate according to the previously mentioned methods.[68] To ensure accuracy in judging fluid needs, most children receiving IV therapy are on strict intake and output, including diaper weighing.

How do fluid requirements differ in a neonate? Their fluid requirements are greater proportionately because of their higher percentage of total body water; therefore, infants are at greater jeopardy for both fluid overload and dehydration. Also, electrolyte status must be followed closely by laboratory tests to determine whether the neonate is in a state of isotonic versus hypertonic dehydration. Actual water requirements vary between a newborn, a low-birth weight infant, and a high-risk infant. The exact amounts of calories, water, and electrolytes required depend on the newborn's gestational age, body stores, and metabolic rates. The smaller and more immature the infant is, the greater is the total body water content. For example, the water content of a 28-week gestational age infant is 85% of total body weight, as compared to the term infant, whose water content is only 70%.[39] To arrive at specific fluid requirements, all these factors are accounted for, and a strict intake and output record is maintained.

Other factors that affect fluid requirements in the neonate include many therapeutic devices affecting metabolic rates. For example, radiant warmers and single-walled incubators may be effective in maintaining the infant's temperature, but this temperature elevation in turn increases the infant's insensible fluid losses. Phototherapy, though effectively used in the treatment of hyperbilirubinemia in the neonate, will increase insensible fluid losses and cause water requirements to be greater.[38] These various losses must be included when determining fluid replacement. If the child's fluid requirements are not met, a number of physiologic and metabolic states may occur, including evidence of weight loss in association with hyperosmolality, hypernatremia, and increased hematocrit, as well as evidence of metabolic acidosis, dehydration, and frequently, in infants, multiple apnea spells and increased bilirubin.

Conversely, administration of excess fluid, either IV or, occasionally, as a result of respiratory support systems, can be associated with edema, congestive heart failure, patent ductus arteriosus, and even bronchopulmonary dysplasia in the neonate.[41]

Accurate intake requires precision in IV administration. It is paramount that the flow of IV fluids be delivered at a constant rate. Even the smallest error can cause serious problems, especially in the compromised child. Rates in pediatrics generally vary from 5 to 80 mL/h depending on the size of the child. Adolescent fluid requirements are similar to those for adults, ranging from 100 to 175 mL/h. Intake and output are monitored hourly; fluids are delivered via gravity or by electronic infusion device for more accuracy through a peripheral or central IV device.

Intravenous Antibiotic and Medication Therapy

Multiple drug therapy is more the norm than the exception in today's high-acuity pediatric patient. A recent survey by this author noted that about 170 IV medications are administered to pediatric patients at St. Christopher's Hospital for Children in Philadelphia; about 60 or more of these medications are used for home IV therapy in children. A large portion of these drugs includes antibiotics, antivirals, and antifungals administered IV for such conditions as meningitis, osteomyelitis, Lyme disease, joint infections, prophylaxis before and after abdominal surgery, bacterial and fungal central line infections, systemic herpes, and sepsis.

Neonates are generally at greater risk of becoming septic, possibly caused by an acquired congenital disorder resulting in intestinal obstruction, immaturity in lung compliance resulting in respiratory distress syndrome, immaturity of the gastrointestinal tract resulting in necrotizing enterocolitis, and immaturity of the immune system. All these problems mandate antibiotic coverage by the IV route because of the neonate's immature gastrointestinal system and decreased tolerance to the systemic effect of the infection.

Pharmacokinetic parameters must be considered when administering IV medications to a child. These parameters include absorption, distribution, metabolism, and excretion, and each is affected by patient maturity and disease process.[47] Absorption of an IV drug depends on adequacy of the IV access and the length of delivery time; IV absorption is usually immediate. Distribution occurs when a drug, having entered the circulatory system, (it takes about 1 minute for blood to circulate through a child's body[72]), is distributed to the tissues. Most drugs are distributed via the extracellular fluid, others via binding with protein or fat molecules. Because the neonate has a higher level of total body water than the adult (80% versus 60%), water-soluble drugs, such as theophylline, have to be given at higher doses.[47] Neonates and malnourished children have decreased levels of plasma proteins, and drugs that bind to protein, such as nafcillin (Unipen), may be given in lower doses to these children. Some drugs may also compete with binding sites on the albumin molecule, displacing bilirubin from these sites in neonates, and increasing risk of hyperbilirubinemia. These drugs include salicylates, sulfonamides, phenytoin (Dilantin), furosemide (Lasix), and sodium benzoate.[25] Many commercially available medications and drug diluents contain sodium benzoate in the form of the preservative benzyl alcohol; this preservative has been linked to toxicity and death in premature infants, and care should be taken to stock only preservative-free diluents in the nursery and neonatal intensive care unit.[50] Because neonates have less subcutaneous fat, medications that are lipid soluble, such as diazepam (Valium), should be given in smaller doses. The liver plays a large part in drug metabolism. In the neonate with an immature hepatic system or the child with liver disease, decreased liver function may cause altered metabolism of such drugs as phenobarbital, phenytoin, and carbamazepine.[25] Many drugs are excreted via the renal system. Again, less efficient renal function caused by immaturity in the neonate or disease process in the older child, may result in decreased excretion of drugs, with longer half-life, and possibility of toxicity. In these patients, penicillins and aminoglycosides are given at greater dosage intervals (every 12 or 18 hours versus every 6 or 8 hours). In children with cystic fibrosis, where extrarenal clearance pathways eliminate drugs more quickly, IV aminoglycosides, such as tobramycin (Nebcin), must be given at two to three times the normal dose.[47]

Intravenous medications may be administered to children using a variety of methods, including manual IV push, volume-control set, syringe pump, or retrograde infusion. Sample minimal dilution guidelines are provided in Table 21-4. Each method is applicable to specific drugs and desired therapeutic outcome. Before and after IV administration of certain drugs, levels of medication in the blood are tested to determine the safe dosage range for therapeutic effectiveness. These levels are known as *trough level*, or the lowest drug level drawn just before giving a scheduled dose, and *peak level*, or the highest drug level, drawn 30 minutes after the drug and postflush have infused.[40] Monitoring of these levels and the clinical status of the patient and being aware of pharmacokinetic parameters will provide a good picture of the effects of IV medication administration in the child.

Dosages for pediatric patients are individualized and usually calculated in milligrams per kilogram for most IV drugs, milligrams per square meter for chemotherapy, and micrograms per kilogram for IV drugs used for resuscitation and advanced pharmacologic life support. A rule of thumb is that most drugs are packaged in single adult-sized doses, so a portion of a vial is usually needed for a child's dose. If more than two vials of a drug are needed for a single pediatric dose, calculations should be rechecked.

Of great concern to many practitioners is the correct administration of IV medications given to a child during advanced life support. Some institutions use bedside charts, particularly in pediatric critical care areas, which list the individual doses of

TABLE 21-4
Maximum Recommended Concentrations and Minimum Recommended Administration Times for the Administration of Antibiotics to the Fluid-Restricted Patient

Antibiotics	Recommended Final Concentration for Administration	Recommended Duration of Infusion	Antibiotics	Recommended Final Concentration for Administration	Recommended Duration of Infusion
Acyclovir	7 mg/mL	1–3 h	Miconazole	6 mg/mL	30–60 min
Amikacin	6 mg/mL	15–30 min	Nafcillin[4]	50 mg/mL	10–30 min
Ampicillin[4]	50 mg/mL	10–30 min	Penicillin G	Infants: 50,000 U/mL	10–30 min
Amphotericin B[1,2]	0.1 mg/mL	2–4 h			
Azlocillin[4]	50 mg/mL	15–30 min		Large Child:	
Aztreonam	20 mg/mL	20–60 min		100,000 U/mL	
Carbenicillin[4]	50 mg/mL	10–30 min	Pentamidine	2.5 mg/mL	1 h
Cefazolin[4]	50 mg/mL	10–30 min	Pipiricillin[4]	50 mg/mL	10–30 min
Cefotaxime[4]	50 mg/mL	10–30 min	Ticarcillin	50 mg/mL	10–30 min
Cefoxitin[4]	50 mg/mL	15–30 min	Tobramycin	2 mg/mL	15–30 min
Ceftazidime[4]	50 mg/mL	15–30 min	Trimethoprim/ Sulfamethoxazole	1 mL in 15–25 mL (5 mL = 80 mg TMP, 400 mg SMX)	60 min
Ceftriaxone[4]	50 mg/mL	10–30 min			
Cefuroxime[4]	50 mg/mL	15–30 min	Vancomycin[3]	5 mg/mL	60 min
Cephalothin[4]	50 mg/mL	15–30 min	Vidarabine	0.45 mg/mL	12–24 h
Chloramphenicol	50–100 mg/mL	10–30 min	**Experimental**		
Clindamycin	6–12 mg/mL	15–30 min	Fluctosine hour[5] (Do not dilute)	10 mg/mL	30 min–1 h
Erythromycin	5 mg/mL	20–30 min			
Gentamicin	2 mg/mL	15–30 min			
Imipenem— Cilastatin	5 mg/mL	30–60 min	Ganciclovir (DHPG)	10 mg/mL	1 hour
Methicillin[4]	50 mg/mL	15–30 min	Rifampin	6 mg/mL	< 3 h
Metronidazole	5–8 mg/mL	60 min	Trimetrexate	4 mg/mL	30 min
Mezlocillin[4]	50 mg/mL	10–30 min			

The main determinant of the maximum recommended concentration of antibiotics for IV administration is the development of phlebitis. The table lists the maximum recommended concentration for infusion of antimicrobial agents. Infusions exceeding these guidelines may cause the development of severe phlebitis and loss of the IV site. Administration of medication faster than the infusion times listed below may lead to an increase in adverse drug reactions.

Table Notes:

1. Amphotericin B is incompatible with saline.

2. Amphotericin B (Fungizone IV) must be given by *SLOW* IV infusion (see package insert). Side effects may be reduced, however, by using a shorter infusion time.

3. Vancomycin should not be infused over < 60 min due to the association of a characteristic rash over the head and neck with more rapid infusion rate.

4. The concentration of beta-lactam drugs (penicillins and cephalosporins) may be increased from 50 mg/mL to 100 mg/mL when administered to large children in whom excessive volumes of fluid would be required with the 50 mg/mL concentration.

5. May infuse over a longer period of time if the fluid volume necessitates.

(From: Farrington, E. (1990). Pediatric drug information. *Pediatrics* 16 (3): 310)

Section Editor's Note:

- If an antibiotic has been noted to be irritating to the veins, the concentration may be decreased to no more than half of what is recommended.

- When infusing antibiotics via a central line, a concentration of twice that listed above may be used to reduce the fluid volume administered to a patient.

resuscitative drugs for the weight of that child. In addition, large, multidose charts listing doses of drugs and sizes of equipment used in a pediatric code may be posted in the emergency or treatment room areas. This information is extremely helpful to nursing and medical personnel who work with adult patients and are not readily familiar with these dosages from experience. Tables 21-5 and 21-6 list pediatric life support medications, dosages, and infusions.

Cancer Therapy

Because of research, discovery of new drug combinations, and aggressive therapy, the mortality rate for children with cancer has decreased greatly since the 1960s. Common cancers in children include leukemia, neuroblastoma, rhabdomyosarcoma, Wilms' tumor, retinoblastoma, lymphomas, Hodgkin's disease, and brain tumors. These cancers are treated with a team approach that includes physicians, clinical nurse specialists, staff nurses, social workers, child-life therapists, pharmacists, surgeons, and home IV and hospice nurses. Childhood cancer is treated with a combination of surgery, radiation, chemotherapy, and biologic response modifiers. Children are usually randomized to be treated according to certain protocols, which are the subject of widespread, ongoing, multicenter research studies. Such aggressive therapy usually requires adequate long-term IV access because attempts to administer a vesicant drug by peripheral IV in an agitated child can result in extravasation injury to the child and occupational exposure to a toxic drug for the nurse. Tunneled catheters, implanted ports, and PICCs are common access devices used in pediatric oncology

---

TABLE 21-5
Intravenous Drugs for Pediatric and Neonatal Resuscitation

Drug	Dose
Sodium bicarbonate (8.4%)	1.0–2.0 mEq/kg
	1.0–2.0 mL/kg
Epinephrine (1:10,000)	0.1 mL/kg
	0.01 mg/kg
Atropine (0.4 mg/mL)	0.02 mg/kg
	Min dose = 0.15 mg
	Max dose = 2.0 mg
Naloxone (Narcan) (0.4 mg/mL)	0.1 mg/kg
	Min dose = 0.5 mg
	Max dose = 2.0 mg
Dextrose 10% via peripheral IV	5.0 mL/kg
Dextrose 25% via central IV	2.0 mL/kg

(Adapted from *Emergency pediatric and neonatal resuscitation reference,* courtesy of Robert Brown, RN, MSN, PNP, Nurse Manager, Emergency Department and Transport Team; and nursing staff of Pediatric/Neonatal Transport Team, St. Christopher's Hospital for Children, Philadelphia, 1991.)

TABLE 21-6
Infusions for Pediatric and Neonatal Resuscitation

Medication	Preparation (add amounts calculated to D_5W to = 100 mL)	Dose	Range
Dopamine µg/kg/min		1 mL/h = 1 µg/kg/min	2.0–15.0
Dobutamine µg/kg/min	(6 × kg) mg		2.0–15.0
Epinephrine	(0.6 × kg) mg	1 mL/h = 0.1 µg/kg/min	0.1–1.0 µg/kg/min
Norepinephrine			
Lidocaine	(60 × kg) mg	1 mL/h = 10 µg/kg/min	10.0–50.0 µg/kgmin
	up to 20 kg: (0.6 × kg) mg	1 mL/h = 0.1 µg/kg/min	0.1–1.0 µg/kg/min
Isoproterenol	20–40 kg: (0.3 × kg) mg	1 mL/h = 0.05 µg/kg/min	
	40 kg and up: (0.12 × kg) mg	1 mL/h = 0.02 µg/kg/min	

patients. The function of various antineoplastic agents and administration guidelines are discussed in Chapter 20; dilution guidelines for pediatric chemotherapy are found in Table 21-7.

Parenteral Nutrition Therapy

Parenteral nutrition is discussed in Chapter 16. The major breakthrough in parenteral feedings occurred in the late 1960s when Stanley J. Dudrick and his colleagues at the University of Pennsylvania reported their results with central venous hyperalimentation. The success of Dudrick's early experiments with subclavian catheters led to further success with human infants and adults who could not be fed adequately by the enteral route because of severe gastrointestinal disorders.

Dudrick devised a simple statement of criteria that differentiates patients who potentially can benefit from TPN therapy into categories. These categories include those patients who cannot eat, will not eat, or cannot eat enough.[63] TPN should be used only in patients having inadequate gastrointestinal function, thereby disallowing feeding by the enteral route (especially because TPN costs are high). Partial parenteral nutrition (PPN) can provide a supplemental source of nutrition for short periods of time in children who eat but do not eat adequate amounts for growth. TPN is becoming one of the most important therapeutic parameters in the successful management of certain pediatric diseases. The widespread use of TPN has sustained numerous children while their gastrointestinal tracts develop enough absorptive capacity to tolerate basal caloric requirements.

Pediatric patients receiving PPN and TPN usually fall into two major categories: those with either congenital or acquired anomalies of the gastrointestinal tract or

TABLE 21-7
Chemotherapy Dilution Guidelines for Pediatric Patients

Drug	Strength	Administration
Alkylating agents	3.3 mg/mL (10% ethanol)	IV infusion slowly over 30–60 min, burning of vein if infused too rapidly
BCNU (Carmustine)		
Cyclophosphamide (Cytoxan)	20 mg/mL	IV push or infusion
Dacarbazine (DTIC)	10 mg/mL	IV injection or infusion over 15–30 min
Mechlorethamine (Mustargen, nitrogen mustard)	1 mg/mL	IV push
Triethylene thiophosphoramide (Thiotepa)	15-mg vial (5 mg/0.6 mL)	IV push, intravesical in 30–60 mL of distilled water
Antibiotics	0.5 mg/mL	IV push infusion over 10–15 min
Dactinomycin (actinomycin D, Cosmegen)		
Doxorubicin (Adriamycin)	2 mg/mL	IV push or infusion over 3–15 min
Mithramycin (Mithracin)	0.5 mg/mL	IV push or infusion
Mitomycin (Mutamycin, mitomycin C)	0.5 mg/mL	IV push or infusion
Streptozocin (Zanosar)	100 mg/mL	IV push or infusion
Antimetabolites	20 mg/mL or 50 mg/mL	IV push or infusion, subcutaneous, intrathecal
Cytarabine (Cytosar-U, Ara-C)		
Methotrexate (MTX, Mexate)	Injection prescribed amount 10 mL	IV push, IV infusion
Miscellaneous	1 mg/mL	IV push or infusion
Cisplatin (Platinol)		
Vinca alkaloids	1 mg/mL	IV push, infusion in D_5W or NS
Vinblastine (Velban)		
Vincristine (Oncovin)	1 mg/mL	IV push, infusion rapidly

Sparrow Hospital Division of Nursing Statement of Policy for Pediatric Chemotherapy Dilutions: A. Pediaric IV push chemotherapeutic drugs will be admixed to establish a minimum volume of 3 mL. B. The following guidelines will be used when admixing and administering IV pediatric chemotherapeutic drugs.
(From CRNIs role in pediatric chemotherapy administration. [1986]. *Journal of the National Intravenous Therapy Association, 9,* 467. Used with permission of J. B. Lippincott and Intravenous Nurses Society.)

those with intractable diarrhea syndromes. The gastrointestinal tract anomalies that generally require TPN include intestinal obstruction (obstruction in the intestinal lumen), gastroschisis (a congenital fissure in the wall of the abdomen that remains open), and necrotizing enterocolitis (necrosis of the small or large bowel caused by sepsis or hypoxia). The most dramatic treatment requires major resection of both small and large bowel and TPN may be needed for several weeks, sometimes months.[61] Other pediatric diseases that may require IV nutrition include cystic fibrosis, renal failure, congenital heart disease, cancer, and Crohn's disease. With the addition of TPN into their therapy regime, affected children can be expected to gain weight normally with only parenteral nutrients. In addition, TPN supplies enough calories to maintain the positive nitrogen balance required for normal growth and development. Criteria used to identify children for parenteral nutrition include greater than 5% weight loss, serum albumin level below 3 g/dL, growth ratio below fifth percentile when height and weight are plotted on growth charts, and total lymphocyte count less than 1000/mm³ (excluding granulocytopenic patients).[27]

Solutions are generally made by hospital or home IV agency pharmacy staff, and the admixture of solutions is done under a laminar airflow hood. The general constituents for TPN—amino acids, a dextrose calorie source, electrolytes, minerals, trace elements, and vitamins—provide amounts of nutrients sufficient to promote growth and maintain a positive nitrogen balance. Nitrogen balance is maintained through the amino acids intake; calories are obtained by glucose. IV fat preparations are currently used to supply essential fatty acids. Electrolytes are usually added to the TPN solution in amounts established for IV maintenance requirements. Calcium, magnesium, phosphorus, and other minerals are incompletely absorbed from the gastrointestinal tract. Therefore, the parenteral needs for minerals are significantly lower than oral needs, and the amounts in the TPN solution rarely exceed half the usual oral amounts. Trace elements may be needed and are now included in commercial solutions; vitamins are added according to children's recommended daily allowances. (*Note:* The yellow color of the TPN solution results from the addition of multivitamins. Because multivitamins limit the shelf-life of TPN to 24 hours, home TPN patients are taught to add vitamins and other medication additives such as heparin).

Pediatric requirements for IV nutrition follow general guidelines and are based on protein, calorie, and fluid needs per kilogram of body weight. See Table 21-3 for specific requirements for children of various ages.

Amino acids provide protein for growth. General pediatric recommendations for daily protein intake in the child are listed in Table 21-3. One gram of protein should deliver at least 30 calories.[62] Protein is administered in the strength of 10% amino acid solution in children and 6% amino acid solution in neonates. The less concentrated solution is used in neonates because it more closely approximates amino acid concentration of the healthy breast-fed infant.

Carbohydrate is infused in the form of dextrose, which provides energy for body tissues. If carbohydrate supply is inadequate, the body will break down protein or fat to provide metabolic needs. Dextrose provides the main calorie source; recommended daily amounts are 20 to 30 g/kg in children weighing less than 10 kg and 25 to 30 g/kg in children weighing more than 10 kg.[62] Because the dextrose in TPN is hydrated, it provides not 4, but 3.4 kcal/g. For example, 100 mL D_5W contains 5 g dextrose, or 17 kcal; 100 mL $D_{10}W$ contains 10 g dextrose, or 34 kcal. The strength of dextrose that can be administered peripherally in a child is 10% to 12.5%.[62] Greater concentrations, given through a peripheral IV, can cause sclerosis, phlebitis, and extravasation injury if infiltration occurs. Although concentrated dextrose is needed to provide calories, the volume of fluid needed to dilute very concentrated dextrose is prohibitive to fluid balance in children, especially neonates. Higher concentrations of dextrose (up to 25%) in less volume of fluid may be delivered via central catheter.

The other source of nonprotein calories is lipids, delivered as a fat emulsion. Originally, fat infusion was kept to a minimum, only 2% to 10% of daily calorie intake, because it was thought that higher fat intake resulted in pulmonary changes.

This hyperlipemia is now thought to have been brought on by rapid infusion rate, not amount of intake, so a slower infusion rate over a longer period of time is now the rule, and fat intake now comprises 40% to 60% of total calories required daily.[62]

Fat emulsions come in strengths of of 10%, with 1.1 kcal/mL and 20%, with 2 kcal/mL. Both may be infused peripherally or centrally. Fats are essential for neurologic development in the infant; however, fatty acids may displace bilirubin from albumin, causing a rise in bilirubin level and an increased risk of kernicterus.[29] Accurate bilirubin levels should be drawn 4 hours after the fat emulsion has infused; if lipid infusion is continuous, the blood sample should be centrifuged before bilirubin assay.[29]

The second major area of responsibility for the nurse is in the delivery of TPN by a constant and proper infusion rate. The amount and rate of flow are governed by the optimal sugar utilization as determined by the renal threshold and the patient's specific requirements. If too little fluid is given, the sugar will be well below the threshold and the maximum caloric intake will not be reached. If too much solution is given, the renal threshold is exceeded and a sugar spill will be noted in the urine. The infusion rate should be checked frequently, at least every hour. Urine Tes-Tapes should be done after every void in neonates. A positive 2+ urine × 2 or a 3+ or 4+ urine requires immediate nursing intervention. If this occurs, the physician should be notified; a serum glucose determination may be ordered and the infusion rate may be adjusted or insulin may be added, depending on the patient's needs. Electronic infusion devices are helpful aids in monitoring desired rates, especially in children. For this reason, TPN is always administered to the pediatric patient via an electronic infusion device.

When a child is first started on TPN, the percentage of dextrose infused is gradually increased from 5% to a maximum of 20% to 25% via central line, according to the caloric needs and tolerance of the child. Infusions may run over 24 hours for the very sick hospitalized child or may be gradually cycled down by 4-hour increments daily, maintaining the same volume infusion over less time. Cycling down to about 12 hours daily of TPN infusion allows far more freedom for the child, particularly the child on home TPN, who may infuse at night while asleep, and still follow a fairly normal life-style of school and activities. Portable infusion pumps, widely used in home IV therapy, also allow more freedom, do not require an IV pole, and can be placed in an unobtrusive carrying case. Weaning on and off the TPN solution used to be popular practice, allowing time for the pancreas to adjust to the change in glucose levels; this weaning process is unnecessary, except in special situations.

Depending on caloric expenditure based on stress levels, lipids may be provided prophylactically biweekly or daily to supplement caloric requirements. Administration of piggyback lipids through a nonfiltered system is common in hospital practice today. The lipids must be connected as close to the venous junction as possible.

Electrolytes, vitamins, minerals, and trace elements are provided in accordance with the child's daily requirements. Sample pediatric TPN solution mixtures are provided in Table 21-8.

The third area of nursing responsibility is patient assessment. The nurse monitors the patient's physical status frequently and screens, intervenes, and reports abnormal findings of temperature spikes, inappropriate glucose spills, chills, rashes, irritability, decreased level of consciousness, and so forth. Any observable abnormality is immediately reported to the physician. Serum levels of various chemistry and

TABLE 21-8
Routine TPN Stock Solution*

Solution	Starter Strength (mL)	Full Strength (mL)
Amino acid solution (8.5%)	100	165
D/W 50%	125	220
NaCl (2.5 mEq/mL)	5	5
$MgSO_4$ (4 mEq/mL)	2	2
Ca gluconate (0.45 mEq/mL)	9	13
KPO_4 (4.4 mEq/k/mL) 3 mmol P/mL)	1	1.5
KCl (2 mEq/mL)	3	2
MVI	2	2
H_2O	252	89
Total volume	500	500
kcal/mL	0.49	0.86
Glucose concentration	12.5%	22%
Protein concentration	1.7 g/100	2.8 g/100

*Trace elements added: $ZnSO_4$, $CuSO_4$, $MnSo_4$, $CrCl_2$, and Fe^{3+}. Weekly supplementation (IM injection): vitamin K, folate, and vitamin B_{12}.

(Prepared by and for Children's Medical Center, Dallas, July 1980.)

hematology tests are assessed daily for the first week and then decreased to a weekly schedule for the stable hospitalized or home TPN patient. Figure 21-19 gives a schedule for assessing these parameters.

The fourth major area of nursing intervention in a child receiving TPN is psychological support. Most TPN patients are infants who are acutely ill and deprived of maternal warmth and comfort. Even though a child on central TPN may be NPO, cuddling and holding the child should assist in meeting maternal needs. Also, allowing parents every opportunity to participate in their child's care is extremely important. First, the nurse should assess the family's level of comprehension about TPN and intervene by offering support in their areas of weakness and insecurities to decrease parental anxiety. As soon as the decision is made to place a child on TPN, it is best to use the preoperative teaching methodology of explaining purpose, procedures, and potential complications. Of course, all further questions can be handled on a daily basis. Permitting this open channel of communication not only supplies parents with the knowledge needed to become involved, but assists them in comprehending the purpose of TPN and why adherence to the protocol of TPN therapy is so important.

Disadvantages to TPN stem from potential complications. Every nurse must fully understand the possible complications of TPN therapy, including the symptoms of each specific complication. Complications are subdivided into three categories: catheter insertion, postinsertion, and metabolic.

TPN FLOW SHEET

Day Starting TPN	BASELINE	1	2	3	4	5	6	7	8	9	10	11	12	13	14	15	16	17	18	19	20	21	22	23	24	25	26	27	28
DATE																													
Weight	•	•	•	•	•	•	•	•	•	•	•	•	•	•	•	•	•	•	•	•	•	•	•	•	•	•	•	•	•
* Length/H.C.	•	•																				•							
Protein/kg/24 hr	•	•	•	•	•	•	•	•	•	•	•	•	•	•	•	•	•	•	•	•	•	•	•	•	•	•	•	•	•
mL/kg/24 hr	•	•	•	•	•	•	•	•	•	•	•	•	•	•	•	•	•	•	•	•	•	•	•	•	•	•	•	•	•
Cal. kg/24 hr	•	•	•	•	•	•	•	•	•	•	•	•	•	•	•	•	•	•	•	•	•	•	•	•	•	•	•	•	•
Na/K	•	•	•	•	•	•	•	•			•				•			•			•	•			•				•
Co₂/Cl	•	•	•	•	•			•			•				•			•			•	•			•				•
BUN	•	•	•		•			•							•			•			•	•							•
Creatinine	•				•										•														
Glu	•	•	•	•	•	•	•	•	•		•				•			•			•	•			•				•
Ca/Phos	•							•							•						•								
TP/Alb	•							•							•						•								
Mg/Zn	•														•														
SGOT/SGPT	•							•							•						•								
GGT	•							•							•						•								
Bili T/D	•							•							•						•								
Triglyceride	•							•							•						•								
Cholesterol	•							•							•						•								
HGB/MCV	•							•							•						•								
Retic	•							•														•							
NUTRITIONAL ASSESSMENT	•																												
Absolute Lymphocyte CT	•																												
Transferrin	•																												
Skin Testing	•																												
Skin Folds	•																												
INFECTION																													
Culture sent & results																													
Chest X-ray (Central line only)	•							•							•						•								

* Indicates study should be done
* Length-Weekly if 2 years - HC-Weekly if 1 year

Catheter Insertion Complications

1. Infection
2. Malposition
3. Perforation of structures (ie, artery, vein, lymph nodes, lung)

Postinsertion Complications

1. Infection
2. Thrombosis
3. Superior vena cava syndrome

Metabolic Complications

1. Hyperglycemia
2. Hypoglycemia
3. Electrolyte imbalance
4. Mineral disorder
5. Hyperammonemia
6. Hyperbilirubinemia

Most of these complications can be treated or even prevented. Maintaining high-caliber aseptic techniques when handling the TPN line reduces the potential risk of sepsis. Certain metabolic complications are preventable through close nursing monitoring although some predisposing metabolic abnormalities may require immediate medical intervention. With the incremental advances in technology and the formation of nutrition support teams, even the most prominent complication, sepsis, has decreased to acceptable rates. In the practice of TPN therapy, the catheter sepsis rate in children may rise as high as 10% because of the increased risks and general behaviors of children (eg, teething children have been known to bite the TPN catheter). See Chapter 16 for more information on nutrition support.

Pediatric Transfusion Therapy

Indications and techniques for transfusing blood and blood products to children are similar to those described for adults in Chapter 17. The major differences between adults and children include decrease in blood volume from neonate to adult, maturation of the immune system with regard to blood typing, blood counts through various stages of development, and requirements for transfusion therapy. Table 21-9 lists blood volumes for various ages. A transfusion procedure unique to the neonate is exchange transfusion, as described later in this segment.

The red blood cell of the infant is nucleated at birth and has a reduced half-life (23.3 days) in contrast to that of the adult (26–35 days).[42] Synthesis of fetal hemoglobin (HbF) declines rapidly after birth when adult hemoglobin (HbA) rises concomitantly. The higher affinity for oxygen of HbF facilitates transfer of oxygen from mother to fetus in utero, but persistence of HbF after birth may result in respiratory

◀ **FIGURE 21-19** Total parenteral nutrition flow sheet, St. Christopher's Hospital for Children, Philadelphia, PA. (From Goldberg, M., & Tyrala, E. [1981]. *Parenteral nutrition guide,* [3rd ed.], pp. 42–43. Used with permission of the authors.)

TABLE 21-9
Blood Volumes at Various Ages

Premature infant	105 mL/kg
Term infant	80 mL/kg
3 months to adult	70–75 mL/kg

(From Luban, N., & Keating, L. [Eds.]. [1983]. *Hemotherapy of the infant and premature* [pp. 5–65, 69–80, 95–124]. Arlington, VA: American Association of Blood Banks; Nathan, D., & Oski, F. [Eds.]. [1981]. *Hematology of infancy and childhood* [pp. 1491–1500]. Philadelphia: W. B. Saunders.)

---

distress and tissue hypoxia in the neonate because of the inability of HbF to release oxygen to the tissues.[37] Manipulations of the infant, such as suctioning and IV starts, as well as crying, can increase peripheral leukocyte counts. Neutropenia, not neutrophilia, in the newborn, is a more common indicator of sepsis. Platelet counts do not differ greatly from neonate to adult, but neonates may easily develop thrombocytopenia from extrinsic sources.

The immune system of the neonate matures during infant stages of development. Circulating antibodies are derived from the mother during the last several prenatal weeks; therefore, premature infants have a less efficient humoral immunity. As a baby is exposed to outside antigens, antibody production begins, and for the first several days of life, mother's serum is used for compatibility testing. In infants older than 1 week and those previously transfused, compatibility testing is done on the blood of the baby. Group O red blood cells that are Rh negative or the same Rh as the infant are frequently used. In addition, red blood cells are tested for cytomegalovirus (CMV) and are only given to neonates if CMV negative. The freshest cells possible are used to avoid potassium load in young infants.

Specific indications for transfusion therapy are outlined extensively in Chapter 17. In general, indications for transfusion therapy in children include acute hemorrhage, anemia, abnormal component function or component deficiency, and removal of harmful substances, such as bilirubin, during exchange transfusion.

The most common blood components given to children are packed red blood cells, platelets, and fresh frozen plasma, as well as plasma derivatives given for congenital or acquired lack or dysfunction of that component. These products are administered in milliliters per kilogram; dosages are based on the volume limits of the child and the desired therapeutic outcome.

Reduction in the blood volume of a child by 30% to 40% produces clinical evidence of shock. When 20% of blood volume is lost and may recur, transfusion is also indicated.[54] Central venous pressure is the best indicator for restoration of blood volume to normal; pulse rate is a less reliable guide, and 24 to 36 hours may pass before hemoglobin reflects the true extent of blood loss. Reduced hemoglobin and hematocrit 3 to 6 hours after hemorrhage suggests loss of 20% to 25% of blood volume, whereas normal hemoglobin 6 hours after hemorrhage suggests that substantial blood loss has not occurred.[54] A red blood cell mass deficit occurs with chronic anemia, and transfusion with packed cells is not indicated until hemoglobin level drops below 6 g/dL.[54] Assessment of the patient's cardiopulmonary status and activity level, along with hemoglobin, should be considered before transfusion because an unstressed child can tolerate hemoglobin values of 3 to 6 g/dL without signs of heart failure. Also, because the most common form of anemia seen in children is iron deficiency anemia (which is rarely treated with transfusion), other treatments may be more indicated, including iron therapy, folic acid, or vitamin B_{12}.

Decreased production or altered function of platelets is usually caused by maternally induced disorder (ie, aspirin intake prenatally), congenital disorder, acquired disorder (ie, idiopathic thromocytopenic purpura [ITP]), or chemotherapy-induced thrombocytopenia. Indications for transfusion of platelets, plasma, and plasma components are similar to those in adults, and Table 21-10 lists some parameters for blood component therapy in children.

Infusion of IV gamma globulin or IV IgG warrants specific mention because the use of this plasma derivative in children has grown substantially since the 1980s, when safe, effective IV preparations became licensed in the United States. Before that time, children with humoral immunodeficiencies were treated with intramuscular injections or infusions of plasma. The large volume of intramuscular IgG required adequate muscle mass, it was uncomfortable because injected volume was large, and IgG levels rose slowly and were only maintained for a short time before another injection was needed to help bolster infection-fighting capabilities. Larger doses of IgG can be given via the IV route, thus maintaining adequate serum levels with more convenient administration. Approved indications for IV IgG include deficiencies of the humoral immune system and ITP, and this product is being studied as a means of heightening the immune response in many other adult and pediatric disorders, such as AIDS, neonatal sepsis, and cystic fibrosis.[20]

Treatment of immunodeficiency requires monthly infusions of from 100 to 400 mg/kg for life; acute ITP is treated with 400 mg/kg up to 1 g/kg until platelet rise is noted.[65] In children, a viral infection often precludes onset of ITP, and 80% to 90% of children exhibit spontaneous remission in 6 to 12 months. Platelet count in ITP lowers because antibody-coated platelets are destroyed by splenic phagocytes, and IV

TABLE 21-10
Blood Component Therapy for Pediatric Patients

Blood Product	Indication	Dosage/Rate
Red blood cells (packed)	Treatment of anemia without volume expansion	10 mL/kg, not to exceed 15 mL/kg at 2–5 mL/kg/h
Platelets	To control bleeding associated with deficiency in platelet number or function	1 U (50–70 mL)/7–10 kg body weight Run over 30 min to maximum of 4 h; IV push or drip
Fresh frozen plasma	Occasionally volume expansion in acute blood loss	Acute hemorrhage: 15–30 mL/kg as indicated.
	To increase levels of clotting factors in children with demonstrated deficiency	Clotting deficiency: 10–15 mL/kg at 1–2 mL/min

(Adapted from *Transfusion therapy guidelines for nurses.* [1990]. National Blood Resource Education Program, Public Health Service, National Institutes of Health, U.S. Department of Health and Human Services.)

IgG is prescribed to elevate platelet counts so that potentially fatal episodes of hemorrhage can be avoided. Palliation of other childhood disease entities, such as neonatal sepsis, cystic fibrosis, and bacterial infection in human immunodeficiency-positive children, is the topic of ongoing research, largely because of the ability of gamma globulin to be administered by the IV route in the neonate to the adolescent.

Blood and blood products in children may be administered via a 27-, 26-, or 24-gauge peripheral IV in neonates and via a 24- or 22-gauge IV in older children. An infusion pump, capable of infusing blood, is recommended for transfusion therapy in children; in neonates, blood may be prefiltered by the blood bank and then infused from a syringe on a syringe pump. Pediatricians request blood and blood products in milliliter per kilogram increments, instead of units, because a single unit of packed red blood cells may equal the entire blood volume of several infants. In children, volume and fluid balance considerations negate the simultaneous infusion of saline, particularly in neonates; instead, the peripheral or central IV device must be flushed with 1 to 3 mL saline before and after the transfusion. Rate of blood transfusion may be very slow or even staggered with boluses of dextrose in neonates. Five to 10% of red cell volume should be infused slowly over the first 15 minutes, then the rate increased to an hourly IV rate tolerated by the child.[37]

Specific physical assessment areas indicative of hematologic function in children include color changes in skin, lips, conjunctiva, mucous membranes, and nails, such as blue for cyanosis, pale for anemia, or yellow for jaundice. Look at fingernails and toenails for clubbing, skin for petechiae, and mucous membranes for bleeding. Blood oozing from old venipuncture sites is often a precursor to onset of disseminated intravascular coagulation (DIC). When a tourniquet is placed on an extremity, evidence of petechiae distal to the tourniquet may be indicative of ITP or other platelet disorders.

In addition to physical assessment, history should include previous exposure to toxins (which may be a cause of aplastic anemia) and any previous transfusions, including the reason and patient reaction. Psychological support of the family is indicated, in addition to education about transfusion therapy and alternatives, if available. Agency policy is necessary regarding refusal of transfusion by a parent or guardian, and state laws differ on this topic; in most cases, a waiver must be signed if transfusion is refused.

In an *exchange transfusion*, most or all of the infant's blood is replaced with compatible red blood cells and plasma from one or several donors. In the early 1950s, exchange transfusion was first used for management of HDN; with the introduction of anti-D immune globulin (Rhogam) in the 1960s, the number of infants with this disease greatly declined. Indications for exchange transfusion include HDN, caused by Rh or ABO incompatibility, DIC, sepsis, respiratory distress syndrome, and polycythemia or "thick blood syndrome," where some of the infant's blood is removed and replaced with plasma. The most common indication for exchange is HDN. Two causes of HDN include Rh incompatibility, where the second Rh+ baby of an Rh– mother is affected when anti-D antibodies in the mother, developed in response to the first pregnancy, cross the placenta and destroy the red blood cells of the second baby. At birth, the infant will be anemic and exhibit increased levels of unconjugated (indirect) bilirubin. Deposition of excess bilirubin in the brain can cause kernicterus, a type of encephalopathy. Exchange transfusion is considered when bilirubin levels increase more than 1 mg/dL each hour, or reach 15 to 16 mg/dL in the neonate and 20 mg/dL in the full-term infant.[29] Although hemolytic disease from ABO incompatibility is more common, it is usually mild enough to be treated with phototherapy or a single blood transfusion, until the infant's liver matures enough to clear bilirubin out of the blood. ABO incompatibility occurs most frequently when a type O mother carries an A or B fetus.[54] In ABO incompatibility, the direct Coombs' test may be only weakly positive, whereas with Rh incompatibility, the Coombs' test is strongly positive. In contrast to Rh disease, ABO HDN may occur in the first infant.

Red blood cells alone, or in conjunction with fresh frozen plasma, may be used for exchange transfusion. To treat Rh HDN, type O, Rh blood crossmatched with the mother is used; for ABO HDN, use Rh compatible, type O blood.

A double-volume or two-volume exchange is usually performed where exchange transfusion is equal to twice the patient's blood volume. This replaces about 85% of the newborn's blood and lowers the bilirubin level in blood by about 50%, but does not have any effect on extravascular bilirubin. Albumin may be administered before the exchange to bind bilirubin, allowing a greater amount to be removed during the procedure. Ideally, two vascular access sites are used to allow simultaneous withdrawal and infusion, including sites such as the umbilical vessels and peripheral or central veins. If only one access is available, the push–pull method is used. Calcium and dextrose levels are closely monitored during the exchange because blood preservatives may cause levels to decrease. Complications can include those related to the catheter, discussed earlier in the chapter, as well as those related to transfusion therapy.

ALTERNATIVE SITE PEDIATRIC IV THERAPY

Much of routine IV therapy has moved out of the hospital and into the home or subacute care facility or outpatient infusion center. Although prior segments of this chapter have included information on home IV therapy, to not include a mention of alternate site therapy would be remiss. Disorders treated at home or other location with IV modalities include, but are not limited to, cystic fibrosis; hemophilia; bone, soft tissue, and joint infections; neonatal sepsis; gastrointestinal disorders; immunologic dysfunction; and oncologic disorders and treatment sequellae.[18,60]

Therapies administered IV in the home or alternate site include fluids, antibiotics or antifungals, parenteral nutrition, chemotherapy, analgesics, chelating agents, and blood components.

Pediatric patients will usually receive one or more doses in a controlled environment to verify that there is no adverse reaction. With TPN, the therapy is usually cycled to infuse over several hours before discharge home or transfer to alternative site care. Intermediate- to long-term catheters are often used for IV therapy at home to avoid the trauma and possible omitted therapy for frequent peripheral IV site changes. Aquavene peripheral IVs, midline, PICC, and tunneled or implanted central devices are those of choice for home or alternate site care.

Readiness, willingness, and ability of the patient and family and extensive teaching with demonstrated feedback should be documented before patient discharge and be ongoing during the patient's course of treatment until service is discontinued.

Outcome data on pediatric home care, lacking in published literature, is another opportunity for nursing research. The pediatric home infusion nurse must be an experienced IV practitioner, as might be indicated by the CRNI status, as well as an expert in recognition and treatment of pediatric normal and abnormal states. Pediatric home care is now the fastest growing portion of the home care market.[18,60]

SUMMARY OF PEDIATRIC CARE

As outlined in INS Standards of Practice, an IV nursing team is an integral part of nursing care for the pediatric patient. Because children vary from neonate to adolescent in physiologic as well as developmental level, special consideration and increased time may be necessary to provide efficacious IV therapy. Consultation to staff nurses regarding safe drug administration and transfusion therapy to children is an integral part of the pediatric IV team function. Assisting families with choice of venous access, providing skilled insertion of that device, as well as follow-up care and teaching have become integral roles for IV nurses. Both IV teams and nutrition support teams have demonstrated lower complication rates and increased quality of care.

In conclusion, specific principles in caring for pediatric patients receiving IV therapy have been discussed, as well as the fluid and nutritional requirements and diseases that necessitate pediatric IV therapy. By familiarizing nurses with this current information, it is hoped that their understanding of the complexities involved in caring for a child receiving IV therapy will be deepened.

REFERENCES

1. Arbeiter, H. I., & Greengard, J. (1944). Tibial bone marrow infusions in infancy. *Journal of Pediatrics, 25*, 1.
2. Batton, D. G., Maisels, J., & Applebaum, P. (1982). Use of peripheral intravenous cannulas in premature infants: A controlled study. *Pediatrics, 70*, 488.
3. Berner-Howry, L. B., McGillis-Bindler, R., & Tso, Y. (1981). *Pediatric medications* (pp. 3–28). Philadelphia: J. B. Lippincott.
4. Bossert, E. & Beecroft, P.C. (1994). Peripheral intravenous lock irrigation in children: Current practice. *Pediatric Nursing, 20*, 346–355.
5. Broviac, J. W., Cole, J. J., & Schribner, B. H. (1973). A silicone rubber atrial catheter for prolonged parenteral alimentation. *Surgery, Gynecology and Obstetrics, 136*, 602.
6. Brown, A. S., Hoelzer, D. J., Piercy, S. A. (1979). Skin necrosis from extravasation of intravenous fluids in children. *Plastic and Reconstructive Surgery, 64*, 145–150.
7. Bryant, B. G. (1990). Drug, fluid, and blood products administered through the umbilical artery catheter: Complication experiences from one NICU. *Neonatal Network, 9*, 27–46.
8. Camp-Sorrell, D. (1990). Advanced central venous access, selection, catheters, devices, and nursing management. *Journal of Intravenous Nursing, 13*, 361–370.
9. Chathas, M. K. (1986). Percutaneous central venous catheters in neonates. *Journal of Obstetric, Gynecologic, and Neonatal Nursing, 15*, 324–331.
10. Clarke, T. A., & Reddy, P. G. (1979). Intra-venous infusion technique in the newborn. *Clinical Pediatrics, 18*, 550–554.
11. Corey, B. E. (1989). Major complications of central lines in neonates. *Neonatal Network, 7*, 17–28.
12. Danek, G. D., & Noris, E. M. (1992). Pediatric IV catheters: Efficacy of saline flush. *Pediatric Nursing, 18*, 111–113.
13. Decker, M. D., & Edwards, K. M. (1988). Central venous catheter infections. *Pediatric Clinics of North America, 35*, 579–612.
14. Dolcourt, J. L., & Bose, C. L. (1982). Percutaneous insertion of Silastic central venous catheter in neonates. *Pediatrics, 70*, 484.
15. Drinker, C. K., Drinker, K. R., & Lund, C. C. (1922). The circulation in the mammalian bone marrow. *American Journal of Physiology, 62*, 1–92.
16. Farrington, E. (Section editor). (1990). Pediatric drug information. *Pediatric Nursing, 16*, 310.
17. Fay, M. J. (1983). The special challenges of pediatric IVs. *Dimensions of Critical Care Nursing, 2*, 24.
18. Ferris, E. W. (1990). A neonatal home intravenous therapy program. *Journal of Intravenous Nursing, 13*, 383–387.
19. Flemmer, L., & Chan, J. S. L. (1993). A pediatric protocol for management of extravasation injuries. *Pediatric Nursing, 19*, 355–358.
20. Frey, A. M. (1991). The immune system. Part II. Intravenous administration of immune globulin. *Journal of Intravenous Nursing, 14*, 397–405.
21. Garland, J.S., Dunne, M., Havens, P., Hintermeyer, M., Bozzette, M. A., Wincek, J., Bromberger, T.,

& Seavers, M. (1992). Peripheral intravenous catheter complications in critically ill children; a prospective study. *Pediatrics, 89,* 1145–1150.

22. Geidell-Oellrich, R., Murph, M. R., Goldberg, L. A., & Aggarwal, R. (1991). The percutaneous central venous catheter for small or ill infants. *American Journal of Maternal Child Nursing, 16,* 92–96.

23. Glaesser, P. N., & Losek, J. D. (1986). Emergency intraosseous infusions in children. *American Journal of Emergency Medicine, 4,* 35.

24. Graef, J., & Cone, T. (1977). *Manual of pediatric therapeutics.* Boston: Little, Brown.

25. Guhlow, L. J., & Kolb, J. (1979). Pediatric IVs: Special measures you must take. *RN, 42,* 40–52.

26. Guyon, G. (1989). Pharmacokinetic considerations in neonatal drug therapy. *Neonatal Network, 7,* 9–12.

27. Haas-Beckert, B. (1987). Removing the mysteries of parenteral nutrition. *Pediatric Nursing, 13,* 37–41.

28. Hadaway, L. (1990). A midline alternative to central and peripheral venous access. *Caring, 9,* 45–50.

29. Hahler-D'Angelo, J., & Welsh, N. P. (Eds.). (1988). Pediatric drug and IV therapy. In *Medication administration and IV therapy handbook* (pp. 305–307). Springhouse, PA: Springhouse.

30. Hanrahan, K. S., Kleiber, C., & Fagan, C. L. (1994). Evaluation of saline for IV locks in children. *Pediatric Nursing, 20,* 549–552.

31. Harris, L. C., Rushton, C. H., & Hale, S. J. (1987). Implantable infusion devices in the pediatric patient: A viable alternative. *Journal of Pediatric Nursing, 2,* 174–183.

32. Heiney, S. P. (1991). Helping children through painful procedures. *American Journal of Nursing, 91,* 24.

33. Holcombe, B., Forloines-Lynn, S., & Garmhausen, L. W. (1992). Restoring patency of long-term central venous access devices. *Journal of Intravenous Nursing, 15,* 36–41.

34. Ingram, J., Weitzman, S., Greenberg, M. L., Partin, P., & Filler, R. (1991). Complications of indwelling venous access lines in the pediatric hematology patient: A prospective comparison of external venous catheters and subcutaneous ports. *American Journal of Pediatric Hematology/Oncology, 13,* 130–136.

35. Revised intravenous nursing standards of practice. (1990). *Journal of Intravenous Nursing* (Suppl.), S46, 47, 67.

36. Kanter, R. K., Zimmerman, J. J., Straus, R. H., & Stoeckel, K. (1986). Pediatric emergency intravenous access: Evaluation of a protocol. *American Journal of Diseases of Children, 140,* 133.

37. Kasprisin, C. A. (1985). Transfusion therapy for the pediatric patient. In R. Rutman & W. Miller (Eds.), *Transfusion therapy* (pp. 179–185). Rockville, MD: Aspen.

38. Kitterman, J., Phibbs, R., & Tooley, W. (1970). Catheterization of umbilical vessels in newborn infants. *Pediatric Clinics of North America, 17,* 895–896.

39. Klaus, M. H., & Fanaroff, A. (1979). *Care of the high risk neonate* (2nd ed.). London: W. B. Saunders.

40. Korth-Bradley, J. M. (1991). A pharmacokinetic primer for intravenous nurses. *Journal of Intravenous Nursing, 14,* 124.

41. Levitt, E. (1980). Neonatal IV therapy. *Journal of the National Intravenous Therapy Association, 3,* 169.

42. Luban, N., & Keating, L. (Eds.). (1983). *Hemotherapy of the infant and premature* (pp. 5–65, 69–80, 95–124). Arlington, VA: American Association of Blood Banks.

43. Manley, L., Haley, K., & Dick, M. (1988). Intraosseous infusion: Rapid vascular access for critically ill or injured infants and children. *Journal of Emergency Nursing, 14,* 63.

44. Marcoux, C., Fisher, S., & Wong, D. (1990). Central venous access devices in children. *Pediatric Nursing, 16,* 123–133.

45. Markels, S. (1990). Impact on patient care: 2652 PIC catheter days in the alternative setting. *Journal of Intravenous Nursing, 13,* 347.

46. Mattson, D., & O'Connor, M. (1986). Transilluminator assistance in neonatal venipuncture. *Neonatal Network, 4,* 43.

47. Matyskiela-Frey, A. M. (1985). Pediatric dosage calculations. *Journal of the National Intravenous Therapy Association, 8,* 373–379.

48. McMullen, A., Fioravanti, I. D., Pollack, V., Rideout, K., & Sciera, M. (1993). Heparinized saline or normal saline as a flush solution in intermittent intravenous lines in infants and children. *Maternal/Child Nursing, 18,* 78–85.

49. Meyenfeldt, M., Stapert, J., DeJong, P., Soeters, P. B., Wesdorp, R. I., & Greep, J. M. (1980). TPN catheter sepsis: Lack of effect of subcutaneous tunneling of PVC catheters on sepsis rate. *Journal of Parenteral and Enteral Nutrition, 4,* 514–517.

50. Meyer, H. M. (1982, May 28). *Letter to Hospital Pharmacists.* Rockville, MD: U.S. Department of Health and Human Services, Federal Drug Administration.

51. Miccolo, M. A. (1990). Intraosseous infusion. *Critical Care Nurse, 10,* 35–47.

52. Milliam, D. (1995). The use of anesthesia in IV therapy. *Journal of Vascular Access Devices, 1,* 22–29.

53. Mofenseon, H. C. (1988). Guidelines for in-

traosseous infusions [Letter to the editor]. *Journal of Emergency Medicine, 6,* 145–146.

54. Nathan, D., & Oski, F. (Eds.). (1981). *Hematology of infancy and childhood* (pp. 1491–1500). Philadelphia: W. B. Saunders.

55. Piercy, S. (1981). Children on long term IV therapy. *Nursing 81, 11,* 66–69.

56. Plesko, L. (1989). Streamlined catheterization. *Neonatal Intensive Care, 2,* 36, 38.

57. Poole, M. A., Ross, M. N., Haase, G. M., & Odom, L. F. (1991). Right atrial catheters in pediatric oncology: A patient/parent questionnaire study. *American Journal of Pediatric Hematology/Oncology, 13,* 152–155.

58. Rosetti, V., Thompson, B., Miller, J., Mateer, J. R., & Aprahamian, C. (1985). Intraosseous infusion: An alternative route of pediatric intravenous access. *Annals of Emergency Medicine, 14,* 885–888.

59. Shulman, R. J., Pokorny, W. J., Martin, C. G., Pettit, R., Baldaia, L., & Roney, D. (1986). Comparison of percutaneous and surgical placement of central venous catheters in neonates. *Journal of Pediatric Surgery, 21,* 348–350.

60. Schuman, A. J., (1990). Homeward bound: The explosion of pediatric home care. *Contemporary Pediatrics, 7,* 26–29, 32–47, 50–54.

61. Teitell, B. C. (1978). *The role of the pediatric TPN nurse with pediatric oncology patients.* Paper presented at ASPENS Third Clinical Congress.

62. Testerman, J. E. (1989). Current trends in pediatric total parenteral nutrition. *Journal of Intravenous Nursing, 12,* 152–162.

63. Third National Cancer Survey. Nutritional Cancer Institute. (1977). *CA: A Cancer Journal for Clinicians,* 27. American Cancer Society.

64. Thompson, V. (1994). An IV therapy teaching tool for children. *Pediatric Nursing, 20,* 351–355.

65. *Transfusion therapy guidelines for nurses.* (1990). National Blood Resource Education Program, Public Health Service, National Institutes of Health, U.S. Department of Health and Human Services.

66. Turkel, H. (1983). Intraosseous infusions [Letter to the editor]. *American Journal of Diseases of Children, 137,* 706.

67. Viall, C. D. (1990). Your complete guide to central venous catheters, *Nursing 90, 20,* 34.

68. Watson, E. H., & Lowery, G. H. (1958). *Growth and development of children.* Chicago: Year Book Medical Publishers.

69. Weeks-Lozano, H. (1991). Clinical evaluation of Per-Q-Cath for both pediatric and adult home infusion therapy. *Journal of Intravenous Nursing, 14,* 249–256.

70. Weibley, T. T., & Fraze, D. E. (1985). Intravenous Teflon catheter cannulation in the premature infant. *Neonatal Network, 3,* 29–33.

71. Wickham, R. S. (1990). Advances in venous access devices and nursing management strategies. *Nursing Clinics of North America, 25,* 345–364.

72. Zenk, K. E. (1986) Administering IV antibiotics to children. *Nursing 86, 16,* 50–52.

REVIEW QUESTIONS _____

1. When starting an IV in a toddler, the best approach would be:
   a. "Let's go and start your IV now."
   b. "You were bad, so we're going to give you a needle."
   c. "Where do you want your IV?"
   d. "Can we start your IV now?"

2. The scalp would be an ideal site for IV access in which of the following children?
   a. neonate with sepsis
   b. 2-month-old with hydrocephalus
   c. 20-month-old with leukemia
   d. 16-month-old in respiratory arrest

3. The IV catheter gauge ideal for most pediatric patients is which of the following?
   a. 16
   b. 18
   c. 20
   d. 24

4. The ideal place to start an IV in a child is:
   a. at the bedside
   b. in the treatment room
   c. in the mother's lap
   d. in the home of the patient

5. After two attempts at IV access during resuscitative efforts, the following site should be used:
   a. intraosseous
   b. intrathecal
   c. intra-arterial
   d. intracardiac

6. An IV site unique to the neonatal population is the:
   a. scalp
   b. foot
   c. abdomen
   d. umbilicus

7. For long-term intermittent access in an adolescent, the central access device of choice would be the:
   a. Broviac catheter
   b. Hickman catheter
   c. subclavian catheter
   d. implanted port

8. The best method for calculating fluid therapy for a child is:
   a. caloric method
   b. weight method
   c. age method
   d. meter squared method

9. Criteria for infusion of TPN include:
   a. low serum albumin
   b. high lymphocyte count
   c. growth ratio below 50th percentile
   d. low protein/fat ratio

10. The purpose of neonatal exchange transfusion is to:
    a. elevate neutrophil count
    b. prevent congestive heart failure
    c. lower bilirubin level
    d. change blood type

CHAPTER 22

Intravenous Therapy in an Older Adult Patient

Key Terms

Aging process	Patient education	Site monitoring
Blood vessels	Physiologic	Skin
Fluid balance	changes	Venipuncture
Immune system	Senses	

AN AGING POPULATION

Advances in medical science and technology have caused resultant changes in life span; sources estimate that by the year 2000, older patients will represent 13% of the population and over two-thirds of the of the American population will be age 65 or older.

The "frail" old will constitute 12% of the elderly and health care professionals will require an increased awareness of the changes associated with the aging process and the special needs of this patient population.[1,2,6]

Aging occurs on the cellular, organic, and systemic levels. Major system changes affecting infusion therapy practice and delivery of care to this patient include those related to homeostasis, cardiovascular systems, and skin and connective tissue. Normal aging changes affecting fluid balance and related nursing implications are featured in Table 22-1.

TABLE 22-1
Normal Aging Changes Affecting Fluid Balance: Related Nursing Implications

Physiological Component	Normal Aging Changes	Nursing Implications
Total body water	Approximately 6% reduction in total body water	Increased risk for fluid volume deficit
	Decrease in ratio of intracellular to extracellular fluid	
Renal function	Reduction in weight by 50 g between ages 40 and 80	Greater difficulty in eliminating heavy solute loads (drugs, glucose, protein, electrolytes)
	Loss of 30% to 50% of glomeruli by age 70	
	Thickening of glomerular and tubular basement membranes	Slower conservation of fluids in response to fluid restriction
	46% decrease in glomerular filtration rate from age 20 to 90 (maximum serum creatinine increase is to 1.9 mg/100 mL)	
	Decrease in ability to concentrate urine (maximum ability to concentrate urine is 1.022–1.026)	
Regulatory functions	Decrease in secretion of aldosterone from adrenal cortex	Diminished ability to conserve sodium and excrete potassium
	Decreased response of zona glomerulosa	
	Decreased response of distal tubule to vasopressin	Reduced ability to correct an acid-base imbalance
	Decreased ability to form and excrete ammonia	Increased risk for hyperglycemia and osmotic diuresis
	Decreased glucose tolerance	Decreased ability to recognize a fluid deficit
	Decreased sensation of thirst	
Skin changes	Decreased skin elasticity	Skin turgor is poor indicator of state of hydration
	Atrophy of sweat glands	Skin is less effective in cooling body temperature
	Diminished capillary bed	
Cardiovascular function	Decreased baroreceptor sensitivity	Diminished ability to manage hypotension associated with shock
	Decreased cardiac output (1% per year from age 20–80)	
	Decreased stroke volume (0.7% per year from age 20–80)	Increased frequency of peripheral edema
	Decrease in renal plasma flow from 600 mL/min in 2nd decade to 300 mL/min by 8th decade	Increased risk for orthostatic hypotension, dizziness, falls
	Decreased elasticity of arteries	
	Increased vascular rigidity causing increased peripheral resistance	
Respiratory function	Decreased compliance of chest wall	Increased difficulty in regulation of pH if experiencing major illness, surgery, burns, or trauma
	Decreased elasticity of lung tissue	
	Decreased number of alveoli	
	Decreased strength of expiratory muscles	
	Decreased normal partial pressure of oxygen	
Gastrointestinal function	Decreased volume of saliva	Mouth may be dryer
	Decreased volume of gastric juice	Increased risk for hypoatremia and hypokalemia during vomiting and gastric suction
	Decreased calcium absorption	

With permission from Metheny, N. M. [1996]. Fluid and Electrolyte Balance [3rd ed., p. 352]. Philadelphia: J. B. Lippincott-Raven.

PATIENT ASSESSMENT

The usual assessment measures used in determining fluid balance often require adjustment when providing care to the older adult. For example, testing skin turgor on the forearm is no longer a valid measure because skin loses elasticity with age. Skin turgor is best assessed in the older patient by tenting the tissue on the forehead or over the sternum because alterations in skin elasticity are less marked in those sites.[4]

Total body water is reduced by 6%, creating a potential for development of fluid volume deficit. Gastrointestinal changes such as decreased volume of saliva, gastric juice, and calcium absorption cause the mouth to be drier and increase potential for sodium and potassium deficit during episodes of vomiting and gastric suction.

Cardiovascular changes are also profound, contributing to a slower response to the stress of blood loss, fluid depletion, shock, and acid–base imbalances. Changes in renal and cardiac status create a patient potentially at great risk for development of infusion-related complications.

Senses

Changes in sensation affect the patient's response to treatment; changes in vision, hearing, and tactile sensation may alter communication. After the age of 50, subtle changes in the hearing process result in difficulty in differentiating sounds. For example, the older patient often cannot hear someone speaking within otherwise normal range because of the outside influence of loud music or traffic sounds.[5,7] Assistive devices, such as hearing aids, eyeglasses, and visual aids may be needed to teach an older patient the skills associated with infusion therapy. Because of decreased tactile sensation, infiltration might go unnoticed, contributing to the potential for developing tissue necrosis, infection, or compartment syndrome.[4]

The Immune System

In aging, the normal immune system becomes hyporesponsive to foreign antigens and hyperresponsive to self.[7] This may contribute to decreased resistance to infection, increased autoimmunity, and development of other immune disorders.

Skin Changes

The skin, the body's first defense against disease, changes in texture, depth, and integrity. After age 60, epidermal cell replacement decreases, resulting in a marked thinning of the epidermis and an increase in fragility of the skin's surface. The result is dry, transparent, paper-thin tissue that tears easily and heals slowly. Changes in the dermis create a loose, wrinkling effect. The skin becomes pale, and nerve endings are less sensitive. The patient is at risk for thermal injuries. Subcutaneous fat cells decrease, resulting in changes to the superficial fascia, including decreased production of sebum and sweat.[4]

Vascular System

The blood vessels in the older patient are affected by chronic disease and the changes associated with atherosclerosis and arteriosclerosis. Vessels are fragile with small, thin-walled surface capillaries easily observed across the extremities and chest of the older patient.

Psychological Changes

A confused patient, or one suffering ill effects of senile dementia, will respond differently to treatment. Teaching may become complicated because the patient has difficulty in differentiating recent and remote memory. You may find that the patient forgets what was taught the previous day, but remembers all of the details of early childhood.

CONSIDERATIONS IN PROVIDING INTRAVENOUS THERAPY

Access and Equipment

Careful consideration should be given to the type of treatment ordered, the duration of therapy, and availability of IV access. A biocompatible catheter material is preferred, including such products manufactured from silicone, elastomeric hydrogels, and others (see Chapters 10 and 11). The smallest gauge possible for the therapy being delivered should be used and consideration should be given to the type of catheter–tubing connection used; some products are more irritating to frail skin and must frequently be padded to avoid injury to the skin surface and underlying tissue.

When a central venous access device is needed for long-term therapy, the type of device should be carefully determined. Consideration should be given to the patient's living circumstances, availability of a family or other support system, the ability to manipulate the equipment involved, and to maintain a secure, intact dressing.[5]

Flow Control

Flow control devices should be used liberally in the older adult to avoid the potential danger of overhydration and resultant fluid imbalances. Pump infusion pressures should be carefully monitored, and as with all patients, the device used should be biomedically safe and meet and exceed standards developed by ECRI, formerly the Emergency Care Research Institute, and internal safety committees (see Chapter 10).

An electronic flow control device should be an accessory to quality patient care and not a substitute for ongoing monitoring. Refer to technical information provided by the manufacturer of equipment and institutional guidelines for use. The alarm on a pump with a fixed pressure of 4 lb psi will activate when the peripheral venous pressure reaches 200 mm Hg (1 psi = 50 mm Hg). This setting can result in serious harm to the patient when infiltration occurs; the alarm will sound only after the damage has been noted. An infiltrated site exerts a mean pressure gradient at 100 mm Hg or 2 psi. Pumps that continue to infuse or that do not have a free-flow alarm system harbor potential danger to the older patient.[5]

Site Selection

Principles of site selection applied to the younger patient (see Chapter 21) may also be used to determine appropriate venous access in the older patient. Assessment of available peripheral venous access is necessary. Avoiding bruised, fragile veins and conserving veins for future use are major considerations. Secure adequate lighting and ensure patient comfort.

Although a tourniquet may be used, it also may not be necessary. Excessive distention of the veins may contribute to bloodback damage and subsequent tearing of the venous wall and hematoma. Palpate the veins carefully to determine state of health and condition. Corded veins may be indicative of thickening, occluded vein walls and valve blockage. Threading a catheter into such vessels may be difficult; venous stasis and dependent edema may result. Principles of site selection also apply to the older patient.[5]

Technique

Skin tension is determined by assessing the direction or axis of the vessel. Ensure traction by placing the thumb directly along the vein axis 2 to 3 inches below the intended venipuncture site. The palm and fingers of the traction hand hold and stabilize the patient's extremity. The index finger of the traction hand can then be used to further stretch the skin above the intended venipuncture site. Traction should be maintained throughout the procedure.[3]

Determine the directional line of the vessel. If the vein is very small, venous distention may be inadequate and imagery techniques may be used.

A small-gauge IV catheter should be selected and should be positioned bevel up. The catheter should be aligned parallel to the vein track, brought close to the skin directly above the insertion site. A lower angle will decrease vein trauma on insertion.[2-5]

The direct or indirect technique may be applied (see Chapter 7); however, for patients with small, fragile veins, the clinician may find the two-step technique more beneficial. If the veins are extremely fragile, and if a tourniquet has been used, it may be helpful to release the tourniquet as soon as blood return is evident to avoid dam-

---

TABLE 22-2
Special Techniques in the Older Adult Patient

---

1. Avoid the use of a tourniquet in those with fragile veins or those taking anticoagulant drugs or steroids.

2. When a tourniquet has been used, release it quickly to decrease backflow of blood.

3. Multiple tourniquets may be used.

   a. Apply the first on the mid-upper arm; stroke the arm downward toward the hand. After 1–2 min, a second tourniquet is placed just below the antecubital fossa. Continue to stroke the lower forearm.

   b. Small veins will begin to be visible due to forced blood distention. A third tourniquet may be applied after 1–2 min at a point just above the wrist. Release the first tourniquet at the mid-upper arm and evaluate the inner wrist, thumb, knuckles, and finger for venous distention.

4. In the edematous patient, use antomic landmarks to determine appropriate venipuncture sites. Displace subcutaneous edema to either side; a flattened area will permit easier vein visualization. A tourniquet may not be needed.

5. Gently tap the vein to distend; do not slap.

6. Consider use of transillumination to visualize veins.

7. Insert the catheter with a steady, firm motion.

8. Consider preflushing the catheter in patients with spidery, capillary-like veins.

9. A one-handed technique will enable the nurse to maintain proper skin tension.

age from high-pressure backflow of blood from the catheter insertion point. The "hooded" technique may also help to reduce vein damage. In this approach, the catheter is advanced forward over the bevel tip into the vein. This action retracts the stylet tip inside the catheter. Then, the catheter is threaded into the vein by grasping the hub of the catheter and advancing the catheter and stylet as a unit up the vein. This procedure minimizes the possibility of perforating the vein during threading. Maintain stabilization and skin tension throughout the process. Table 22-2 list the special techniques required in an older adult.

Maintenance and Monitoring

Securing, dressing, and stabilizing the IV catheter are unique challenges when providing infusion care to the elderly patient. Although the catheter should be secure, use of excessive tape is discouraged because of the fragile condition of the patient's skin. Adaptations to taping technique should be used as needed. The use of additional protection such as a skin polymer solution should be considered. The polymer solution is best applied in a concentric circle from the center to the periphery and allowed to air dry before applying the dressing.[5]

The elderly patient may be unaware of the surroundings, and the nurse should make every effort to ensure safety with the infusion device. Care should be taken when armboards or restraints are used. The IV tubing should be long enough to provide adequate range of motion, but not so long as to dangle on the floor or get caught on the bedside or IV pole. A luer locking device provides added protection. Surgical stretch mesh gauze may also be used to cover the IV site, providing stability and protecting the catheter from snagging bed garments. Roll-type gauze should be avoided, consistent with institutional guidelines and established practice standards.[5]

The IV site should be evaluated at regularly established intervals and as needed to ensure patency. Site rotation is recommended every 48 hours; however, deviations from the standard may be acceptable if they are documented. If a routine site change is not performed due to limited access or the patient's clinical condition, a full description of the site, dressing change, and reasons for not completing the site rotation should be documented in the clinical record.

REFERENCES

1. American Association of Retired Persons. (1985). *A profile of older Americans*. Washington, DC: U.S. Department of Health and Human Services.
2. Matteson, R. N. (1991). *Gerontological nursing concepts and practice* (pp. 2–29). Philadelphia: W. B. Saunders.
3. Mellema, S. J., & Poniatowski, B. C. (1989). Geriatric IV therapy. *Journal of Intravenous Nursing, 11*(1), 56–62.
4. Metheny, N. M. (1996). *Fluid and electrolytes* (3rd ed., 352–357). Philadelphia: Lippincott-Raven.
5. Intravenous Nurses Society. (1990). *Revised standards of practice*. Philadelphia: J. B. Lippincott.
6. Taylor, S. (1992). Lost in the system. *Journal of Intravenous Nursing, 15*, 52–56.
7. University of North Texas, Center for Study in Aging. (1992). Lecture Materials.

REVIEW QUESTIONS

1. Which of the following techniques ensures venous distention in the older adult patient?
   a. Eliminate use of a tourniquet.
   b. Multiple tourniquets may be used.
   c. Gently tap the vein.
   d. Always use a tourniquet in the patient receiving steroids.

2. Normal changes occurring in aging affect which of the following:
   a. skin
   b. senses
   c. immune system
   d. vascular system

3. Dry, transparent surfaces are associated with which of the layers of the skin?
   a. dermis
   b. epidermis
   c. superficial fascia
   d. deep fascia

4. The alarm on a pump with a fixed pressure of 4 lb psi will sound when the peripheral venous pressure reaches how many mm Hg?
   a. 100
   b. 150
   c. 200
   d. 250

5. Excessive distention of the veins may contribute to which of the following:
   a. difficult palpation
   b. corded veins
   c. bloodback damage
   d. hematoma formation

CHAPTER 23

Alternate Site Therapy

Key Terms

Accreditation	Competition	Medicaid
Alternate site	First dosing	Medicare
Candidates	ICD-9 codes	Payer source
Certification for	Infusion center	Plan of care
home care	Managed care	Reimbursement

GROWTH OF HOME CARE

The growth of home infusion therapy and alternative site treatment has opened countless opportunities for IV nurses nationwide. This growth is the product of social, economic, and political forces that have shaped our overall system for delivering health care, including the inception of diagnosis-related groups and the Tax Equity and Fiscal Responsibility Act of 1982 (TEFRA). Factors contributing to the growth of home care are found in Table 23-1.

HOME INFUSION PROGRAMS

Home infusion programs may function under the auspices of any number of parent organizations. State and county health departments are the most commonly used example of governmental agencies providing home health care services. Visiting nurse associations have always been providers of extensive Medicare services to clients in need. Proprietary agencies provide services on a fee-for-service basis or managed care contract to private individuals. Until 1981, such companies were precluded from participation in the Medicare program. Agencies under the controlling authority of local

> ──────────────────────────
> **TABLE 23-1**
> **Factors Contributing to the Growth of Home Care**
> ──────────────────────────
> 1. Aging population
> 2. Increased technology
> 3. Changes in payer sources
> 4. Growth of managed care
> ──────────────────────────

hospitals or conducted as joint ventures are generally hospital-based programs. Proprietary agencies have followed the pattern of many health care organizations nationwide, creating megacompany, full-service, national providers of patient care, pharmaceutical, and medical supply goods and services.

NURSING SUPPORT

Nursing support begins at the time of hospitalization with the key words "discharge planning." Never before has this been truer, as patients move from the security of the inpatient environment to assume responsibility for self-care in the comfort of residences. The IV nurse's role includes initial patient assessment, review of body systems, development of nursing diagnosis, review of current and past medical history, psychosocial assessment, evaluation of available support systems, assessment of functional limitations, environment, and cognitive and technical skills.

Continuing activities include assessment of a patient's compliance with the therapeutic regimen, patient training, monitoring and evaluation, psychosocial support, and 24-hour home emergency access. Care provided by a credentialed professional is preferred by some organizations.

The *home care coordinator* is involved in identification of appropriate candidates for home infusion therapies. The inpatient teaching program is consistent with the type of therapy ordered and includes line management, dressing changes, flushing, hookup and disconnect, handling of equipment, aseptic technique, emergency interventions, recognition of signs and symptoms of possible complications, handling of inventory, and pump management. Specific teaching packets should be provided. Patients are not medical professionals; a teaching plan specific to the patient's individualized needs is essential. Language barriers often inhibit otherwise successful teaching programs. Every effort should be made to address the patient in language he or she best understands. Figures 23-1 and 23-2 provide examples of IV teaching in various languages. Final coordination with the supplier is made before discharge to ensure safe, timely arrival of pump, solutions, and related equipment.

THE PHARMACIST

In some parts of the country, the pharmacist participates in home visits; the role and responsibility of this level of professional varies. In general, the pharmacist is responsible for reviewing medical records for current and past medical, nutritional, and

| ¿Cómo está? Soy la enfermera encargada de administrarle el suero intravenoso. |
| ▲ HELLO, I AM YOUR I.V. NURSE. (FEMALE) |

| Como esta? Soy el enfermero encargado de administrarle el suero intravenoso. |
| ▲ HELLO, I AM YOUR I.V. NURSE. (MALE) |

| Vengo a revisarle la aguja del suero intravenoso. |
| ▲ I AM HERE TO CHECK YOUR I.V. |

| Voy a aplicarle el suero intravenoso. |
| ▲ I AM HERE TO START YOUR I.V. |

| Le cambiaremos la aguja intravenoso de lugar cada (2) - (3) dias. |
| ▲ WE CHANGE THE I.V. SITE EVERY (2) - (3) DAYS. |

| Le duele en donde tiene inyectada la aguja intravenosa?   Si   No |
| ▲ DO YOU HAVE PAIN AT YOUR I.V. SITE?   YES   NO |

| Tengo que cambiarle el lugar de la aguja intravenosa debido a que: |
| ▲ I NEED TO   CHANGE YOUR I.V. TODAY BECAUSE OF: |

| (a) le duele, | (b) tiene inflamacion, | (c) tiene la piel roja, | (d) es un procedimiento de rutina. |
| ▲ (A) PAIN | (B) SWELLING | (C) REDNESS | (D) ROUTINE |

| Si le duele o si se le inflama el lugar donde tiene la aguja del suero intravenoso, hagaselo saber a la enfermera. |
| ▲ IF PAIN OR SWELLING BEGINS, TELL YOUR NURSE. |

SPANISH

FIGURE 23-1   Language for IV patient teaching: Spanish. (Courtesy: Jaclyn Tropp, CRNI)

medication history; reviewing laboratory data; obtaining and correlating physician orders; and preparing, dispensing, and delivery medications, solutions, supplies, and equipment to the patient's place of residence.

POLICIES AND PROCEDURES

Impact of Accreditation

Policies and procedures for the provision of home infusion services must be consistent with published practice standards. Guidelines are provided by two accrediting bodies: the Joint Commission on Accreditation of Healthcare Organizations (JCAHO) and the Community Health Accreditation Program (CHAP) of the National League for Nursing (NLN). Table 23-2 compares JCAHO and CHAP.

Procedures must be comprehensive and address all infusion therapies provided as well as the governing body and management of the organization. Reviewers from both the accrediting bodies and the Medicare program (if a Medicare-certified agency) may inspect agency documents without prior notification. The home infusion therapy program must be consistent with the organization's philosophy and pur-

Guten Tag/ Abend, ich bin die Krankenschwester zuständig für die Infusion.
▲ HELLO, I AM YOUR I.V. NURSE. (FEMALE)

Guten Tag/ Abend, ich bin der Krankenpfleger zuständig für die Infusion.
▲ HELLO, I AM YOUR I.V. NURSE. (MALE)

Ich muss Ihre Infusion kontrollieren.
▲ I AM HERE TO CHECK YOUR I.V.

Ich muss Ihnen eine Infusion geben.
▲ I AM HERE TO START YOUR I.V.

Wir wechseln die Infusionsstelle alle (2) - (3) Tage.
▲ WE CHANGE THE I.V. SITE EVERY (2) - (3) DAYS.

Haben Sie Schmerzen an der Infusionsstelle?	Ja	Nein
▲ DO YOU HAVE PAIN AT YOUR I.V. SITE?	YES	NO

Ich muss heute Ihre Infusionsstelle wechseln, wegen:
▲ I NEED TO CHANGE YOUR I.V. TODAY BECAUSE OF:

(a) Schmerzen	(b) Schwellung	(c) Rötung	(d) Routinemässig
▲ (A) PAIN	(B) SWELLING	(C) REDNESS	(D) ROUTINE

Wenn Schmerzen auftreten oder Rotung beginnt, teilen Sie das bitte der Krankenschwester mit.
▲ IF PAIN OR SWELLING BEGINS, TELL YOUR NURSE.

GERMAN

FIGURE 23-2 Language for IV patient teaching: German. (Courtesy: Jaclyn Tropp, CRNI)

pose. A qualified professional must be responsible for the direction, coordination, and general supervision of all professional services. Infusion nursing care must be provided by a registered professional nurse; must be in accordance with the client's plan of treatment; and must include comprehensive health and psychosocial evaluation, monitoring of the client's condition, teaching and training activities in the self-administration of medications given IV, subcutaneously, or intraspinally, and provide for the overall well-being of the client. Necessary drugs, biologics, equipment, and supplies may be provided directly by the organization or by arrangement. Services must be coordinated with a designated case manager for each client who is responsible for ensuring those services described in Table 23-3.

STAFF DEVELOPMENT

Infusion therapy case managers are selected for their expertise and experience. The ability to provide intensive care services to patients in their places of residence is essential. The job description and evaluation process for this nursing professional must

TABLE 23-2
Comparing CHAP and JCAHO

	CHAP	JCAHO
Number of accredited providers		
Home care organizations	100	3500
Infusion providers	0	1500
Cost of accreditation	$1300–24,000	$3000–10,000
Accredits networks	No*	Yes
Accredits ambulatory centers	Yes	Yes
Year accrediting for home care facilities began	1965	1988

*Effective mid 1995.

Adapted with permission from Epstein, D. (1995). Struggling for Recognition. *Infusion* 1(7)36–37.

encompass the need for further development and education to remain abreast of the latest technologies, equipment, and infusion therapy procedures. Nurses providing home infusion therapy should work with mentors who can enable them to grow personally and professionally within their chosen fields.

The resources of professional societies and the role that such organizations play in staff development cannot be overlooked. These societies provide the collegiality and professional camaraderie that enable nurses to grow in this rapidly changing field. IV nursing professionals should be encouraged to participate in such organizations on national and local levels. They should be encouraged to publish case studies about their success stories in home infusion care and to share their knowledge and expertise with others. Table 23-4 lists available resources.

TABLE 23-3
Responsibility of the Case Manager

1. Initial assessment of the individual, family, and home environment
2. Development of a plan of care
3. Appropriate referral and follow-up
4. Coordination of services
5. Implementation of the plan of care
6. Ongoing evaluation
7. Plan for termination of care

TABLE 23-4
Available Resources

American Association of Blood Banks (AABB)
American Hospital Association (AHA)
American Society of Health-System Pharmacists™ (ASHP)
American Society for Parenteral and Enteral Nutrition (ASPEN)
Association for Practitioners in Infection Control (APIC)
Case Management Society of America (CMSA)
Centers for Disease Control and Prevention (CDC)
Community Health Accreditation Program (CHAP)
Intravenous Nurses Society (INS)
Joint Commission on Accreditation of Healthcare Organizations (JCAHO)
National Association of Vascular Access Networks (NAVAN)
National Association for Home Care (NAHC)
National Home Infusion Association (NHIA)
Oncology Nursing Society (ONS)

HOME INFUSION THERAPIES

The majority of IV procedures provided in the hospital can likewise be provided in the home. Home infusion therapies are diverse and encompass many modalities for patient care, including antibiotics and anti-infectives, nutritional support, hydration, pain management, antiemetics, antineoplastics, blood and component therapy, venous sampling, IV drugs such as cardiovascular agents, growth hormones, colony-stimulating factors, and tocolytics.

Antibiotics and Anti-infectives

Antibiotic and anti-infective therapies are an established procedure in the confines of one's home. Newer technology and the development of more potent ß-lactam antibiotics have facilitated the growth of this treatment modality. To qualify for service, the patient should be medically stable, the infection should be one that can be treated on an outpatient basis, the patient should be compliant, and reliable venous access should be available. As with any drug, the first dose should be administered in a monitored clinical setting.

First Dosing

This is a controversial subject and a controlled setting remains the location of choice for first-dose administration. Today, however, this practice has changed considerably, and first doses of medication are more frequently administered in the patient's residence. This change may be attributed to changes in technology and pharmaceuticals as well as the increased availability of credentialed professional caregivers.

The patient who is scheduled to receive a first dose in the home should have a thorough allergy profile and history and the risks should be weighed. An appropriate order for emergency anaphylaxis should be provided and the medication should be immediately available.

Allergic reactions may occur with subsequent doses of medication as well. The home IV nursing clinician must be able to identify and differentiate allergic responses from anaphylactic reactions. The ability to differentiate such responses is an important component of the patient teaching plan. Components of an anaphylactic kit include epinephrine, diphenhydramine, hydrocortisone, acetaminophen, sodium chloride solution, IV administration set, needles, and syringes.

Nutritional Support

The advent of home parenteral nutrition (HPN) in the 1960s enabled physicians to support intestinally handicapped patients for indefinite time periods. Technical barriers to HPN have diminished over time. Advanced products, catheters, and technologies have enabled us to provide advanced nutritional support to patients with appropriate diagnoses. If the patient is receiving care under the Medicare program, the test of permanence must be met, and the patient must be in need of HPN for 90 days or more.

Usually administered as a cyclic infusion in the home setting, the patient receives a full day's requirement of fluid, glucose, lipid, and other nutrients over a shorter 10- to 12-hour period. (See Chapter 16 and Box 23-1. The use of intradialytic parenteral nutrition (during hemodialysis) has been limited due to reimbursement concerns. This type of treatment is usually given over a 3- to 4-hour period, three to four times weekly at the time of dialysis.

Hydration

The ability to maintain fluid balance in the patient in the place of residence is the goal of home hydration therapy. Hydration may also be given to augment the HPN program by providing supplemental potassium or insulin, or be implemented to prehy-

---

Box 23-1
Applicable Diagnoses for Home Total Parenteral Nutrition

Kwashiorkor

Nutritional marasmus

Other severe protein–calorie malnutrition

Malnutrition

Unspecified vitamin deficiency or other nutritional deficiency

Disorders for amino acid transport and metabolism

Intestinal disaccharidase deficiencies malabsorption

Disorders of lipid metabolism

Disorders of fluid, electrolyte, and acid–base balance

Cystic fibrosis

Disorders involving the immune mechanism

Anorexia nervosa

Nutritional and metabolic cardiomyopathy

Obstruction of duodenum

Regional enteritis

Idiopathic proctocolitis

Chronic liver disease and cirrhosis

Postsurgical nonabsorption

Cancer cachexia

drate the patient in need of a cardiac fluid challenge or antineoplastic agent. Long-term administration of multiple electrolyte solutions is also possible.

Pain Management

Continuous or intermittent self-administration of IV analgesics in the home allows those in need to remain with their families with a degree of comfort not previously available. Manufacturers have kept pace with demands for more sophisticated equipment to ensure safe administration of these drugs in an unmonitored environment. Pain medications may be administered by a patient-controlled analgesia or portable pump, through IV, intrathecal, epidural, subcutaneous, or other routes of administration (see Chapter 19). The most frequently encountered medications are morphine sulfate, meperidine, and hydromorphone.

A common concern among patients and families is one of addiction. Patients and caregivers should be assured that addiction is a minimal concern and that bolus dosing should be administered as needed.

Antiemetics

Antiemetic protocols aimed at intermittent infusion have facilitated the care of the patient in need of antineoplastic therapies and ensured patient comfort to a new level of care. A diversity of protocols provide antiemetic infusions as a single-agent treatment or combined with HPN therapies.

Antineoplastics

Chemotherapeutic agents are administered to patients in their homes by various IV systems. Nonvesicant chemotherapeutic agents are often given through peripheral cannulas, either short- or intermediate-term products. Vesicant and nonvesicant agents are being administered by centrally placed catheters, implanted catheters, and implanted pumps. Complex antineoplastic regimens are now administered more frequently in the home environment (see Chapter 20).

Blood and Component Therapy

Transfusions of blood and blood components are now performed on home patients. Compatible blood is taken to the home and transfused under the direction of a professional nurse. Policies and procedures for this type of service entail development of methods of securing the component, billing for service, remaining with the patient for the duration of the transfusion, emergency measures, transport of the blood/blood product, and follow-up. As with all therapies, the same level of care provided to patients in the inpatient setting is provided to patients in their residences (see Chapter 17).

Tocolytic Therapies

Recent studies using continuous subcutaneous infusion of terbutaline have proved it to be safe and cost effective in the treatment of premature labor. Home therapy is administered via a portable infusion pump, programmed to administer a continuous basal rate (0.05 mg/h), scheduled bolus doses (0.25 mg) four to six times daily for peak periods of contractions, and unscheduled bolus doses (0.25 mg) should the patient experience two contractions in 10 minutes or four contractions in 60 minutes. The subcutaneous site is rotated every 72 to 96 hours. Terbutaline therapy is usually discontinued at 37 weeks' gestation.

Venous Sampling

Venous sampling for all types of laboratory testing is available in home infusion programs. Peak and trough levels, chemistry panels for the HPN patient, white blood cell counts for the oncology patient, and other tests may be performed. Venous samples may be drawn through peripheral venipuncture, existing line, or central line sampling. As with all home procedures, care must be taken to ensure the safe handling and disposal of medical waste.

Drug Administration

Intravenous drug administration is a rapidly growing area of home infusion therapy. IV drugs administered in the home care setting include cardiovascular drugs, antihypertensive agents, heparin, interferon, colony-stimulating factors, chelation therapy (deferoxamine), growth hormone, gamma globulin, and others. Again, first dosing should occur in a clinically monitored environment. Emergency drugs should be readily available, and protocols for their use should be established in written policies and procedures.

CANDIDATES FOR HOME INFUSION

The criteria used for patient selection play a key role in the success or failure of a home infusion therapy program (Table 23-5).

Once the referral to home care has been made, a referral checklist should be developed (Figure 23-3). Then, an initial patient assessment should be performed, followed by clarification of orders, development of the patient's plan of care, interdisciplinary communications, and orientation of the patient to the service being provided.

Diagnosis

The home infusion therapy ordered must be consistent with the patient's diagnosis and ability to be treated in an alternative care setting. Common diagnoses for antibiotic therapy include osteomyelitis, otitis media, sinusitis, cryptococcal meningitis, pneumonia, subacute bacterial endocarditis, primary bacteremia, cellulitis, urinary tract infection, pyelonephritis, septic arthritis, histoplasmosis, peritonitis, toxic shock syndrome, Lyme disease, rickettsial infection, acquired immunodeficiency syndrome-related opportunistic infections, and others.

All types of cancer patients are appropriate candidates for home infusion of antineoplastic agents, especially combination protocols. Many third-party payers restrict reimbursement for antineoplastic agents to the alternative care setting and have set limits on inpatient treatments. Even if treatment is initiated on an inpatient basis, the protocol that was started or the investigational treatment may be continued in the home care setting. Related infusion therapies for the oncology patient might include nutritional support, IV pain management, antiemetics, leucovorin rescue regimens, and intraperitoneal protocols. Table 23-6 lists potential home infusion diagnoses and suggested therapies.

TABLE 23-5
Criteria for Patient Selection

1. Appropriate diagnosis
2. Medical stability
3. Venous access
4. Evaluation of drug therapy
5. Laboratory profile
6. Presence of a support system
7. Technical criteria, including desire and willingness to receive therapy at home, educability, manual dexterity, appropriate home environment (telephone, electricity, hot and cold water, refrigeration, and a clean work area for medication preparation)
8. Financial resources

Medical Stability

Medical stability is essential if patients are to perform all required procedures themselves. If a patient is not medically stable but has medical approval for home care, a family member may assume full responsibility for performing all techniques. A backup person may be needed, depending on the individual home situation. Policies and procedures outlining medical stability must be developed and approved by the home care provider's medical board. Such a policy might indicate that the patient must be afebrile for the 24-hour period before discharge, or if febrile, the patient must be on antibiotics that have been started as an inpatient. The patient should have a comprehensive assessment before leaving the hospital.

Vascular Access

Vascular access appropriate to the planned course of treatment is essential if the home infusion program is to be a success. Home nutritional support is best given through an acceptable central venous access route. When IV nurses are involved in product selection, the patient's clinical needs will be met. Use of a dual-lumen port or tunneled line is helpful and should be encouraged. Measures must be in place to deal with the potential for cannula occlusion, and appropriate drugs such as urokinase should be readily available. Teaching protocols for line management will vary with the type of access involved. Teaching plans must be patient specific and address all areas of maintenance and self-care.

Drug Therapy

Often the type of drug therapy ordered will determine the appropriateness of a candidate for the home infusion program. Most drugs given in the inpatient setting are also acceptable in a home infusion program. Dobutamine, for example, requires frequent electrocardiographic monitoring; this may easily be accomplished in a full-service home care program.

Text continues on page 599

Home Infusion Referral Checklist

Home Care Provider:

[   ] ————————————————

[   ] ————————————————

		DATE/INITIAL
INFORMATION TO:		
A.	DISCHARGE PLANNER INFORMED	————
B.	IV TEAM INFORMED	————
C.	HOME AGENCY INFORMED:	————

Name of agency ————————————————

Address ————————————————

Phone # ———————————— FAX # ————————

Local contact ————————————————

D.   LOCAL PHYSICIAN IDENTIFIED (if applicable)   ————

Name ————————————————

Address ————————————————

Phone # ———————————— FAX # ————————

TYPE OF REFERRAL:

A.   Parenteral nutrition   ————

B.   Enteral nutrition   ————

C.   IV antibiotics   ————

D.   Pain management   ————

E.   Nupogen   ————

F.   Chemotherapy   ————

G.   Catheter care   ————

H.   Other ————————————————   ————

TEACHING COMPLETED:

A.   HOME INFUSION ————————————————   ————

B.   SUBCLAVIAN/CATHETER CARE   ————

[   ] Port   Type ————————————

[   ] Hickman/Groshong   [   ] Subclavian   [   ] Other ————————

Lumens ————————

SUPPLIES NEEDED FROM HOSPITAL UPON DISCHARGE:

————————————————————————

————————————————————————

————————————————————————

————————————————————————

DELIVERY DATE ————————————   START OF INFUSION ————————

DATE OF REFERRAL FROM PHYSICIAN ————————   DATE OF DISCHARGE ————————

SIGNATURE/INITIAL ——————————— ————   TITLE ————————————

————————————— ————   ————————————

————————————— ————   ————————————

FIGURE 23-3   Home infusion referral checklist.

TABLE 23-6
Potential Home Infusion Diagnoses and Suggested Therapies

Diagnosis/ICD9 Description Code	ICD9 Code	Suggested Therapy	Diagnosis/ICD9 Description Code	ICD9 Code	Suggested Therapy
Abscess, general	682.9	Antibiotic	Diabetes	250.0	Antibiotic
Abscess, brain	324.0	Antibiotic	Diabetes with gangrene	250.7	Antibiotic
Abscess, pelvic	614.4	Antibiotic	Diabetic ulcer	250.8	Antibiotic
Achalasia, digestive organs congenital	751.8	TPN	Diarrhea, chronic	558.9	TEN/TPN
Achalasia, esophagus	530.0	TPN	Diarrhea, infectious	009.2	TEN/TPN
Acquired immune deficiency syndrome	279.3/D43	Anti-infective/TPN	Disease, pelvic inflammatory chronic	614.4	Antibiotic
Actinomycosis	039.9	Anti-infective	Embolism, pulmonary	415.1	Antithrombolytic
Adhesions, intestinal with obstruction	560.81	TPN	Encephalitis, viral	049.9	Anti-infective
Amyotonia	728.2	Antibiotic/TPN	Encephalitis, viral, arthropod borne	064.0	Anti-infective
Anemia	285.9	Blood	Endocarditis, infectious	421.0	Antibiotic
Aphagia	783.0	TEN	Enteritis, viral	008.6	Anti-infective
Arthritis, bacterial	040.89	Antibiotic	Enteritis, bacterial	008.5	Antibiotic
Arthritis, infective	711.9	Antibiotic	Fibrosis, cystic	277.0	Antibiotic/TEN/TPN
Asthma	493.9	Aminophylline	Fistula, abdomen	569.8	TEN/TPN
Atresia, alimentary organ or tract	751.8	TPN	Fracture, open	829.1	Antibiotic
Bacteremia	790.7	Antibiotic	Fungal disease	117.9	Anti-infective
Bacteremia caused by organism	038.8	Antibiotic	Gangrene	785.4	Antibiotic
Blastomycosis	116.0	Anti-infective	Gonococcal joint infection	098.5	Antibiotic
Blood transfusion	V58.2	Blood	Gonococcal pelvis infection chronic	098.39	Antibiotic
Bronchiectasis	494.0	Antibiotic	Hemophilia	286.0	Blood products
Bronchitis	491.0	Antibiotic	Herpes simplex, complicated	054.8	Anti-infective
Cachexia caused by cancer	199.1	TEN/TPN	Histoplasmosis	115.9	Anti-infective
Cachexia caused by malnutrition	261.0	TEN/TPN	Hodgkin's disease	201.9	Chemotherapy
Candidiasis	112.9	Anti-infective	Human immunodeficiency virus	044.9	Anti-infective/TEN/TPN
Carcinoma	194.3	Chemotherapy	Hyperalimentation	783.6	TPN
Celiac disease	579.0	TEN/TPN	Hyperemesis gravidarum	643.0	TPN/Hydration
Cellulitis	682.9	Antibiotic	Hypogammaglobulinemia	279.0	Gamma globulin
Chemotherapy	V58.1	Chemotherapy	Ileus	560.1	TPN
Coccidioidomycosis	114.9	Anti-infective	Infarct, bowel	557.0	TPN
Colitis	558.9	TEN/TPN	Infection	136.9	Antibiotic
Colitis, ulcerative	556.0	TEN/TPN	Infection, atypical mycobacteria	031.9	Antibiotic
Congestive heart failure	428.9	Dobutamine	Infection, bacterial	041.9	Antibiotic
Cooley's disease	282.4	Deferoxamine mesylate	Infection, brain	323.9	Antibiotic
Crohn's disease	555.9	TEN/TPN	Infection, cytomegalovirus	771.1	Anti-infective
Crush injury with infection	929.9	Antibiotic	Infection, skin	686.9	Antibiotic
Cryptococcoses	117.5	Antibiotic	Ischemic, bowel	557.1	TPN
Cytomegalovirus	363.2	Antibiotic	Ixodiasis	134.8	Antibiotic
Deficiency, α_1-antitrypsin	277.6	Prolastin	Kaposi's sarcoma	173.9	Chemotherapy
Deficiency, antihemophilic factor	286.0	Blood product	Labor, premature	644.2	Tocolytics
Deficiency, growth hormone	253.3	Growth hormone	Leukemia	208.9	Chemotherapy
Deficiency, immunoglobulin	279.0	Gamma globulin	Leukemia, acute myelogenous	205.9	Chemotherapy
Decubitus ulcer	707.0	Antibiotic	Lymph node removal	088.8	Chemotherapy
Degenerative heart disease	429.1	Dobutamine	Lymphoma	202.8	Chemotherapy
Dehydration	276.5	Hydration	Malabsorption	579.9	TEN/TPN

(continued)

TABLE 23-6 *(Continued)*

Diagnosis/ICD9 Description Code	ICD9 Code	Suggested Therapy	Diagnosis/ICD9 Description Code	ICD9 Code	Suggested Therapy
Malnutrition	263.9	TEN/TPN	Obstruction, intestine	560.9	TPN
Melanoma	172.9	Chemotherapy	Osteomyelitis	730.2	Antibiotic
Meningitis	322.9	Antibiotic	Otitis, external malignant	380.14	Antibiotic
Metaplasia, agnogenic myeloid	289.8	Antibiotic/TEN	Pain, bone	733.9	Pain
Mycobacterium avium-intracellulare	031.0	Antibiotic	Parkinson's disease	332.0	TEN/TPN
Mycosis	117.9	Anti-infective	Pneumonia	486.0	Antibiotic
Myeloma	203.0	Chemotherapy	Pneumonia, Pneumocystis carinii	136.3	Anti-infective
Myocarditis	429.0	Antibiotic	Prematurity	765.1	PEN
Neoplasm	199.1	Chemotherapy	Prostatitis	601.9	Antibiotic
Neoplasm, alimentary tract	159.9/197.8	Chemotherapy	Pseudomonas	250.8/682.6	Antibiotic
Neoplasm, bone	170.9/198.5	Chemotherapy	Pseudo-obstruction, intestinal	564.8	TPN
Neoplasm, breast	174.9/198.81	Chemotherapy	Pulmonary disease, chronic obstructive	416.9	α_1-Proteinase inhibitor
Neoplasm, digestive organs	159.9/197.8	Chemotherapy	Purpura, idiopathic thrombocytopenic	287.3	Biologics
Neoplasm, esophagus	150.9/197.8	Chemotherapy	Pyelonephritis	590.8	Antibiotic
Neoplasm, intestine	159.0/197.8	Chemotherapy	Septicemia	038.9	Antibiotic
Neoplasm, large intestine	153.9/197.5	Chemotherapy	Short-bowel syndrome	579.2	TPN
Neoplasm, larynx	161.9	Chemotherapy	Sinusitis, chronic	473.9	Antibiotic
Neoplasm, lung	162.9/197.0	Chemotherapy	Stomatitis	528.0	PEN
Neoplasm, metastatic	275.4	Chemotherapy	Thalassemia	282.4	Deferoxamine mesylate
Neoplasm, neck	195.0/198.89	Chemotherapy	Thrombophlebitis	451.9	Anticoagulants
Neoplasm, prostate	185.0	Chemotherapy	Wound, complicated	879.8	Antibiotic

CD = International Classification of Diseases; PEN = partial enteral nutrition; TEN = total enteral nutrition; TPN = total parenteral nutrition.
(Courtesy: Terry, J., ed. (1995). *INS Intravenous Therapy: Clinical principles and practice.* Philadelphia: W.B. Saunders.)

Laboratory Profile

Procedures must be in place for routine laboratory work-ups and transmission of reports of such studies to the ordering physician. Changes in laboratory values, including panic values, should be reported immediately and adjustments made in the treatment plan consistent with the patient's clinical condition. Laboratory testing for the HPN patient might include twice-weekly chemistry profiles, transferrin levels, and application of an anergy panel (Multitest) 2 days before resuming antineoplastic therapy. The patient receiving antibiotic or antifungal agents might require routine peak and trough levels, blood cultures, and white blood cell counts.

Support System

The patient's life-style is an important consideration. If removed from a controlled hospital environment, will the patient be responsible for avoiding potentially dangerous situations? Does the patient live alone or with a family member who can provide the emotional support needed for a successful course of treatment? The home setting should be evaluated for safety, availability of clean and dry storage for supplies or refrigeration for drugs and supplies, and sufficient space to permit privacy while performing procedures. Safe ambulation, adequacy of outlets, convertors, and battery power for ambulatory drug delivery systems are all important factors to be considered. Emotional stability and individual level of motivation with a desire to be involved in self-care are essential to the success of treatment.

Educability

Principles of adult learning must be considered when assessing appropriateness for home infusion therapy. The patient should be capable of learning and performing all procedures. Ideally, with the educational process initiated at the time of admission and early identification of potential home infusion candidates, the teaching process will be enhanced and learning levels will be high. Illiteracy may be overcome by audio or audiovisual training programs.

Visual Acuity

Visual acuity is required for maintaining sterility and avoiding potential touch contamination of supplies. Magnifying or reading glasses may be required.

Manual Dexterity

Manual dexterity is needed to manipulate supplies and equipment used in the infusion without touch contamination. Manipulation of supplies, Luer connections, junction securement devices, needleless connectors, and Huber needles may present a problem to the patient with arthritis or another degenerative disorder.

Financial Resources

Before acceptance, a patient's insurance benefits are assessed for home care coverage. Although many patients have outstanding health care benefits for inpatient care, the benefits for home infusion therapy may be limited or nonexistent. Reimbursement for home care services is covered in depth at the close of this chapter.

PLAN OF TREATMENT

The physician, as gatekeeper, writes the plan of treatment for the patient in need of home infusion therapy. The individualized plan, in addition to routine infusion orders, should also define functional limitations, goals of treatment, and duration of treatment; for some modalities, a letter of medical necessity is required.

SELECTING A HOME INFUSION PROVIDER

Discharge planners, home care coordinators, and social workers are involved in the process of selecting a home infusion provider. If the hospital offers its own service or a preferred provider arrangement exists, this process is facilitated. Otherwise, the selection may be an ordeal unless specific criteria have been developed and parameters are followed.

The home infusion provider should be involved in the training process; continuity of care from hospital to home is enhanced when the relationships are developed early and when the patient and family members have a high degree of confidence in the professional responsible for training and support services. The inpatient training program should be started as early as possible. Training should be individualized and consistent with the patient's needs and the type of therapy or modalities ordered. Training includes line management, dressing changes, infusion techniques, flushing, handling of equipment, sterility, recognition of signs and symptoms of possible complications, handling of inventory, and pump management. Teaching packets and visual aids should be provided whenever possible. A teaching plan for the patient should be developed, reviewed, and signed and a copy should become a part of the patient's clinical record. A second copy should accompany the patient to the place of residence. Teaching level and return demonstrations should be validated (Figure 23-4).

If hospitalized, the patient should safely demonstrate the ability to perform all required procedures to comply with the regimen. If therapy is initiated in the home, adequate time must be taken to ensure patient compliance with the therapeutic regimen. The patient must have the necessary knowledge for the prevention, recognition, and appropriate action required for any potential complication. The home infusion provider should review the patient's Bill of Rights, Responsibilities for Participation in the Home Infusion Program, and the Assignment of Benefits documents. Final coordination is made before discharge. The nurse should visit the patient on the day of discharge. Supplies should be checked, inventoried, and stored in an appropriate designated area. Support should be provided to the patient and family during initial procedures and throughout the duration of treatment. The documentation process should be reviewed with the patient and procedures established for daily monitoring and ongoing support. A monthly report and report of case conferences should be sent to the physician; the hospital may also request copies of these forms. Open lines of communication will enable the infusion provider to meet the patient's current and ongoing needs for care and will ensure a high degree of confidence on the part of the referral source.

Service

The home care program chosen must be a full-service program, one that is able to meet the patient's total needs for nursing, supplies, delivery, inventory, and storage. Such needs should be considered expectations and should be consistent with the highest standards of accrediting organizations. The service must be available on a 24-hour basis, with response time limited to 30 minutes or less.

EQUIPMENT NEEDS

Equipment needs in the home infusion program will vary with the type of therapy ordered and the need for electronic infusion instrumentation. When a single modality, such as antibiotic therapy, has been ordered, the supply needs are simple. More complex regimens, such as HPN, require additional supplies and equipment. Various electronic instruments are available for infusion purposes in the alternative care setting. Backup support should be available on a 24-hour basis in the event of pump or product failure. *Text continues on page 605*

New England Critical Care

PATIENT TEACHING CHECKLIST/ CERTIFICATION OF INSTRUCTION

PATIENT NAME: _____

CAREGIVER: _____

TYPE OF THERAPY: _____

DATE: _____

CONTENT (Check all that apply) (Fill in blanks as indicated)	THEORY/SKILL REVIEWED (INITIAL/DATE)	RETURN DEMONSTRATION COMPLETED (INITIAL/DATE)	SUMMARY/COMMENTS RE: PATIENT/CAREGIVER'S SUCCESS WITH TEACHING
1. Reason for Therapy_____			
2. **Drug/Solution**_____			
☐ Dose _____			
☐ Schedule _____			
☐ Label Accuracy _____			
☐ Storage _____			
☐ Container Integrity _____			
☐ Side Effects _____			
3. Aseptic Technique _____			
☐ Handwashing _____			
☐ Prepping Caps/Connections _____			
☐ Tubing/Cap/Needle Changes _____			
4. Access Device Maintenance _____			
Type/Name: _____			
☐ Device/Site Inspection _____			
☐ Site Care/Dsg. Changes _____			
☐ Catheter Clamping _____			
☐ Maintaining Patency _____			
☐ Saline Flushing _____			
☐ Heparin Locking _____			
☐ Fdg. Tube Declogging _____			
☐ Self Insertion of Device _____			
5. Drug Preparation _____			
☐ Premixed Containers _____			
☐ Compounding ☐ Recipe _____			
☐ 3:1 Lipid Transfer _____			
6. Method of Administration _____			
☐ Gravity _____			
☐ **Pump (Name):** _____			
☐ Continuous ☐ Intermittent _____			
☐ Cycle/Taper: _____			
7. Administration Technique _____			
☐ Pump Rate/Calibration _____			
☐ Priming Tubing ☐ Filter _____			
☐ Filling Syringe _____			
☐ Loading Pump _____			
☐ Access Device Hookup/Disconnect _____			
☐ Head Elevation _____			
8. Potential Complications _____			
☐ Pump Alarms/Troubleshooting _____			
☐ Phlebitis/Infiltration _____			
☐ Clotting/Dislodgement _____			
☐ Infection ☐ Air Embolus _____			
☐ Breakage/Cracking _____			
☐ Electrolyte Imbalance _____			
☐ Fluid Balance _____			
☐ Glucose Intolerance _____			
☐ Aspiration _____			
☐ N/V/D/Cramping _____			
☐ Other: _____			

FIGURE 23-4 Patient teaching checklist. (Reprinted with permission from Oncology Nursing Press. Coker, M., & Lampert, A. [1990]. *Oncology Nursing Forum, 17*[6], 923–925.)

CONTENT (Check all that apply) (Fill in blanks as indicated)	THEORY/SKILL REVIEWED (INITIAL/DATE)	RETURN DEMONSTRATION COMPLETED (INITIAL/DATE)	SUMMARY/COMMENTS RE: PATIENT/CAREGIVER'S SUCCESS WITH TEACHING
9. Self Monitoring: _____			
☐ Weight ☐ Temperature _____			
☐ I & O ☐ Urine S & A _____			
☐ Fingersticks _____			
☐ Other: _____			
10. Supply Handling/Disposal _____			
☐ Disposal of Sharps _____			
☐ Disposal of Supplies _____			
☐ Cleaning Pump _____			
☐ Changing Batteries _____			
☐ Blood/Fluid Precautions _____			
☐ Chemo/Spill Precautions _____			
11. ☐ Electrical Safety _____			
12. Contact Information Given to Patient Re: _____			
☐ Inventory Checks _____			
☐ Deliveries _____			
☐ Nursing _____			
☐ Reimbursement _____			
☐ Service Complaints _____			
13. Written instructions/phone numbers given to patient ☐ Yes ☐ No			
If No/Why: _____			

NURSE'S INITIAL	SIGNATURE	NURSE'S INITIAL	SIGNATURE

CERTIFICATION OF INSTRUCTION

I agree that I have been instructed as described above and understand that the above functions will be performed in the home, outside a hospital or medically supervised environment.

_____   _____
PATIENT/LEGAL GUARDIAN SIGNATURE   DATE

_____   _____
CAREGIVER'S SIGNATURE (IF NOT PATIENT)   DATE

_____ RN _____   _____
WITNESS (NECC NURSE)   DATE

COMPLIANCE

Positive outcomes should be the treatment goal—restoring the patient to a functional capacity and enabling the patient and family to return to a functional level consistent with the stage of disease and its process are essential. Outcome measurements, based on those developed by JCAHO and CHAP, enhance the level of care provided and ensure excellence. Ongoing monitoring of the patient's status is needed; compliance with the protocol is evaluated and documented. The compliant patient administers the drugs and treatments as ordered; follows aseptic practice; reports signs and symptoms of complications; monitors and records weights, temperature, urine glucose determinations, and other parameters; and delights in the ability to provide self-care.

PATIENT'S ROLE IN HOME CARE

The patient is responsible for specific aspects of this care, including compliance, monitoring, line management, operation of electronic infusion equipment, and other duties.

The patient should be made aware of the relationship with the home infusion provider, the right to consent for service, release of medical information, and financial responsibility for the services provided.

INFECTIOUS WASTE MANAGEMENT

Within the home care program, provisions must be made for handling infectious patient waste. The Environmental Protection Agency (EPA), a federal regulatory board, has developed many advisories regarding infectious waste. With passage of the Medical Waste Tracking Act of 1988, Congress mandated to the EPA the investigation and development, if needed, of guidelines for handling home-generated medical waste. The home care provider should establish policies and procedures for handling such waste, particularly when patients reside in more remote, less accessible areas of the country. Prepackaged kits are available from a number of manufacturers and include sharps disposal systems as well as the more sophisticated ChemoBLOC Spill Kit (Figure 23-5).

REIMBURSEMENT

Reimbursement for home infusion therapies is somewhat complex and depends on the nature of the business itself. For example, a Medicare-certified home health agency may bill for supplies associated with a Medicare Part A visit; the same agency may not bill under Part A for HPN. When a managed care company is involved, services are provided on a per diem basis.

Third-Party Payers

Third-party payers for home infusion therapies include Medicare, Medicaid, commercial insurance, health maintenance organizations (HMOs), preferred provider organizations (PPOs), and managed care companies. The HMOs, PPOs, and managed care payers make determinations on a case-by-case basis and generally do not go "out of contract." An overview of various payment plans for therapies may be found in Table 23-7.

FIGURE 23-5 Home health care kit for final disposal of ChemoBLOC container. (Courtesy of U.S. Clinical Products, Dallas, TX)

INFUSION THERAPY CENTERS

Growth

Although home care has had a tremendous impact on a reduction in length of hospital stay, the ambulatory infusion center has also provided an alternative setting for treatment.

Management

The infusion center may be affiliated with a physician's individual or group practice, be a part of a hospital-based program, or be a free-standing private center. Regardless of the management of the organization, it is imperative that a continuum of care be maintained to ensure positive IV patient outcomes.

TABLE 23-7
Home Intravenous Infusion Coverage

Payer	Antibiotic	Chemo	Hydration	Pain	HPN
Medicare A	—	Yes	—	No	—
Medicare B	No	Yes	No	Yes	No
Medicaid	—	Yes	—	Yes	Yes
PEN	No	No	No	No	Yes
HMO/PPO	Yes	Yes	Yes	Yes	Yes
Commercial	Yes	Yes	Yes	Yes	Yes
CHAMPUS	Yes	Yes	Yes	Yes	Yes

CHAMPUS, Civilian Health and Medical Programs for Uniformed Services; HPN, home parenteral nutrition; HMO, health maintenance organization; PPO, preferred provider organization; PEN, parenteral/enteral nutrition program.

Candidates for Infusion Center Treatment

Candidates for this treatment setting are the same as those who are candidates for home infusion care. Additionally, because the center has the inhouse support of a full-time pharmacist, and usually immediate access to a licensed physician, the patient with a potential for development of untoward responses is safely treated.

Physical Layout

The physical layout is ideally in a medical office building, either adjacent to or near an inpatient hospital. A small laboratory, IV admixture room, education and training area, medical records station, nourishment area, and individualized patient rooms are the standard. The patient is seated in a recliner-type chair, with access to IV teaching videotapes or other movies during the treatment. Laboratory parameters are reviewed, along with physician's orders. If needed, additional laboratory studies are obtained and processed. The patient is offered juices and appropriate snacks during the visit to the center. A nurse manager, assigned to and familiar with the patient, assesses vital signs, performs a complete assessment, and initiates treatment, which may take from 30 minutes to 4 hours or more.

Reimbursement

Reimbursement for outpatient infusion procedures is provided by Medicare, Medicaid, and other third-party payers, including managed care programs.

BIBLIOGRAPHY _____

Baldwin, D. (1992). Management of IV hazardous materials and hazardous wastes in the work environment. *Journal of Intravenous Nursing, 15*(2), 50.

Beason, R., Bourguignon, J., Fowler, D., & Gardner, C. (1992). Evaluation of a needle-free intravenous access system. *Journal of Intravenous Nursing, 15*(1), 11–13.

Cherney, A. (1995). Ambulatory infusion centers: Should you or shouldn't you? *Infusion 1*(7), 17–19.

Epstein, D. (1995) Struggling for recognition: Meet CHAP—the "other" accrediting body. *Infusion 1*(7), 36–37.

Grace, L. A., & Tomaselli, B. J., (1995). Intravenous therapy in the home. In J. Terry (Ed), *Intravenous therapy clinical principles and practice* (pp. 510–514). Philadelphia: W. B. Saunders.

HME group wants industry-specific accreditation program. (1995). *Home Health Line, 20*(44), 4.

Malloy, J. A. (1990). Home care accreditation through Joint Commission on Accreditation of Healthcare Organizations. *Journal of Intravenous Nursing, 13*(3), 185–187.

Moeser, L. C. (1991). Anaphylaxis: A preventable complication of home infusion therapy. *Journal of Intravenous Nursing, 14*(2), 114.

Weinstein, S. (1987). Regulatory concerns: Home care. *Journal of the National Intravenous Therapy Association, 10*(3), 175–184.

Weinstein, S. (1984). Intravenous therapy within the scope of home health services. *Journal of the National Intravenous Therapy Association, 7*(1), 39.

REVIEW QUESTIONS

1. The growth of home care is attributed to which of the following factors?
   a. aging population
   b. technology
   c. reimbursement
   d. baby boomers

2. A patient teaching checklist should includes instruction in which of the following:
   a. aseptic technique
   b. access/device maintenance
   c. compliance
   d. potential complications

3. Policies and procedures for the provision of home infusion services must be consistent with:
   a. published Standards of Practice
   b. JCAHO guidelines
   c. CHAP criteria
   d. ASHP standards

4. A case manager is responsible for which of the following activities?
   a. initial assessment
   b. development of a care plan
   c. appropriate referral and follow-up
   d. ongoing evaluation

5. Home infusion therapies may include:
   a. antibiotics
   b. parenteral nutrition
   c. hydration
   d. antiemetics

6. The first dose of an antibiotic drug should be given:
   a. in the home
   b. in a monitored environment
   c. by the patient
   d. by a professional

7. Patients are deemed appropriate candidates for home infusion therapy after assessment of:
   a. venous access
   b. drug therapy
   c. laboratory profile
   d. educability

8. Common diagnoses for antibiotic therapy include:
   a. Lyme disease
   b. osteomyelitis
   c. otitis media
   d. bronchitis

9. The plan of treatment in a home care program is written by the:
   a. pharmacist
   b. nurse
   c. physician
   d. branch manager

10. Treatments available at an ambulatory infusion center include which of the following:
    a. antifungal therapy
    b. pain management
    c. transfusion
    d. IV gamma globulin

$\mathcal{A}$ PPENDIX A

Licensed Practical/Vocational Nurse-Delivered Therapies

Many IV teams nationwide have recognized the valuable contribution that a licensed practical/vocational nurse (LPN/LVN) may make as a member of an IV team. Other institutions have created a career ladder and development for the LPN/LVN articulating to the professional registered nurse (RN) role.[2]

A survey, completed in 1991, provided a source of information relevant to the role of the LPN/LVN related to IV therapy. The survey found that the role of the LPN/LVN had changed dramatically during the past 10 years. From state to state, the issue of the role of this level of caregiver in infusion therapy is under scrutiny.

Twenty states have identified that the LPN/LVN has a designated role in IV therapy; however, the scope of practice is left up to each individual state agency. States with these expanded role guidelines are identified in Box A-1.[1]

The 26 states that identify the role of the LPN/LVN to include IV therapy, but who delegate the responsibility of education, competency, and role delineation to each agency, are found in Box A-2.[1]

Four states indicate that the role of the LPN/LVN is not in the maintenance or initiation of IV therapy. These are identified in Box A-3.[1]

The health care system in the United States is consistently challenged to deliver the highest level of care to the greatest number of people at the lowest cost. Nurse managers are now more than ever before involved in managing the fiscal responsibility for their areas in addition to patient care. With an emphasis on re-engineering and restructuring the workload, many hospitals have added LPN/LVN and nurse extender positions at a lower cost than that of the professional RN. Given the acute nature of IV therapy, and the need for a highly trained professional to deliver this intense level of care, the workload for IV nurses has expanded dramatically, both within and outside the hospital setting. The RN may be responsible for mentoring an LPN/LVN in the IV nursing practice, consistent with the guidelines of the scope of practice for that level of caregiver.

The Intravenous Nurses Certification Corporation (INCC) recently explored the possibility of providing an entry-level credential to those LPN/LVNs who had achieved success in a standardized curriculum and who possessed the body of knowl-

Box A-1
States With Expanded Role Guidelines

Alabama

Arizona

California

Colorado

Delaware

District of Columbia

Florida

Idaho

Louisiana

Maine

Maryland

Mississippi

Missouri

Nevada

New Hampshire

New York

North Carolina

Pennsylvania

South Carolina

Wyoming

Box A-2
States That Identify the Role of the LPN/LVN in IV Therapy*

Alaska

Arkansas

Connecticut

Georgia

Illinois

Indiana

Kansas

Kentucky

Massachusetts

Michigan

Minnesota

Montana

New Mexico

Ohio

Oklahoma

Oregon

Rhode Island

South Dakota

Tennessee

Texas

Utah

Vermont

Virginia

Washington

West Virginia

Wisconsin

*All delegate the responsibility of education, competency, and role delineation to each agency.

Box A-3
States That Do Not Include IV Therapy in the Role of the LPN/LVN

Hawaii

Iowa

Nebraska

New Jersey

edge and clinical skills to pass an examination administered by the INCC. This process has now been completed.

Currently, LPN/LVN responsibilities are limited by the guidelines of individual state nursing boards and institutional policy. In general, LPN/LVN responsibilities do not include administration of IV medications, blood products, and antineoplastic agents. Routine duties include monitoring, dressing and tubing changes, and site maintenance.

REFERENCES

1. Phillips, L. D. (1993). *Manual of IV therapeutics* (pp. 547–548). Philadelphia: F. A. Davis.
2. Intravenous Nurses Society. (1990). *Revised intravenous nursing standards of practice*. Philadelphia: J. B. Lippincott.

$\mathcal{A}$PPENDIX B

Standards of Practice: Nutrition Support Nurse

American Society for Parenteral and Enteral Nutrition (A.S.P. E.N.)

INTRODUCTION

A.S.P.E.N. is a professional society whose members are health care professionals—physicians, nurses, dietitians, pharmacists, and nutritionists—who are dedicated to optimum nutritional support of patients in health care settings and at home.

The diversity of A.S.P.E.N.'s professional membership reflects the basic importance of good nutrition to optimal health and the multidisciplinary team approach to sound nutritional support.

These Standards have been developed, reviewed, and approved by the following A.S.P.E.N. groups: Standards Committee, Nurses' Committee, Executive Committee, and Board of Directors.

These Standards of Practice for Nutrition Support Nursing should be used in conjunction with the following A.S.P.E.N. publications:

Definitions of Terms Used in A.S.P.E.N. Guidelines and Standards

Standards for Nutrition Support, Hospitalized Patients

Standards for Nutrition Support, Home Patients

Standards of Practice, Nutrition Support Dietitian

Standards of Practice, Nutrition Support Pharmacist

A.S.P.E.N. has developed these standards to promote the health and welfare of those patients in need of enteral and parenteral nutrition. The standards represent a consensus of A.S.P.E.N.'s members as to that minimal level of practice necessary to assure safe and effective enteral and parenteral nutrition care. A.S.P.E.N. disclaims any liability to any health care provider, patient, or other persons affected by these standards.

SCOPE OF PRACTICE

Role. Nutrition Support Nursing is the care of individuals with potential or known nutritional alterations. Nurses who engage in specialized nutrition support use specific expertise to enhance the maintenance and/or restoration of an individual's nutritional health. Physiological, metabolic, and behavioral principles, as well as technological advances, are considered when interventions that use the nursing process are planned. The nursing process includes ongoing assessment and planning of care, the provision of care, and an evaluation of the individual's response to the care delivered.

The Nutrition Support Nurse may function as a member of a multidisciplinary nutrition support service, team, or committee that coordinates the provision of specialized nutrition support in the hospital, home, or other settings. Because the care delivered by other health care professionals interfaces with Nutrition Support Nursing, common practice areas are approached from a collegial point of view.

Nutrition Support Nursing encompasses all nursing activities that promote optimal nutritional health. Nursing interventions are based upon scientific principles. These interventions are revised when changes occur in the individual's situation and/or when research data can be translated into new or different clinical practice. The scope of practice includes but is not limited to: direct patient care; consultation with nurses and other health professionals in a variety of clinical settings; education of patients, students, colleagues, and the public; participation in research; and administrative functions.

Goals. Nutrition Support Nursing uses nursing expertise to optimize the maintenance or restoration of an individual's nutritional health. Identification of measurable outcomes requires data collection and frequent assessment. The Nutrition Support Nurse participates in the development and review of standards of care for nutrition support for the institution or provider. The following outcomes are specific to the individual who requires nutrition support nursing care:

- The individual demonstrates the anticipated responses to nutrition support interventions.
- The individual/family demonstrates a knowledge of nutritional requirements and self-care measures to meet these requirements.
- The individual experiences no preventable complications resulting from nutritional support interventions or related nursing care.
- The individual/family uses nutrition support methods that maintain or improve nutritional status.

CHAPTER I. ASSESSMENT

The Nutrition Support Nurse, in collaboration with other members of the health care team, assesses the individual who is or may become malnourished for adequacy of nutritional status.

Required Characteristics

    1.1. The Nutrition Support Nurse shares in the responsibility of assuring that an appropriate nutritional assessment has been performed. This assessment may include the following parameters:

        1.1.1. Current weight

        1.1.2. History of weight changes (rapidity of changes, presence of edema or ascites)

        1.1.3. Height (plus head circumference in infants)

        1.1.4. Age

        1.1.5. Sex

        1.1.6. Clinical signs of malnutrition

        1.1.7. Laboratory evidence of malnutrition

        1.1.8. Nutrient intake prior to admission, including type and amount of supplements

        1.1.9. Food intolerance and allergies

        1.1.10. Mechanical or physiological changes that affect (a) ingestion, digestion, absorption, or metabolism or (b) nutrient needs, *eg,* infancy, adolescence, or pregnancy

        1.1.11. Psychological changes that affect nutrient intake

        1.1.12. Acute and/or chronic diseases or conditions

        1.1.13. Medications/ substances with potential for drug/drug, drug/nutrient, or nutrient/nutrient interactions

        1.1.14. Social, cultural, and religious factors that affect food preferences, ability to purchase and prepare food, and food intake patterns

        1.1.15. Activity level

        1.1.16. Periodic reassessment of any of the above

CHAPTER II: THERAPEUTIC PLAN

The Nutrition Support Nurse, in collaboration with other health care professionals and the individual/family, participates in the development of a therapeutic plan of care for the individual.

Required Characteristics

    1.1. There is documentation of a nursing plan, policy, and/or procedure/protocol for nutritional care which is compatible with the multidisciplinary therapeutic plan of care.

    1.2. There is documentation that the individual/family has been informed of and/or participated in developing the nursing plan of care.

    1.3. The nursing plan of care considers goals of therapy, discharge planning, and individual/family education needs.

CHAPTER III: IMPLEMENTATION

Nursing interventions in collaboration with other health care professionals ensure that the individual receives the prescribed feeding formulation in a safe, accurate, and cost-effective manner, using an appropriate delivery system and access device.

Required Characteristics

    1.1. The Nutrition Support Nurse participates in the development and review of procedures/protocols and policies related to the administration of feeding formulations and to the management of access devices.

    1.2. The Nutrition Support Nurse participates in quality assurance activities related to the administration of feeding formulations and to the management of access devices.

    1.3. The Nutrition Support Nurse participates in educational activities, for nursing staff and other members of the health care team, that are related to the administration of feeding formulations and the management of access devices.

    1.4. Nursing interventions for the individual/family are appropriate to prevent or manage any side effects or complications related to (a) the feeding formulation or its administration, and/or (b) the access device.

    1.5. The Nutrition Support Nurse participates in selection and monitoring of delivery systems appropriate for the administration of feeding formulations.

CHAPTER IV: PATIENT MONITORING

The Nutrition Support Nurse, in collaboration with other members of the health care team, monitors and evaluates the individual's response to nutrition support therapy.

Required Characteristics

    1.1. The medical record includes documentation of the Nutrition Support Nurse's evaluation of the individual's responses to nursing interventions and overall progression with regard to the plan of care.

CHAPTER V: PROMOTION OF SELF-CARE

The Nutrition Support Nurse, in collaboration with other health care professionals, assists the individual/family to maintain a level of independent care that is both safe and appropriate.

Required Characteristics

    1.1. There is documentation that the Nutrition Support Nurse provided and evaluated interventions to assist the individual/family toward maximum self-care.

    1.2. There is documentation that the individual/family participated in the development of short- and long-term goals and in decisions about related resources needed after discharge from acute care.

    1.3. There is documentation that the individual/family has acquired the necessary self-care skills.

CHAPTER VI: RESEARCH AND EDUCATION

The Nutrition Support Nurse has acquired current knowledge in the area of nutrition support and participates in continuing education.

Required Characteristics

    1.1. The Nutrition Support Nurse participates in educational offerings.

    1.2. The Nutrition Support Nurse incorporates current and appropriate research findings into clinical practice.

(Reprinted with permission of A.S.P.E.N.)

Standards of Practice: Standards for Home Nutrition Support

American Society for Parenteral and Enteral Nutrition (A.S.P. E.N.)

INTRODUCTION

A.S.P.E.N. is a professional society whose members are health care professionals—physicians, nurses, dietitians, pharmacists, and nutritionists—dedicated to optimum nutrition support of patients during hospitalization and rehabilitation.

A.S.P.E.N.'s diverse professional membership emphasizes the basic importance of good nutrition to good medical practice and the multidisciplinary team approach to sound nutrition.

These Standards have been developed, reviewed, and approved by the following A.S.P.E.N. groups: Standards Committee, Executive Committee, and Board of Directors.

The following terms were defined during the revision of the home nutrition support standards and are used in these standards.

1. Home nutrition therapy—the provision of nutrients and any necessary adjunctive therapeutic agents to patients by administration into the intestine or stomach or by intravenous infusion for the purpose of improving or maintaining a patient's nutrition status in the home environment.

2. Referring physician—the physician who develops and retains the ultimate authority for the patient's treatment plan.

3. Physician/nutrition support team—physician or nutrition support team under the guidance of a physician.

4. Treatment plan—orders established and signed by the referring physician for the care of the home patient (*ie*, the medical orders including: nutrients, medications, activity orders, access site orders, etc.).

5. Care plan—a plan of professional clinical activities developed by the home nutrition therapy provider to implement the treatment plan.

6. Home nutrition therapy provider—the organizations providing the nutrients, medications, supplies, equipment, and professional clinical services to a home nutrition therapy patient in accordance with these standards.

7. Feeding formulation—a ready-to-administer mixture of nutrients.

These Standards of Practice for Home Nutrition Support should be used in conjunction with the following A.S.P.E.N. publications:

Definitions of Terms Used in A.S.P.E.N. Guidelines and Standards

Standards for Nutrition Support, Hospitalized Patients

Standards of Practice, Nutrition Support Dietitian

Standards of Practice, Nutrition Support Pharmacist

Standards of Practice, Nutrition Support Nursing

Standards of Practice, Nutrition Support Physician

A.S.P.E.N. has developed these standards to promote the health and welfare of those patients in need of enteral and parenteral nutrition. The standards represent a consensus of A.S.P.E.N.'s members as to that minimal level of practice necessary to assure safe and effective enteral and parenteral nutrition care. A.S.P.E.N. disclaims any liability to any health care provider, patient, or other persons affected by these standards.

ORGANIZATION STANDARDS

Standard 1. The referring physician/nutrition support team (NST) responsible for home nutrition support shall be clearly identified and their roles defined.

1. The physician who has expertise in home parenteral and enteral nutrition support is primarily responsible for the patient's nutrition care. The physician acts in concert with a registered nurse, a dietitian, and a registered pharmacist. Each of these health care professionals shall have appropriate education, specialized training, and experience in home parenteral and enteral nutrition.

2. Home nutrition support services shall be initiated, modified, supervised, evaluated, and coordinated by the physician/NST.

Standard 2. The physician/NST caring for home parenteral and enteral nutrition patients shall be guided by written policies and procedures specifically designed to address the needs of the home patient or the patient in transition to home care.

1. There shall be written policies and procedures concerning the scope and provision of home parenteral and enteral nutrition services.

2. These written policies and procedures shall be developed by the physician/NST in conjunction with other professionals, as appropriate.

3. These policies and procedures shall be reviewed at least every 3 years and revised as appropriate to reflect optimal standards of care.

4. Written policies and procedures shall include but not be limited to:
    4.1 The roles, responsibilities, and 24-hour availability of care from the physician/NST and home nutrition therapy provider.

4.2 Defined criteria for patient eligibility and selection, which might include: medical suitability; rehabilitative potential; social and economic factors; and educational, psychological, and emotional factors pertinent to the patient and others who are significantly involved in this care.

4.3 A mechanism for referral to a knowledgeable and experienced home nutrition therapy provider for acquisition and delivery of enteral or intravenous nutrients, equipment, and supplies, with consideration for patient's freedom of choice.

4.4 Education of patient/caregiver.

4.5 A mechanism for patient monitoring (*eg*, frequency of follow-up contact, laboratory studies, response to nutrition therapy, and physical examination).

4.6 A mechanism for referral to consultative medical services and services of other professionals (*eg*, psychologists and social workers) and non-professionals (*eg*, patient support groups), as appropriate.

4.7 Reimbursement mechanisms for payment for services, equipment, and supplies.

4.8 Preparation, storage of, and techniques for administering a feeding formulation in the home.

    4.8.1 Feeding schedules.

    4.8.2 Care of feeding tubes and equipment for patients receiving enteral formulas.

    4.8.3 Care of catheters and tubing for patients receiving intravenous nutrition.

    4.8.4 Care and maintenance of electronic infusion devices.

    4.8.5 Care and maintenance of feeding formulations.

4.9 Prevention, management, and timely response to complications in the home, and emergency consultation with professional staff.

4.10 A mechanism for timely communication and collaboration among the physician/NST, home nutrition therapy provider, patient, caregiver, and other health care professionals involved.

4.11 A mechanism for quality assurance, which shall include but not be limited to mortality, hospital readmission, and complications.

Standard 3. Home parenteral and enteral nutrition services shall be documented.

1. Medical records shall be maintained for every patient receiving home parenteral and enteral nutrition and shall include but not be limited to:

    1.1 Designation of a physician with expertise in parenteral and enteral nutrition having primary responsibility for patient's home nutrition care.

    1.2 All pertinent patient diagnoses and prognoses, including long- and short-term treatment objectives.

    1.3 A nutrition assessment and medical evaluations, with follow-up as appropriate.

    1.4 Scope and results of initial and ongoing education of patient/caregiver.

    1.5 Treatment plan shall include orders established and signed by the referring physician for care of the patient (which include medical orders for nutrients, medications, activity level, access-site care).

    1.6 A care plan including consideration of functional limitations of the patient, activities permitted, psychosocial needs, suitability of home environment for provision of home nutrition services, and name(s) of other individual(s) who will assist in care of the patient if required.

    1.7 A current medication profile including prescription and nonprescription drugs, home remedies, and known allergies or sensitivities.

    1.8 Signed and dated progress notes for each contract between the patient and physician/NST or home nutrition therapy provider (*eg*, home visit, clinic visit, telephone contact, and rehospitalization). Progress notes shall report response to nutrition therapy including but not limited to results of serial monitoring, complications, and revisions in the therapeutic regimen.

    1.9 Signed and dated progress notes for each contact between the home nutrition therapy provider and the physician/NST including but not limited to results of serial monitoring, complications, and revision in the therapeutic regimen.

  1.10 A summary statement at termination of nutrition therapy including but not limited to the reason for terminating treatment, complications, patient outcome, and followup.

Standard 4. The home parenteral and enteral nutrition treatment and care plan shall be reviewed, evaluated, and updated regularly by the physician/NST to determine overall appropriateness, effectiveness, and safety.

1. Evaluation of patient's need for and response to home parenteral and enteral nutrition shall be the responsibility of the physician/NST.

2. This review and evaluation shall be performed and documented periodically as dictated by patient's medical and nutrition status.

3. The treatment and care plan shall be revised based on the review, and changes shall be communicated and implemented.

PATIENT SELECTION STANDARD

Standard 5. Indications and contraindications for home parenteral and enteral nutrition are as follows:

1. The patient shall be carefully evaluated prior to selection for home parenteral and enteral nutrition.

    1.1 A patient who is a candidate for home enteral nutrition should be unable to meet nutrient requirements by voluntary oral intake. A patient who is a candidate for home parenteral nutrition should be unable to meet nutrient requirements via the gastrointestinal tract safely and adequately.

    1.2 The patient's home environment should be such that the physician, in consultation with the appropriate social worker or other health professional, concludes that home therapy is more appropriate than long-term institutional care.

    1.3 The treatment and care plan should be designed to achieve the home parenteral or enteral nutrition objectives.

  1.4 The patient's home environment should be appropriate for the safe use of home parenteral or enteral nutrition support.

  1.5 The patient/caregiver should be willing and able to perform home parenteral or enteral nutrition support procedures.

  1.6 The patient/caregiver should be knowledgeable about therapeutic expectations, risks, benefits, and responsibilities (financial and other) of home parenteral or enteral nutrition and should agree to participate.

2. The patient/caregiver should understand the rationale, risks, benefits, and therapeutic options regarding nutrition support.

3. The patient and/or family should understand the cost of equally suitable nutrition support approaches and alternatives, insurance coverage, and financial responsibilities.

4. An evaluation of the nutrient needs of the patient shall be performed prior to the initiation of home parenteral or enteral nutrition support.

  4.1 Nutrition requirements shall take into account the patient's disease state, nutrition status, activity level, and growth requirements.

  4.2 The anticipated duration and route of nutrient administration shall be determined.

  4.3 The goals for home parenteral or enteral nutrition support shall be established in consideration of the immediate and long-term needs of the patient.

TREATMENT PLAN STANDARDS

Standard 6. The home parenteral and enteral nutrition treatment plan shall be determined and documented prior to the initiation of treatment and on an ongoing basis.

1. Elements of the treatment plan should include but are not limited to:

  1.1 Nutrition goals.

  1.2 Prescribed nutrients (type and dose of calories, protein, fluid volume, vitamins, minerals, trace elements, and electrolytes).

  1.3 Infusion times and rates.

  1.4 On-and-off tapering schedule.

  1.5 Specialized techniques of preparation and administration in the home setting.

  1.6 Care of access device, equipment, solutions, and formulas.

  1.7 Prescriptions for home parenteral or enteral solutions, medications, items, etc.

  1.8 Clinical monitoring (see Standard 13).

  1.9 Laboratory monitoring (see Standard 13).

  1.10 When appropriate, methods for transition from parenteral to enteral or oral nutrition and from enteral or oral nutrition.

2. Short-term goals should be developed and may include resolution of disease progression, wound healing, progression to enteral support, and oral nutrition.

3. Long-term goals should be developed and may include maintenance of normal nutrition and rehabilitation to physical and social independence.

4. Objectives should be developed prior to the initiation of nutrition support and on an ongoing basis as needed dependent on medical and nutrition evaluations.

Standard 7. The route(s) selected to provide home parenteral or enteral nutrition support shall be appropriate to meet assessed nutrient requirements and achieve treatment plan goals and objectives.

1. The safest, most cost-effective route that meets the patient's needs and preferences should be used.
2. The physician/NST should recognize that as the patient's therapy progresses, the optimal feeding mode may change and may, at times, include a combination of oral, enteral and parenteral feedings.
3. Use of the enteral route is preferred for patients who have a functioning and accessible gastrointestinal tract that can be safely used.

Standard 8. The selected home parenteral or enteral formula shall be appropriate for the disease process and compatible with other medications, therapy, and access route, and shall meet nutrient needs.

1. The formulation selection and modification should be directed by the physician/NST.
2. The patient should be given a copy of the prescriptions for the feeding formulation and other medications.

IMPLEMENTATION STANDARD

Standard 9. The access device and infusion method shall be appropriate for home use.

1. Selection of the access device should be based on safety and efficacy, and consideration should be given to patient preference.
2. The placement of parenteral and enteral devices should be performed or supervised by a physician proficient in such placement.
   2.1 Parenteral access
       2.6.1 Central venous lines or implanted ports should be placed by a physician.
       2.6.2 Peripherally inserted central catheter (PICC) lines should be placed by a physician or a nurse (where allowed by state nursing licensure boards).
   2.2 Enteral access
       2.2.1 Nasogastric tubes should be placed by a health care professional or patient/caregiver who has been properly trained and is proficient in such placement.
       2.2.2 Nasoduodenal or nasojejunal tubes must be placed by a physician or a health care professional designated by the physician.
       2.2.3 Percutaneous enterostomy (gastrostomy or jejunostomy) tubes must be placed by a physician or under the guidance of a physician; subsequent replacement may be done by a health care professional

or patient/caregiver proficient in such placement, as designated by the physician.

3. Policies and procedures shall be established to address access to implanted ports and central venous lines, and reintroduction of each type of feeding tube.

4. The nutrient infusion method or electronic infusion device selected should be suitable for home use.

   4.1 Selection should be based on safety and cost-effectiveness.

   4.2 Consideration should be given to patient preference, volume to be infused, type of regimen (cyclic, continuous, or intermittent), and activity level of the patient.

Standard 10. The patient/caregiver shall receive education and demonstrate competence in the preparation and administration of home parenteral and enteral nutrition support.

1. The patient/caregiver receiving home parenteral nutrition should be instructed in:

   1.1 Proper storage of formulated and admixed parenteral feeding formulations.

   1.2 Inspection of home parenteral nutrition containers and contents.

   1.3 Aseptic technique required for the admixture procedure and administration via access device.

   1.4 Compatibility and stability of nutrition and coadministered solutions under refrigeration or at room temperature.

   1.5 Infusion method.

   1.6 Use of parenteral infusion equipment.

   1.7 Proper disposal of used containers, tubing, and needles.

   1.8 Drug–nutrient and nutrient–nutrient interactions.

   1.9 Medication information and administration.

2. The patient/caregiver receiving home enteral nutrition should be instructed in:

   2.1 Proper storage for ready-to-feed or formula that requires mixing.

   2.2 Inspection of enteral products for contents and expiration date.

   2.3 Clean technique for preparation of formula, administration, and reuse of supplies and equipment.

   2.4 Stability of formula at room temperature.

   2.5 Infusion method.

   2.6 Use of enteral feeding equipment.

   2.7 Timing, method of administration, and compatibility of any medications via enteral access.

   2.8 Drug–nutrient and nutrient–nutrient interactions.

   2.9 Medication information and administration.

   2.10 Product hang time.

3. Educational material tailored to the patient and the therapy is provided to the patient/caregiver for use at home.

4. Patient/caregiver education should include periodic reassessment and retraining as needed.

Standard 11. The patient/caregiver shall receive education and demonstrate competence in access route care.

1. The patient/caregiver receiving parenteral infusions should be trained in:
   1.1 Aseptic techniques to access and maintain the access device.
   1.2 Connecting and disconnecting the intravenous tubing to the catheter.
   1.3 Post-infusion flushing to prevent catheter occlusion.

2. The patient/caregiver receiving enteral feedings should be trained in:
   2.1 Clean techniques for handling the tube.
   2.2 Maintaining the access site.
   2.3 Flushing the tube to maintain patency.

Standard 12. The patient/caregiver shall receive education and demonstrate competence in the recognition and appropriate response to complications.

1. Patient/caregiver should be able to recognize and respond to indications of potential metabolic complications.

2. Patient/caregiver should be able to recognize mechanical and procedural problems that include but are not limited to:
   2.1 Catheter or tube occlusion, leakage, breakage, or dislodgement.
   2.2 Equipment malfunction or breakage.
   2.3 Infusate contamination or precipitate or inhomogeneity.

3. Patient/caregiver should be able to recognize and report any signs/symptoms of a localized or systemic infectious process.

4. Patient/caregiver should know when and whom to contact when complications occur.

PATIENT MONITORING STANDARD

Standard 13. The patient shall be monitored for therapeutic efficacy, adverse effects, and clinical changes that may influence specialized nutrition support.

1. Protocols should be developed for periodic review of the patient's clinical and biochemical status.

2. Routine monitoring should include:
   2.1 Continued need to therapy.
   2.2 Nutrient intake.
   2.3 Review of current medications.
   2.4 Signs of intolerance to therapy.
   2.5 Weight changes.
   2.6 Biochemical, hematologic, and other pertinent data including clinical signs of nutrient deficiencies and excesses.
   2.7 Adjustment to therapy.
   2.8 Changes in lifestyle.
   2.9 Psychosocial problems.
   2.10 Changes in the home environment.

3. Assessment of the patient's major organ functions should be made periodically.

4. Psychosocial aspects of the patient/caregiver should be reassessed periodically.

TERMINATION OF THERAPY STANDARD

Standard 14. Prior to discontinuation of parenteral or enteral nutrition support one of the following criteria shall be applicable:

1. Parenteral nutrition should not be discontinued until nutrient requirements can be met by enteral or oral nutrition.

2. Enteral nutrition should not be discontinued until nutrient requirements can be met by oral nutrition.

3. Parenteral or enteral nutrition support should be discontinued whenever the patient's medical condition, especially complications, so indicates.

4. Parenteral or enteral nutrition support should be terminated when the physician and patient judge that the patient no longer benefits from the therapy. The decision to discontinue support must be made according to accepted community standards of medical care and in compliance with applicable law.

(Reprinted with permission of A.S.P.E.N.)

APPENDIX D

ASHP Therapeutic Position Statement on the Institutional Use of 0.9% Sodium Chloride Injection to Maintain Patency of Peripheral Indwelling Intermittent Infusion Devices

Am J Hosp Pharm. 1994; 51:1572-4

STATEMENT OF POSITION

0.9% Sodium chloride injection is a safe and effective means for maintaining catheter patency of peripheral indwelling intermittent infusion devices (PIIIDs) in adults. ASHP supports the use of 0.9% sodium chloride injection in preference to heparin-containing flush solutions (heparin flush) in the institutional setting, on the basis of clinical evidence indicating that 0.9% sodium chloride injection (1) is as effective as heparin flush in maintaining the patency of PIIIDs when blood is not aspirated into the device, (2) is safer to use than heparin flush because of less potential for adverse effects, (3) avoids drug incompatibilities associated with heparin flush, and (4) is a

---

Approved by the ASHP Board of Directors April 27, 1994. Developed by the Commission on Therapeutics

The correct bibliographic citation for this document is as follows: American Society of Hospital Pharmacists. ASHP therapeutic position statement on the institutional use of 0.9% sodium chloride injection to maintain patency of peripheral indwelling intermittent infusion devices. *Am J Hosp Pharm.* 1994; 51:1372-4.

Index terms: American Society of Hospital Pharmacists; Catheters; Costs; Devices; Guidelines; Heparin; Incompatibilities; Injections; Organizations; Pharmacy, institutional; Protocols; Sodium chloride; Toxicity cost-effective alternative to heparin flush. Because of limited available scientific evidence to date, this recommendation is not applicable to children under the age of 12 years, patients in the home or other outpatient settings, catheters used for central venous or arterial access (including peripherally, inserted central catheters and midline catheters), or the maintenance of patency in indwelling venipuncture devices used to obtain blood samples. Further research on PIIID patency in the aforementioned patient populations and settings is warranted.

BACKGROUND

PIIIDs, commonly referred to as "heparin locks," are used to provide convenient intravenous (i.v.) access in patients who require intermittent i.v. administration of medications without a continuous infusion of i.v. fluids. The advantages of PIIIDs include patient mobility and comfort and reduced fluid load.[1-4] PIIIDs most commonly consist of an intravenously inserted catheter attached to a short external cannula with a resealable injection port that is designed to facilitate multiple needle entries; thus, these devices eliminate the unnecessary trauma of multiple venipunctures.[4]

A problem frequently encountered with a PIIID is the loss of patency because of clot formation within the catheter. To prevent clot formation, catheters are commonly flushed after each administration of i.v. medication and every 8 to 12 hours when the device is not in use.[5] Because of heparin's anticoagulant effects, dilute solutions of heparin in 0.9% sodium chloride injection (e.g., 10–100 units/mL) have traditionally been used to periodically flush and fill these devices and hence to prevent the formation of clots. Dilute heparin solutions are used to maintain patency while avoiding the systemic effects associated with therapeutic doses of heparin.[6] The optimum concentration of heparin and whether the drug is needed at all have not been established.[4,7-11]

Efficacy. Studies indicate that 0.9% sodium chloride injection alone is as effective as heparin-containing solutions in maintaining PIIID patency.[5,9,10,12-19] In several randomized, double-blind studies in which PIIIDs composed principally of fluoroethylene propylene (FEP-Teflon) were used, 0.9% sodium chloride injection for flushing was associated with patency rates similar to those achieved with flush solutions containing 10 or 100 units of heparin sodium per milliliter.[13-15] The frequency of phlebitis associated with the use of these solutions was also similar.[7-11,13-15] The type of solution used to maintain PIIID patency may not be as important as the positive pressure maintained in the i.v. line by the capped (sealed) injection device, which appears to prevent blood reflux and clot formation in the device.[10-11] Several studies provide a scientific basis for using heparin,[6,20,21] but most published research supports 0.9% sodium chloride injection as an effective alternative to heparin flush in maintaining the patency of PIIIDs. Limited data from children four weeks to 18 years of age suggest no difference between 0.9% sodium chloride injection alone and 0.9% sodium chloride injection with heparin 10 units/mL in maintaining device patency.[22] Until further controlled studies are conducted in this patient population, heparin, if it is used, should be administered in the smallest amount necessary to maintain patency of the device. One survey showed that it is common practice to flush catheter devices in neonates with heparin 1–2 units/mL.[23]

Adverse effects of heparin flush therapy. Heparin, even when used in small doses, may elicit adverse reactions in some patients. The potential for bleeding complications increases when patients receive multiple, unmonitored heparin flushes.[24] Repeated injections of heparin even in small doses can alter activated partial thromboplastin time results.[25] Allergic reactions are an inherent risk of using heparin. Although rare, heparin flush-associated thrombocytopenia and hemorrhage have been reported.[24,26–28] The risks of these adverse effects may be avoided by using 0.9% sodium chloride injection instead of heparin flush.

Drug incompatibility. Heparin has been shown to be incompatible with many commonly used i.v. drugs.[29] If heparin flush has been used to maintain the patency of a PIIID and a drug must be administered that is incompatible with heparin, it is necessary to flush the catheter with 0.9% sodium chloride injection before and after administering the incompatible drug and then to refill the PIIID with heparin. This procedure is commonly referred to as "SASH" (sodium chloride—administration [of drug]—sodium chloride—heparin).[30] The use of 0.9% sodium chloride injection as a flushing agent avoids the numerous drug incompatibilities associated with heparin and obviates the need for SASH.

Cost implications. Enhanced quality of patient care should be the primary reason for deciding to use 0.9% sodium chloride injection for flushing. Secondarily, the choice of 0.9% sodium chloride injection may avoid substantial costs associated with drugs, related supplies, and staff time.[11]

SUMMARY

Because of current therapeutic evidence supporting the efficacy of 0.9% sodium chloride and the inherent risks associated with heparin, ASHP believes the use of 0.9% sodium chloride injection is appropriate for maintaining the patency of PIIIDs in adults in institutional settings.

REFERENCES

1. Millam DA. Intermittent devices. *NITA.* 1981; 4(Mar.–Apr.):142–5.
2. Larkin, M. Heparin locks. *NITA.* 1979; 2(May–Jun):18–9.
3. Thomas RB, Salter FJ. Heparin locks: their advantages and disadvantages. *Hosp Formul.* 1975; 10:536–8.
4. Deeb EN, Di Mattia PE. How much heparin in the lock? *Am J IV Ther.* 1976; 3(Dec–Jan):22–6.
5. Tuten SH, Gueldner SH. Efficacy of sodium chloride versus dilute heparin for maintenance of peripheral intermittent intravenous devices. *Appl Nurs Res.* 1991; 2:63–71.
6. Hanson RL, Grant AM, Majors KR. Heparin-lock maintenance with ten units of sodium heparin in one milliliter of normal saline solution. *Surg Gynecol Obstet.* 1976; 142:373–6.
7. Garrelts JC. White clot syndrome and thrombocytopenia: reasons to abandon heparin i.v. lock flush solution. *Clin Pharm.* 1992; 11:797–9.
8. Weber DR. Is heparin really necessary in the lock and, if so, how much? *DICP Ann Pharmacother.* 1991; 25:399–407.
9. Barrett PJ, Lester RL. Heparin versus saline flushing solutions in a small community hospital. *Hosp Pharm.* 1990; 25:115–8.
10. Dunn DL, Lenihan SF. The case for the saline flush. *Am J Nurs.* 1987; 87:798–9.
11. Goode CJ, Titler M, Rakel B et al. *Nurs Res.* 1991; 40:324–30.
12. Fry B. Intermittent heparin flushing protocols. A standardization issue. *J. Intraven Nurs.* 1992; 15(May–Jun):160–3.

13. Epperson EL. Efficacy of 0.9% sodium chloride injection with and without heparin for maintaining indwelling intermittent injection sites. *Clin Pharm.* 1984; 3:626–9.

14. Garrelts JC, LaRocca J, Ast D et al. Comparison of heparin and 0.9% sodium chloride injection in the maintenance of indwelling intermittent IV devices. *Clin Pharm.* 1989; 8:34–9.

15. Hamilton RA, Plis JM, Clay C et al. Heparin sodium versus 0.9% sodium chloride injection for maintaining patency of indwelling intermittent infusion devices. *Clin Pharm.* 1988; 7:439–43.

16. Shearer J. Normal saline versus dilute heparin flush: a study of peripheral intermittent IV devices. *NITA.* 1987; 10:425–7.

17. Miracle V, Fangman B, Kayrouz P et al. Normal saline vs. heparin lock flush solution: one institution's findings. *Ky Nurse.* 1989; 37(Jul–Aug):1, 6–7.

18. Ashton J, Gibson V. Summers S. Effects of heparin versus saline solution on intermittent infusion device irrigation. *Heart Lung.* 1990; 19: 608–12.

19. Hook ML, Ose P. Heparin vs. normal saline. *J Intraven Nurs.* 1990; 13:150.

20. Cyganski JM, Donahue JM, Heaton JS. The case for the heparin flush. *Am J Nurs.* 1987; 87:796–7.

21. Holford NH, Vozeh, S, Coates P et al. More on heparin lock. *N Engl J Med.* 1977; 296:1300–1. Letter.

22. Lombardi TP, Gundersen B, Zammett LO et al. Efficacy of 0.9% sodium chloride injection with or without heparin sodium for maintaining patency of intravenous catheters in children. *Clin Pharm.* 1988; 7:8332–6.

23. Romanowski GL, Zenk KE. Intravenous flush solutions for neonates. Paper presented at 26th Annual ASHP Midyear Clinical Meeting. New Orleans, LA: 1991 Dec 10.

24. Passannante A, Macik BG. Case report: the heparin flush syndrome: a cause of iatrogenic hemorrhage. *Am J Med Sci.* 1988; 296(Jul):71–3.

25. AHFS Drug Information 93. McEvoy GK, ed. Heparin sodium. Bethesda, MD: American Society of Hospital Pharmacists; 1993: 833.

26. Heeger PS, Backstrom JT. Heparin flushes and thrombocytopenia. *Ann Intern Med.* 1986; 105: 143.

27. Doty JR Alving BM, McDonnell DE et al. Heparin-associated thrombocytopenia in the neurosurgical patient. *Neurosurgery.* 1986; 19:69–72.

28. Cines DB, Tomaski A, Tannenbaum S. Immune endothelial-cell injury in heparin-associated thrombocytopenia. *N Engl J Med.* 1987; 316: 581–9.

29. Trissel LA. Handbook on injectable drugs. 7th ed. Bethesda, MD: American Society of Hospital Pharmacists; 1992.

30. Intravenous Nurses Society. Intravenous Nursing Standards of Practice. *J Intraven Nurs.* 1990; 13:S77–8.

Glossary

ABO system—a basic hereditary blood group system; it denotes a patient's blood group

Adjuvant chemotherapy—the use of drugs in addition to surgery and/or radiation therapy administered to eradicate metastatic disease

Agglutination—clumping of red blood cells when incompatible bloods are mixed

Agglutinin—an antibody causing agglutination with its corresponding antigen

Alkylating agents—agents that kill cells by cross-linking DNA strands (ie, disturbing the normal structure) in the DNA molecule

Alopecia—the loss of hair from the body and/or the scalp

Alternate site care—care that is delivered beyond the confines of an inpatient facility

Analogue—a compound that resembles another in structure (eg, fluorouracil is an analogue of uracil)

Anorexia—absence or loss of appetite for food

Antibody—a substance present in the plasma that incites immunity; is capable of reacting with the specific antigen that caused its production

Anti–free-flow administration set—stops when removed from the electronic infusion device, yet allows gravity flow when the user takes action

Antigen—an immunizing agent capable of inducing the body to form antibodies

Antimetabolites—anticancer drugs that substitute for or block the use of an essential metabolite

Antimicrobial—an agent that destroys or prevents development of microorganisms

Antimicrobial ointment—a semisolid preparation used to prevent the pathogenic action of microbes

Antineoplastic agent—a medication or treatment for cancer

Antitumor antibiotics—anticancer drugs that interfere with cellular production of DNA and/or RNA

Arterial pressure monitoring—monitoring of arterial pressure through an indwelling arterial catheter connected to an electronic monitor

Arteriovenous (AV) fistula—the surgical anastomosis of an artery and vein

Arteriovenous (AV) grafts—the insertion of a synthetic device connecting a vein and an artery

Aseptic technique—mechanisms employed to reduce potential contamination

Assay determination—decision based upon an analysis and/or examination

Auscultation—process of listening for sounds in the body

Autologous—products or components of the same individual

Bacteria—microorganisms that may potentiate a diseased state

Benchmarking—comparing one's systems to others

Blood grouping—the testing of red blood cells to determine antigens present and absent

Body surface area—surface area of the body determined through use of a nomogram; important when calculating dosages

Bone marrow—the inner spongy tissue of a bone where red blood cells, white blood cells, and platelets are formed

Cancer—the general name for more than 100 diseases in which abnormal cells grow out of control; a malignant tumor

Cannula—a hollow tube made of plastic or metal; used for accessing the vascular system

Catheter—a hollow tube made of plastic for accessing the vascular system

Cell kill—the number of cancer cells killed at a given dose by an antineoplastic drug

Chemical incompatibility—a change in the molecular structure or pharmacologic properties of a substance, which may or may not be visually observed

Chemotherapy—the treatment of cancer patients with chemical agents designed to kill cancer cells

Cognitive—behaviors that place primary emphasis on the mental or intellectual processes

Cold agglutinin—a red blood cell agglutinin that acts at relatively low temperature; part of a disease process caused by a transient infectious disease; may be idiopathic

Color coding—system developed by manufacturers that identifies products/medications by the use of a color system. These color code systems are not standardized and may vary with manufacturer.

Compartment syndrome—compression of circulation evidenced by impaired pulses, compromised circulation, and pain

Compatibility—capable of being mixed and administered without undergoing undesirable chemical and/or physical changes or loss of therapeutic action

Compatibility test—all tests performed on donors and recipients to determine compatibility of blood; also known as the cross-match

Complement—a group of proteins in normal blood serum and plasma that in combination with antibodies causes the destruction of particular antigens

Contamination—introduction of pathogens or infectious material from one source to another

Corrective action—a defined plan to eliminate deficiencies

Cross contamination—movement of pathogens from one source to another

Curative—therapy that is either healing or corrective

Cutdown—surgical procedure for exposure and cannulation of a vein

Delayed reaction—adverse effect occurring after 48 hours and up to 180 days post-transfusion

Delivery system—a product(s) that allows for the administration of medication. These systems can be integral or have component parts. Delivery systems encompass all products used, from the solution container down to the cannula.

Disinfectant—an agent that eliminates all microorganisms except spores, generally used on inanimate objects

Distal—furthest from the heart; furthest from point of attachment; below previous site of cannulation

Distention—increase in size due to pressure within

Document—a record written or printed that contains original, official, or legal information

Documentation—a recording in written or printed form containing original, official, or legal information

Dome—a plastic component used in hemodynamic monitoring

Dose-limiting toxicity—the degree of toxicity that dictates the maximum amount of drug that safely can be administered

Electronic infusion device—an electronic instrument that is used to regulate the flow rate of the prescribed therapy. These are often referred to as EIDs.

Embolus—a blood clot or other foreign substance that is carried in the blood stream. It has the potential to impede and/or obstruct circulation.

Epidemiology—the division of medical science concerned with defining and explaining the interrelationships of the host, agent, and environment in causing disease

Epidural—located on or over the dura mater

Epithelialized—the growth of epithelial cells over a wound or over and around a catheter site

Erythema—redness of the skin

Extravasation—inadvertent administration of vesicant solution/medication into surrounding tissue

Filter—a porous device used to prevent the passage of undesired substances

Free-flow—nonregulated, inadvertent administration of fluid

Fungi—vegetable cellular organisms that subsist on organic matter

Gram negative bacteria—organisms remaining unstained by the Gram's method; such as *Kleb-*

siella, *Escherichia coli, Pseudomonas, Serratia,* etc., associated with infusate contamination and arterial catheters

Gram positive bacteria—organisms holding the dye after being stained by the Gram's method; such as *Staphylococcus epidermidis, Staphylococcus aureus,* etc., associated with venous catheter contamination

Hematocrit—an expression of the volume of red cells per unit of circulating blood

Hemodynamic pressure monitoring—the measurement of pulmonary artery pressure, arterial pressure, cardiac output, etc., via an electronic monitor

Hemoglobin—the iron-containing pigment of red blood cells functioning primarily in the transport of oxygen from the lungs to the tissues of the body

Hemolysis—rupture of the red cell membrane causing the release of hemoglobin

Hemorrhage—abnormal discharge of blood, either external or internal

Hemostasis—cessation of the flow of blood through a port or vessel

HLA system—human leukocyte antigens; a complex array of genes that are involved in immune regulation and cell differentiation

Hypercalcemia—serum calcium concentrations above normal levels

Hypertonic—solution more concentrated than that with which it is compared; a fluid having a concentration greater than the normal tonicity of plasma

Hyperuricemia—uric acid blood concentrations above normal levels

Hypotonic—solution less concentrated than that with which it is compared; a fluid having a concentration less than the normal tonicity of plasma

IgA—immunoglobulin A; a class of immunoglobulins in body secretions

IgG—immunoglobulin G; a class of immunoglobulins or circulating antibodies in the blood that frequently cause sensitization

IgM—immunoglobulin M; a class of immunoglobulins or circulating antibodies in the blood that are capable of binding complement

Immediate reaction—adverse effect occurring immediately or up to 48 hours post-transfusion

Immunocompromised—having decreased resistance to disease

Immunoglobulin—a protein with antibody activity

Immunohematology—the study of blood and blood reactions

Implanted port/pump—vascular access device placed totally beneath the skin surface by surgical procedure

Incident—an unusual occurrence that requires documentation and action because of potential or implied consequences

Incompatible—incapable of being mixed or used simultaneously without undergoing chemical or physical changes or producing undesirable effects

Infection—invasion of the body by living microorganisms

Infiltration—the inadvertent administration of non-vesicant solution/medication into surrounding tissues

Infusate—parenteral solution administered into the vascular system

Integumentary—cutaneous; dermal

Intermittent intravenous therapy—administered at prescribed intervals with periods of infusion cessation

Intraosseous—within the cavity of a bone that is filled with marrow

Intrathecal—inside the spinal cord

Intrinsic contamination—contamination during product manufacture

Isolation—the separation of potentially infectious persons and/or materials

Isotonic—solution having the same concentration as that with which it is compared (*ie*, plasma)

Laminar flow hood—a contained work area in which the air flow within a confined area moves with uniform velocity along parallel flow lines with a minimum of eddies

Latex injection port—a resealable rubber cap designed to accommodate needles for administration of solutions into the vascular system

Leukopenia—total number of leukocytes in the circulating blood less than normal, the lower limit of which generally is regarded as $5000/\mu/L$

Lumen—the interior space of a tubular structure, such as a blood vessel or cannula

Lymphedema—swelling of an extremity caused by obstruction of the lymphatic vessel(s)

Malignancy—uncontrolled growth and dissemination of a neoplasm

Medical act—procedure performed by a licensed physician

Metastasis—the spread of cancer to sites distant from the site of origin

Microabrasion—break in skin integrity which may predispose the patient to infection

Microaggregate—microscopic collection of particles such as platelets, leukocytes and fibrin, that occurs in stored blood

Microaggregate blood filter—filter that removes potentially harmful microaggregates and reduces non-hemolytic febrile reactions

Microorganisms—extremely minute living matter which can only be seen with the aid of a microscope

Monoclonal antibody—antibody produced by a clone of cells derived from a single cell in large quantities for use against a specific antigen

Morbidity—number of infected persons or cases of infection in relation to a specific population

Mortality—ratio of number of deaths in a population to number of individuals in that population

Multiple-dose vial—medication bottle designed to be entered more than one time that is hermetically sealed with a rubber stopper

Nadir—the lowest level to which a blood count drops in response to an antineoplastic agent

Needle—a slender, pointed, hollow metal device

Neoplasm—a new growth or tumor, either benign or malignant

Nitrosoureas—anticancer drugs that produce metabolites that attack DNA in a manner analogous to alkylating agents

Nonpermeable—able to maintain integrity

Nonvesicant—intravenous medications, including but not limited to medications administered for cancer, which generally do not cause damage or sloughing of tissue

Occlusion—a cannula blockage due to precipitation and/or clot formation

Oncology—the study of tumors

Osmolarity—number of solutes contained in solution measured in milliosmoles per liter

Outcome—the interpretation of documented results

Palliative—treatment that may be provided for comfort and/or temporary relief of symptoms and does not cure

Palpable cord—a vein that is rigid and hard to the touch

Palpation—examination by touch

Parenteral—denoting any route other than the alimentary canal, such as intravenous

Parenteral nutrition—nutrients that are administered intravenously, comprised of carbohydrates, proteins, and/or fats, and additives such as electrolytes, vitamins, and trace elements

Paresthesia—abnormal spontaneous sensations (*eg,* burning, prickling, tingling, or tickling without physical stimulus)

Particulate matter—relating to or composed of fine particles

Pathogens—disease-producing microorganisms

Percutaneous puncture—puncture performed through the skin

Peripheral—pertains to veins of the extremities, scalp, and external jugular

Peripheral neuropathy—dysfunction of postganglion nerves, ranging from paresthesia to paralysis

Phlebitis—inflammation of a vein; may be accompanied by pain, erythema, edema, streak formation, and/or palpable cord. Rated by a standard scale (see phlebitis topic). A possible precursor to sepsis

Phlebotomy—withdrawal of blood from a vein

Physical incompatibility—an undesirable change that is visually observed

Plant alkyloids—anticancer drugs derived from plants, such as the periwinkle (vincristine and vinblastine)

Positive pressure—maintaining a constant, even force within a lumen to prevent reflux of blood; achieved while injecting by clamping or withdrawing needle from cannula

Post-infusion phlebitis—inflammation of a vein occurring after cannula removal

Pounds per square inch (psi)—a measurement of pressure, psi equals 50 mm Hg or 68 cm H_2O

Preservative-free—contains no added substance capable of inhibiting bacterial contamination

Process—actual performance and observation of performance based on compliance with policies, procedures, and professional standards

Product integrity—intact, uncompromised product; condition suitable for intended use

Proximal—nearest to the heart; closest to point of attachment; above previous site of cannulation

Pruritis—itching

Psychomotor—behaviors that place primary emphasis on the various degrees of physical skills and dexterity as they relate to the thought process

Purulent—containing or producing pus

Push—direct injection of a medication into a vein or access device

Quality indicator—a systematic process for monitoring, evaluating, and problem solving

Radiopaque—able to be detected by radiographic examination

Rh system—a blood group system denoting the presence or absence of D (Rh) red cell antigen

Risk management—process that centers on identification, analysis, treatment, and evaluation of real and potential hazards

Roller bandage—a roll of gauze or other material used for protecting an injured part, for immobilizing a limb, for keeping dressings in place, etc.

Sclerotic—fibrous thickening of the wall of the vein resulting in decreased lumen size. On palpation, usually feels hard to the touch

Semi-quantitative culture technique—a laboratory protocol used for isolating and identifying microorganisms

Sensitization—the initial exposure of an individual to a specific antigen that results in an immune response

Sepsis—The presence of infectious microorganisms or their toxins in the blood stream

Single-use vial—medication bottle intended for one-time use that is hermetically sealed with a rubber stopper

Skin-cannula junction—point at which the cannula enters the skin

Statistics—the science of collecting, classifying, and interpreting information based on the numbers of things

Stomatitis—sores on the inside of the mouth

Structure—describes the elements on which the program is based. These elements include resources such as federal and state laws, professional standards, position descriptions, patient rights, policies and procedures, documentation forms, quality controls, corrective action programs, etc.

Stylet—a rigid metal object within a catheter designed to facilitate insertion

Surfactant—material whose properties reduce the surface tension of fluid

Surveillance—the active, systematic, ongoing observation of the occurrence and distribution of disease within a popoulation and of the events or conditions that increase or decrease the risk of such disease occurrence

Tamper-proof—impossible to alter

Thrombocytopenia—decreased thrombocytes or platelets

Thrombolytic agent—a pharmacologic agent capable of dissolving blood clots

Thrombophlebitis—inflammation of the vein with clot formation

Thrombosis—formation of a blood clot within a blood vessel

Trace elements—minute amounts of essential elements present in the body

Transfusion reaction—any adverse effect to the transfusion of whole blood or its components or derivatives

Transparent semipermeable membrane (TSM)—a sterile dressing that allows visualization, is water resistant, and is air permeable

Trendelenburg—a position used to increase venous distention in which the head is lower than the feet

Tunneled catheter—a central catheter designed to have a portion lie within a subcutaneous passage before exiting the body

Valsalva maneuver—the process of making a forceful attempt at expiration with the mouth, nostrils, and glottis closed

Vascular access—means of approaching or entering the vascular system

Venipuncture—puncture of a vein for any purpose

Vesicant—intravenous medication that causes blisters and tissue injury when it escapes into the surrounding tissue(s)

Volumetric—relating to measurement of or by volume

Answers to Questions

Chapter 1 _____

No Questions

Chapter 2 _____
1. B
2. D
3. D
4. D
5. C
6. A
7. B
8. D

Chapter 3 _____
1. D
2. D
3. A
4. A
5. B

Chapter 4 _____
1. D
2. C
3. C
4. A
5. B, C
6. D
7. D
8. D
9. D
10. A

Chapter 5 _____
1. D
2. D
3. A

Chapter 6 _____
1. A, B
2. A, C
3. A
4. A, B, C, D
5. A
6. B
7. A, B, D
8. A
9. A, B
10. D

Chapter 7 _____
1. A
2. B
3. A, B, C, D
4. B
5. C
6. A
7. B
8. A, B, C
9. A, B, C, D
10. A, B, C

Chapter 8 _____
1. A, C
2. D
3. A, B, D
4. A

5. A, B
6. A, B
7. A, B, C
8. D
9. C
10. B

Chapter 9 _____
1. A
2. B
3. A
4. C
5. C
6. B
7. D
8. B
9. A
10. C

Chapter 10 _____
1. B
2. B
3. C
4. C
5. D
6. A, B, C, D
7. C
8. B
9. A
10. C

Chapter 11 _____
1. A
2. B

3. A
4. B
5. C
6. D
7. B, C
8. D
9. C
10. C

Chapter 12

1. C
2. A, B, C
3. A
4. A
5. A
6. D
7. A
8. B
9. C
10. D

Chapter 13

1. B
2. D
3. A
4. A, B, D
5. A, C
6. A, B
7. A, B, C
8. A
9. A, B, C
10. A

Chapter 14

1. A, B, C
2. D
3. A
4. A, B, C
5. B
6. A
7. A
8. B
9. A
10. A

Chapter 15

1. A
2. B
3. C

4. A, B, C
5. A
6. A
7. B
8. A
9. A, B, C, D
10. A

Chapter 16

1. C
2. B
3. A
4. D
5. D
6. C
7. C
8. D
9. A
10. D

Chapter 17

1. A
2. C
3. A, B
4. D
5. B
6. C
7. A
8. C
9. C
10. A

Chapter 18

1. B
2. B
3. C
4. A, B
5. A, B, C
6. A, B, D
7. A, B, C, D
8. A
9. A, B, D
10. D

Chapter 19

1. A, B, C, D
2. A
3. A, B
4. A

5. A, B
6. A, B, C, D
7. C, D
8. C
9. A
10. A, B, C, D

Chapter 20

1. D
2. A, B, C, D
3. A
4. B
5. D
6. A
7. A, B, C, D
8. D
9. D
10. B

Chapter 21

1. A
2. A
3. D
4. B
5. A
6. D
7. D
8. A
9. A
10. C

Chapter 22

1. B, C
2. A, B, C, D
3. B
4. C
5. D

Chapter 23

1. A, B, C
2. A, B, D
3. A, B, C, D
4. A, B, C, D
5. A, B, C, D
6. B, D
7. A, B, C, D
8. A, B, C
9. C
10. A, B, C, D

Index

Note; *Page numbers followed by f indicate figures; those followed by t indicate tables.*